Venous Thromboembolism:
An Evidence–Based Atlas

Edited by
Russell D. Hull, M.B.B.S, M.Sc.
Director, Clinical Trials Unit
Department of Medicine
Foothills Hospital
University of Calgary
Calgary, Alberta, Canada

Gary E. Raskob, M.Sc.
Department of Biostatistics
and Epidemiology, and
Department of Medicine
University of Oklahoma
Health Sciences Center
Oklahoma City, Oklahoma
USA

Graham F. Pineo, M.D.
Director, Clinical Trials Unit
Department of Medicine
Calgary General Hospital
University of Calgary
Calgary, Alberta, Canada

**Futura Publishing
Company, Inc.**
Armonk, NY

Library of Congress Cataloging-in-Publication Data

Venous thromboembolism : an evidence-based atlas / edited by Russell
   D. Hull, Gary E. Raskob, Graham F. Pineo.
        p.   cm.
     Includes bibliographical references and index.
     ISBN 0-87993-633-9
     1. Thromboembolism.   2. Thrombophlebitis.   I. Hull, Russell.
   II. Raskob, Gary E.   III. Pineo, Graham F.
     [DNLM: 1. Thromboembolism. WG 610 V4647 1996]
     RC697.V465   1996
     616.1'45—dc20
     DNLM/DLC
     for Library of Congress   95-39036
                                                                      CIP

                                                                 Rev.

Copyright 1996
Futura Publishing Company, Inc.

Published by
Futura Publishing Company, Inc.
135 Bedford Road
Armonk, NY   10504-0418

LC#95-39036
ISBN#0-87993-633-9

Every effort has been made to ensure that the information in this book is as up-to-date
and as accurate as possible at the time of publication. However, due to the constant developments in medicine, neither the authors, nor the editors, nor the publisher can accept any legal or any other responsibility for any errors or omissions that may occur.

Printed in the United States of America.

This book is printed on acid-free paper.

Foreword

In the vast majority of circumstances, venous thromboembolism (VTE) occurs as a complication of other disorders. It has long been recognized as a potentially lethal complication of surgical procedures and medical illnesses, especially when associated with immobility, and the incidence increases sharply with increasing age. For these reasons, nearly all practicing physicians (with the possible exception of pediatricians), will find this new text on VTE to be relevant to their daily clinical practice.

Since VTE occurs in such a diverse patient population, it is not surprising that the major investigators in this field are drawn from a wide array of specialties: hematology, cardiology, pulmonary disease, neurology, surgery, epidemiology. This unique broadly-based group of investigators has made an enormous impact on our understanding of VTE in the last several decades.

Perhaps the most important insight has been the recognition that venous thrombosis, especially of the deep venous system and pulmonary embolism (PE), are manifestations of the same underlying disorder: venous thromboembolism. In earlier texts, thrombophlebitis was often listed as a risk factor for PE. We now recognize that PE and thrombophlebitis are manifestations of the same basic underlying disorder: venous thrombosis.

The risk factors for venous thrombosis are widely recognized. Most relate to Virchow's triad of stasis, venous injury, and hypercoagulability. It is my belief that the most critical risk factor is the one we are least able to document: a hypercoagulable state. I believe that most patients with VTE have a hypercoagulable state; the other risk factors are conditions that may precipitate venous thrombosis in patients with an underlying hypercoagulable state. Most patients who take oral contraceptive agents, most patients who undergo surgical procedures, and most patients who have acute myocardial infarction do not develop venous thrombosis. I believe that those who do, have an underlying hypercoagulable state. When we are able to accurately identify patients with a hypercoagulable state, we will be able to concentrate prophylaxis on those patients who are at the greatest risk of VTE.

Great strides have been made in the noninvasive diagnosis of deep venous thrombosis utilizing impedance plethysmography and duplex ultrasound. The use of these techniques also helps to determine which patients with suspected PE are at risk of recurrent PE and, therefore, require anticoagulant therapy. The use of these noninvasive tests for deep venous thrombosis is especially critical in patients suspected of pulmonary embolism who have nondiagnostic lung scans.

The principal treatment for VTE continues to be anticoagulation. Recent studies have improved the monitoring of heparin therapy to permit earlier and more consistent achievement of therapeutic levels. One of the most significant advances in the treatment of VTE is improved monitoring of warfarin treatment. The use of the International Normalized Ratio (INR) corrects prothrombin time ratios that are obtained from thromboplastin reagents that vary in their intensity. It has been demonstrated that adjusting the dose of warfarin to prolong the INR to 2.0 to 3.0 times control is effective, and greatly reduces the bleeding complications of warfarin treatment. In patients in whom anticoagulation treatment is contraindicated, or proves to be ineffective, IVC filters, which can be introduced intravenously, are effective in preventing recurrent PE.

It is intended that this text, with authors representing a wide variety of disciplines, will be very useful to clinicians who deal with the problems of prevention, detection, and treatment of venous thromboembolism.

James E. Dalen, M.D.
Vice Provost for Health Sciences
Dean, College of Medicine
University of Arizona
Tucson, Arizona 85724

Preface

The unique features of this book are defined by the title "Venous Thromboembolism — An Evidence-Based Atlas." The book is being presented in an atlas format to enhance the quality of the reproductions on patient studies in the final chapter. The case studies are derived from database of over 600 patients presenting to a large thromboembolism consultation service. Many of these patients participated in a series of randomized clinical trials, most of which have been published in the peer-reviewed literature. As clinical practice changed in response to these and other Level 1 clinical trials, the approach to the diagnosis and management of venous thromboembolism changed and this is reflected in the various case studies. Furthermore, the technology related to investigation of patients presenting with suspected pulmonary embolism or deep-vein thrombosis improved dramatically with time and these changes are evident in reproductions of the various investigative procedures; in particular the improvements in ventilation and perfusion lung scans. The atlas demonstrates specific features of the clinical presentation, diagnosis and treatment of patients with venous thromboembolism including an orderly presentation of photographs of the diagnostic studies. It is our hope that these patient studies will help consolidate a number of the points made in the preceding chapters with respect to the diagnosis and treatment of venous thromboembolism. Levels of evidence have been applied to all clinical trials relating to diagnostic tests or the prevention and treatment of venous thromboembolism; thus the title "Evidence-Based Atlas."

With this evidence-based approach we have identified a large number of high-quality clinical trials that have been performed. At the same time we have demonstrated the numerous areas where further trials will be required. Our approach to rules of evidence for clinical trials is summarized in Chapter 3 by Gary Raskob. These rules were largely defined by Dr. David Sackett and colleagues at McMaster University and they are achieving wide application. Firm recommendations can be made on Level 1 studies which provide the clinical anchor. However there are certain situations where Level 1 trials may not be possible and our intention is not to distract from the efforts and achievements of investigators performing clinical trials which do not quite reach the Level 1 status. Nonetheless, it has become clear that the findings of Level 1 trials, if consistent will rapidly become the standard of clinical practice. Therefore in reviewing this book, firm recommendations regarding approaches to the prevention and treatment of venous thromboembolism or the application of diagnostic tests are best made where Level 1 evidence is available.

Venous Thromboembolism has been compiled by an international panel of experts providing the reader with concise and current reviews of the various topics. The book should be of interest to general internists and primary care physicians as well as subspecialists involved in the care of patients with thrombotic disorders. We hope the evidence-based approach used in this book will help the reader readily identify where clinical practice is based on firm grounds as opposed to personal opinions and intuition.

The authors would like to thank the following individuals for their assistance in the preparation of this book; Karen Fettes, Lori Genert, Toni McGee, Darlene McKeage, Lori Nairn, Marisa Reibin and Marion Rooney. Dr. Naomi Anderson provided valuable editorial assistance. The art work for the book cover was provided by Kathryn Pineo.

Russell Hull
Gary Raskob
Graham Pineo

Dedication

Dedicated to all of the patients and colleagues who participated in the clinical trials.

Contributors

Melvin A. Andersen, MD
Department of Pathology
Calgary General Hospital
Bow Valley Centre
Calgary, Alberta
Canada

Fred A. Anderson, Jr., PhD
Department of Surgery
University of Massachusetts Medical Center
Worcester, Massachusetts

Jack E. Ansell, MD
Department of Medicine
Boston University School of Medicine
Boston, Massachusetts

William R. Auger, MD
University of California-San Diego Medical Center
Division of Pulmonary and Critical Care Medicine
San Diego, California

Brent R. Bagg, RT
Respiratory Technology
Holy Cross Hospital
Calgary, Alberta
Canada

Linda Barbour, MD, MSPH
University of Colorado
Health Sciences Center
Denver, Colorado

Brian G. Birdwell, MD
Department of Medicine
College of Medicine
University of Oklahoma
Health Sciences Center
Oklahoma City, Oklahoma

Mark A. Bisesi, MD
Department of Radiology
Michigan State University
B220 Clinical Center
East Lansing, Michigan

Lars C. Borris, MD
Venous Thrombosis Group
Department of Orthopaedics
Aalborg Hospital
Aalborg, Denmark

Harry R. Büller, MD, PhD
Centre for Hemostasis, Thrombosis
Atherosclerosis & Inflammation Research
Academic Medical Centre
University of Amsterdam
Amsterdam, The Netherlands

Cedric J. Carter, MB
Department of Laboratory Medicine
Acute Care Unit
University Hospital
Vancouver, British Columbia

G. Patrick Clagett, MD
Vascular Surgery
University of Texas Health Sciences Center
Dallas, Texas

Alexander T. Cohen, MBBS
Thrombosis Research Institute
Emmanuel Kaye Bldg.
London, England

Philip C. Comp, MD, PhD
Department of Medicine
University of Oklahoma
Health Sciences Center
Oklahoma City, Oklahoma

Jacqueline Conard, PhD
Laboratoire Central d'Hématologie
Hopital de L'Hotel Dieu
Paris, France

James E. Dalen, MD
College of Medicine
University of Arizona
Tucson, Arizona

Bruce L. Davidson, MD, MPH
328 South Juniper Street
Philadelphia, Pennsylvania

Sherri S. Durica, MD
Department of Medicine
College of Medicine
Health Sciences Center
Oklahoma City, Oklahoma

Bo Eklof, MD, PhD
Straub Clinic and Hospital
Honolulu, Hawaii

C. Gregory Elliott, MD
Pulmonary Division
LDS Hospital
University of Utah School of Medicine
Salt Lake City, Utah

William Feldstein, BSc, MBA
Clinical Trials Unit
University of Calgary
Calgary, Alberta
Canada

Gordon T. Ford, MD
Respiratory Care
Calgary General Hospital
University of Calgary
Calgary, Alberta
Canada

Alexander S. Gallus, MB
Department of Hematology
Flinders Medical Centre
Bedford Park, South Australia
Australia

James N. George, MD
Department of Medicine
University of Oklahoma
Oklahoma City, Oklahoma

Alexander Gottschalk, MD
B-220 Clinical Center
Michigan State University
East Lansing, Michigan

David Green, MD, PhD
Rehabilitation Institute of Chicago
Northwestern University
Chicago, Illinois

David A. Hanley, MD
University of Calgary
Health Sciences Centre
Calgary, Alberta
Canada

Marie-Helene Horellou, MD
Laboratoire Central d'Hématologie
Hopital de L'Hotel Dieu
Paris, France

Menno V. Huisman, MD, PhD
Academisch Ziekenhuis Leiden
General Internal Medicine
Leiden, The Netherlands

Russell D. Hull, MBBS, MSc
Department of Medicine
Foothills Hospital Health Sciences Center
University of Calgary
Calgary, Alberta
Canada

Vijay V. Kakkar, FRCS
Thrombosis Research Institute
Emmanuel Kaye Bldg.
London, England

Mark A. Kelley, MD
Department of Medicine
Division of Critical Care and Pulmonary Medicine
University of Pennsylvania Medical Center
Philadelphia, Pennsylvania

Maria M.W. Beaumont-Koopman, MD, PhD
Department of Vascular Medicine
Academic Medical Center
Amsterdam, The Netherlands

Michael R. Lassen, MD
Department of Orthopedics
Hillerod Hospital
Hillerod, Denmark

Anthonie W.A. Lensing, MD, PhD
Center for Thrombosis
Hemostasis and Atherosclerosis Research
Academic Medical Center
Amsterdam, The Netherlands

Marcel Levi, MD
Center for Thrombosis
Hemostasis and Atherosclerosis Research
Academic Medical Center
Amsterdam, The Netherlands

Kenneth Moser, MD
University of California-San Diego Medical Center
San Diego, California

Jeffrey Pickard, MD
University of Colorado
Health Sciences Center
Denver, Colorado

Graham F. Pineo, MD
Clinical Trials Unit
Calgary General Hospital
University of Calgary
Calgary, Alberta
Canada

Martin H. Prins, MD
Center for Thrombosis
Hemostasis and Atherosclerosis Research
Academic Medical Center
Amsterdam, The Netherlands

Gary E. Raskob, MSc
Department of Biostatistics and Epidemiology
College of Public Health
Department of Medicine
College of Medicine
University of Oklahoma
Oklahoma City, Oklahoma

Professor Meyer M. Samama, MD, PhD
Laboratoire Central d'Hématologie
Hopital de L'Hotel Dieu
Paris, France

Arthur A. Sasahara, MD
Venture Head, Thrombolytics Research
Abbott Laboratories
Abbott Park, Illinois

G.V.R.K. Sharma, MD
Veterans Affairs Medical Center
Department of Cardiology
West Roxbury, Massachusetts

Paul D. Stein, MD
Henry Ford Hospital
Levine Health Enhancement Center
Detroit, Michigan

Jan W. ten Cate, MD, PhD
Centre for Hemostasis, Thrombosis
Atherosclerosis & Inflammation Research
Academic Medical Centre
University of Amsterdam
Amsterdam, The Netherlands

Alexander Graham G. Turpie, MD
Hamilton General Hospital
McMaster Clinic
McMaster University
Hamilton, Ontario
Canada

Karen A. Valentine, MD, PhD
Department of Medicine
Clinical Trials Unit
Foothills Hospital Health Sciences Center
University of Calgary
Calgary, Alberta,
Canada

Edwin J.R. van Beek, MD, PhD
Department of Radiology
Academic Medical Centre
University of Amsterdam
Amsterdam, The Netherlands

Sidney M. Viner, MD
Intensive Care Unit-G4
Calgary General Hospital
University of Calgary
Calgary, Alberta
Canada

H. Brownell Wheeler, MD
Department of Surgery
University of Massachusetts Medical School
Worcester, Massachusetts

Contents

SECTION I

Epidemiology, Pathophysiology, and Natural History

1

Epidemiology and Pathophysiology of Venous Thromboembolism

Cedric J. Carter, Frederick A. Anderson, Jr., H. Brownell Wheeler

INTRODUCTION

The epidemiology of a disease such as venous thromboembolism involves the study of the distribution and determinants of this disease in the human population. It addresses general questions such as the type of population that acquires the disease, in what circumstances, when, and how? Results are often expressed in terms of rates for a defined or general population.

Pathophysiology of venous thromboembolism concerns itself with the study of specific mechanisms that may cause or mediate this disease. These studies can involve humans, animals, organisms, *in vitro* systems, or more recent concepts such as computer modelling of disease processes.

Pathophysiological studies are often initiated following epidemiologic observations but occasionally discrete pathophysiological observations can generate the hypotheses that become the basis of epidemiologic studies. An example of the former, was the clinical observation that prolonged immobility was a risk factor for the development of venous thrombosis. This led to the development of the various animal stasis models that have been used to investigate the pathophysiology of venous thrombosis. The converse was the biochemical discovery of Protein C. From a physiological point of view it was possible to postulate that a deficiency of this protein should predispose to venous thrombosis. Subsequent epidemiologic studies confirmed this hypothesis. Thus it can be seen that epidemiology and pathophysiology of a disease are intimately related and depending on the rigidity of the definition, the terms clearly overlap.

In order to obtain a better understanding of a disease process there are advantages in considering the epidemiologic and pathophysiological aspects from an integrated rather than a separate viewpoint. The main area of inter-

action is in the understanding of the currently identified risk factors for venous thromboembolism.

GENERAL METHODOLOGY

Despite the apparent differences between the epidemiologic and the pathophysiological approaches to the study of a disease, the fundamental research philosophies are very similar. Both processes involve the formation of a hypothesis and the concept of establishment of causation, when there are observed differences or similarities of any observed or generated end points. Perhaps the most obvious differences in scientific style are the reliance of epidemiology on human population material and the tendency for most epidemiologic studies to be observational rather than interventional. The observational nature of epidemiologic studies has led to a variety of specific investigative and interpretive maneuvers that are not commonly used in pathophysiological investigations. Some of these aspects are described below.

BACKGROUND TO EPIDEMIOLOGIC METHODS

Epidemiologic studies may be descriptive and concerned with the distribution and/or progression of a disease. They may be analytic and/or involved with the investigation of hypotheses suggested by descriptive studies. Finally they may be experimental or interventional. This may involve the evaluation and interpretation of the effects of preventive or therapeutic procedures or the modification of putative risk factors.

In descriptive studies, events are often expressed as rates for a defined population. It is important to make a distinction between the prevalence and incidence of a disease. Prevalence refers to the frequency of a disease at a given point in time. Incidence refers to the rate at which new cases of a disease occur in a defined period. For the purposes of understanding a disease process, the incidence is a more useful index. It incorporates a component of temporality that is important when trying to assess causal associations.

Obviously accuracy of diagnosis is a key issue in the description of rates of a disease. For venous thromboembolism this is discussed in detail in Chapter 12. It should be noted that in some cases the rigor of diagnostic accuracy that can be accepted for epidemiologic studies may be lower than that needed for individual patient management. For descriptive studies of rates, highly specific and sensitive tests are required, but for determining a hierarchy of risk factors, a less rigorous diagnostic test can still give useful information. This divergence from the strict diagnostic requirements for therapeutic interventions require that bias in the diagnostic test apply to all groups under investigation. It is also important that relative rather than absolute information is required, and that a large study sample is available to ameliorate some of the obligate loss of efficiency that occurs with suboptimal diagnostic methods. These are important concepts since there are an increasing number of studies where hard diagnostic endpoints, such as ascending contrast venography, are not feasible or in some cases no longer considered ethical.

In addition to considerations concerning diagnostic methods, an important aspect of epidemiologic studies is the strength of the study design. In terms of structure the weakest form of study is a descriptive study. The main problem is the lack of any formal control group. These studies may suggest strong associations, for example, the association between age and vascular disease, however these simple associations need careful and further investigation.

A very popular type of epidemiologic investigation is the case-control study. In this instance a group of people with the disease of interest, eg. venous thrombosis, is identified together with a group of individuals who clearly do not have the disease of interest. Various data are collected on both groups, for example age, recent surgery, medication exposure, and the relative frequency with which these putative risk factors occur in both cohorts. If one cohort has a marked excess in the frequency of a particular "risk" factor, then this supports a potentially causal relationship.

This type of study has some major attractions. Because the cases are selected it is possible to ask questions concerning diseases that have a low frequency in the population. If a disease has a very low frequency, then a descriptive population study would have to be huge before apparent associations could be detected. If however there are means of extracting these cases from the population, such as from a national disease register, then a case-control study is possible. A key issue is the selection of the appropriate control group or groups. It is

very important to be sure that the controls really are free of the disease of interest. It is also often important to match for certain primary demographic features, provided these are not the questions of interest. In general the sort of items that one might want to match would be broad characteristics such as age and sex. There is a potential problem with over matching of cases and controls. This can destroy real associations. Case-control studies are retrospective. This gives rise to methodological problems including the accuracy of diagnostic end points, completeness of data retrieval, and other sources of bias.

Cohort-analytic studies are usually a more powerful study design. They share the concept of the evaluation of the presence of risk factors between identified cases and controls but have the fundamental difference that cases and controls are identified prospectively with respect to exposure. They are then followed longitudinally to determine the frequency of outcomes. This type of design permits a more accurate documentation of exposure. Classic retrospective case-control studies often have to rely on recollection of exposure, for example the period of exposure to a noxious agent or medication.

The main problem with cohort-analytic studies is that the cases are self-selected and may have intrinsic characteristics that may be absent in the control group. Estimates of the importance of a particular risk factor in both case-control and cohort-analytic studies are usually expressed as a form of ratio. In cohort-analytic studies this can be calculated directly. For example one can make a statement that women taking the contraceptive pill are twice as likely to experience venous thrombosis as nontakers. This would be expressed as a relative risk of 2:0. Using this figure as a basis, and by the correlation of this type of exposure to the incidence of thrombosis in the general population, one can also derive an attributable risk. This is a numerical estimate of the impact of the risk factor on the general population. For the determination of health care policy, attributable risk is often the most important statistic.

In case-control studies it is not possible to directly calculate the clinical impact of a risk factor. It is possible to derive an indirect estimate of risk, termed the relative odds. The clinical impact of relative odds cannot be directly translated to a population, but relative odds are useful in supporting the strength of an association relative to other risk factors.

For determining the importance of associations, the preferred approach is to use multivariate rather than univariate analyses. This is important since it allows for the dissection of the effects of linked risk factors, whereas univariate analysis will not. When one uses multivariate analytic methods to evaluate apparent risk factors, the relative importance of some of the traditional deep-vein thrombosis (DVT) risk factors greatly diminishes. The contribution of obesity to the development of venous thrombosis is an example of this and will be discussed in more detail later.

The most powerful form of study design to evaluate epidemiologic associations is a randomized-controlled clinical trial. In its most evolved form this is most commonly associated with determination of efficacy and safety of therapeutics, but in specific circumstances this approach can be used to evaluate either individual or multiple risk factors. An example of an individual risk factor that might be evaluated is the role of estrogen preparations as causal agents for venous thrombosis. An example of the concept of testing multiple risk factors would be to randomize patients with a particular disease to either inpatient or outpatient management.

This type of design provides very powerful information but its application is often limited by a series of practical considerations. For example, you cannot randomize primary demographic components such as age or sex. Controlled-randomized studies usually represent the final confirmation of associations suggested by descriptive, case-control, or cohort-analytic studies.

Irrespective of the study methodology employed, a key issue is whether identified risk factors have a causal association with the disease of interest or whether they merely represent some kind of epidemiologic marker. This is particularly difficult to evaluate with nonexperimental studies. To facilitate the examination of potentially causal associations, a series of guidelines have been developed. These guidelines include the examination of the strength of association, in general relative risks or odds ratios should be greater than 2.0, and demonstration of consistency. The latter is supported by multiple studies showing a similar association. Other factors include the specificity, the presence of a biological gradient, the temporality, and the biological plausibility of any observed associations. The exact weighting of these factors will clearly vary according to the risk factor under investigation.

BACKGROUND TO THE PATHOPHYSIOLOGY OF VENOUS THROMBOSIS

A venous thrombus is an intravascular mass composed of the constituents of blood. Although much of the research interest in coagulation has focussed on the prevention of bleeding, a much more important issue is why blood, which can rapidly clot, actually remains liquid? There appears to be three primary determinants, an intact undamaged venous endothelium, normal amounts of both the pro and antithrombotic plasma proteins, and normal blood rheology. These concepts, although enumerated over a hundred years ago, remain the basis of our understanding of the pathophysiology of venous thrombosis. Recent progress has been based on the ability to quantify the constituent components of these primary determinants.

Vessel Wall Anatomy and Physiology

Normal veins comprise an endothelial layer, a medial layer, and an outer adventitial layer. In comparison to arteries the internal elastic lamina is thin or absent and the medial layer is rich in collagen but has little muscle tissue. Compared to arteries, congenital variations of venous anatomy are common. A unique feature of the larger veins is the presence of venous valves. These are more frequent in distal vessels, for example seven to 15 pairs may occur in the tibial veins but only two to four pairs may be present in the proximal venous system. Intact valves ensure that the high pressures generated by contraction of muscle in the lower limb, propel the venous blood against the effect of gravity back to the heart.

Two aspects of vessel wall are important in the genesis of venous thrombi, endothelial cell function, and venous anatomy. The latter will be discussed below in the rheology section.

The endothelium provides the direct interface with the blood. Endothelial cells have a synthetic function and produce prothrombotic substances that support platelet-vessel wall interactions, the initiating process in both venous and arterial thrombosis. These substances include von Willebrand factor, type IV collagen, and fibronectin.[1-3] Also synthesized is Plasminogen Activator Inhibitor Type I (PAI-1) which inhibits natural fibrinolysis and is therefore prothrombotic.[4] Other prothrombotic proteins synthesized or released by endothelium include tissue factor and factor VIIIc.[5,6]

Various antithrombotic substances are synthesized or released from intact endothelium. These include the antiplatelet substance PGI_2, several glycosaminoglycans which mediate the effects of Antithrombin and Heparin Cofactor II, the profibrinolytic Tissue Plasminogen Activator (TPA), and thrombomodulin, the cofactor for thrombin's activation of the natural anticoagulant Protein C.[6-10] The natural state of endothelium is for the antithrombotic component described above to have the greater effect. When endothelium is challenged by physical or chemical damage, the prothrombotic components may predominate. For functional as well as anatomical reasons endothelial cell function is integrated with the coagulation system.

Coagulation Physiology

The coagulation system, with its interface the endothelium, has to sustain two physiological functions. These are: 1) That essential organs receive an uninterrupted supply of blood-born nutrition and 2) That any breach in the vascular integrity will be rapidly repaired. These requisites are clearly competing and the key issue is the maintenance of an appropriate balance between these needs.

The current concept is that the initiation of a thrombus starts with an enhanced platelet-vessel-wall interaction. This is clear in the case of arterial disease where thrombus *in situ* is almost always associated with macroscopic changes in the vessel wall. Although vessel wall lesions are sometimes present in venous thrombosis it is postulated that even macroscopically normal venous endothelium, when associated with venous thrombosis, is abnormal.[11] The initial platelet-endothelial interaction will cause platelet adherence which is rapidly followed by platelet aggregation. In experimental thrombosis models, platelet aggregation and release can occur within 10 seconds of endothelial injury. This is followed by early fibrin formation at around 30 seconds and a visible hemostatic plug at 2–3 minutes.[12] Platelet-coagulation interactions are complex. Although the classical coagulation cascade has traditionally involved a role for factor XII, it now seems that initiation of the intrinsic coagulation pathway starts at factor XI.[13] Platelets can directly participate in this process but it has also been demonstrated that thrombin can directly activate factor XI.[13] Activated factor XI can activate factor IX which in turn participates in the "Tenase complex" of factors VIII, IX, and X. This complex is thought to be assembled on the surface of activated platelets thereby providing a secondary link between initial and subsequent thrombotic forces.

There is a second and perhaps more important pathway that will activate the "Tenase complex." This involves the extrinsic pathway. Tissue factor is a ubiquitous membrane lipoprotein consisting of an azoprotein and an associated phospholipid. Tissue factor combines with factor VII to provide an alternative means of interacting on a phospholipid surface to convert factor X to Xa.[14]

The activated factor X whether generated from this complex or via the intrinsic pathway as described above, is then involved in the "prothrombinase complex" which generates thrombin. Again the platelet surface is the template for this interaction. Thrombin once generated has multiple thrombotic functions including the conversion of fibrinogen to fibrin and a feedback activation of factor XI which reactivates the intrinsic pathway.[13] Thrombin will also aggregate platelets and interact with fibrinolysis. Factor XIII when activated by thrombin to factor XIIIa will crosslink and stabilize fibrin.[15] In this form fibrin is relatively resistant to fibrinolysis. The only obvious antithrombotic effect of thrombin is when it binds to thrombomodulin and activates Protein C.

If one calculates the apparent kinetics of the intrinsic pathway, particularly on the basis factor XII being the initiating coagulation protein, then the pathway appears to be too slow to be of physiological importance. Recent studies seem to have resolved some of these issues. It now appears that the Tissue Factor pathway is the rapid prohemostatic response pathway. Cellular damage activates this pathway and generates the thrombin required to support primary hemostasis. The generated thrombin also feeds back to factor XI to initiate the intrinsic pathway. At first sight it would appear that if this mechanism was the major participant in thrombus formation, then people with intrinsic factor deficiencies such as hemophilia A would not bleed. Again this paradox has been resolved by the discovery of an inhibitor of the extrinsic pathway. The current name for this inhibitor is the Tissue Factor Pathway Inhibitor (TFPI).[16] After the initial burst of prohemostatic activity has occurred TFPI shuts down the extrinsic pathway but coagulation continues through autoactivation of factor XI through thrombin. By analogy with other inhibitors of coagulation such as Antithrombin, Protein C, or Protein S, it might be expected that TFPI deficiency would predispose to thrombosis. To date despite a variety of clinical studies, low levels of TFPI have not shown a correlation with the development of venous thrombosis. Unopposed thrombin generation has the potential to cause massive thrombosis and it is clear that this system must be modulated. In fact, control of the prothrombotic forces occurs at a variety of levels. A primary feature of the coagulation cascade is the serial activation of inactive precursor coagulation proteins by a hydrolytic cleavage by a serine protease. Each precursor, for example factor XI when activated to factor XIa, becomes a serine protease and activates the next precursor protein, for example factor IX. Serine proteases are most efficiently inhibited by Antithrombin (previously called antithrombin III).[17] Factors V and VIII although part of the coagulation cascade and activatable by the serine protease thrombin, do not become serine proteases. They act as coagulation cofactors that facilitate serine protease-zymogen precursor interactions. These two proteins are modulated by a different inhibitory principle via activated Protein C and its cofactor Protein S.[18] On a biochemical basis one might predict that deficiencies in these inhibitory proteins would predispose to thrombosis and this is the case. So far most of these proteins appear to show some clinical penetrance even when they occur as congenital heterozygous cases. They will cause spontaneous thrombosis but will also clearly summate with other risk factors. The exception to this concept is the TFPI system described above. More complete aspects of conditions such as Protein C, Protein S, and Antithrombin deficiency are discussed in much greater detail in Chapter 36.

If the inhibitory mechanisms described above fail to modulate thrombus formation, the final defense against the deleterious effects of unwanted thrombosis is the fibrinolytic system. There are two major components, the cellular system and the plasma mediated system. Macrophages and neutrophils can both ingest fibrin and may be important in the extracellular environment but their importance intravascularly is not clear.[19] The bulk of fibrinolysis within the vessel is thought to be mediated through the generation of plasmin. Current theory suggests that many of the stimuli which initiate thrombosis will also cause the release of tissue plasminogen activator

(TPA) from endothelial cells.[20] Also released will be its natural inhibitor PAI-1. Provided TPA is in a functional excess, it will bind to fibrin and after a conformational change become a very efficient converter of inactive plasminogen, to the highly fibrinolytically active plasmin. Plasminogen is closely associated with fibrin and plasmin will be generated *in situ*. Any free plasmin is rapidly neutralized by α-2-antiplasmin.[21] There are various abnormalities of the fibrinolytic system that will predispose to thrombosis. Some patients show a suboptimal TPA release. Some patients release increased amounts of PAI-1. In rare instances abnormal fibrinogens will give rise to abnormal fibrin which will not catalyze TPA activity or may be resistant to the action of plasmin. Chapter 36 contains further details of the specific conditions.

Blood Rheology

The third component of the classic prothrombotic triad is the blood rheology. This is a complex area and at a theoretical level involves a substantive understanding of fluid mechanics. This means that with a few exceptions little work has been done in this area by physicians. There are, however, some basic observations that are of importance in the understanding of the development of venous thrombosis.

Interest in blood viscosity and blood clotting is not recent. Poiseuille published a series of experiments on the relationship of blood viscosity and thrombosis in 1842.[22] The constituents of blood itself are of interest. Important variables include the hematocrit and fibrinogen levels. The geometry and elastic properties of the vessel are an area of active investigation. Most interest has focussed on the arterial system where a wide range of shear forces are present. In veins, shear rates are low compared to arteries, but red cell aggregates and the non-Newtonian character of normal blood at low shear rates, result in a relatively high blood viscosity. This means that decreases in venous perfusion pressure will tend to decrease shear rates and to increase blood viscosity. These conditions should predispose to thrombosis since high local concentrations of procoagulant material can accumulate rather than being diluted and subsequently cleared in the liver. In addition to these general observations on venous rheology there may be some specific areas of importance. Both venographic and postmortem studies have demonstrated that thrombi often appear to have started in the venous valve pockets. Experimental studies have demonstrated vortices in valve pockets.[23] These conditions favor multiple platelet-endothelial cell interactions and provide a reasonable theoretical basis for the initiation of venous thrombus. Subsequent growth and proliferation would be enhanced by stasis in conjunction with other modulators of the coagulation process including the natural inhibitors and the fibrinolytic system.

EPIDEMIOLOGIC STUDIES: IDENTIFICATION OF RISK FACTORS AND PATHOPHYSIOLOGICAL CORRELATES

General Epidemiology

In 1986 a National Institutes of Health Consensus Conference estimated that as many as 50,000 people die annually from (PE) pulmonary embolism and that between 300,000 and 600,000 hospitalizations each year in the United States are associated with PE and/or DVT.[24] Such estimates are largely based upon extrapolations of data obtained in individual hospitals and, despite the clinical importance of DVT and PE, the fundamental epidemiology of these disorders has not been adequately described.

The most basic information on thromboembolic disease is the simple estimation of the incidence. The two main areas of interest are the incidence of PE and of deep venous thrombosis of the lower limb. The interest in the former is in part because it is a significant cause of death, and in part because it is a marker of the success or failure of various antithrombotic measures. Lower limb thrombosis is of interest because it appears to be the most commonly detected type of venous thrombosis, and because of its close relationship with pulmonary emboli.

The weakest link in the determination of the incidence of venous thromboembolic disease is the attempt to obtain reliable estimates in the general as opposed to the hospital population. One of the basic principles of any disease survey is the ability to accurately determine the diagnosis. As will be apparent from Section III of this book, this is a key issue for incidence studies.

A source of information on incidence of fatal venous thromboembolic disease are death certificate returns in countries that keep centralized records. Using the International Classification of Disease classifications, Hume et al, obtained an estimate for fatal PE of 21,000 deaths in England and Wales in 1967.[25] This would give an incidence of 40 per 100,000 per annum, a not so inconsequential figure. This figure is in general agreement with extrapolations from other countries' national statistics. The problem that one has to consider is the components that go into this source of estimate. One immediate problem is that, even for many of the fatal PEs, only a clinical diagnosis was available. Autopsy rates have declined under the misapprehension that premortem diagnostic technology has lessened the value of the traditional autopsy. Even if there are autopsy data there is a problem of adjudication as to whether detected pulmonary emboli were actually the cause of death or just an associated agonal event. A third confounding problem is the legislative requirements as to how deaths are recorded. In some circumstances the requirement is to record the underlying disease, for example cancer or congestive heart failure, as the cause of death and the information regarding PE is not apparent.

There have been several large hospital series examining some of the issues.[26,27] These are not recent studies and date back to the time when autopsies were often mandatory in academic institutions. These hospital-based series showed that major emboli, of which up to two-thirds were ascribed as being fatal, were present in approximately 10 percent of fatalities. The proportion of pulmonary emboli that were defined as being fatal was very much influenced by the vigilance of the detection process.[28]

Utilizing large national databases, such as the National Hospital Discharge Survey, several investigators have estimated the rates of venous thromboembolism in U.S. hospitals.[29,30] In 1985, based on an estimated 120,000 hospital discharge diagnoses of PE and 187,000 diagnoses of DVT, the prevalence rate of PE was estimated to be 51 per 100,000 and 79 per 100,000 for DVT;[29] however, such data must be interpreted with appropriate caution due to several potentially important sources of bias, including variations in coding practices, limitations in the number of secondary diagnoses coded, and inclusion of diagnoses that were ultimately ruled-out. In addition, these databases do not allow analysis of time or severity dependent factors, for example, identification of first episodes of venous thromboembolism or inclusion of the results of objective diagnostic testing. Although expensive and time-consuming, focused review and independent validation of patient charts is the only systematic and accurate method of obtaining these data.

There have been several attempts to assess the frequency of DVT in the general population. These studies have suffered from many of the limitations described in the documentation of PE. One early attempt was the Tecumseh Community Health study.[31] This was a prospective study, but the value of the information obtained is limited because of the use of non-objective diagnostic criteria. A population-based study performed in Scandinavia had similar limitations.[32] Notwithstanding these criticisms, both these studies indicated that 2.5% to 5% of the population had experienced venous thrombosis. Direct figures on incidence were not reported. These studies have to be distinguished from hospital studies where, unless one has a relative captive population, one is subject to major referral bias.

There have been three recent studies that have addressed the incidence of venous thromboembolic disease on a community basis. The first study, known as the Worcester DVT Study, was performed in the United States and was based on the Worcester, MA metropolitan statistical area that encompasses a population of 380,000.[33] Information on the diagnosis of DVT and PE was retrieved retrospectively from hospital records.

Advantage was taken of the presence of a computer-based hospital discharge coding system that included a wide variety of ICD codes. In order not to miss cases a broad range of codings were used and subsequently validated by careful review of individual patient charts. Patients were assigned to a diagnosis of acute DVT or PE, either as a first or repeat episode. Attention was paid to various risk factors that were based on earlier studies. Estimates of the incidence of DVT and PE related to the population served by the participating hospitals.

There were several confounding factors that were addressed as much as is possible in a retrospective descriptive survey. One issue was whether the population was community-based. Postal codes were used to exclude patients from outside the catchment area for the study. What could not be controlled, were patients who had elected to take their medical problems to alternate centers, although it should be noted that given the quality of the participating institutions, the major problem was likely to be referred-in rather than referred-out patients. A second issue was the question of the use of clinical diagnoses. On examination of the charts, 84% of DVT cases had an objective diagnosis suggesting that this was not a major bias. The overall incidence of the first episode of DVT was 56 per 100,000 per annum. The incidence of PE was 23 per 100,000 per annum. If one compares the DVT figures from the Worcester DVT Study to an incidence estimate derived from the Tecumseh Study, or its equivalent Scandinavian study, the results are quite similar. Not unexpectedly various apparent risk factors were identified including age, recent surgery, malignancy, and obesity (Table 1). It should be noted that Worcester DVT Study was a descriptive study with no control group and multivariate techniques were not applied to this data. Despite these criticisms this is the best estimate of the magnitude of the problem of DVT and PE currently available in the North America (Table 2).

Table 1
Risk Factors in 405 Patients with an Initial Episode of Deep-Vein Thrombosis (DVT) and/or Pulmonary Embolism (PE)

Risk Factors	DVT (n = 274)	PE (n = 131)
Age ≥ 40 years	85%	89%
Cancer	32%	27%
Congestive Heart Failure	15%	31%
Chronic Obstructive Pulmonary Disease	18%	34%
Diabetes	14%	15%
Fracture	13%	11%
Myocardial Infarction	3%	9%
Obesity	39%	38%
Stroke	2%	8%
Surgery	19%	19%
Trauma	1%	3%

* Adapted from Anderson et al,[33]

Table 2
Deep-Vein Thrombosis and/or Pulmonary Embolism Treated in Acute Care Hospitals

	Incidence Per 100,000 Population Per Year	U.S. Cases in 1986 (estimated)
Attack rate of DVT/PE	107 (100-117)*	257,972
Recurrent DVT/PE	36 (32-40)*	86,760
First episode DVT/PE	71 (65-78)*	171,178
First episode DVT (only)	48 (43-54)*	115,726
First episode PE (with or without DVT)	23 (19-27)*	55,452

* 95% confidence intervals
Adapted from Anderson et al,[33]

Concomitant with this study was a prospective study performed in the community of Malmo, Sweden.[34] In this community all people with suspected venous thrombosis are referred to in one institution and, at the time of the report, contrast venography was the primary method of objective diagnosis. Compared to the American study the population served was slightly smaller at 281,000. A total of 1009 patients were referred for venography for suspected venous thrombosis and in 366 cases DVT was confirmed. The observed prevalence of DVT was 160 per 100,000 per annum. If one allows for the inclusion of recurrent DVT episodes, then the incidence is strikingly similar to the Worcester study. What was very different was the incidence of PE at approximately two per 100,000 per annum. This may reflect the fact that the point of entry for the Swedish Study was symptomatic venous thrombosis, whereas the Worcester study also included patients who had been specifically investigated for PE. Again this was a descriptive study and conclusions with respect to any associations must be limited. Perusal of the data indicates the anticipated risk factors such as age, recent surgery, trauma, and malignancy were evident.

The third community-based study is ongoing at the Mayo Clinic. This retrospective study, based on the well-known Rochester Epidemiology Project, is designed to include all residents of Olmstead County, MN who were diagnosed with DVT or PE between 1966 and 1990. Results published to date include estimates of the incidence of DVT and PE for the time period 1966 to 1970.[35,36]

The complete inpatient and outpatient medical records of all patients suspected of having DVT or PE were reviewed and classified as definite (pulmonary angiogram, venogram or autopsy), probable (noninvasive tests), or clinical DVT or PE. Initial data from 1966 to 1970 indicate that the annual incidence of DVT/PE was 120 per 100,000 (95% CI 108–131). Despite the strengths of this study, data from 1966 to 1970 contain a high proportion of clinically diagnosed DVT and PE, reflecting the absence of noninvasive tests for DVT/PE prior to 1970.[37] Incidence rates were 43 per 100,000 for definite and prob-

able DVT/PE and 76 per 100,000 for clinical DVT/PE during this time period.

Using all the available information from the five studies described above an estimate of the incidence of DVT in the general population would appear to be in the region of 60 to 180 cases per 100,000 per annum. Estimates for the incidence of PE are less reliable and the retrospective estimate from the Worcester DVT Study of 23 per 100,000 per annum is not unreasonable (Table 2).

Case-Fatality and Survival Rates

In addition to the incidence of disease, epidemiology is also concerned with the rates of both in-hospital death (short-term survival rate) and the rate of death following hospital discharge (long-term survival rate), in patients with the target disease. As discussed previously, attribution of death to PE poses a dilemma for epidemiologists and clinicians. Nevertheless, both the Worcester study and the Mayo Clinic study estimated the case-fatality and long-term survival rates following an episode of venous thromboembolism.[33,36]

Autopsy data are the basis for most estimates of the frequency of death due to PE. The current autopsy rate in U.S. hospitals is approximately 14% (and is often less than 5% in nonteaching hospitals).[38] Autopsy technique is a critical factor that strongly influences the proportion of cases where PE is found. It is often difficult to establish the clinical importance of pulmonary embolism in patients who die with cancer or other serious underlying illness. Estimates of the prevalence of PE in patients who die in the hospital range as high as 67%.[26] However, most investigators agree that PE is a significant contributor to 10% to 15% of all hospital deaths. A recent autopsy review in a large teaching hospital documented massive fatal pulmonary embolism in 6% of deceased patients.[39] Since published autopsy studies of PE have been conducted in large teaching hospitals, which typically include patients with more severe illness, it is unknown whether these data can be extrapolated to nonteaching hospitals, where the severity of illness is usually lower; however, the Worcester DVT Study reported no significant difference between nonteaching and teaching hospitals in the proportion of discharges with a diagnosis of venous thromboembolism.[33]

In-Hospital Case-Fatality Rates

In the Worcester DVT Study there were 405 patients with a first recognized (incident) episode of venous thromboembolism of whom 47 (12%) died in the hospital. The case-fatality rates for DVT and PE were 5% and 2% respectively. The in-hospital case-fatality rates increased with increasing patient age. Among patients less than 40 years, 2% died during the acute hospital phase. This increased to 10% in patients 40 to 59 years, 11% in patients 60 to 79 years, and 16% in patients 80 years of age or older.

Pulmonary embolism was listed on the death certificate as a contributing cause of death in 20 (43%) of 47 patients who died in the hospital with an antemortem diagnosis of venous thromboembolism. Based on data from medical records, autopsies were performed in 14 (30%) of 47 patients and PE was confirmed in 12 of 14 cases. Pulmonary embolism was listed as the primary cause of death in five patients and as a secondary cause of death in seven patients.

In the Mayo Clinic study[36] 413 patients were identified with incident episodes of DVT or PE occurring between 1966 and 1970. In 115 patients (28%), PE was first diagnosed at autopsy or the patient had a rapidly fatal event with death occurring within one day of the onset of symptoms. This is more than twice the short-term fatality rate reported for patients in the Worcester study, perhaps reflecting a significantly higher autopsy rate during 1966–1970 in Ohlmstead County, MN. These data may also reflect a true decrease in the short-term case fatality rate for PE between 1966–1970 and 1985–1986.

Long-Term Prognosis

In the Worcester DVT Study all 358 patients discharged alive after an initial episode of venous thromboembolism were followed over the subsequent two to three and one-half year period. A total of 108 (30%) of these 358 patients died during this period. The overall long-term case-fatality rate in patients with PE was 25% whereas 32% of patients with DVT died during the follow-up period. Long-term survival was significantly associated with age (Figure 1). The age-specific survival curves were statistically significantly different from one another by the log rank test. Neither sex nor whether the event was DVT or PE was an important predictor of long-term survival.[33]

Pulmonary embolism was listed on the death certificate as a contributing cause of death in four of 108 patients who died during a two to three and one-half year period, following discharge from the hospital with an antemortem diagnosis of venous thromboembolism. Of 108

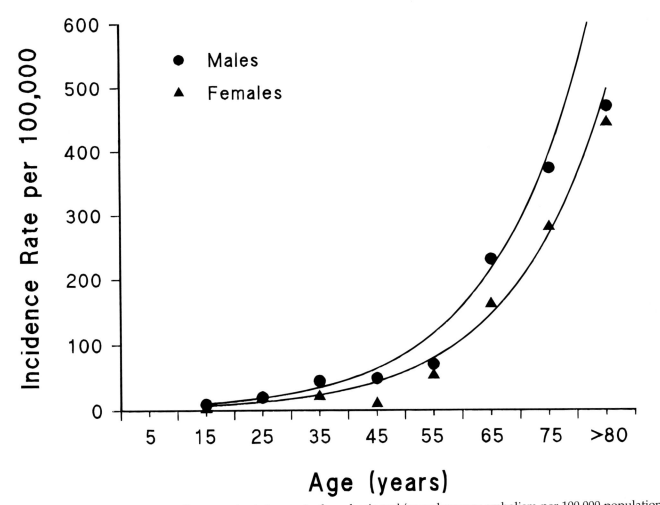

Figure 1. Incidence rate of clinically recognized deep-vein thrombosis and/or pulmonary embolism per 100,000 population. The increase in rates for both males and females is well approximated by an exponential function of age. The modeled rate for males (upper curve) is significantly higher (p < 0.05) than that for females (lower curve). (From Anderson FA, Jr et al: Archives of Internal Medicine 151:935, 1991).

patients who died following hospital discharge, 11 underwent autopsy. No pulmonary emboli were found.

The Mayo Clinic study evaluated the long-term survival of 298 patients with an initial episode of DVT/PE, survival was 95% at 30 days, 88% at one year, 74% at five years, 62% at ten years, 54% at 15 years, and 43% at 20 years. Observed survival was significantly lower for patients with PE than for patients with DVT.[36]

Survival data from both the Worcester study[33] and from the Mayo Clinic study[36] indicate that the greatest mortality following hospitalization for a recognized episode of venous thromboembolism occurs within the first 12 months after discharge. A strength of the Mayo study was the selection of a control group of age and sex matched 1970 Minnesota residents. From this comparison, it was estimated that there was a 15% long-term reduction in predicted survival among patients with DVT/PE.

Due to the low rate of autopsy, the mortality from venous thromboembolism remains uncertain. The 12% in-hospital case-fatality rate observed in the Worcester DVT Study for patients with recognized venous thromboembolism is sobering, but not unanticipated. The 28% short-term fatality rate observed in the Mayo Clinic study may reflect a poorer outcome due to the more limited resources for diagnosis and treatment available in the late 1960s. It may also reflect a more complete assessment of the true fatality rate based on a higher rate of autopsy during the late 1960s. The 30% long-term case fatality rate within 3 years of hospital discharge observed in the Worcester Study may be the inevitable result of terminal co-morbidities, such as myocardial infarction or cancer; however, the Mayo Clinic study showed that there was a 15% excess of deaths in patients who had an incident episode of DVT/PE compared to age and sex matched control patients, suggesting a causal association between DVT/PE and decreased long-term survival.

Incidence rates are important in defining the scope and impact of a health problem. The planning of specific preventive or treatment measures requires a delineation of risk factors, and an elucidation of the probable pathophysiological mechanisms involved in the genesis and propagation of thrombosis.

RISK FACTOR EVALUATION AND PATHOPHYSIOLOGY

Most of the information relating to risk factors and pathophysiology are based on hospital surveys. This is partly based on convenience but also relates to various clinical maneuvers or clinical conditions that are associated with a very high incidence of thrombosis. By dissecting the components of various situations that are associated with hospital thrombosis a considerable understanding of the pathophysiology can be obtained.

One intrinsic problem of interpretation of hospital-

Table 3
Prevalence of Risk Factors for Venous Thromboembolism Among Hospitalized Patients

Risk Factor	(%)	# Risk Factors (Mean ± SD)
Age ≥ 40 years	59.1	2.1 ± 1.0
Obesity	27.6	2.4 ± 1.0
Major Surgery	22.8	2.3 ± 1.1
Prolonged Immobilizaton	14.2	3.0 ± 1.1
Cancer	9.3	2.8 ± 1.0
Congestive Heart Failure	7.8	2.8 ± 0.9
Myocardial Infarction	2.9	3.3 ± 0.9
Fracture (Hip or Leg)	2.2	3.7 ± 1.3
History of Venous Thromboembolism	1.8	3.0 ± 1.0
Trauma	1.6	2.1 ± 1.5
Stroke	1.5	3.3 ± 1.3
Estrogen Replacement Therapy	0.4	2.0 ± 0.8

* Adapted from Anderson et al.[40]

based thrombosis is the quantitation of the contribution of apparent risk factors (Table 1). People who go to the hospital are often elderly. They often have multiple risk factors and hospital interventions are often complex[40] (Table 3). For example surgical procedures involve anesthesia, prolonged perioperative immobility, the administration of various medications that may affect the coagulation or vessel wall, the type of surgery itself, and a variety of postoperative risk factors. All these items are in addition to primary preoperative risk factors. The problem is that these items are not independent and they are often interdependent. Simple univariate analysis cannot address these issues. Multivariate techniques are a partial solution, but closely linked risk factors cannot be easily separated and quantified.

Surgery and Trauma

One of the major initial stimuli for the investigation of the etiology of DVT was the occurrence of pulmonary emboli after major surgical procedures. Autopsies confirmed the presence of venous thrombi in fatal embolism cases and demonstrated the association between DVT and embolism. It became apparent that various clinical groups were particularly liable to this type of complication. Once the ability to reliably detect thrombi in vivo became available, then the true magnitude of the problem became apparent.

Orthopedic Surgery and Trauma

The strongest association between surgery and DVT demonstrated so far is in cases of orthopedic surgery or direct trauma to the lower limbs. Venographic studies show an incidence of venous thrombosis in tibial fractures or knee surgery that range from 50% to 65%.[41–43] The continued validity of these figures has been confirmed in the placebo arm of a recent clinical trial of antithrombotic prophylaxis for knee surgery where there was a 65% thrombosis rate.[44] This information is so consistent that an untreated control arm in orthopedic antithrombotic clinical trials is no longer considered ethical. Fractured hips show a similar high incidence of venous thrombosis. In general for hip replacement the incidence of venous thrombosis is generally a little lower, ranging from 35% to almost 50%.[45,46] The early observations on the incidence of thrombosis in both hip and knee surgery were descriptive. More recently the placebo arms of randomized trials of low-molecular-weight heparin prophylaxis have confirmed that, despite the general advances in patient care, the historic rates of thrombosis remain high.[47]

With respect to the pathophysiology, orthopedic patients show certain seminal features. One observation is that the site of the injury or surgical procedure is a very strong determinant of the site of the thrombus. Thus the major thrombi tend to be in the operated side and at the site of local vessel damage, for example the femoral vein after hip replacement or the popliteal region after knee surgery. This certainly fits with the concept of altered endothelial function being a determinant. Rheological factors may also be involved. These may be of a general nature in terms of venous stasis from immobility caused by the general anesthetic. It is of interest that regional anesthesia has a lower DVT rate in hip surgery. In addition to general stasis there may also be local disorganization of flow relating to tissue edema or vessel repositioning. The third component in the traditional triad is also present in that there are coagulation changes. Some are of a general nature and associated with all major surgeries. These reflect changes in acute phase reactants such as fibrinogen or factor VIII. There is also a decrease in fibrinolytic activity. It has been suggested that these changes are prothrombotic although a true causal relationship has not been demonstrated. There is also a release of prothrombotic material in the form of tissue factor directly from the area of surgical trauma. This is perhaps exemplified by the induction of disseminated intravascular coagulation after gun shot wounds to the head. In orthopedic procedures such as hip replacement there is considerable tissue damage and presumably tissue factor release. This may explain a component of the observed relationship between the extent of surgery or trauma and the incidence of thrombosis. In the trauma field this is seen in the higher rate of DVT with intratrochanteric hip fractures compared to subcapital fractures.[48] It appears that orthopedic surgery provides a prototypic model for risk factor delineation and pathophysiological explanations. The high frequency of events in the absence of aggressive antithrombotic prophylaxis also permits observations on the association between proximal DVT and PE. This has been confirmed by autopsy studies. In the traditional surveys fatal emboli are reported to have occurred in up to 10% of cases of hip surgery. Recent figures are much lower, but fatal embolism still appears to have a case-frequency of 2.0% to 3.0%.[49]

General, Urologic and Gynecological Surgery

Patients undergoing abdominothoracic surgery are another important group who incur postoperative thrombotic complications. In orthopedics, hip and knee replacement cases form a relatively discrete operative group and the rates of thrombosis are fairly consistent. In abdominothoracic surgery there are a wide range of types and severities of surgeries in a very diverse patient population. This is reflected in the wide range of thrombosis rates which can vary from close to zero in a young patient undergoing minor elective surgery, to 33% or more in elderly patients undergoing major surgery for malignancy. Early descriptive studies took advantage of the availability of radiofibrinogen leg scanning. This is a highly sensitive technique for screening for thrombosis and in particular for the distal leg region.

Since abdominothoracic surgery is a large patient group, much of the evidence regarding risk factors has been obtained from their study. If one uses a multivariate analytic technique and applies this to the large surgical surveys, a variety of risk factors become apparent. These include age, magnitude of the surgical procedure, the presence of malignancy, the duration and type of anesthetic, the use of hormonal preparations, and previous thrombosis.[50] The exact impact for an individual patient will depend on the exact type of procedure, but if one had to pick the most general significant risk factor it would be a history of previous thrombosis. Since these specific risk factors apply to all types of surgical and nonsurgical patients they will be described in more detail later.

In urological surgery postoperative venous thrombosis presents particular problems. Proctectomy is a common procedure in the elderly patient. It is potentially a very hemorrhagic procedure. The traditional open proctectomy has an incidence of venous thrombosis of approximately 30% as detected by leg scanning and the clinical trials of low-dose subcutaneous heparin to prevent thrombosis, have showed only modest efficacy. In contrast, independent descriptive studies showed that the transurethral procedure has an incidence of postoperative venous thrombosis of less than 10% despite the presence of a high number of cases of malignancy.[51,52] Unfortunately there was not a random assignment to either open or the transurethral procedure, so direct conclusions are limited, but it appears that the less invasive transurethral procedure may be one way of modifying the thrombotic risk. This epidemiological approach is particularly useful in situations where suitable or simple prophylactic measures are not available.

A similar procedural difference is seen in gynecologic surgery. Following vaginal hysterectomy the incidence of thrombosis may be as low as 7%, but following abdominal hysterectomy observed rates may be two-fold higher.[53] This fits in with a general hypothesis that the magnitude of tissue damage contributes to the thrombotic risk, although it should be acknowledged that more extensive surgery also will be associated with other risk factors such as prolonged immobilization.

Epidemiological studies on surgical patients have proven highly useful for the identification of risk factors and in developing ideas on the pathophysiology, but many of the studies cited above are from 20 years ago. A variety of changes have occurred that have decreased the opportunity to study these aspects of venous thrombosis. Radiofibrinogen leg scanning has fallen from favor, partly due to cost, but also because of concerns about virus transmission. Regional anesthesia is now more common, and there are a new range of endoscopic or laprascopic procedures that induce very little general morbidity. Finally, and perhaps most importantly, the demonstration of the efficacy of various perioperative antithrombotic regimens has meant that there are often no placebo arms in randomized trials of antithrombotic prophylaxis. In general surgery the overall thrombosis rates are now almost universally considerably less than 10%. The modern surgical milieu with respect to the study of the epidemiology of venous thrombosis is therefore one of rapidly diminishing returns.

Pregnancy and the Puerperium

The decrease in maternal deaths from hemorrhage, sepsis, and eclampsia has emphasized the significance of venous thromboembolism as a major cause of morbidity and mortality in pregnancy. The current importance is supported by various national statistics including the Confidential Enquiries into Maternal Deaths in England and Wales. These reports are published regularly and provide a historical perspective on the problem of fatal embolism.[54–56]

The above series of reports provide reasonably reliable and often autopsy-confirmed data on PE, but venous thrombosis has proven more difficult to study. Early studies often relied on clinical diagnosis. This was in part due to a reluctance to use conventional contrast venography because of fetal radiation concerns. Accepting the limitations of these studies, various estimates for venous thrombosis have been obtained. If one expresses these events per delivery then the rates are in the region of three per each thousand deliveries. Although it is not always easy in terms of establishing the temporal relationship, many of these thromboses relate to the delivery period where the risk may be 20-fold the antepartum risk. This is not surprising in that delivery is in many ways analogous to major surgery.

In the earlier studies that were summarized by Drill and Calhoun there was no strong evidence to support a difference in risk among the antepartum trimesters.[57]

Unfortunately, anecdotal statements that the third trimester was a higher risk period has led to the use of more aggressive antithrombotic prophylaxis for high risk cases during this trimester. This practice has been challenged by the results of a new prospective survey using objective documentation of the presence of DVT.[58] This study indicates an approximately equal risk for each trimester. The other interesting aspect raised by this study is the question of laterality of venous thrombosis in pregnancy. The right common iliac vein crosses from the aorta across the left common iliac vein. On the basis of venographic appearances the functional compression that this anatomy causes, has been suggested as an etiological factor in left leg venous thrombosis. Certainly in pregnancy this appears to be the case in that 58 of the 60 DVTs diagnosed in the above study were on the left side.[58]

If one uses the national statistics cited above to examine deaths due to PE during or after pregnancy, then for the last 20 years there have been between 25 and 50 cases per 10,000 deliveries or pregnancies.[59] This is half the rate of the previous decade. Overall postpartum deaths are similar to the rate of antepartum deaths although if one corrects for a monthly incidence, again the excess of postpartum thrombosis deaths is evident. The most striking figures are the rates after cesarean section. On a percentage basis the rates of fatal embolism are twice those associated with vaginal delivery. Obviously there are a variety of reasons why women have cesarean sections and it would be incorrect to attribute all the increase in postpartum embolism to the caesarean procedure alone. A similar pattern for venous thrombosis is seen between vaginal and caesarean deliveries, but again the same limitations on interpretation apply. The final issue relating to the puerperium is the period of increased thrombotic risk after delivery. The first week postpartum has the highest incidence of PE but the risk appears to extend out to six weeks. It has been suggested that the period of prophylaxis for high risk cases should therefore be extended out to six weeks but it should be noted that since PE is a sequel to DVT, and these data relate to untreated cases, a full six weeks prophylaxis may not be necessary.

With respect to the pathophysiology of pregnancy related thrombosis there are a variety of potential risk factors present. The concept of anatomical compression of the left iliac vein has been referred to above.[58] The surgical trauma component of delivery and in particular cesarean section is evident. There are some other changes that relate to the rheology of pregnancy. In normal pregnancy there is considerable hemodilution. The biological function of this process is not clear, however the obstetric literature shows that failure to hemodilute causes both intrauterine growth retardation, but also has a strong association with the development of preeclampsia.[60,61] This suggests that hemodilution may protect against thrombosis in pregnancy. Certainly, immediately at postpartum the hemodilution effect is lost and there is relative hemoconcentration. There are also a variety of changes in various coagulation factors and inhibitor levels during pregnancy.[62] It is tempting to speculate that high fibrinogen levels, or conversely decreases in AT-III or Protein S levels, have a causal relationship to pregnancy associated thrombosis, but to date these acquired changes have not been shown to have a close association with any thrombotic events.

Cardiac Disease

The relationship between surgery and thrombosis has been extensively studied but the same degree of interest has not been applied to medical conditions. In general the highest rates of medically related thrombosis have occurred in major medical conditions. It is likely that in the absence of objective testing the cause of the adverse outcome has been attributed to the primary diagnosis. This is a very different clinical environment compared to the situation where apparently successful elective surgery is suddenly jeopardized by unexpected PE.

Despite the different clinical investigative environment, there are clear indications that in certain circumstances venous thrombosis is a problem. Early studies using leg scanning showed a 20% to 40% incidence of DVT with acute myocardial infarction.[63,64] It was of interest that patients in whom myocardial infarction was not confirmed, only had a 10% incidence suggesting some commonality of process between the arterial and venous thrombosis.[65,66] A biological gradient was also observed between the extent and severity of the myocardial infarction and the development of DVT.

There are a variety of potential explanations for the association between myocardial infarction and venous thrombosis. Recent studies have provided strong evidence for a role for thrombin both in preinfarction angina and myocardial infarction itself.[67] This generalized prothrombotic stimulus associated with additional risk factors such as immobility provide a biological explanation for the clinical observations.

Probably the most important issue is whether these historic high frequencies of venous thrombosis are still present. In keeping with the importance of myocardial infarction to communal health, there have been a whole variety of management improvements that will almost certainly minimize the clinical impact of DVT in these cases. Following the studies mentioned above, heparin prophylaxis has become a standard recommendation. In addition, patients will often receive full-dose heparin and in many cases this will be preceded by a course of fibrinolytic therapy. These positive antithrombotic measures have occurred in conjunction with the introduction of medications controlling vascular tone, myocardial rhythm, and cardiac output. If surveillance for DVT was reintroduced today it is likely that the incidence of DVT would now be much lower than in the classical early studies. Autopsy data show a strong relationship between congestive heart failure and pulmonary emboli. The incidence of emboli may be as high as 5%. Congestive failure has a variety of etiologies. It tends to occur in elderly patients with comorbid conditions. It is associated with relative immobility and it is unclear whether the congestive failure has a primary causative role in the development of DVT.

Neurological Disease

A consistent finding over the past 20 years has been a high incidence of deep venous thrombosis in stroke patients. There is strong laterality to the paralyzed limb where rates are ten-fold those of the active limb.[68] The role of paralysis as an etiological factor is supported by the equal rates of thrombosis observed in venographic studies of both limbs in paraplegia.[69] The current recommendations are for active prophylaxis against venous thrombosis for stroke cases and recent randomized clinical trials have compared novel heparins and heparinoids to, in most series, a placebo group. The DVT rates in the untreated cohorts range from 28% to 50% and are very similar to the earlier results which were largely based on leg-scan surveillance.[46] On the basis of the laterality the predominant pathophysiological factor seems to relate to stasis. In the denervated limb it may be more than simple immobility, in that there will be a loss of venous tone, plus there may well be vessel damage due to inadvertent trauma to the paralyzed limb.

GENERAL RISK FACTORS

There are a variety of risk factors for thrombosis that are not disease specific, and are best discussed from a broader perspective.

Malignancy

The early report by Trousseau suggested a link between cancer and venous thrombosis. There have been many subsequent case reports and descriptions.[70,71] In general, no effort was made to establish the strength of this apparent association. More recently autopsy studies have confirmed the earlier reports, however postmortem findings by definition are a late look at the problem.[26] Of more interest is the relationship between cancer and thrombosis during life, and the question as to whether the detection of unexplained DVT is an indication to screen for occult malignancy. There have been a series of cohort analytic studies where cancer rates were compared for surgical procedures in patients with and without cancer. These have included gynecological surgery, laparotomy and abdominothoracic surgery cases.[50,53] The cancer cases have an increased risk of thrombosis of two to three-fold compared to the cancer-free cohort. These results are consistent but in most series only limited matching for other risk factors was possible and, although the association is probably correct, the magnitude of the risk may be an overestimate.

There is a considerable amount of biological literature to suggest mechanisms for cancer induced thrombosis. Several constituents of tumors are highly thrombogenic in experimental thrombosis models. The best characterized is a cysteine protease that can directly activate factor X.[72] Tissue factor has been demonstrated in some tumors including small-cell carcinoma of the lung but has also been found to be increased in peripheral blood macrophages in patients with tumors.[73] More recently other tissue factor-like substances have been described.[74] The other source of biological information on a link between DVT and cancer has been the demonstration of procoagulant markers in the plasma of patients with cancer.[75] Such markers as fibrinopeptide A (FPA) appear to show a relationship to the tumor burden.

If there really is a causal relationship between cancer and thrombosis, then with a sufficiently large sample, it should be possible to show an excess of cancer cases in patients presenting with venous thrombosis. Thrombosis may precede the clinical appearance of the cancer and an appropriate study should involve prospective surveillance of the DVT positive and negative cases. One such study confirmed an increased risk of cancer in the DVT positive cases, with relative risks showing a striking age dependency.[76] The youngest cohort showed a relative risk for cancer of 19:0 for the DVT cases. These differences remained even after correction for confounding risk factors such as the oral contraceptive.

A second more recent study has addressed the same issue. In this study 250 patients with documented symptomatic DVT were followed for 2 years.[77] Cancer was detected during follow-up in only two of the 105 cases of secondary thrombosis, compared to 11 in the 145 idiopathic thrombosis cases. These studies were both community-based and provide the strongest epidemiological support obtained so far for an association between cancer and venous thrombosis.

Age

A consistent feature of vascular disease in general is the positive association of thrombosis with increasing age. Because of the perceived disease impact, most attention has been paid to arterial and cardiac disease, but a very similar magnitude of effect is present for venous thrombosis. In the two community-based surveys discussed previously, the effects of age were striking. In the Malmo study, thrombosis was almost absent below the age of 20 but had reached an incidence of 800 per 100,000 by the ninth decade.[34] Obviously increasing age is associ-

ated with the acquisition of other risk factors including malignancy and exposure to trauma. Unfortunately this aspect, which is amenable to multivariate analytic procedures, was not addressed in this study.

In the American study from Worcester, a similar age effect was observed.[33] In this series, PE was analyzed separately and showed a very similar age effect. Both PE and DVT when plotted against age showed an exponential increase (Figure 2). This study was able to compare the age dependency of community cases of venous thrombosis to hospital-based cases. The hospital cases showed a more linear age effect. This was attributed to the higher incidence of additional risk factors in this population.

There are two hospital-based surveys that examined the effect of age on surgery associated venous thrombosis.[50,71] These studies applied multivariate analysis, and were able to show that increasing age appeared to persist as a risk factor, after correction for concomitant risk factors such as previous thrombosis or type of surgery.

Obesity

Obesity has been recognized as one of the traditional risk factors for postoperative venous thrombosis. Early studies using univariate analysis showed obesity to carry a two-fold risk of venous thrombosis for general surgery patients.[71] There are other studies that show less or no effect. One obvious problem relates to the definition of obesity that varies from study to study on an anthropological and cultural basis.

Using multivariate analytic techniques, the contribution of obesity to postoperative thrombosis appears to be confounded by it's association with the type and severity of operation.[50]

In the American community survey, using the criterion for obesity of body weight of 20% greater than the population median, 39% of the DVT cases were designated as being obese.[33] There is no direct control group in descriptive studies but this does not appear to be a particularly remarkable figure. A random sample of hospitalized patients revealed a 28% prevalence of obesity using the same definition.[40] In a recent French study, Samana reported an odds ratio of 2:11 for the risk of DVT in obese patients.[79]

If one combines the hospital-based studies with the limited community data, then modest obesity itself seems to contribute relatively little risk, compared to the other important factors such as age, previous DVT, major surgery, or cancer.

Previous Venous Thromboembolism

Two hospital-based studies using radiofibrinogen leg scanning show that a previous history of deep venous thrombosis is associated with a two- to three-fold increase in postoperative thrombosis.[50,71] In the study where mul-

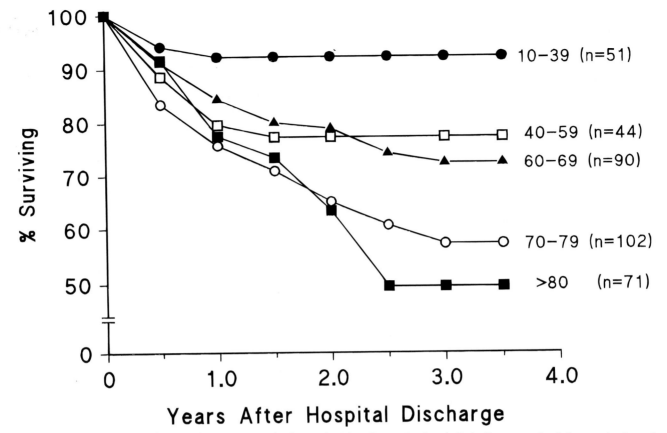

Figure 2. Age-specific survival rates in 358 patients discharged with a first episode of clinically recognized deep-vein thrombosis and/or pulmonary embolism. (From Anderson FA, Jr, et al: Archives of Internal Medicine 151:936, 1991).

tivariate analysis was used this was shown to be an independent risk factor.[50]

More recently a French study identified a history of previous DVT or PE as the most important primary risk factor (odds ratio 7:9), in a case-control study of 636 DVT cases and 635 controls.[79] The Scandinavian community-based study obtained a history of previous thromboembolic disease in 14% of the 336 cases of DVT detected in their study.[34] The 700 negative venography cases did not have the frequency of previous thrombosis determined, so a case-control analysis was not possible, but on the published incidence of DVT in this and the American study it would appear that previous history cases were over-represented. This remains a difficult area to study. Confirmation of recurrent DVT is often difficult.[80] Aggressive antithrombotic prophylaxis for previous DVT histories has preempted further surgery studies.

Immobilization

Prolonged bed rest was identified as a positive association with autopsy-proven venous thrombosis and PE. The largest series reported a six-fold increase in thrombosis rates for patients on strict bed rest for longer than a week.[81] These were a mixed group of hospitalized patients and incorporated a high proportion of high-risk cases. A more discrete group of patients are the neurolog-

ical patients mentioned earlier. In these patients the thrombus causing the stroke would be anticipated to cause very little systemic disturbance, and the overall situation is probably one primarily of stasis.

Cinephlebography has confirmed the importance of calf-muscle contraction in the avoidance of venous pooling in the soleal veins. The latter are the most common sites of immobilization-associated thrombosis. This information has given rise to a series of mechanical devices to prevent venous stasis. In many cases the efficacy of these devices is equivalent to pharmacological prophylaxis. This data provides experimental support for the concept that immobilization is an independent risk factor for thrombosis.

Blood Groups

Thirty years ago before the advent of a modern molecular biology technique, there was a great interest in establishing genetic linkages between biological markers and various clinical conditions. The classic examples were ABO blood group linkage with duodenal ulcer and gastric carcinoma or between Blood Group-A and factor-VIII levels. After an initial report from Boston, a series of other studies supported the observation that Blood Group-O was under-represented in nonobstetric venous thrombosis. In contrast, Blood Group-O was present in excess in obstetric thrombosis.[83,84] Biological explanations of these observations have not been forthcoming and interest in the field has waned. However, in the Malmo study of community-diagnosed thrombosis the observation was made yet again of excess cases of Blood Group-A.[34]

Ethnicity

In parallel with the epidemiological data on ethnic differences in the incidence of arterial disease, various studies have shown different rates of surgically related venous thrombosis between various racial groups. The concern was that these differences may reflect local health conditions rather than primary differences in genetic predisposition. The limited studies that compare different ethnic groups in the same location implicate environmental aspects to be more important.[85,86]

Oral Contraceptives and Hormonal Replacement Therapy

The absolute risk of venous thrombosis or PE to an individual due to the contraceptive pill is low, however, the ubiquitous use of these medications makes quantitation of thrombogenicity important. The range of study methodologies employed over the past 30 years have included case reports, descriptive studies, cohort analytic studies, and finally one randomized clinical trial. Recent studies have again reverted to simple descriptions. End points have also varied considerably from death with postmortem examination to clinical diagnosis. All studies have included serious methodological flaws.

The early case report studies originated from Britain. The first study was a case-control study based on death certificate and postmortem evidence of PE. The relative odds of a contraceptive user dying of PE were 8:3.[87] A second case-control study was published the same year and used hospital discharge diagnoses of DVT or pulmonary embolus. This study showed relative odds of 6:4.[88] A similar study from the United States showed relative odds of 4:1.[89] The above studies largely addressed the question of idiopathic thrombosis but studies have looked at the risk of oral contraceptive-associated secondary thrombosis, and generated relative odds of 3:9 and 2:7 respectively.[90,91] There was one further case-control study from Boston addressing idiopathic thrombosis and this study showed relative odds of 11.[92]

All these studies showed a consistent adverse effect on venous thrombosis from the contraceptive pill that could account for approximately 25 cases per 100,000 per annum. A common feature of these studies was the high dose of estrogen. In most instances the dose was at least 100 micrograms of ethanol estradiol or a pharmacological equivalent. A further U.S. study published in 1975, supported an earlier report that patients receiving preparations of less than 100 micrograms had half the risk of

thrombosis than their higher-dose cohort.[93] This concept has received some support from a descriptive study from Scandinavia where sub 50 microgram preparations appeared to show a lesser risk.[94] The data in this study have since been reexamined and it appears as if the earlier conclusions may have been confounded by an age effect.[95]

As described in the section on general methodology, descriptive studies lack a control group and case-control studies are subject to a variety of biases. Despite the logistic problems associated with prospective studies there have been two cohort analytic studies. The larger study reported from England compared 23,000 oral contraceptive users with a similar group of nonusers. This study showed a relative risk for venous thrombosis among users of 4:2.[96] A second smaller U.S. study involving 16,000 users demonstrated a relative risk of approximately 7:0 for current users.[97] Neither of these studies was blinded in terms of assessment of the diagnosis and there may have been some diagnostic suspicion bias, but this is unlikely to invalidate the overall direction of the observed effect.

A properly conducted randomized and blinded trial is the epidemiologist-preferred design to evaluate risk factors. There has been one randomized but unblinded trial to evaluate the adverse effects of oral contraceptives.[98] Unfortunately, the trial involved relatively few subjects and despite the strong primary design, had problems of validation of end points and it gave equivocal results.

On balance, the oral contraceptive pill, even in its current low-dose form, appears to still carry a risk of venous thromboembolic disease. The lack of recent studies and the judicious avoidance of its use in apparent high risk patients, means that assessment of the true magnitude and current risk is not possible, but it is likely to be smaller than that reported in the two large cohort analytic studies. Despite numerous attempts there has been no success in developing a convincing biological rationale for the thrombogenicity of the contraceptive pill and dosage lowering has been on an empirical basis.

The other major use of estrogenic compounds in the community is for postoophorectomy or postmenopausal hormonal replacement. There has been considerable confusion regarding the thrombogenicity of the various estrogenic preparations. The most commonly used preparation is stated to contain 0.625 mg of natural estrogen, however this is the pharmacological equivalent of only 5 micrograms of ethanol estradiol, a very small dose. Venous thrombogenicity has been examined in two case-control studies. Both showed no association between low-dose estrogen replacement and thrombosis.[99,100]

SUMMARY

Epidemiological studies have proven useful in several areas of study of thrombosis. Although in many cases the actual cause of the thrombosis is not entirely clear, it has proven possible to either avoid or modify risk factors. Much of the original epidemiological work is now largely of historical interest, but the information has proven to be highly useful in selecting suitable physical and pharmacological agents, that have dramatically reduced the rates of surgery related thrombosis

REFERENCES

1. Jaffe EA. Endothelial cells and the biology of factor VIII. N Engl J Med 1977;296:377–383.
2. Jaffe EA, Minick R, Adelman B, et al. Synthesis of basement membrane collagen by cultured endothelial cells. J Exp Med 1976;144:209–225.
3. Jaffe EA, Mosher DF. Synthesis of fibronectin by cultured human endothelial cells. J Exp Med 1978;147:1779–1791.
4. Hekman CM, Loskutoff DJ. Endothelial cells produce a latent inhibitor of plasminogen activators that can be activated by denaturants. J Biol Chem 1985;260:11581–11587.
5. Stemerman MB, Pitlick FA, Dembitzer HB. Electron microscopic immunohistochemical identification of endothelial cells in the rabbit. Circ Res 1976;38:146–156.
6. Jaffe EA, Nachman RL, Becker CG, Minick CR. Culture of human endothelial cell derived from umbilical veins: Identification by morphologic and immunologic criteria. J Clin Invest 1973;52:2745–2756.
7. Weksler BB, Marcus AJ, Jaffe EA. Synthesis of prostaglandin I_2 (prostacyclin) by cultured human and bovine endothelial cells. Proc Natl Acad Sci 1977;74:3922–3926.
8. Wight TN. Vessel proteoglycans and thrombogenesis. Prog Hemost Thromb 1980;5:1–39.
9. Levin EG, Loskutoff DJ. Cultured bovine endothelial cell produce both urokinase and tissue-type plasminogen activators. J Cell Biol 1982;94:631–636.
10. Dittman WA. Thrombomodulin: Biology and potential cardiovascular applications. Trends Cardiovasc Med 1991;1:331–336.
11. Ashford TP, Frieman DG. Platelet aggregation at sites of minimal injury: an electron microscopic study. Am J Pathol 1969;53:599–603.
12. Wester J, Sixma JJ, Geuze JJ, Heinjen HFG. Morphology of the hemostatic plug in human skin wounds: transformation of the plug. Lab Invest 1979;41:182–192.
13. Gailani D, Broze GJ. Factor XI activation in a revised model of blood coagulation. Science 1991;253:909–912.
14. Jesty J, Spencer AK, Nemerson Y. The mechanism of activation of factor X: kinetic control of alternative pathways leading to the formation of activated factor X. J Biol Chem 1974;249:5614–5622.
15. Lorand L, Losowsky MS, Miloszewski KJM. Human factor XIII: Fibrin-stabilizing factor. Prog Hemost Thromb 1980;5:245–290.
16. Novotny WF, Girard TJ, Miletich JP, Broze GJ. Purification and characterization of the lipoprotein-associated inhibitor from human plasma. J Biol Chem 1989;264:18832–18837.
17. Rosenberg RD, Damus PS. The purification and mechanism of action of human anti-thrombin heparin co-factor. J Biol Chem 1973;248:6490–6505.
18. Walker FJ. Regulation of bovine activated protein C by protein S: the role of the cofactor in species specificity. Thromb Res 1981;22:321–327.
19. Moroz LA. Decreased blood fibrinolytic activity after aspirin ingestion. N Engl J Med 1977;296:525–529.
20. Collen D. On the regulation and control of fibrinolysis. Thromb Haemostas 1980;43:77–89.
21. Aoki N. Natural inhibitors of fibrinolysis. Prog Cardiovasc Dis 1979;21:267–286.
22. Poiseuille JL. Recherches experimentales sur le mouvement des liquids dans les tubes de tres-petites diametres. Compt Rend 1842:1167–1177.
23. Karino T, Goldsmith HL. Aggregation of human platelets in an annular vortex distal to a tubular expansion. Microvasc Res 1979;17:217–237.
24. Consensus conference: prevention of venous thrombosis and pulmonary embolism. JAMA 1986;256:744–749.
25. Hume M. The incidence and importance of thromboembolism. In: Hume M, Sevitt S, Thomas DP, eds. Venous Thrombosis and Pulmonary Embolism. Cambridge: Harvard University Press,1970;1–20.
26. Morrell MT, Dunill MS. The post-mortem incidence of pulmonary embolism in a hospital population. Br J Surg 1968;55:347–352.
27. MacIntyre IMC, Ruckley CV. Pulmonary embolism-A clinical and autopsy study. Scot Med J 1974;19:20–24.
28. Freiman DG, Suyemoto J, Wessler S. Frequency of thromboembolism in man. N Engl J Med 1965;272:1278–1280.
29. Gillum RF. Pulmonary embolism and thrombophlebitis in the United States, 1970–1985. Am Heart J 1987;114:1262–1264.
30. Lilienfeld DE, Godbold JH, Burke GL, Sprafka JM, Pham DL, et al. Hospitalization and case fatality for pulmonary embolism in the twin cities: 1979–1984. Am Heart J 1990;120:392–395.
31. Coon WW, Willis PW, Keller JB. Venous thromboembolism and other venous disease in the Tecumseh Community Health Study. Circulation 1973;48:839–846.
32. Gjores JE. The incidence of venous thrombosis and its sequelae in certain districts in Sweden. Acta Chir Scand 1956;111(Suppl 206):16–24.
33. Anderson FA, Wheeler HB, Goldberg RJ, et al. A population-based perspective of the hospital incidence and case-fatality rates of deep vein thrombosis and pulmonary embolism. The Worcester DVT Study. Arch Int Med 1991;151:933–938.
34. Nordstrom M, Lindblad B, Berqvist D, Kjellstrom T. A prospective study of the incidence of deep-vein thrombosis within a defined urban population. J Int Med 1992;232:155–160.
35. Silverstein MD, Mohr DN, Heit JA, Petterson T, O'Fallon WM. Incidence of deep vein thrombosis and pulmonary embolism: a population-based study. Society of General Internal Medicine. 1993;6(abstract).
36. Silverstein MD, Heit JA, Mohr DN, Petterson T, O'Fallon WM, et al. Long-term survival following deep vein thrombosis or pulmonary embolism: a population-based study. Society of General Internal Medicine. 1993;6(abstract).
37. Wheeler HB, Anderson FA, Jr. Use of noninvasive tests as the basis for treatment of deep vein thrombosis. In: Bernstein EF, ed. Vascular Diagnosis. 4th ed. St.Louis: C.V. Mosby Company, 1993:1894–1912.
38. Hill RB, Anderson RE. The autopsy: medical practice and public policy. Boston: Butterworths, 1988:153.
39. Dismuke SE, Wanger EH. Pulmonary embolism as a cause of death: The changing mortality in hospitalized patients. JAMA 1986;255:2039–2042.
40. Anderson FA, Jr., Wheeler HB, Goldberg RJ, Hosmer D, Forcier A. Prevalence of risk factors for venous thromboembolism among hospital patients. Arch Int Med. 1992;152:1660–1664.
41. Hjelmstedt A, Bergvall U. Incidence of thrombosis in pa-

tients with tibial fractures. Acta Chir Scand 1968;134; 209–218.

42. Cohen SH, Ehrlich GE, Kaufman MS, Cope C. Thrombophlebitis following knee surgery. J Bone Joint Surg 1973;55(1):106–111.

43. Hull R, Delmore TJ, Hirsh J, et al. Effectiveness of an intermittent pulsatile elastic stocking for the prevention of calf and thigh vein thrombosis in patients undergoing elective knee surgery. Thromb Res 1979;16:37–45.

44. Leclerc J, Desjardins L, Geerts W, Jobin F, Delorme F, et al. A randomized trial of enoxaparin for the prevention of deep vein thrombosis after knee surgery. Thromb Haemost 1991;65:(Suppl):753.

45. Hull RD, Raskob GE. Prophylaxis of venous thromboembolic disease following hip and knee surgery. J Bone Joint Surg 1986;68:146–150.

46. Collins R, Scrimgeour A, Yusuf S, Peto R. Reduction in fatal pulmonary embolism and venous thrombosis by perioperative administration of subcutaneous heparin. N Engl J Med 1988;318:1162–1173.

47. Hirsh J, Levine MN. Low molecular weight heparin. Blood 1992;79:1–17.

48. Field ES, Nicolaides AN, Kakkar VV, Crellin RQ. Deep-vein thrombosis in patients with fractures of the femoral neck. Br J Surg 1972;59:377–379.

49. Coventry MB, Nolan DR, Beckenbaugh RD. Delayed prophylactic anticoagulation: a study of results in 2012 total hip arthroplasties. J Bone Joint Surg 1973;55:1487–1492.

50. Nicolaides AN, Irving D. Clinical factors and the risk of deep venous thrombosis. In: Nicolaides AN,ed. Thromboembolism: Aetiology, Advances in Prevention and Management. Lancaster, England: MTP Press 1975; 193–204.

51. Nicolaides AN, Field ES, Kakkar VV, Yates-Bell AJ, Taylor S, et al. Prostatectomy and deep-vein thrombosis. Br J Surg 1972;59:487–488.

52. Mayo M, Halil T, Browse NL. The incidence of deep vein thrombosis after prostatectomy. Br J Urol 1971;43:738–742.

53. Walsh JJ, Bonnar J, Wright FW. A study of pulmonary embolism and deep vein thrombosis after major gynaecological surgery using labelled fibrinogen-phlebography and lung scanning. J Obstet Gynaecol Br Commonw 1974;81:311–316.

54. Department of Health and Social Security (1986). Report on Confidential Enquiries into Maternal Deaths in England and Wales, 1979–1981. HMSO, London.

55. Department of Health (1989). Report on Confidential Enquiries into Maternal Deaths in England and Wales, 1982–1984. HMSO, London.

56. Department of Health, Welsh Office, Scottish Home and Health Department and Department of Health and Social Services, Northern Ireland (1991). Report on confidential enquiries into maternal deaths in the United Kingdom 1985–87. HMSO, London.

57. Drill VA, Calhoun DW. Oral contraceptives and thromboembolic disease. JAMA 1968;206:77.

58. Ginsberg JS, Brill-Edwards P, Burrows RF, et al. Venous thrombosis during pregnancy: Leg and trimester of presentation. Thromb Haemostas 1992;67:519–520.

59. Bonnar J. Epidemiology of venous thrombosis in pregnancy and the puerperium. In: Greer IA, Turpie AGG, Forbes CD, eds. Haemostasis and Thrombosis in Obstetrics and Gynaecology. London: Chapman and Hall, 1992;257–266.

60. Buchan PC. Pre-eclampsia-a hyperviscosity syndrome. Am J Obstet Gynecol 1982;142:111–112.

61. Lang DG, Lowe GDO, Walker JJ, et al. Blood rheology in pre-eclampsia and intrauterine growth retardation; effect of blood pressure reduction with labetalol. Br J Obstet Gynaecol 1984;91:438–443.

62. Forbes CD, Greer IA. Physiology of haemostasis and the effect of pregnancy. In: Greer IA, Turpie AGG, Forbes CD, eds. Haemostasis and Thrombosis in Obstetrics and Gynaecology. London: Chapman and Hall, 1992;1–25.

63. Maurer BJ, Wray R, Shillingford JP. Frequency of venous thrombosis after myocardial infarction. Lancet 1971;(ii):1385–1387.

64. Kotilainen M, Ristola P, Ikkala E, Pyorala K. Leg vein thrombosis diagnosed by ^{125}I-fibrinogen test after acute myocardial infarction. Ann Clin Res 1973;5:365–368.

65. Murray TS, Lorimer AR, Cox FC, Lawrie TDV. Leg-vein thrombosis following myocardial infarction. Lancet 1970;(ii):792–793.

66. Nicolaides AN, Kakkar VV, Renney JTG, Kidner PH, Hutchinson DCS, et al. Myocardial infarction and deep-vein thrombosis. Br Med J 1971;1:432–434.

67. Theroux P, Latour J-G, Leger-Gauthier C, De Lara J, et al. Fibrinopeptide A and platelet factor levels in unstable angina pectoris. Circulation 1987;75:156–162.

68. Warlow C, Ogston D, Douglas AS. Deep venous thrombosis of the legs after strokes. Br Med J 1976;1:1178–1181.

69. Bors E, Conrad CA, Massell TB. Venous occlusion of the lower extremities in paraplegic subjects. Surg Gynecol Obstet 1954;99:451–454.

70. Coon WW. Epidemiolgy of venous thromboembolism. Ann Surg 1977;186:149–164.

71. Kakkar VV, Howe CT, Nicolaides AN, Renney JTG, Clarke MB. Deep vein thrombosis of the leg. Is there a "high risk" group? Am J Surg 1970;120:527–530.

72. Gordon SG, Cross BA. A factor X-activating cysteine protease from malignant tissue. J Clin Invest 1981;67:1665–1671.

73. Rickles FR, Hancock WW, Edwards RL, Zacharski LR. Antimetastatic agents 1. Role of cellular procoagulants in pathogenisis of fibrin deposition in cancer and use of anti-coagulants/ or antiplatelet drugs in cancer treatment. Semin Thromb Hemostas 1988;14(1):88–94.

74. Maruyama M, Yagawa K, Hayashi S, et al. Presence of thombosis-inducing activity in plasma from patients with lung cancer. Am Rev Resp Dis 1989;140:778–781.

75. Rickles FR, Edwards RL, Barb C, et al. Abnormalities of blood coagulation in patients with cancer: fibrinopeptide A generation and tumour growth. Cancer 1983;51:301–307.

76. Goldberg RJ, Seneff M, Gore JM, et al. Occult malignant neoplasms in patients with deep venous thrombosis. Arch Int Med 1987;147:251–253.

77. Prandoni P, Lensing AWA, Buller HR, et al. Deep-vein thrombosis and the incidence of subsequent symptomatic cancer. N Engl J Med 1992;327:1128–1133.

78. Hills NH, Pflug JJ, Jeyasingh K, Boardman L, Calnan JS. Prevention of deep vein thrombosis by intermittent pneumatic compression of calf. Br Med J 1972;1:131–135.

79. Samama MM, Simmoneau G, Wainstein JP, De Vathaire F, Huet Y, et al. Sirius Study: Epidemiology of risk factors of deep venous thrombosis (DVT) of the lower limbs in community practice. Thromb Haemostas 1993;69(6):797A.

80. Hull RD, Carter CJ, Jay RM, et al. The diagnosis of acute, recurrent, deep-vein thrombosis: a diagnostic challenge. Circulation 1983;67:901–906.

81. Gibbs NM. Venous thrombosis in the lower limbs with particular reference to bedrest. Br J Surg 1957;45:209–229.

82. Almen T, Bylander G. Serial phlebography in the normal lower limb during muscular contraction and relaxation. Acta Radiol 1962;57:264–272.

83. Jick H, Stone D, Westerholm B, et al. Venous Thromboembolic disease and ABO blood type. Lancet;i: 539–542.

84. Westerholm B, Wiechel B, Eklund G. Oral contraceptives, venous thromboembolic disease, and ABO blood type. Lancet 1971;ii:664.

85. Thomas WA, Davies JPN, O'Neal RM, Dimakulangan AA. Incidence of myocardial infarction correlated with venous thrombosis and pulmonary thrombosis and embolism. Am J Cardiol 1960;5:41–47.

86. Joffe SN. Racial incidence of post operative deep vein thrombosis in South Africa. Br J Surg 1974;61:982–983.

87. Inman WHW, Vessey MP. Investigation of death from pulmonary, coronary, and cerebral thrombosis and embolism in women of child-bearing age. Br Med J 1968;1:193–199.

88. Vessey MP, Doll R. Investigation of relation between use of oral contraceptives and thromboembolic disease. Br Med J 1968;1:199–205.

89. Sartwell PE, Masi AT, Arthes FG, et al. Thromboembolism and oral contraceptives: an epidemiologic case-control study. Am J Epidemiol 1969;90:365–380.

90. Vessey MP, Doll R, Fairburn AS, et al. Postoperative thromboembolism and the use of oral contraceptives. Br Med J 1970;2:123–126.

91. Greene GR, Sartwell PE. Oral contraceptive use in patients with thromboembolism following surgery, trauma, or infection. Am J Public Health 1972;62:680–685.

92. Boston Collaborative Drug Surveillance Program. Oral contraceptives and venous thromboembolic disease, surgically confirmed gall bladder disease and breast tumours. Lancet 1973;i:1399–1404.

93. Stolley PD, Tonascia JA, Tockman MS, et al. Thrombosis with low-estrogen oral contraceptives. Am J Epidiol 1975;102:197–208.

94. Bottinger LE, Boman G, Eklund G, et al. Oral contraceptives and thromboembolic disease; effects of lowering oestrogen content. Lancet 1980;i:1097–1101.

95. Kierkegaard A. Deep vein thrombosis and the oestrogen content in oral contraceptives-an epidemiological analysis. Contraception 1985;31:29–41.

96. Royal College of General Practioners' Oral Contraception Study. Oral contraceptives, venous thrombosis, and varicose veins. J R Coll Gen Pract 1978;28:393–399.

97. Porter JB. Oral contraceptives and nonfatal vascular disease-recent experience. Obstet Gynecol 1982;59:299–302.

98. Fuertes-De La Haba A, Curet JO, Pelegrina I, et al. Thrombophlebitis among oral and nonoral contraceptive users. Obstet Gynecol 1971;38:259–263.

99. Boston Collaborative Drug Surveillance Program. Surgically confirmed gall bladder disease, venous thromboembolism, and breast tumours in relation to postmenopausal estrogen therapy. N Engl J Med 1974;290:15–19.

100. Devor M, Barrett-Connor E, Renvall M, Feigal D, Ramsdell J. Estrogen replacement therapy and the risk of venous thrombosis. Am J Med 1992;92:275–282.

2

The Natural History of Venous Thrombosis and Pulmonary Embolism

Menno V. Huisman

INTRODUCTION

In the acute phase of venous thrombosis, once a thrombus has formed in veins it can resolve, extend or embolize, depending on the balance between the body's intrinsic fibrinolytic system and the forces of thrombogenesis. On a more chronic basis, the thrombus may organize and become incorporated into the wall of the veins, thus giving rise to the development of a chronic post-thrombotic condition. Pulmonary embolism (PE) can resolve or become attached to the pulmonary arteries, in which case chronic thromboembolism with pulmonary hypertension may then result. Finally, both deep-vein thrombosis (DVT) and PE may recur even with adequate treatment.

Before the introduction of anticoagulant therapy, studies reported a mortality rate for PE of about 10% in hospitalized patients with clinically overt venous thrombosis.[1] With the introduction of heparin[2] and dicumarol[3] it has become routine practice to treat patients with venous thrombosis and PE with anticoagulants, and as a consequence only the true natural history of isolated calf-vein thrombosis and asymptomatic thromboembolism—as may occur in postoperative patients—can be derived from recent studies. This is because there is still debate on the need to treat isolated calf-vein thrombosis,[4] or reluctance to apply thrombotic prophylactic therapy perioperatively in patients at high risk for bleeding complications.[5] The natural history of postoperative thrombosis is discussed in Section II of this book.

From careful long-term follow-up studies, it has become clear that the natural history of venous thromboembolism is dependent on the presence of temporary or permanent risk factors. Carson et al, followed 399 patients with treated PE for one year and demonstrated a 1-year mortality rate of 24%.[6] Cardiac disease, infection and cancer were the cause of death in almost three quarters of patients. This contrasts with a one-year mortality rate rang-ing from 3 to 9% in patients without pre-existing cardiac or pulmonary disease.[7,8]

Prandoni and colleagues followed a large series of 352 consecutive patients with proximal-vein thrombosis[9] and observed a one-year mortality rate of 16%. Patients with persistent risk factors faced significantly higher mortality rates (risk ratio for malignancy 7.7). Another important finding of this study was that patients with temporary risk factors such as surgery, trauma or immobilization, had a significantly lower risk for recurrent venous thromboembolism (RR 0.45 to 0.58), than patients with persistent risk factors such as cancer or inherited, or acquired thrombophilia (RR 1.48 and 2.0 respectively).

Although it is now increasingly recognized that venous thrombosis and PE are closely related[10] and can be viewed as one disease, traditionally they have been described and treated as distinctive separate disorders. The natural history of venous thrombosis and PE are therefore discussed separately.

VENOUS THROMBOSIS

Venous thrombosis of the leg can occur in the superficial veins, the deep calf veins, the popliteal vein or the more proximal veins (femoral, deep formal or iliac vein).

Although no formal studies on the natural history of superficial venous thrombosis exist, the course of this disease is usually benign and self limiting. Occasionally deep extension can occur, especially if superficial-vein thrombosis is located in the upper thigh, from which it may extend through the saphenofemoral junction.

Deep-Vein Thrombosis

Deep-vein thrombosis can be arbitrarily divided into distal or calf-vein thrombosis—when the thrombus is

From *Venous Thromboembolism: An Evidence-Based Atlas* edited by Russell Hull, Gary Raskob, Graham Pineo © 1996, Futura Publishing Co., Armonk, NY.

confined to the calf veins—and proximal-vein thrombosis—when there is thrombus extension into or proximal to the popliteal level.

CALF-VEIN THROMBOSIS

The clinical management of calf-vein thrombosis is controversial. Calf-vein thrombosis is described in more detail in chapter 37.

No Anticoagulant Treatment

Philbrick et al, performed an analytic review of 20 papers with calf-vein thrombosis.[4] In this important review, four studies investigating the natural history of untreated calf-vein thrombosis, which reported on the early complications, are described.[11–15] Kakkar et al,[11] and Doouss,[12] screened postoperative patients for DVT with ^{125}I fibrinogen uptake testing, and used venography for confirmation to show that DVT originally confined to the calf, extended proximally in 23% and 5.6% of the patients respectively. In both studies the thrombosis was asymptomatic. The occurrence of PE was reported—and said to be 40% to 50% of patients whose thrombi had extended proximally—but the diagnosis of PE was based either on signs and symptoms[11] or on a lung scan without specific criteria for PE.[12] It is noteworthy that PE in these two studies was only suspected in those patients in whom proximal extension of the thrombosis had occurred. Hull and colleagues,[13] and Moser et al,[14] prospectively followed patients with calf-vein thrombosis and showed that none of the patients with isolated calf-vein thrombi had complications while left untreated,[14] or treated only with low-dose heparin.[13] In a study of 426 outpatients with clinically suspected DVT, Huisman et al, reported an abnormal impedance plethysmography (IPG) indicating proximal-vein thrombosis in 117 patients at presentation.[15] Of the 309 patients with an initially normal IPG, 20 (6.5%) became abnormal over the next 10 days. If the incidence of calf-vein thrombosis at presentation is estimated to be 15%, then the extension rate over ten days would be around 40%. The 289 patients with repeatedly normal IPGs were followed for three months and in this period only one patient (0.2%) returned with proximal-vein thrombosis.[15]

A more recent study in symptomatic, postoperative patients reported a 15% extension of calf-vein thrombosis and a 5% incidence of a high-probability lung scan abnormalities in patients who had no symptoms of PE.[16] In this study however, no baseline lung scan had been done, thus leaving doubt as to whether the demonstrated high probability lung scan had already existed at presentation.

It can be concluded from these studies that proximal extension of calf-vein thrombosis can occur. The difference in rates can be ascribed to different study methods.

The complication rate of PE is low and it is unclear whether the reported scan abnormalities are clinically relevant. Moreover nearly all emboli arise from thrombi in the proximal veins, many of which originate in the calf and progress into the proximal veins before embolizing.[17]

Initial Anticoagulant Therapy

Two studies have reviewed patients with isolated calf DVT who were treated with heparin for one or two weeks but received no secondary prophylactic treatment. Kakkar and Lawrence repeated venography after five to seven days and saw a 10% propagation rate despite intravenous heparin therapy.[18] Lagerstedt et al,[19] performed a randomized clinical trial in 51 patients and observed among patients treated for only five days with intermittent intravenous heparin, a symptomatic recurrence (confirmed by plasmin scan and subsequent venography) in eight patients (29%; 95% C.I. 13–49%), of whom five had proximal extension of the thrombus. None of the patients treated with heparin and oral anticoagulants for three months had a recurrence. One patient treated only initially with heparin developed a clinically-suspected PE, confirmed by repeated perfusion-ventilation lung scanning. In this patient no repeat venography was done to document proximal extension of calf DVT. In a randomized trial comparing low dose subcutaneous heparin therapy—5000 IU subcutaneously three times a day—versus warfarin in the long-term treatment of DVT, Hull et al, demonstrated that only patients with proximal-vein thrombi had recurrences. None of the 32 patients with isolated calf-vein DVT recurred, suggesting that treatment with low-dose heparin might be sufficient for calf DVT.[13]

Doyle et al, performed serial lung scans within 48 hours of initiation of heparin treatment and after seven days of treatment.[20] Thirty-three percent of patients with isolated calf-vein thrombi had a high probability defect that was indicative of silent PE, while an additional 49% of patients had non-high probability defects. These results confirmed the results of studies by Bentley et al,[21] and Browse et al,[22] who found asymptomatic perfusion abnormalities in 55% to 66% of patients with calf-vein thrombosis.

Initial and Long-term Anticoagulant Treatment

The risk of thrombus extension in patients with calf-vein DVT who are treated with initial heparin and subsequent anticoagulant therapy is very low. In three studies, this risk was shown to be 1/168 patients.[13,22,23]

Five studies involving 180 patients with calf-vein DVT assessed the risk of PE and identified eight patients (4.4%).[13,21,24,25,25a] However, for six of these patients, no clear description of the diagnosis of PE was given.[24,25,25a] The well-designed study by Hull et al, found no emboli.[13] Bentley et al, demonstrated an area of ventilation-perfusion mismatch in two of the 11 patients who initially had normal lung scans.[21] One of these patients had proximal extension of the calf DVT. None of the eight reported emboli was fatal.[13,21,24,25,25a]

Recurrence of calf DVT during long-term anticoagulant therapy is also an infrequent finding. Two studies[13,19] revealed no recurrences during low-dose heparin and warfarin therapy respectively. Holmgren et al,[26] and Schulman et al,[27] reported recurrences during one-year follow-up in two of 23 and one of 23 patients respectively. In a recently published randomized study by Shulman, patients with isolated calf DVT had 11.8% recurrence rate over two years when treated for six weeks with warfarin versus 5.8% when treated with warfarin for six months.[28]

PROXIMAL-VEIN THROMBOSIS

No Anticoagulant Treatment

There are no recent studies describing the outcome of untreated proximal-vein thrombosis, because in these patients anticoagulant treatment is considered mandatory. This is partly based on early anecdotal reports in the 1930s, which described patients who were successfully treated for venous thrombosis with heparin,[29,30] while in the 1950s Bauer claimed that he encountered only five thromboembolic deaths among 937 cases with venous thrombosis.[31] Indirect but decisive evidence came from a landmark prospective study in patients with PE. No patients on anticoagulants died, as compared with 26 percent of the patients who did not receive anticoagulation.[32] More recently, prospective studies have demonstrated that in patients with proximal thrombosis, suboptimal treatment leads to a 20%–49% incidence of recurrent venous thrombosis.[13,19,33] Finally, it is known that 40% to 51% of patients admitted with proximal-vein thrombosis have a high-probability lung scan, representing firm evidence of the presence of PE.[14,20,34]

Initial Anticoagulant Therapy

Clinically recurrent venous thrombosis or PE during initial heparin treatment is a rare event provided that adequate doses of heparin are administered—especially in the first 24 hours of treatment. This was demonstrated in two randomized studies comparing different anticoagulation schemes for patients with proximal-vein thrombosis.[33,35] The first study compared intravenous with intermittent subcutaneous heparin in the initial treatment of 115 patients with proximal-vein thrombosis.[35] Eleven of 57 patients (19.3%) randomized to the subcutaneous heparin group had recurrent thromboembolic events during 3 months follow-up, of which five occurred in the first week of treatment (8.8%), as opposed to three thromboembolic events (one of which (1.7%)) occurred in the first week in 58 patients who got intravenous heparin. Ten of the 11 patients with recurrent venous thromboem-

bolism in the subcutaneous heparin group as well as the patient in the intravenous heparin group who developed a recurrence, had a subtherapeutic anticoagulant response. The relative risk of recurrent venous thromboembolism was 15 times higher in patients with inadequate anticoagulation during the first 24 hours or more.[35] In the other study, patients were randomized to oral anticoagulants only or intravenous heparin and oral anticoagulants in the initial treatment of proximal-vein thrombosis.[33] Nine of the 60 patients (15%) receiving oral anticoagulants only had recurrent thromboembolic events during three months follow-up, of whom three (5%) occurred during the first week of treatment. In the group receiving intravenous heparin followed by oral anticoagulants only one patient (1.6%) had a recurrent event (during the first week of treatment).

Although clinical recurrence of venous thromboembolism during the first week of treatment is an infrequent finding if patients who get adequate heparin treatment, asymptomatic extension of proximal-vein thrombosis and asymptomatic PE can occur. In the study by Brandjes et al, 4 of 49 (8.2%) evaluable patients in the group receiving intravenous heparin and oral anticoagulants, had evidence of asymptomatic extension of venous thromboembolism (one with extension of venous thrombosis and three patients with new high-probability defects on lung scanning).[33] In contrast, in the group receiving anticoagulants only, 21 of 53 (39.6%) evaluable patients had evidence of asymptomatic extension (15 patients with venographic extension of thrombosis and seven patients with new high-probability defects on lung scanning; one patient had both extension of thrombosis and a new defect on lung scanning), thus further substantiating the failure of oral anticoagulants to inhibit the thrombotic process from the start of treatment.

Other studies have demonstrated asymptomatic extension of treated proximal-vein thrombosis in up to 20% of patients[36,37] and new high-probability defects in 10% of patients.[21]

Initial and Long-term Anticoagulant Therapy

After initial treatment with heparin, patients with proximal-vein thrombosis are treated with oral anticoagulants, traditionally for a period of three months. This treatment, called secondary prophylaxis, is considered necessary to render the thrombus less thrombogenic and thus reduce the risk of recurrent thrombosis and/or PE. The incidence of recurrent venous thromboembolism during secondary prophylaxis can be derived from various studies which evaluated less intensive regiments—i.e., low-dose subcutaneous heparin,[13] or a different period of oral anticoagulants, i.e., 6 weeks[26–28,38] or 6 months.[28] In the study comparing low-dose heparin—5000 I.U. subcutaneous three times daily, with standard oral anticoagulant treatment,[13] the recurrence rate of venous thromboembolism was 47% (9/19) during three months follow-up in patients with proximal-vein thrombosis; eight patients had recurrent venous thrombosis, shown by a new intraluminal defect on venography, one patient had PE. None of the patients who received oral anticoagulants had a recurrence.[13] Other studies reported a recurrence rate of venous thromboembolism during three months of anticoagulant treatment, varying from 0.7% over 6 weeks[28] to 7% over 3 months.[10]

The incidence or recurrent venous thromboembolic disease after long-term anticoagulants have been given, can be indirectly derived from the study by Shulman et al.[28] He demonstrated an annual risk between 5% and 6% percent. This in agreement with the study by Prandoni and colleagues, who followed a cohort of 352 patients with proximal-vein thrombosis and demonstrated a cumulative incidence of recurrent VTE, after two and five years of 15% and 22% respectively.[9]

In both studies, the importance of temporary versus permanent risk factors was established. Patients with temporary risk factors, i.e., after operation, during prolonged immobilization or in the postpartum period, had an overall recurrence rate after 2 years follow-up of only 6.6%, whereas the recurrence rate was 18% over the same period in patients with one or more permanent risk factors, ie, cancer, inherited thrombophilia (protein C, protein S, or antithrombin deficiency, activated protein C resistance or lupus anticoagulant).[9,28] Biological evidence for these observations comes from studies in which it was shown that in patients with inherited thrombophilia or cancer which contributed to their hypercoagulable state—there is a procoagulant state with increased level of markers of activation of the coagulation process. In cancer patients, these changes are even more marked because these patients are often bedridden or receiving chemotherapy.[39,39a]

PULMONARY EMBOLISM

Historically it has been difficult to define the incidence and natural history of PE, because the diagnosis was often based on clinical criteria and lethality of PE and was uncertain due to considerable inaccuracy inherent in death certificates and even autopsy reports.[40] Besides, PE often develops without symptoms and as a result the natural history of these silent emboli is unclear, although it remains a major cause of hospital mortality.[41]

From pathophysiological investigations it has been postulated that the first minutes to hours after arrival of the embolus in the pulmonary vasculature, pertain to the greater risk to the patient.[42] A sudden increase in right ventricular afterload can lead to dysfunction of the right ventricle with resulting decrease in cardiac output, hypotension, shock, arrhythmias, syncope or cardiac arrest. In many patients, reopening of the occluded pulmonary vascular segment occurs within minutes to hours or days,

depending on the spontaneous remodelling and/or fibrinolytic dissolution on the embolus.[40] This was demonstrated by serial right heart catheterization in 15 patients treated for major PE.[43] Pulmonary artery pressures decreased toward normal within 10 to 21 days, but in only one patient was it completely normalized. At angiography some resolution of PE was seen within the first week and moderate to near complete resolution at 10 to 21 days after the index episode.[43] These observations were confirmed by serial lung scans in patients involved in the Urokinase Pulmonary Embolism Trial (UPET).[44] The rate of resolution of lung scan defects in treated patients was 36%, 52%, 73% and 76% after 5 days, 14 days, 3 months and 1 year respectively.[44]

Untreated patients who survive their initial episode of PE run a great risk of fatal and nonfatal recurrent PE. This was demonstrated in the landmark trial by Barritt and Jordan.[32] In a prospective randomized trial, five of the 19 (26%) patients who were not treated for PE died of fatal recurrent PE confirmed by autopsy; the time of death in these patients was 1, 2, 12, 14 and 21 days respectively after the first PE.[32] No death due to PE occurred in the patients treated with intermittent intravenous heparin followed by oral anticoagulants. Moreover five patients in the nontreated group had signs and symptoms of recurrent PE versus none in the treated group, thus yielding a 53% total recurrence rate of fatal and nonfatal PE in the nontreated patient group. This figure is likely to be an overestimate, due to the nonspecific diagnosis of clinically suspected nonfatal PE.

Since this trial, which conclusively demonstrated the need for anticoagulant treatment in thromboembolic disease, several studies using objective endpoints have provided data on the recurrence rates during anticoagulant therapy and long-term follow-up. In the UPET, intravenous heparin was compared with urokinase as the initial treatment for patients with PE. The recurrence rate of venous thromboembolism was 17% in patients treated with heparin, while it was 11% in the urokinase treated group.[44] This recurrence rate, however, was partly based on new lung scan defects as demonstrated by follow-up lung scanning rather than on the development of new symptoms. The two-week mortality rate in the UPET trial was 10% whereas the 6-month mortality rate of the whole group was 13%.[44] In a report by Alpert and colleagues there was a 17% mortality rate but PE itself accounted for the cause of death in only 3% of the patients.[45] In two other studies, the reported one-year mortality in patients without pre-existing cardiac or pulmonary disease ranged from 3% to 9%.[8,46]

Carson et al, reported the natural history of 399 patients with documented PE, of whom 94% were treated, mostly with conventional anticoagulation.[6] Clinically suspected recurrent PE, confirmed by objective tests, occurred in 33 (8.3%) of the patients in the study. These recurrences developed soon after the initial event of PE, 16 of the 33 patients (48%; 4% of the 399 patients) had recurrences within 1 week of their initial PE.

Of the patients with a recurrence, 15 (45%) died during the one-year follow-up, with PE as the cause of death in nine patients. Ten patients (2.5%) died of recurrent PE, eight within the first week (2%) and nine did so within two weeks. According to the authors of this landmark natural history study of PE, (other investigators have described a similarly high-risk period for DVT),[13,47] the first 4 to 6 weeks of therapy is a vulnerable period, when thromboembolic recurrence is most common, and if it occurs, is associated with a high death rate.

Even when patients survive the acute episode of PE their long-term prognosis is largely dependent on underlying conditions. This was clearly demonstrated in the same study by Carson et al.[6] At the one-year follow-up, 95 (23.8%) of these 399 patients had died; in these patients the most frequent causes of death were cancer (in 34.7%), infection (22.1%), cardiac disease (16.8%) and pulmonary disease (5.3%). These rates are in agreement with another follow-up study by Kuijer et al, who followed 193 patients who had PE and received standardized treatment with intravenous heparin and oral anticoagulants for 3 months.[48] The 6 month mortality rate was 16.6%, of which only 6.7% was attributed to recurrent PE.

Although the overall majority of patients with PE recover and have resolution of the pulmonary emboli[43,44] a small percentage of patients (0.1%) are subject to embolic recurrences and, when major occlusion of the main pulmonary arteries and lobar arteries occur, may develop chronic pulmonary hypertension and even cor pulmonale, in months or years.[42]

POSTPHLEBITIC SYNDROME

The precise incidence of the postphlebitic or postthrombotic syndrome is not well established. This is mainly because of a lack of long-term prospective follow-up studies, the lack of predefined criteria for the postthrombotic syndrome and the long delay between the initial episode of thrombosis and the appearance of postphlebitic symptoms. It has been reported to vary between 20% and 100%.[49–54,60]

The postphlebitic signs and symptoms may include persistent swelling, pain, pigmentation and induration around the ankle and the lower third of the leg and ultimately, venous ulceration. The postphlebitic syndrome is caused by venous hypertension, which itself occurs by the combination of recanalization of thrombi, leading to patent but scarred veins, or persistent outflow obstruction, due to large thrombi and venous incompetence as a consequence of incompetent valves.[54–56] This venous hypertension leads to increased pressure in the deep calf veins and renders incompetent the calf-perforating veins. As a consequence, flow is directed from the deep into the superficial system, leading to edema and impaired viability of the dermis. This can ultimately lead to ulceration.[57]

In two follow-up studies in patients with proximal-vein thrombosis it has been demonstrated that outflow obstruction, as measured by impedance plethysmography—is frequently relieved either by presumed collateral circulation or recanalization in 30%, after three weeks and up to 70% after 3 months.[58,59] According to two studies evaluating venous valve function after thrombosis, valvular incompetence is a more important predictor for the postphlebitic syndrome than is outflow obstruction.[54,60] In a third study, valvular incompetence was shown to be a frequent finding after DVT. It was present in 17% after one week, 37% after 1 month and 69% after 1 year. In a control group, reflux was uncommon (6%).[61]

Except for patients with massive thrombosis in the iliofemoral veins where persistent swelling may ensue, the signs and symptoms of the acute thrombosis may completely disappear and recur only months or years after the event.

In a long-term follow-up study by Brandjes et al, 194 consecutive outpatients with a first episode of proximal-DVT were randomized to wear made-to-measure graded compression stockings or no stockings.[62] Patients were followed prospectively for a minimum of 5 years. A mild to moderate postphlebitic syndrome defined according to a predefined symptom score that included subjective symptoms such as pain on walking or standing, edema, or heaviness as well as objective symptoms, such as increase in circumference of the calf and/or ankle, the presence of pigmentation, newly formed varicosities, or phlebitis—occurred in 19 (20%) of the 96 patients in the group that wore stockings, and in 46 (47%) in the 98 patients without stockings. Surprisingly, the majority of patients who developed the postphlebitic syndrome did so within 2 years. A total of 11 (11.5%) patients in the stocking-wearing group and 23 (23.5%) patients wearing no stockings developed severe postphlebitic complaints. The severe postphlebitic complaints also developed within two years.[62] Prandoni and colleagues, followed in an unpublished study, 216 patients after treatment for DVT thrombosis for a mean period of 45 months.[63] The postthrombotic syndrome was defined according to predefined criteria. It occurred in 64 (30%) of the patients: the syndrome was severe in 15 patients (7%), moderate in nine and mild in 40 (18.5%). On the other hand, more than 70% of the patients did not develop any manifestation during a period of almost 4 years. The risk for developing postthrombotic complaints was greatly increased when patients had a recurrent thrombosis. Of the 190 patients without recurrent DVT, 12 developed severe postthrombotic symptoms, whereas 12 of the 26 patients with recurrent DVT developed severe symptoms. Whether patients with isolated calf-vein thrombosis are at less risk of developing postphlebitic symptoms is uncertain. In a small study, patients with proximal-vein thrombosis had frequently had greater disability and a much higher frequency of venous claudication than patients with more distal-vein thrombosis.[64] Prandoni et al, however showed that the level and extent of the original thrombosis had no relation to the occurrence and severity of the postthrombotic syndrome.[63]

Although the number of patients in the subgroups are somewhat limited, postthrombotic symptoms developed in 26%, 20%, 26%, 31% and 15% of patient with thrombi in the calf only, popliteal vein only, popliteal and femoral, all of the proximal veins and femoral and iliac vein respectively.[63] Interestingly, two studies evaluated both legs with calf DVT and control legs not involved with calf DVT.[51,65] These studies showed that while there was evidence of chronic venous disease in the legs that had calf DVT in 8% and 20% respectively, the rates of the control legs were 7.1% and 13% respectively.

Finally, it has been postulated that treatment of DVT with thrombolytic drugs could potentially reduce the development of the postphlebitic syndrome, possibly by resolving of outflow obstruction caused by the thrombus. However, clinical trials have not been able to demonstrate this.[66] Kakkar and Lawrence, assessed venous function after an average of 5.8 years and revealed no less morbidity among patients who had been treated with thrombolytic treatment.[67]

REFERENCES

1. Ziliacus H. On the specific treatment of thrombosis and PE with anticoagulants, with particular reference to the post thrombotic sequelae. Acta Med Scand 1946;171(Suppl): 1–221.
2. Murray DWG, Jacques LB, Perrett TS, Best CH. Heparin and the thrombosis of veins following injury. Surgery 1937;2:163–187.
3. Stahman MA, Huebner CF, Ling KP. Studies on the hemorrhagic sweet clover disease V. Identification and synthesis of the hemorrhagic agent. J Biol Chem 1941;138:513–527.
4. Philbrick JT, Becker DM. Calf deep venous thrombosis. A wolf in sheep's clothing? Arch Intern Med 1988;148: 2131–2138.
5. Gallus AS, Salzman EW, Hirsh J. Prevention of venous thromboembolism. In: Hemostasis and Thrombosis: Basic Principles and Clinical Practice. Third Edition. JB Lippincott Company, Philadelphia. Chapter 68, 1331–1345.
6. Carson JL, Kelley MA, Duff A, et al. The clinical course of pulmonary embolism. N Engl J Med 1992;1240–1245.
7. Macintyre D, Banham SW, Moran F. Pulmonary embolism—a long-term follow-up. Postgrad Med J 1982;58: 222–225.
8. Sutton GC, Hall RJC, Kerr IH. Clinical course and late prognosis of treated subacute massive, acute minor and chronic pulmonary thromboembolism. Br Heart J 1977;39: 1135–1142.
9. Prandoni P, Lensing AWA, Cogo A, et al. The clinical course of deep-vein thrombosis. Thromb Haem 1995;73: 1092.(Abstract)
10. Prins MH, Turpie AGG. Diagnosis and treatment of venous thromboembolism. In: Bloom AL, Forbes CD, Thomas DP, et al (editors). Haemostasis and Thrombosis. Churchill Livingstone, London, UK. 1994. Chapter 63:1381–1417.
11. Kakkar VV, Howe CT, Flanc C, et al. Natural history of postoperative deep-vein thrombosis. Lancet 1969;2:230–232.
12. Doouss TW. The clinical significance of venous thrombosis of the calf. Br J Surg 1976;63:377–378.
13. Hull RD, Delmore T, Genton E, et al. Warfarin sodium versus low dose heparin in the long-term treatment of venous thrombosis. N Engl J Med 1979;301:855–858.
14. Moser KM, LeMoine JR. Is embolic risk conditioned by location of deep venous thrombosis? Ann Int Med 1981;94: 439–444.
15. Huisman MV, Bueller HR, ten Cate JW, et al. Serial impedance plethysmography for suspected DVT in outpatients. The Amsterdam General Practitioner Study. N Engl J Med 1986;314:823–828.
16. Lohr JM, Kerr TM, Lutter KS, et al. Lower extremity calf thrombosis: to treat or not to treat. J Vasc Surg 1991;14: 618–623.
17. Hume M, Sevitt S, Thomas DP. The incidence and importance of thromboembolism. In Hume M, Sevitt S, Thomas DP(eds). Venous Thrombosis and Pulmonary Embolism. Cambridge, Harvard University Press, 1970.
18. Kakkar VV, Lawrence D. Hemodynamic and clinical assessment after therapy for acute deep vein thrombosis: A prospective study. Am J Surg 1985;150(4A):54–63.
19. Laegerstedt CI, Olsson CG, Fagher BO, et al. Need for longterm anticoagulant treatment in symptomatic calf vein thrombosis. Lancet 1985;2:515–518.
20. Doyle DJ, Turpie AGG, Hirsh J, et al. Adjusted subcutaneous heparin or continuous intravenous heparin in patients with acute deep vein thrombosis. A randomised trail. Ann Int Med 197;107:441–445.
21. Bentley PG, Kakkar VV, Scully MF, et al. An objective study of alternative methods of heparin administration. Thromb Res 1980;18:177–187.
22. Browse NL, Clemenson G, Croft DN. Fibrinogen-detectable thrombosis in the leg and pulmonary embolism. Br Med J 1974;1:603–604.
23. Shulman S, Granqvist S, Juhlin-Dannfelt A, et al. Longterm sequelae of calf vein thrombosis treated with heparin or low-dose streptokinase. Acta Med Scand 1986;219:349–357.
24. Kistner RL, Ball JJ, Nordyke RA, et al. Incidence of pulmonary embolism in the course of thrombophlebitis of the lower extremities. Am J Surg 1972;124:169–176.
25. Menzoian JO, Sequeira JC, Doyle JE, et al. Therapeutic and clinical course of deep vein thrombosis. Am J Surg 1983;146:581–585.
25a. Kistner RL, Ball JJ, Nordyke RA, et al. Incidence of pulmonary embolism in the course of thrombophlebitis of the lower extremities. Am J Surg 1972;124:169–176.
26. Holmgren K, Andersson G, Fagrell B, et al. One-month versus six-month therapy with oral anticoagulants after symptomatic deep vein thrombosis. Acta Med Scand 1985;218: 279–284.
27. Shulman S, Lockner D, Jhulin-Dannfelt A. The duration of oral anticoagulation after deep-vein thrombosis: A randomised study. Acta Med Scand 1985;217:547–552.
28. Shulman S, Rhedin AS, Llindmarker P, et al. A comparison of six weeks with six months of oral anticoagulant therapy after a first episode of venous thromboembolism. N Engl J Med 1995;332:1661–1665.
29. Murray D, Jacques L, Perret T, Best C. Heparin and thrombosis of veins following injury. Surgery 1937;2:163–187.
30. Crafoord C. Preliminary report on post-operative treatment with heparin as preventive of thrombosis. Acta Chir Scand 1937;79:407–426.
31. Bauer G. The introduction of heparin therapy in cases of early thrombosis. Circulation 1959;19:108–109.

32. Barritt DW, Jordan SC. Anticoagulant drugs in the treatment of pulmonary embolism: a controlled trial. Lancet 1960;1:1309:1312.

33. Brandjes DPM, Heijboer H, Bueller HR, et al. Acenocoumarol and heparin compared with acenocoumarol alone in the initial treatment of proximal-vein thrombosis. N Engl J Med 1992;327:1485–1489.

34. Huisman MV, Bueller HR, ten Cate JW, et al. Unexpected high prevalence of silent pulmonary embolism in patients with deep venous thrombosis. Chest 1989;95:948–952.

35. Hull RD, Raskob GE, Hirsh J, et al. Continuous intravenous heparin compared with intermittent subcutaneous heparin in the initial treatment of proximal-vein thrombosis. N Engl J Med 1986;1109–1114.

36. Marder VJ, Soulen RL, Atichartakarn V, et al. Quantitative venographic assessment of deep vein thrombosis in the evaluation of streptokinase and heparin therapy. J Lab Clin Med 1977;89:1018–1029.

37. Robertson BR, Nilsson IM, Nylander G. Thrombolytic effect of streptokinase as evaluated by phlebography of deep venous thrombi of the leg. Acta Chir Scand 1970;136:173–180.

38. Research Committee of the British Thoracic Society. Optimum duration of the anticoagulation for deep-vein thrombosis and pulmonary embolism. Lancet 1992;340:873–876.

39. Levine MN, Gent M, Hirsh J, et al. The thrombogenic effect of anticancer drug therapy in women with stage II breast cancer. N Engl J Med 1988;318:404–407.

39a. Bauer K. The hypercoagulable states. In: Williams Hematology 1995. McGraw Hill Inc, USA. Chapter 144:1531–1550.

40. Alpert JS, Dalen JE. Epidemiology and natural history of venous thromboembolism. Progr Cardiovasc Dis 1994;36:417–422.

41. Goldman L, Sayson R, Robbins S, et al. The value of the autopsy in three medical areas. N Engl J Med 1983;308:1000–1005.

42. Moser KM. Venous thromboembolism. Am Rev Resp Dis 1990;141:235–249.

43. Dalen JE, Banas Jr JS, Brooks HL, et al. Resolution rate of acute pulmonary embolism in man. N Engl J Med 1969;280:1994–1199.

44. National Heart, Lung and Blood Institute: Urokinase Pulmonary Embolism Trial—Phase I results. JAMA 1970;214:2163–2172.

45. Alpert JS, Smith R, Carolson J, Ockene IS, et al. Mortality in patients treated for pulmonary embolism. JAMA 1976;236:1477–1480.

46. Macintyre D, Banham SW, Moran F. Pulmonary embolism—a long-term follow-up. Postrgad Med J 1982:58:222–225.

47. Hull RD, Hirsh J, Jay R, et al. Different intensities of anticoagulant therapy in the treatment of proximal-vein thrombosis. N Engl J Med 1982;307:1676–1681.

48. Kuijer PMM, van Beek EJR, Bueller et al. The 6 months outcome of patients with clinically suspected pulmonary embolism. Thromb Haemost 1995;73:1095. (Abstract 745)

49. Bauer G. Roentgenological and clinical study of the sequelae of thrombosis. Acta Chir Scand 1942;86 (Suppl 74):1–110.

50. Gjores JE. The incidence of venous thrombosis and its sequelae in certain districts of Sweden. Acta Chir Scand 1956;206 (Suppl 1):1–88.

51. Browse NL, Clemenson G, Lea Thomas M, et al. Is the postphlebitic leg always postphlebitic? Relation between phlebographic appearance of deep-vein thrombosis and late sequelae. Br Med J 1981;281:1167–1170.

52. Widmer LK, Zemp E, Widmer MT, et al. Late results in deep-vein thrombosis of the lower extremities. VASA 1985;14:264–268.

53. Lindner LK, Edwards JM, Phinney ES, et al. Long term hemodynamic and clinical sequelae of lower extremity deep vein thrombosis. J Vasc Surg 1986;4:436–442.

54. Shull KC, Nicolaides AN, Fernandes F, et al. Significance of popliteal reflux in relation to ambulatory venous pressure and ulceration. Arch Surg 1979;114:1304.

55. O'Donnell TF, Browse NL, Burnand KG, et al. Iliac vein thrombosis: A ten year follow-up study. J Surg Res 1977;22:431.

56. Negus D. The post-thrombotic syndrome. Ann R Coll Surg Engl 1970;47:92.

57. Immelman EJ, Jeffery PC. The postphlebitic syndrome. Pathophysiology, prevention and management. Clin Chest Med 1984;5:537–550.

58. Jay R, Hull RD, Carter C, et al. Outcome of abnormal impedance plethysmography results in patients with proximal vein thrombosis: Frequency of return to normal. Thromb Res 1984;36:259.

59. Huisman MV, Bueller HR, ten Cate JW. Utility of impedance plethysmography in the diagnosis of recurrent deep vein thrombosis. Arch Int Med 1988;148:681–683.

60. Strandness ED Jr, Langlois Y, Cramer M, et al. Long-term sequelae of acute venous thrombosis. JAMA 1983;250:1289.

61. Markel M, Manzo RA, Bergelin RO, et al. Incidence and time of occurrence of valvular incompetence following deep vein thrombosis. Wien Med Wschr 1994;144:216–220.

62. Brandjes DPM, Heijboer H, de Rijk M, et al. The effect of graded compression stockings on the development of the post-thrombotic syndrome in patients with proximal venous thrombosis. Thromb Haemost 1991;65;1131. (Abstract 1568)

63. Prandoni P, Lensing AWA, Polistena P, et al. Symptomatic deep-vein thrombosis and the post-thrombotic syndrome. Thromb Haem 1993;69:1211. (Abstract 2379)

64. Cockett FB, Lea Thomas M, Negus D. Iliac vein compression—its relation to iliofemoral thrombosis and the post-thrombotic syndrome. Br Med J 1967;2:14.

65. Lindhagen A, Bergqvist A, Hallbook T, et al. Venous function five to eight years after clinically suspected deep venous thrombosis. Acta Med Scand 1985;217:389–395.

66. Trubestein G. Can thrombolytics prevent post-phlebitic syndrome and thromboembolic disease? Haemostasis 1986;3 (Suppl):38–50.

67. Kakkar VV, Lawrence D. Hemodynamic and clinical assessment after therapy for acute venous thrombosis: A prospective study. Am J Surg 1985;150(4A):54–63.

3

Evidence-Based Recommendations for the Diagnosis and Treatment of Thromboembolic Disease: Rules of Evidence for Assessing Literature

Gary E. Raskob

INTRODUCTION

In recent years, clinicians have been increasingly encouraged to practice "evidence-based" medicine, that is the evaluation of evidence from clinical trials as the basis for clinical decisions and patient care.[1] This often requires a change from the traditional approach in which pathophysiological understanding and clinical experience form the basis for clinical decisions. To practice evidence-based medicine, the clinician must understand and apply formal rules of evidence for evaluating the clinical literature.[1] In the past 15 years, scientific criteria for clinical studies evaluating new diagnostic tests[2-4] and treatments[5-8] have been defined, and rules of evidence for assessing the literature and making clinical recommendations have been developed.[9,10]

The wealth of data from rigorously designed clinical trials evaluating new approaches for treatment and diagnosis, makes thromboembolic disease particularly suited to the practice of evidence-based medicine. In this chapter, the study-design requirements for evaluating new diagnostic approaches and new therapies in the context of thromboembolic disease are reviewed. Rules of evidence for assessing the clinical literature are outlined; these rules are used throughout the remainder of the book to qualify the strength of evidence supporting specific recommendations. Firm recommendations are made only when they can be supported by "level I" evidence: without such evidence, firm recommendations are not made, and in such instances, the alternative clinical approaches are described.

DIAGNOSIS: STUDY-DESIGN REQUIREMENTS FOR DIAGNOSIS

Many diagnostic tests have been introduced into clinical practice and accepted enthusiastically. However, upon further evaluation, they have proved to be limited in terms of clinical application, or even useless. The noncritical acceptance of a diagnostic test for thromboembolic disease has serious implications. Patients with false-positive results may receive unnecessary, potentially harmful treatment, and patients with false-negative findings may have necessary and highly effective treatment withheld. In the past, the evaluation of diagnostic tests has often been based on studies that have failed to include the essential design features required to avoid bias. In more recent years, essential design features for such studies have been defined[2-4] and applied in the setting of diagnostic tests for thromboembolism.

The essential study design features for studies evaluating diagnostic tests are the following:

1. The study should include a consecutive series of patients.

2. All patients should undergo both the test under evaluation and the diagnostic reference test ("gold standard") in order to determine the four indices of diagnostic efficacy: sensitivity, specificity, positive predictive value, and negative predictive value.

3. The test should be evaluated in a broad spectrum of patients, both with and without the disease of interest, with varying severity of the disease, and with a variety of comorbid conditions which are commonly confused with the disease of interest.

From *Venous Thromboembolism: An Evidence-Based Atlas* edited by Russell Hull, Gary Raskob, Graham Pineo © 1996, Futura Publishing Co., Armonk, NY.

4. The results of the test under evaluation and the reference test should be interpreted independently and without knowledge of the results of the other test, or of the patient's clinical or ancillary test findings.

5. A sufficient number of patients should be studied to draw valid conclusions, based on 95% confidence intervals, for the indices of sensitivity, specificity, and positive and negative predictive values.

6. There should be studies including long-term follow-up to determine the safety of withholding treatment in patients with negative results by the test under evaluation.

It is important that consecutive patients be evaluated in order to avoid selection bias and that a broad spectrum of patients should be included to provide valid estimates of sensitivity, specificity, and predictive values. The study should include patients with comorbid conditions that may produce false-positive or false-negative results to determine the usefulness of the test in various patient subgroups. Failure to evaluate the test in a broad spectrum of patients may result in falsely high indices of efficacy.[4]

"Work-up" bias should be avoided. This bias occurs when the results of the test under evaluation influence the decision to perform the reference ("gold standard") test. Work-up bias can be avoided by performing both the test under evaluation and the reference test in all patients. Interpretation bias occurs when knowledge of the result of one test influences the interpretation of another test. Interpretation bias can be avoided if the new test and the reference test are interpreted independently, without knowledge of the other result, and without knowledge of the patient's clinical findings or ancillary test results.

The final step in the process of evaluating a new diagnostic test is to confirm the clinical validity of a negative result. Clinical validity can be determined by long-term follow-up of consecutive patients in whom treatment has been withheld due to negative test results. This approach has been used to validate negative findings by objective testing for deep-vein thrombosis,[11–15] for pulmonary embolism,[16,17] and for thallium scanning in patients with chest-pain.[18]

The validity of a new test can also be assessed by a randomized comparison with a "gold standard" test and assessment of the clinical outcome in patients managed on the basis of either the "gold standard" or the new test. This approach can be used if the disease being studied is responsive to treatment, and if inadequate management leads to clinical complications (eg, recurrent thromboembolism) which can be objectively measured. These complications can be used as outcome measures for comparing the diagnostic efficacy of the two approaches. This randomized trial approach has been used to evaluate diagnostic tests in patients with clinically suspected venous thrombosis.[13,15]

LEVELS OF EVIDENCE FOR DIAGNOSTIC STUDIES

Diagnostic studies are classified as level I evidence if the essential design features outlined above are met. To qualify as level I evidence, there must be either an independent, blind comparison with a reference test and long-term follow-up to assess clinical validity of negative results, or a randomized comparison with a reference test measuring clinical outcome in patients on long-term follow-up. In either case, a sufficient number of patients should be included to provide valid conclusions based on the 95% confidence intervals for sensitivity, specificity, and predictive values, and for the clinical outcomes. Firm recommendations for diagnosis of thromboembolism can be made only when they are supported by level I evidence. If the study design fails to meet the essential design criteria outlined above, then the study is designated as nonlevel I and recommendations cannot be made based on this data.

ANTITHROMBOTIC THERAPY: STUDY DESIGN REQUIREMENTS

Study designs commonly used in the past to evaluate antithrombotic therapy (such as uncontrolled case-series or studies utilizing historical controls) are subject to many potential biases that may lead to spurious estimates of effectiveness and safety. It is now generally agreed that properly designed and executed clinical trials are necessary, if the effectiveness and safety of new antithrombotic treatments are to be adequately evaluated. The essential design features required to avoid bias have now been defined.[5–8] These essential design features, which have been applied in many clinical trials evaluating antithrombotic therapy, are:

1. The study should be performed prospectively and include a concurrent control group.

2. The patients should be randomly allocated to the alternative treatment groups.

3. It should be demonstrated that the patient characteristics and important prognostic variables are comparable between the alternative groups.

4. Effectiveness and safety should be evaluated by well-defined objective measures; bias in the assessment of outcomes should be avoided.

5. All clinically relevant outcomes should be assessed and reported.

6. The number of patients must be large enough to allow valid conclusions. Appropriate statistical methods should be used to analyze data.

Retrospective studies are susceptible to numerous potential biases, particularly in the selection of patients and the allocation of treatment. Retrospective studies are not adequate for evaluating new therapies. If a study is uncontrolled, it is impossible to determine whether an observed outcome is a true effect of treatment or whether the outcome would have occurred even in the absence of the treatment being evaluated. Studies which use historical (nonconcurrent) controls are subject to potential bias resulting from: (a) changes in the demographic and clinical characteristics of a particular population of patients with time, (b) changes in patient management, and (c) improvements in health care. Therefore, a concurrent control group is required if valid inferences about the relative effectiveness and safety of a new therapy are to be made.

The use of random allocation is the only technique which will ensure that the treatment groups are comparable with respect to the *unknown*, as well as the known, characteristics which influence patient outcome. Although alternate procedures for allocating patients to the treatment groups have been proposed to replace random allocation,[19] none of these procedures can ensure that the treatment groups will be comparable with respect to variables that may influence the patient's outcome but are *unknown* at the time of study. For this reason, random allocation of patients to the treatment groups remains a mandatory requirement if the effectiveness and safety of a new therapy is to be definitively evaluated.[19]

The knowledge of a patient's treatment may influence both the intensity and the result of the search for a particular outcome (known as diagnostic-suspicion bias). Because of this, the assessment of outcome should be performed without the knowledge of the patient's treatment group, and should be based on well-defined objective outcome measures. Ideally, a double-blind design should be used. In this case, neither the patient nor members of the health-care team know which treatment the patient receives. For antithrombotic therapy, double-blind designs have been developed for clinical trials which evaluate treatments requiring laboratory monitoring and dose titration (such as heparin or oral anticoagulant therapy). In such studies, adjustments in the drug regimen would be made by a physician who was not involved in the assessment of patient outcome. The results of laboratory monitoring of coagulation tests, which could reveal the nature of the patient's treatment, would be released only to this designated physician. The remaining members of the health-care team, including the patient's attending physician and those involved in assessing the outcome, would not know which treatment the patient was receiving. This approach has been used successfully to provide double-blind designs in randomized trials evaluating alternative approaches for the initial treatment of venous thrombosis,[20–22] the prevention of venous thrombosis,[23] and long-term anticoagulant therapy for myocardial infarction[24] or atrial fibrillation.[25]

To avoid diagnostic suspicion bias when a double-blind design is not possible, objective tests performed routinely at fixed intervals in all patients can be used. The test results should be interpreted without knowledge of the patient's treatment group, other test results, or the patient's clinical findings. This approach was used successfully to evaluate the effectiveness of alternative regimens for the long-term treatment of venous thrombosis when the nature of the interventions did not allow the use of a double-blind design.[26,27]

A sufficient number of patients should be evaluated to minimize the possibility of two important statistical errors: the alpha error (a false-positive conclusion) and the beta error (a false-negative conclusion). If the number of patients evaluated in a clinical trial is small, even differences in outcome between treatments that are considered clinically important may not be statistically significant.[8] This may lead to the erroneous conclusion that no difference in outcome between treatment exists, when in fact it does (the beta error). A sufficient number of patients should be studied to ensure that the probability of a beta error is low (less than 10%).

To the clinician assessing the results of a clinical trial of therapy, two questions are important:

1. If a statistically significant ($p < 0.05$) difference in outcome between treatments is found, is this difference clinically important?
2. If a statistically significant difference is not found, was the study large enough to exclude the existence of a true, clinically important difference?

The 95% confidence interval for the observed difference in the outcomes of effectiveness or safety between treatments should always be provided.[28] If the minimum clinically important difference, as defined by the reader, lies outside the 95% confidence interval, then the reader can conclude that the existence of a true clinically important difference is unlikely.[7] Using the 95% confidence interval to determine if a clinically important difference has been excluded, allows individual readers to apply their own values for the "minimum clinically important difference."

Data should be appropriately analyzed. If interim analyses are performed during the course of the study, appropriate statistical procedures to account for these multiple analyses should be used. Sub-group analyses should be based on a well-defined, scientific rationale defined before the study begins, and should be kept to a minimum.[29] Ideally, these sub-groups will have been defined by stratifying patients before random allocation to the experimental or control treatment.

LEVELS OF EVIDENCE FOR THERAPY STUDIES

Levels of evidence for clinical studies evaluating antithrombotic therapy have been defined and these have been used to qualify the strength of evidence supporting

Table 1
Levels of Clinical Evidence for Therapy*

Level		Study Design Features
I	Strongest	Large randomized trials with definite results (low chance of alpha or beta error)
II		Small randomized trials with uncertain results (moderate to high alpha or beta error)
III		Non-randomized studies with concurrent controls
IV		Non-randomized studies with historical controls
V	Weakest	Case-series with no controls

* Sackett DL. Rules of evidence and clinical recommendations on the use of antithrombotic agents. CHEST 1989; 95:February supplement: 2s–4s.

a specific clinical recommendation.[9,10] The definitions of levels of evidence are based on the study design as shown in Table 1. The levels I (the strongest) and II are distinguished from levels III, IV and V (the weakest) based on two key design features: (a) the nature of the control group, either concurrent, historical, or absent, and (b) the use of random allocation to the alternative treatment groups. Both levels I and II evidence use a concurrent control group with random allocation of patients to the alternative treatments. The distinction between level I and level II evidence is statistical. Level II evidence has a higher likelihood of either false-positive results (alpha error) or false-negative results (beta error).

There are two factors which determine whether a given randomized trial will be classified as level I or level II. These are (a) the sample size, and (b) the size of the observed treatment effect. There is no arbitrary sample size which distinguishes a level I or level II study. Studies which have relatively small sample sizes but which identify profound treatment effects may provide level I evidence. An example is provided by a randomized trial which evaluated alternative approaches to the long-term treatment of proximal deep-vein thrombosis. There was a clinically striking and statistically significant difference in the rates of recurrent venous thromboembolism in patients treated with warfarin (no recurrence in 17 patients), compared with patients who received low dose subcutaneous heparin (nine recurrences in 19 patients) (p<0.001).[26] This study provides level I evidence for the effectiveness of warfarin in this setting. Conversely, studies with larger sample sizes may be classified as level II if they do not enroll sufficient patients to exclude a clinically important difference in outcomes between treatments. An example is given by two randomized trials that enrolled 200 to 300 patients per group to evaluate long-term oral anticoagulant therapy after myocardial infarction.[30,31] They are classified as level II,[24] because these

studies could not exclude a risk reduction in mortality of 20% in favor of oral anticoagulant treatment (a clinically important difference). Subsequently, larger trials with 400 to 600 patients per group established the effectiveness of long-term oral anticoagulant therapy for improving survival in patients with myocardial infarction.[24,33]

The levels of evidence approach was used by the American College of Chest Physicians (ACCP) working group on antithrombotic therapy to evaluate the literature and make clinical recommendations.[9,10] This approach provides several advantages over previous approaches to the development of clinical recommendations and practice guidelines.[34] First, it avoids recommendations based on "expert" opinion which may be incorrect and potentially harmful. Second, the rules of evidence are explicit, and practitioners can judge for themselves the validity of a specific recommendation based on the evidence cited. Third, those clinical scenarios which lack firm evidence for a particular approach can be identified, and research can be targeted to these areas. This latter point has been demonstrated in the case of oral anticoagulant treatment for patients with nonvalvular atrial fibrillation.[35] At the time of the second ACCP consensus conference, the value of long-term anticoagulant treatment in patients with nonvalvular atrial fibrillation remained uncertain because of a lack of level I evidence. By the time the third ACCP consensus conference was held in 1992, four level I trials had been completed, providing firm evidence for the benefit of oral anticoagulants.[35] This enabled the third conference to make a firm recommendation based on level I evidence.[35]

The levels of evidence approach is used throughout the remainder of this book to qualify the strength of evidence for specific clinical recommendations about therapy.

REFERENCES

1. Evidence-based Medicine Working Group. Evidence-based medicine. A new approach to teaching the practice of medicine. JAMA 1992;268:2420–2425.
2. Department of Clinical Epidemiology and Biostatistics, McMaster University. How to read clinical journals: II. To learn about a diagnostic test. Can Med Assoc J 1981;124:703–710.
3. Jaeschke R, Guyatt G, Sackett DL, for the Evidence-based Medicine Working Group. Users' guides to the medical literature III. How to use an article about a diagnostic test. A. Are the results of the study valid? JAMA 1994;271:389–391.
4. Ransohoff D, Feinstein AR. Problems of spectrum and bias in evaluating the efficacy of diagnostic tests. N Engl J Med 1978;299:926–930.
5. Department of Clinical Epidemiology and Biostatistics, McMaster University. How to read clinical journals: V: to distinguish useful from useless or even harmful therapy. Can Med Assoc J 1981;124:1156–1162.
6. Guyatt GH, Sackett DL, Cook DJ, for the Evidence-based Medicine Working Group. Users' guides to the medical literature II. How to use an article about therapy or preven-

tion. A. Are the results of the study valid? JAMA 1993;270: 2598–2601.

7. Guyatt GH, Sackett DL, Cook DJ, for the Evidence-based Medicine Working Group. Users' guides to the medical literature II. How to use an article about therapy or prevention. B. What were the results and will they help me in caring for my patients? JAMA 1994;271:59–63.

8. Frieman JA, Chalmers TC, Smith H, Kuebler RR. The importance of beta, the type II error, and sample size in the design and interpretation of the randomized controlled trial: survey of 71 "negative" trials. N Engl J Med 1978;299:690–694.

9. Sackett DL. Rules of evidence and clinical recommendations on the use of antithrombotic agents. CHEST 1989;95: February supplement:2s-4s.

10. Cook DJ, Guyatt GH, Laupacis A, Sackett DL. Rules of evidence and clinical recommendations on the use of antithrombotic agents. CHEST 1992;102:October supplement: 305s-311s.

11. Hull R, Hirsh J, Sackett DL, et al. Clinical validity of a negative venogram in patients with clinically suspected venous thrombosis. Circulation 1981;64:622–625.

12. Hull R, Carter CJ, Jay R, et al. The diagnosis of acute recurrent deep-vein thrombosis: a diagnostic challenge. Circulation 1983;67:901–906.

13. Hull R, Hirsh J, Carter CJ, et al. Diagnostic efficacy of impedance plethysmography for clinically suspected deep-vein thrombosis: a randomized trial. Ann Intern Med 1985;102:21–28.

14. Huisman MV, Buller HR, ten Cate JW, Vreelsen J. Serial impedance plethysmography for suspected deep-vein thrombosis in outpatients. The Amsterdam General Practitioner Study. N Engl J Med 1986;314:823–828.

15. Heijboer H, Buller HR, Lensing AW, Turpie AG, Colly LP, et al. A comparison of real-time compression ultrasonography with impedance plethysmography for the diagnosis of deep-vein thrombosis in symptomatic outpatients. N Engl J Med 1993;329:1365–1369.

16. Kipper MS, Moser KM, Kortman KE, Ashburn WL. Long-term follow-up of patients with suspected pulmonary embolism and a normal lung scan. CHEST 1982;82:411–415.

17. Hull R, Raskob G, Coates G, Panju A. Clinical validity of a normal perfusion lung scan in patients with suspected pulmonary embolism. CHEST 1990;97:23–26.

18. Pamelia FX, Gibson RS, Watson DD, et al. Prognosis with chest pain and normal thallium-201 exercise scintigrams. Am J Cardiol 1985;55:920–926.

19. Sackett DL. Readers' guides for therapy: was the assignment of patients to treatment randomized? ACP Journal Club 1991 May/June:A-12.

20. Hull R, Raskob G, Rosenbloom D, et al. Heparin for 5 days compared with 10 days in the initial treatment of proximal venous thrombosis. N Engl J Med 1990;322:1260–1264.

21. Hull R, Raskob G, Pineo G, et al. Subcutaneous low molecular weight heparin compared with continuous intravenous heparin in the treatment of proximal vein thrombosis. N Engl J Med 1992;326:975–982.

22. Brandjes DPM, Heijboer H, Buller HR, De Rijk M, Jagt H, et al. Acenocoumarol and heparin compared with acenocoumarol alone in the initial treatment of proximal-vein thrombosis. N Engl J Med 1992;327:1485–1489.

23. Hull R, Raskob G, Pineo G, et al. A comparison of subcutaneous low-molecular weight heparin with warfarin sodium for prophylaxis against deep-vein thrombosis after hip or knee implantation. N Engl J Med 1993;329:1370–1376.

24. Report of the Sixty Plus Reinfarction Study Research Group. A double-blind trial to assess long-term anticoagulant therapy in elderly patients after myocardial infarction. Lancet 1980;2:989–994.

25. Connolly S, Laupacis A, Gent M, et al. Canadian Atrial Fibrillation Anticoagulation (CAFA) study. J Am Coll Cardiol 1991;18:349–355.

26. Hull R, Delmore T, Genton E, et al. Warfarin sodium vs. low-dose heparin in the long-term treatment of venous thrombosis. N Engl J Med 1979;301:855–858.

27. Hull R, Delmore T, Carter C, et al. Adjusted subcutaneous heparin versus warfarin sodium in the long-term treatment of venous thrombosis. N Engl J Med 1982;306:189–194.

28. Braitman LE. Confidence intervals assess both clinical significance and statistical significance. Ann Intern Med 1991;114:515–517.

29. Oxman AD, Guyatt GH. A consumer's guide to subgroup analysis. Ann Intern Med 1992;116:78–84.

30. Second Report of the Working Party on Anticoagulant Therapy in Coronary Thrombosis to the Medical Research Council. An assessment of long-term anticoagulant administration after cardiac infarction. Br Med J 1964;2: 837–843.

31. Breddin D, Loew D, Lechner K, et al. The German-Austrian trial: a comparison of acetylsalicylic acid, placebo, and phenproucoumon in secondary prevention of myocardial infarction. Circulation 1980;62(suppl 5):6.

32. Cairns JA, Hirsh J, Lewis HD, Resnekov L, Theroux P. Antithrombotic agents in coronary artery disease. CHEST 1992;102: October supplement:456s-481s.

33. Smith P, Arnesen H, Holme I. The effect of warfarin on mortality and reinfarction after myocardial infarction. N Engl J Med 1990;323:147–152.

34. Hirsh J, Haynes B. Transforming evidence into practice: evidence-based consensus. ACP Journal Club 1993 January/February:A-16.

35. Laupacis A, Albers G, Dunn MI, Feinberg WM. Antithrombotic therapy in atrial fibrillation. CHEST 1992; 102:October supplement:426S-433S.

SECTION II

Prevention

4

Overview of Prevention of Venous Thromboembolism

G. Patrick Clagett

INTRODUCTION

Venous thromboembolism remains a major, preventable cause of death and morbidity in hospitalized patients. It has been estimated that pulmonary embolism (PE) causes death in over 100,000 patients each year in the United States and contributes to death in another 100,000.[1] Although many of these patients have terminal illnesses that are complicated by pulmonary embolism, more than one-half have treatable conditions and would enjoy extended longevity were it not for fatal pulmonary embolism. The loss of productive lives and the economic burden imposed by dealing with the consequences of venous thromboembolism in surviving patients demand serious consideration from a public health perspective.

The estimates cited above are from older, crude data. However, they have recently been substantiated in a community-wide study conducted in 16 short-stay hospitals in central Massachusetts, where the annual incidence of verified PE was 23 per 100,000 residents with an in-hospital case fatality rate of 12%.[2] Extrapolation of these data to the entire United States population suggests that approximately 260,000 cases of *clinically diagnosed* venous thromboembolism occur each year in patients hospitalized in acute care hospitals in this country. Undiagnosed PE is a larger problem. Fatal and nonfatal PE are most often clinically silent with the disease being unsuspected in 70% to 80% of patients diagnosed at autopsy.[3,4] Because of the low rate of autopsy in the United States and the failure of the Massachusetts study to include nonacute care facilities such as nursing homes and rehabilitation hospitals, where the incidence of PE may be higher, the actual incidence of venous thromboembolism is far greater. These concerns are justified based on data from population studies in countries where the rate of autopsy is much higher.[5]

RATIONALE FOR PROPHYLAXIS

An important rationale for considering prophylaxis of venous thromboembolism is the clinically silent nature of the disease. Deep-vein thrombosis (DVT) and PE manifest few specific symptoms,[6] and the clinical diagnosis based on physical examination alone is insensitive and unreliable.[7] In addition, to wait until venous thromboembolism becomes clinically apparent and then to treat the condition, exposes susceptible patients to unacceptable risks. The first manifestation of the disease may be fatal PE. Although anticoagulation is a highly effective therapy for venous thromboembolism, the majority of patients who die from PE do so within one-half hour of the onset of symptoms,[8] too soon for anticoagulant therapy to be effective. Unrecognized and untreated DVT may also lead to the long-term sequela of chronic venous insufficiency and the postphlebitic syndrome, as well as predispose patients to future episodes of recurrent venous thromboembolism.

In addition to saving lives and reducing morbidity, health care dollars are saved by broad application of strategies to prevent venous thromboembolism. All cost-effectiveness analyses dealing with this topic have demonstrated that it is far cheaper to employ routine prophylaxis rather than to pay for treatment of clinically recognized venous thromboembolism.[9–14] In a recent study that addressed the prevalence of risk factors for venous thromboembolism in hospitalized patients in the United States, the costs of broad application of prophylaxis to the patients at risk were assessed.[15] The authors estimated that for the 1.18 million patients over the age of 40 years undergoing major operations annually, the cost of prophylaxis, based on $50 to $100 per patient, would be $59 million to $118 million. Effective prophylaxis would prevent 158,000 episodes of DVT and 6000 deaths due to PE. The cost savings would be $119 million to $301 million. In

From *Venous Thromboembolism: An Evidence-Based Atlas* edited by Russell Hull, Gary Raskob, Graham Pineo © 1996, Futura Publishing Co., Armonk, NY.

addition, the authors estimated that there were 6 million patients hospitalized annually for medical and surgical conditions who were at high risk for venous thromboembolism, in that they had at least three clinical risk factors. In extrapolating the data from surgical patients to this larger group, the general application of prophylaxis to these patients might prevent 700,000 episodes to DVT and 25,000 to 33,000 deaths from PE annually. This would represent a savings of $330 million to $660 million.

An alternative to prophylaxis would be to use serial surveillance tests such as impedance plethysmography, labeled fibrinogen scanning, or duplex ultrasonography in high-risk patients.[16,17] Although attractive, this approach is expensive and can be applied to only limited numbers of patients at risk. Most experts believe that broad application of effective methods of prevention is more cost-effective than selective, intensive surveillance.[9,10]

REASONS CITED FOR NOT USING PROPHYLAXIS

Despite convincing evidence of the efficacy of a wide variety of prophylactic agents, surveys conducted in the United States, England, and Sweden document wide practice variations among physicians; approximately one-half of surgeons in these countries use effective prophylaxis in less than one-fifth of their patients.[19–22] A recent study of over 2000 patients with multiple risk factors hospitalized at 16 acute care hospitals showed that only one-third of these patients received prophylaxis.[23] Use of prophylaxis was higher in teaching than nonteaching hospitals, and patients undergoing vascular, abdominal, and orthopedic operations were the most likely to receive prophylaxis. Risk factors for venous thromboembolism were highly prevalent in this population of hospitalized patients; 78% of all patients had one or more risk factors, 48% had two or more, and 19% had three or more.[15] The authors concluded that despite widespread recognition of the problem and the effectiveness of multiple preventive strategies, prophylaxis was woefully underutilized at present.

Why don't physicians use prophylaxis more widely? Many feel that the overall incidence of venous thromboembolism among hospitalized and postoperative patients has decreased over the past decades to the point where the incidence is too low to consider prophylaxis. These individuals will frequently cite informal, retrospective surveys of their own clinical services and the rare occurrence of fatal PE, diagnosed by autopsy at their hospital to bolster this argument. In fact, the incidence of venous thromboembolism has declined in recent years[24] and this may represent some of the success of prophylactic strategies.[25] Even so, the incidence remains too high for a preventable condition and the current estimates of the incidence of fatal PE based on hospital discharge data

suggest the need for wider application of prophylaxis.[26] Furthermore, the difficulties in establishing the antemortem diagnosis of PE has been alluded to as well as the low rate of autopsy in the United States, especially in elderly patients with chronic conditions. Data from countries where autopsy is mandated, indicate that fatal PE remains a significant problem.[5,27] In addition, contemporary data from the central Massachusetts study show that clinically recognized PE is surprisingly common.[2]

Another reason not to use prophylaxis, especially in surgical patients, is the concern about bleeding complications with antithrombotic agents.[22] Countering this argument are the abundant data from overview analyses and placebo-controlled, double-blind randomized trials, that demonstrate no significant increase in major bleeding with the use of low-dose heparin and low molecular weight heparin.[28–30] The incidence of wound hematomas is increased with these agents and this can be a significant problem leading to wound infection, dehiscence and infection of a prosthetic device placed at the time of operation.[28] However, alternative, mechanical methods of effective prophylaxis are available in such patients that carry no bleeding risk. Heparin-induced thrombocytopenia has also been raised as a concern with widespread use of low dose heparin. Critical review of this problem, though, suggests that the incidence with this route of heparin administration is vanishingly rare.[31] The cost of prophylaxis has also been used as an argument against its wider use; however, as cited above, every study addressing this issue has concluded that broad application of prophylaxis is highly cost effective.

The final reason for not using prophylaxis has to do with subjective perceptions of the magnitude of the problem and the effects of prophylaxis in *individual* practices. Because venous thromboembolism is most often clinically silent, the occurrence of overt venous thromboembolism among an individual physician's patients is perceived to be rare.[22] For example, extrapolation of data from meta-analyses suggests that fatal PE might occur in 0.5% to 0.8% of patients undergoing major abdominal surgery over the age of 40 years,[11,28,29] and many of these embolic events would go unrecognized. Similarly, proximal or above knee venous thrombosis would be present in 6% to 7%, and less than 50% of these would be clinically overt and detected. Therefore, an average busy general surgeon whose practice consists of a high volume major abdominal surgery, would not perceive venous thromboembolism to be a significant problem. More importantly, this physician would have little appreciation of the effectiveness of, say, low-dose heparin in reducing the incidence of fatal PE in his/her individual practice from 0.7% to 0.2%, as has been pointed out in meta-analyses dealing with large numbers of patients.[28] Thus, from an individual practice perspective, it would be difficult to appreciate the effectiveness of prophylaxis, whereas failures (patients developing clinically overt venous thromboembolism who receive prophylaxis) would be readily apparent. Additionally, bleeding complications that are clinically overt are not easily forgotten and frequently blamed on prophylaxis. Physician education is the only antidote to these misperceptions.

CLINICAL RISK FACTORS

Application of effective prophylaxis depends upon the knowledge of specific clinical risk factors in individual patients. Clinical risk factors include age greater that 40 years; advanced age (greater than 70 years); prolonged immobility or paralysis; prior venous thromboembolism; cancer; major surgery (particularly operations involving the abdomen, pelvis, and lower extremities); obesity; varicose veins; congestive heart failure; myocardial infarction; stroke; fractures of the pelvis, hip, or leg; and estrogen use.[32–34] In addition, congenital and acquired aberrations in hemostatic mechanisms (prethrombotic states), that are ordinarily predisposed to venous thromboembolism assumes even greater risk when afflicted patients are hospitalized and undergo surgical procedures. Hemostatic abnormalities include antithrombin III deficiency, protein C deficiency, protein S deficiency, dysfibrinogenemia, disorders of plasminogen and plasminogen activation, antiphospholipid antibodies and lupus anticoagulant, heparin-induced thrombocytopenia, myeloproliferative disorders such as polycythemia vera and hyperviscosity syndromes.[35]

In many patients, multiple risk factors may be present and the risks are cumulative. For example, elderly patients with hip fractures undergoing major orthopedic operations who remain immobile in bed after operation, are among the most susceptible to fatal PE. Awareness of the risk of venous thromboembolism in general patient categories and clinical settings, where the risk has been defined by epidemiologic studies, is also important in successful application of prophylaxis.[32] For example, the overall incidence of venous thromboembolism is higher in orthopedic services and in intensive care units than in general medical services. The levels of risk were thromboembolic events based on clinical risk factors and epidemiologic data are shown in Table 1.

APPLICATION OF PROPHYLAXIS

Just as the level of risk varies in individual patients, so too does the effectiveness of various prophylactic approaches. An effective strategy in one type of patient may be relatively ineffective in another. An example is low-dose heparin that is highly effective in moderate risk general surgery patients, but is a poor prophylactic agent in high risk orthopedic patients. In addition to relative effectiveness, the risk of bleeding, other side effects and expense vary with different agents. An underlying philosophy of broad application of prophylaxis, is that many patients will be treated to spare the few who might develop venous thromboembolism. Therefore, costly strategies with significant bleeding potential should be reserved for patients at highest risk. For example, moderate intensity warfarin (INR = 2–3) is an excellent choice in high risk orthopedic patients but would be inappropriate in moderate risk general surgery patients.

The results of prophylactic strategies in various patient groups are shown in Table 2. Effectiveness is defined by the relative risk reduction (% reduction) and DVT, the precursor to PE. These data were derived from pooled analyses of the results of randomized trials published in English up to 1992.[36] The following recommendations in various patient categories were made by a consensus group[36] that critically reviewed these data, applied formal statistical rules of evidence to judge efficacy,[37] ex-

Table 1
Classification of Level of Risk
(Based on Published Data)*

Thromboembolism Event	Low Risk (Uncomplicated surgery in patients under 40 years of age with no other risk factors)	Moderate Risk (Major surgery in patients over 40 years of age with no other clinical risk factors)	High Risk (Major surgery in patients over 40 years of age who have additional risk factors or myocardial infarction)	Very High Risk (Major surgery in patients over 40 years of age plus previous thrombomalignant disease or orthopedic surgery or hip fracture or stroke or spinal cord injury)
Calf Vein Thrombosis (%)	2	10–20	20–40	40–80
Proximal Vein Thrombosis (%)	0.4	2–4	4–8	10–20
Clinical Pulmonary Embolism (%)	0.2	1–2	2–4	4–10
Fatal Pulmonary Embolism (%)	0.002	0.1–0.4	0.4–1.0	1–5

* (Modified from Salzman EW and Hirsh J: Prevention of Venous Thromboembolism. In: Colman RW, Hirsh J, Marder VJ, and Salzman EW (eds): *Hemostasis and Thrombosis: Basic Principles and Clinical Practice*, p. 1253. Philadelphia, J.P. Lippincott, Co. 1987)

Table 2
Effectiveness of Prophylaxis of Venous Thromboembolism According to Patient Category*

Patient Category**	No Prophylaxis		Relative Risk Reduction (%) with Prophylactic Methods							
	Incidence of DVT (%)	95% CI	Low-Dose Heparin	Low-Dose Heparin plus Dihydro-ergotamine	Low Molecular Weight Heparin	Warfarin	Dextran	Aspirin	Intermittent Pneumatic Compression	Elastic Stockings
General Surgery***	25	24–26	68	64	86	59	38	19	61	63
Elective Hip Replacement	50	46–55	32	26	68	63	41	11	60	25
Hip Fracture	43	38–49	9	17	74	43	32	6	?	?
Neuro-Surgery	24	20–28	75	?	?	?	?	?	73	64
Spinal Cord Injury	38	31–46	?	?	?	?	?	?	?	?
Multiple Trauma	48	43–53	?	?	?	?	?	?	?	?
Myocardial Infarction	24	18–30	72	?	?	?	?	?	?	?
Stroke	47	35–48	45	?	79	?	?	?	?	?

* Data obtained from pooled analysis of English Language trials reported through 1992.[36]
** Deep venous thrombosis (DVT) diagnosed by labeled fibrinogen uptake test in general surgical, neurosurgical, myocardial infarction, and stroke patients; by phlebography in elective hip surgery, hip fracture, and multiple trauma patients; and impedance plethysmography in spinal cord injury patients.
*** General surgery patient includes any patient over the age of 40 years undergoing major abdominal surgery (gastrointestinal, gynecologic, and urologic complications).
? Indicates that data is too scant to make reliable estimate of risk reduction.

trapolated results from studies in similar patient groups when data was insufficient, and tempered their recommendations with practical concerns of cost, patient acceptance, physician and nursing compliance.

General Surgery

The overall incidence of thromboembolic end-points in general surgical patients was calculated by pooling data in control patients in published English language trials of prophylactic methods.[28] The overall incidence of DVT as assessed by the labeled fibrinogen uptake test was 25% in control subjects; in trials in which the fibrinogen uptake test was confirmed by phlebography, the incidence was 19%. Most of this represents calf or leg vein thrombosis of questionable clinical significance. The presence of more serious proximal or above-knee DVT was 6% to 7% in patients not treated with prophylaxis. The overall incidence of clinically recognized PE (fatal and nonfatal) was 1.6% and the incidence of fatal PE, 0.8%.[28]

In low-risk general surgery patients who are undergoing minor operations, are less than 40 years of age, and have no clinical risk factors, no specific prophylaxis other than early ambulation is warranted. Elastic stockings, low-dose heparin (given every 12 hours), or intermittent pneumatic compression would be appropriate for moderate risk general surgery patients who are over 40 years of age and are undergoing major operations, but who have no additional clinical risk factors for venous thromboembolism. Low-dose heparin (given every eight hours) or

low-molecular-weight heparin, should be used in higher risk general surgery patients who are over the age of 40 years, undergoing major operations, and have additional risk factors. Low-molecular-weight heparin appears to be slightly better than low-dose unfractionated heparin in preventing venous thromboembolism (Table 2) and may be associated with slightly fewer bleeding complications.[30,38(I)] It is also more convenient and can be administered in a single, daily dosage regimen. However, both strategies are highly successful in preventing venous thromboembolism in general surgical patients, and the marginal advantages of low-molecular-weight heparin may be offset by its higher expense. Low-dose heparin combined with dihydroergotamine is also effective but has been withdrawn from the market in the United States. In higher-risk general surgery patients who are prone to wound complications such as hematoma and infection, dextran or intermittent pneumatic compression would be good alternative choices for prophylaxis. These agents have been proven effective in multiple trials and carry less bleeding risk.[28] In very high-risk general surgery patients with multiple risk factors, pharmacological methods (low-dose heparin, low-molecular-weight heparin, or dextran) may be combined with intermittent pneumatic compression. In selected very high-risk general surgery patients, perioperative warfarin may be an appropriate choice. Aspirin has been found to be ineffective[28] or marginally effective,[39] in preventing venous thromboembolism in general surgery patients and would not be an appropriate strategy.

Orthopedic Surgery

Orthopedic operation and orthopedic trauma are high risk conditions in which the most frequent cause of death is often PE. In patients not treated with prophylaxis, DVT complicates the postoperative course after total hip replacement in approximately 50% of patients.[29,40(I),41(I)] Fatal PE occurs in up to 6% of patients who received no antithrombotic prophylaxis.[42] The mortality of hip fractures without prophylaxis is over 3% and may be as high as 12% with death being most commonly due to fatal PE.[42] After knee replacement surgery, the incidence of DVT is over 50% and may reach 80%.[43(I),44(I),45(IV)]

In patients undergoing total hip replacement, warfarin and low-molecular weight heparin are the most effective antithrombotic agents (Table 2). Although other methods such as low-dose heparin, dextran, aspirin, intermittent pneumatic compression, and elastic stockings reduce the overall incidence of venous thromboembolism, they are less effective and should not be used routinely. Subcutaneous heparin given in adjusted doses to maintain the activated partial thromboplastin time in the upper normal range has also been found to be highly effective.[46(I),47(I)] However, this method of administration is cumbersome, requires close monitoring, and is not commonly used.

Warfarin and low-molecular-weight heparin are the most effective prophylactic agents in patients with hip fractures. Dextran, low-dose heparin, and aspirin are less effective and are not recommended for routine use (Table 2). Placement of a prophylactic inferior vena cava filter may be considered in selected high orthopedic and multiple trauma patients, in whom other forms of prophylaxis would be contraindicated or ineffective.[48,49]

Neurosurgery/Acute Spinal Cord Injury/Multiple Trauma

Patients undergoing elective intracranial neurosurgery are at high risk for venous thromboembolism because they frequently have paralysis, prolonged postoperative immobility, and often have lengthy operations with the lower extremities in a dependent position. In controlled patients not treated with prophylaxis, the average incidence of DVT is approximately 24% (Table 2). Physical methods of prophylaxis in neurosurgical patients have been preferred to anticoagulant therapy because of concern about intracranial bleeding. Intermittent pneumatic compression with or without elastic stockings is the prophylactic method of choice in these patients.

Although the high incidence of DVT in patients with hip and lower extremity fractures is well established, the incidence following other types of trauma is less well-known. The literature is difficult to interpret because trauma patients are heterogeneous with a variety of injuries, and studies reporting a high incidence of DVT may have a large proportion of patients with lower extremity trauma and fractures. A recent review article suggests that trauma patients with no additional risk factors for venous thromboembolism are at relatively low risk.[50] In multiple trauma patients, intermittent pneumatic compression, warfarin, or low-molecular-weight heparin may be effective but data are limited. A recent nonrandomized study suggests that low-dose-heparin is inadequate prophylaxis in patients with multiple trauma.[51] In patients with extensive trauma who have multiple risk factors but who cannot receive other forms of prophylaxis, inferior vena cava filter insertion may be considered, but there are no randomized prospective control studies to verify efficacy.

In patients with acute spinal cord injury, the venographic incidence of DVT has been reported as 18% to 90%, with an average incidence of 38% (Table 2). PE occurs in about 5% of patients following paralysis, due to acute spinal cord injury and the period of greatest risk appears to be during the first two weeks following the injury.[52] Death from PE is rare three months or more after injury. Low-dose-heparin appears to be relatively ineffective in patients with spinal cord injury, whereas low-molecular-weight heparin is clearly efficacious.[53(I),54(I)] Warfarin and intermittent pneumatic compression prophylaxis have not been well studied in these patients, but would probably be effective based on their ability to prevent venous thromboembolism in other high-risk patient groups[55] (Table 2).

Myocardial Infarction/Ischemic Stroke

The overall incidence of DVT is about 24% among myocardial infarction patients not treated with prophylaxis. From available data, low-dose-heparin and full anticoagulation with heparin are effective in reducing the incidence of venous thromboembolism in these patients (Table 2). Because of this and because anticoagulants reduce other thromboembolic events (mural thrombosis and systemic arterial embolism) in these patients without incurring a significant major bleeding risk, liberal use of these agents is appropriate. Although data is limited, mechanical methods of prophylaxis (elastic stockings and intermittent pneumatic compression), would also be useful in myocardial infarction when bleeding risk is great and conventional antithrombotic agents are contraindicated. Fibrinolytic therapy to treat myocardial infarction may also reduce the incidence of DVT complicating this condition.

Stroke patients have a high risk of DVT in the paretic or paralyzed lower extremity. The overall incidence of leg DVT is 47% (Table 2). Low dose heparin and low-molecular-weight heparin have been shown to be highly effective in reducing the incidence of DVT in these patients.[56(I),57(I),58,59] Because of the efficacy of intermittent pneumatic compression in neurosurgical patients, many of whom have hemiparesis, this method should also be beneficial in stroke patients. Elastic stockings may also be of benefit.

CONCLUSION

A wide variety of effective prophylactic methods are available to prevent venous thromboembolism. These methods have been tested in numerous randomized clinical trials of immaculate scientific design. Whether these trials are considered singly or in aggregate in the form of overview analyses, the inescapable conclusion is that the prophylactic strategies considered in this review prevent morbidity and mortality associated with venous thromboembolism. Individual patients can be assigned a level of risk for venous thromboembolism based on clinical risk factors. The choice of prophylactic method is based on the level of risk, the potential for side effects and complications, and the overall costs. With the wide variety of proven prophylactic methods, the most appropriate method can be readily tailored to individual patient's needs, and no patient at significant risk for venous thromboembolism should be left unprotected.

REFERENCES

1. Dalen JE, Alpert JS. Natural history of PE. Prog Cardiovasc Dis 1975;17:259–270.
2. Anderson FA, Wheeler HB, Goldberg RJ, et al. A population-based perspective of the hospital incidence and case-fatality rates of deep vein thrombosis and pulmonary embolism. Arch Intern Med 1991;151:933–938.
3. Goldhaber SZ, Hennekens CH, Evans DA, et al. Factors associated with correct antemortem diagnosis of major pulmonary embolism in a hospital population. Br J Surg 1968;55:347–352.
4. Rubinstein I, Murray D, Hoffstein V. Fatal pulmonary emboli in hospitalized patients. Arch Intern Med 1988;148:1425–1426.
5. Lindblad B, Eriksson A, Bergqvist D. Autopsy-verified pulmonary embolism in a surgical department: analysis of the period from 1951 to 1988. Br J Surg 1991;78:849–852.
6. Huisman MV, Buller H, Jan W, et al. Unexpected high prevalence of silent pulmonary embolism in patients with DVT. Chest 1989;95:498–502.
7. Hirsch J, Hull RD. Diagnosis of venous thrombosis. In: Venous Thromboembolism: Natural History, Diagnosis, and Management. Boca Raton, Fla: CRC Press, 1987;23–28.
8. Donaldson GA, Williams C, Scannell JG, et al. A reappraisal of the application of the Trendelenburg operation to massive fatal embolism: report of a successful pulmonary-artery thrombectomy using a cardiopulmonary bypass. N Engl J Med 1963;268:171–174.
9. Hull R, Hirsh J, Sackett DL, et al. Cost-effectiveness of primary and secondary prevention of fatal pulmonary embolism in high-risk surgical patients. Can Med Assoc J 1982;127:990–995.
10. Salzman EW, Davies GC. Prophylaxis of venous thromboembolism: analysis of cost-effectiveness. Ann Surg 1980;191:207–218.
11. Oster G, Tuden R, Colditz G. Prevention of Venous Thromboembolism after general surgery: cost-effectiveness analysis of alternative approaches to prophylaxis. Am J Med 1987;82:889–899.
12. Oster G, Tuden R, Colditz G. A cost-effectiveness analysis of prophylaxis against DVT in major orthopedic surgery. JAMA 1987;257:203–208.
13. Bergqvist D, Matzsch T. Cost/Benefit aspects on thromboprophylaxis. Haemostasis 1993;23(Suppl 1):15–19.
14. Bergqvist D, Jendteg S, Lindgren B, Matzsch T, Persson U. Economics of general thromboembolic prophylaxis. World J Surg 1988;12:349–355.
15. Anderson FA, Wheeler HB, Goldberg R, Hosmer D, Forcier A. The prevalence of risk factors for venous thromboembolism among hospital patients. Arch Intern Med 1992;152:1660–1664.
16. Barnes RW, Nix ML, Barnes CL, et al. Perioperative asymptomatic venous thrombosis: role of duplex scanning versus venography. J Vasc Surg 1989;9:251–260.
17. Comerota AJ, Katz ML, Greenwald LL, et al. Venous duplex imaging: should it replace hemodynamic tests for DVT? J Vasc Surg 1989;9:251–260.
18. Salzman EW, Hirsh J. Prevention of venous thromboembolism. In: Coleman RW, Hirsh J, Marder VJ, et al, eds. Hemostasis and thrombosis. Philadelphia: JB Lippincott 1987;1252–1265.
19. Conti S, Daschback M. Venous thromboembolism prophylaxis. Arch Surg 1982;117:1036–1040.
20. Morris GK. Prevention of venous thromboembolism: a survey of methods used by orthopaedic and general surgeons. Lancet 1980;2:572–574.
21. Bergqvist D. Prevention of postoperative deep-vein thrombosis in Sweden: results of a survey. World J Surg 1980;4:489–495.
22. Laverick MD, Croal SA, Mollan RAB. Orthopaedic surgeons and thromboprophylaxis. Brit Med J 1991;303:549–550.
23. Anderson FA, Wheeler HB, Goldberg RJ, Gent M. Physician practices in the prevention of venous thromboembolism. Ann Intern Med 1991;115:591–595.
24. Dismuke SE, Wagner EH. Pulmonary embolism as a cause of death: the changing mortality in hospitalized patients. JAMA 1986;255:2039–2042.
25. Ruckley CV, Thurston C. Pulmonary embolism in surgical patients: 1959–79. Brit Med J 1982;284:1100–1110.
26. Lilienfeld DE, Chan E, Ehland J, Godbold JH, Landrigan PJ, et al. Mortality from pulmonary embolism in the United States: 1962–1984. Chest 1990;98:1067–1072.
27. Bergqvist D, Lindblad B. A 30-year survey of pulmonary embolism verified at autopsy: an analysis of 1274 surgical patients. Br J Surg 1985;72:105–108.
28. Clagett GP, Reisch JS. Prevention of Venous Thromboembolism in general surgical patients. Ann Surg 1988;208:227–240.
29. Collins R, Scrimgeour A, Yusuf S, Peto R. Reduction in fatal pulmonary embolism and venous thrombosis by perioperative administration of subcutaneous heparin. N Eng J Med 1988;318:1162–1173.
30. Nurmohamed MT, Rosendaal FR, Buller HR, et al. Low-molecular weight heparin versus standard heparin in general and orthopaedic surgery: a meta-analysis. Lancet 1992;340:152–155.
31. Schmitt BP, Adelman B. Heparin-associated thrombocytopenia: a critical review and pooled analysis. Am J Med Sci 1993;305:208–215.
32. Carter C, Gent M, Leclerc JR. The epidemiology of venous thrombosis. In: Coleman RW, Hirsh J, Marder VJ,

et al, eds. Hemostasis and thrombosis. Philadelphia: JB Lippincott 1987;1185–1198.

33. Coon WW. Epidemiology of venous thromboembolism. Ann Surg 1977;186:149–164.

34. Goldhaber SZ, Savage DD, Garrison RJ, et al. Risk factors for pulmonary embolism: the Framingham study. Am J Med 1983;74:1023–1028.

35. Schafer AI. The hypercoagulable states. Ann Intern Med 1985;102:814–828.

36. Clagett GP, Anderson FA, Levine MN, Salzman EW, Wheeler HB. Prevention of venous thromboembolism. Chest 1992;102:391S-407S.

37. Cook D, Guyatt GH, Laupacis A, Sackett D. Rules of evidence and clinical recommendations on the use of antithrombotic agents. Chest 1992;102:305S-311S.

(I)38. Kakkar VV, Cohen AT, Edmonson RA, et al. Low molecular weight versus standard heparin for prevention of venous thromboembolism after major abdominal surgery. Lancet 1993;341:259–265.

39. Lensing AWA, Hirsh J, Roberts R, et al. Critical review of aspirin in the prevention of postoperative venous thromboembolism. Br Med J. (In press)

(I)40. Turpie AGG, Levine MN, Hirsh J, et al. A randomized controlled trial of a low-molecular weight heparin (Enoxaparin) to prevent deep vein thrombosis in patients undergoing elective hip surgery. N Engl J Med 1986;315:925–929.

(I)41. Gallus A, Raman K, Darby T. Venous thrombosis after elective hip replacement: the influence of preventive intermittant calf compression and of surgical techinique. Br J Surg 1983;70:17–19.

42. Haake DA, Berkman SA. Venous thromboembolic disease after hip surgery. Clin Orthop 1989;242:212.

(I)43. Hull R, Delmore TJ, Hirsh J, et al. Effectiveness of intermittent pulsatile stockings for the prevention of calf and thigh vein thrombosis in patients undergoing elective knee surgery. Thromb Res 1979;16:37–45.

(I)44. Lynch AF, Bourne RB, Rorabeck CH, et al. DVT and continuous passive motion after total knee arthroplasty. J Bone Joint Surg 1988;70:11.

(IV)45. Stulberg BN, Insall JN, Williams GW, et al. Deep-vein thrombosis following total knee replacement. J Bone Joint Surg 1984;66:194.

(I)46. Leyvraz PF, Richard J, Bachmann F. Adjusted versus fixed-dose subcutaneous heparin in the prevention of deep-vein thrombosis after total hip replacement. N Engl J Med 1983;309:954–958.

(I)47. Leyvraz PF, Backmann F, Hoek J, et al. Prevention of deep vein thrombosis after hip replacement: randomized comparison between unfractionated heparin and low-molecular-weight heparin. BMJ 1991;303:531–532.

48. Golueke PF, Garrett WV, Thompson JE, et al. Interruption of the vena cava by means of the Greenfield filter: expanding the indications. Surgery 1988;103: 111–117.

49. Vaughn BK, Knezevich S, Lombardi AV, et al. Use of the Greenfield filter to prevent fatal embolism associated with total hip and knee arthroplasty. J Bone Joint Surg 1989;71:1542.(Abstract)

50. O'Malley KF, Ross SE. Pulmonary embolism in major trauma patients. J Trauma 1990;30:748–750.

51. Ruiz AJ, Hill SL, Berry RE. Heparin, DVT, and trauma patients. Am J Surg 1991;162:159–162.

52. Waring WP, Karunas RS. Acute spinal cord injuries and the incidence of clinically occuring thromboembolism in spinal cord injury. JAMA 1988; 260:1255–1258.

(I)53. Green D, Lee MY, Ito VY, et al. Fixed vs adjusted dose heparin in the prophylaxis of thromboembolism in spinal cord injury. JAMA 1988;260:1255–1258.

(I)54. Green D, Lee MY, Lim AC, et al. Prevention of thromboembolism after spinal cord injury using low-molecular weight heparin. Ann Intern Med 1990;113:571–574.

55. Green, D. Prophylaxis of thromboembolism in spinal cord-injured patients. Chest 1992;102:649S-651S.

(I)56. McCarthy ST, Turner JJ, Robertson D, et al. Low dose heparin as a prophylaxis against deep vein thrombosis after acute stroke. Lancet 1977;2:800–801.

(I)57. Turpie AGG, Levine MN, Hirsh J, et al. A double-blind randomized trial or ORG 10172 low molecular weight heparinoid in the prevention of deep vein thrombosis in thrombotic stroke. Lancet 1987;1:523–526.

58. Prins MH, den Ottolander GJH, Gelsema R, et al. Deep vein thrombosis prophylaxis with a low molecular weight heparin (Kabi 2165) in stroke patients. Thromb Haemost 1987;58(Suppl):117.

59. Turpie AGG, Levine MN, Powers PJ, et al. A double-blind randomized trial of ORG 10172 low molecular weight heparinoid versus unfractionated heparin in the prevention of deep vein thrombosis in patients with thrombotic stroke. Thromb Haemost 1991;65(Suppl):753.

5

Prevention of Venous Thromboembolism in General Surgery

Alexander T. Cohen, Vijay V. Kakkar

INTRODUCTION

General surgery encompasses a broad spectrum of operations and specialities. This chapter will cover the following areas: i) general abdominal surgery, ii) thoracic and cardiothoracic surgery with particular emphasis on cardiac surgery, thoraco-abdominal surgery being included in both these areas, iii) urological surgery including renal transplantation, iv) gynecological surgery, v) female patients in general, vi) surgery for malignancy, vii) the various therapeutic options, viii) anesthetic factors, and ix) the future of thromboprophylaxis.

Being a heterogeneous group, general surgical patients have a wide range of risk of developing postoperative venous thromboembolism (VTE). They therefore highlight the importance of assessing the risk and choosing the appropriate form of thromboprophylactic therapy. Those with benign conditions are generally considered to be of low to medium risk of developing VTE. Those undergoing extensive pelvic or abdominal operations for malignant disease are of high risk. The overall frequency of postoperative deep-vein thrombosis (DVT) is 25% as diagnosed by the I^{125} fibrinogen uptake test and 19% as diagnosed by venography. Proximal DVT occurs in 7% of patients.[1] The frequency of DVT diagnosed by the I^{125} fibrinogen uptake test in various operation groups are recorded in Table 1.[2] The figures are for elective surgery; emergency general surgery is thought to have at least the same risk of VTE. The overall frequency of pulmonary embolism (PE) is 1.6% and fatal pulmonary embolism (FPE) in patients not receiving thromboprophylaxis is 0.8% (0.5%–1%).[1] Effective prophylaxis can significantly reduce the incidence of DVT and PE in general surgical patients.[3] The main barrier to successful thromboprophylaxis is failure to use the available methods in the patients at risk. Continuing education is therefore essential.

RISK FACTORS FOR VENOUS THROMBOEMBOLISM

Risk of thromboembolic disease increases with age, becoming significant in otherwise low-risk patients undergoing general surgery at over 40 years of age. Risk factors for venous thromboembolic disease have been covered in Chapter 4. All general surgical patients should be assessed for thromboembolic risk factors prior to surgery as this determines the therapy. For example, the incidence of thromboembolism in patients in the low-risk group undergoing minor surgical procedures is such that the potential complications and expense of prophylaxis may not be warranted. However, others at low risk as determined by the type of surgery, may in fact be at much higher risk of DVT if they have one or more risk factors. Clinical findings such as varicose veins, obesity and heart failure should be sought, since their presence is associated with an increased risk of VTE and may therefore result in modification of thromboprophylaxis.

GENERAL ABDOMINAL SURGERY

The majority of research has been performed in patients undergoing general abdominal surgery and has included thoracoabdominal procedures such as esophageal operations. Modalities that have been shown to be efficacious include low-molecular-weight heparin (LMWH), unfractionated heparin (UFH) with and without dihydroergotamine, intermittent pneumatic compression (IPC), graduated compression stockings (GCS), oral anticoagulants such as warfarin, dextran and antiplatelet agents. The efficacy varies: LMWH results in a large reduction in the relative risk (RR) of developing DVT (86%), whereas antiplatelet agents have the lowest efficacy giving a 19% reduction of RR.[4]

Minimally invasive surgery is now used for many

From *Venous Thromboembolism: An Evidence-Based Atlas* edited by Russell Hull, Gary Raskob, Graham Pineo © 1996, Futura Publishing Co., Armonk, NY.

Table 1
The Frequency of DVT Diagnosed by the I^{125} Fibrinogen
Uptake Test (modified from Bergqvist 1983 (3))

General abdominal	30%
General surgery for malignancy	40%
Thoracic surgery,	
malignancy	45%
other non-cardiac	30%
cardiac	30%
Gynecological surgery	25%
benign, abdominal hysterectomy	12%
radical abdominal hysterectomy	26%
surgery for ovarian, vulval cancer	45%
Urological surgery	
transvesical prostatectomy	40%
transurethral prostatic resection	10%
Herniorraphy	5%

procedures previously requiring open surgery. Despite this type of surgery resulting in less tissue damage and early mobilization, VTE is known to occur. Crural thromboses have been recorded after rectosigmoid surgery,[5] and other DVT after laparoscopic Nissen fundoplication.[6] In some cases this may be due to increased operation times and to abdominal insufflation causing venous compression. However, clotting activation may be less of a problem as shown in a study on patients undergoing videolaparoscopic surgery for cholecystectomy. Minimally invasive surgery did not induce a significant activation of the clotting system.[7]

THORACIC AND CARDIOTHORACIC SURGERY

Thromboembolism occurs commonly after thoracic surgery, and heparin with and without DHE, has been investigated and found to be efficacious. In patients undergoing major thoracic surgery such as those having thoracotomy for carcinoma of the lung or oesophagus, the incidence of DVT with routine low-dose heparin prophylaxis, 10,000 U daily, remains high, around 25%. Higher doses of heparin, totalling 15,000 U daily, have resulted in a nonsignificant decrease in total DVT frequency, but in a significant reduction in the extent of thrombosis. Despite prophylaxis, DVT is common after oesophagogastrectomy.[8(II)] In 191 patients undergoing thoracic surgery for lung cancer, the prophylactic action of heparin-DHE and of low-dose heparin was compared in a randomized, controlled study. The thrombosis rate measured by I^{125} fibrinogen test was 35% in the control group, 11% in the low-dosage heparin group and 2.5% in the heparin-DHE.[9]

Most studies in the area of cardiac surgery have investigated VTE in patients undergoing coronary artery bypass grafting (CABG).[10] These patients have many risk factors for VTE including stasis, long anesthetics, advanced age, and heart failure, resulting in a high rate of DVT, 30%,[11,12] and a very high rate of PE, 4%.[13,14]

Mechanical methods have been employed most often and compared with no therapy. IPC appeared to be effective in one study[11] and GCS was used in others with variable results.[12,13]

UROLOGIC SURGERY

Venous thromboembolism is the most common cause of death following urological surgery.[15] The incidence of DVT is at least five times higher in those undergoing retropubic prostatectomy compared with transurethral operations. IPC, oral anticoagulants, low-dose heparin with and without DHE, and dextran have been shown to decrease the risk of DVT.[16(II)] The efficacy varies, however. IPC results in a large reduction in the relative risk (RR) of developing DVT (70%) whereas oral anticoagulants have shown variable efficacy.

Deep venous thrombosis occurs frequently in patients undergoing renal transplantation and is more common in those with established risk factors and in those with juvenile diabetes mellitus.[17] In a retrospective study of deep venous thrombosis after renal transplantation, 480 consecutive renal transplant operations were reviewed to obtain the incidence of DVT or PE, or both. Forty (8.3%) thrombotic events were diagnosed, comprising 25 lower limb DVT alone, 11 DVT with PE and four with PE alone. Four deaths were directly attributable to PE, which was the fourth major cause of death in the review period. DVT was more common on the side of the transplant but the difference was not significant.[18] Other studies have shown a higher incidence of fatal PE, occurring in over 4% of patients undergoing renal transplantation.[19]

GYNECOLOGICAL SURGERY

Forty percent of all deaths following gynecological surgery are due to VTE.[20] The National Confidential Enquiry into Perioperative Deaths (NCEPOD) showed that 20% of deaths following hysterectomy were due to VTE.[21] The risk of DVT depends on the type of surgery (Table 1) and overall, fatal PE occurs in 1% of patients. Pelvic and ovarian-vein thrombi are particularly common. Trials in gynecological surgery have shown that oral anticoagulants, low-dose heparin, dextran, and IPC are effective in this situation.[22,23(I),24(I),25(I)] Low-dose heparin with combined DHE may not be more effective than low-dose heparin on its own in this setting.[26(II)] Bleeding is a particular problem and is seen frequently.[24] The site of heparin administration may be a factor as a significant proportion is absorbed via the lymphatic channels. Since incisions, especially transverse ones, divide some of the subcutaneous lymphatics, this may result in a higher local tissue concentration of heparin which may predispose to wound hematoma.[27(I)] Heparin administered subcutaneously to the upper arm, instead of the abdominal wall, is associated with a lower incidence of abdominal wound hematoma.[28]

FEMALE PATIENTS

Women on hormonal therapy or who are pregnant require special consideration. It is important to establish whether women of reproductive age undergoing general surgery are taking the oral contraceptive pill (OCP). In a retrospective study on 5,603 women undergoing surgery, 34 of whom subsequently developed VTE, the incidence of VTE was found to be 1% (12/1244) for pill users, and 0.5% (22/4359) for nonusers.[29] However, it does not follow that women scheduled for surgery should be advised to stop the OCP. These women may be at risk of an unplanned or unwanted pregnancy, with the subsequent risk to both mother and fetus during surgery. Patients with additional risk factors should, in most circumstances, receive thromboprophylaxis, but each case should be assessed individually. Although even low doses of estrogen have been shown to have significant effects on coagulation parameters, the risk of thrombosis seems to be directly related to the dose of estrogen contained in oral contraceptive preparations. The progesterone-only pill does not seem to confer a greater risk of DVT.

Hormone replacement therapy (HRT) may also confer a greater risk of DVT. However, no randomized studies have been performed to confirm this. Although the HRT preparations currently in use contain much lower doses of estrogen than the combined OCP, the increased age of this group of patients makes them more likely to have additional risk factors for postoperative DVT. Consequently, although there is no evidence to suggest that withdrawal of HRT prior to surgery is necessary, this group of patients should probably receive thromboprophylaxis.

Pregnancy is associated with VTE and PE is now one of the leading causes of maternal death in pregnancy and the puerperium. However, routine prophylaxis during an uncomplicated pregnancy is not justified. Obesity, over age 35, parity of three or greater, and prolonged bed rest are additional risk factors and thromboprophylaxis should be considered for these women, especially if they are immobilized for any reason, either in the pre or postpartum period. In most circumstances, thromboprophylaxis should be given to pregnant women undergoing surgery (including cesarean section). Pregnant women with thrombophilia are at greater risk of developing DVT and if possible should be referred to a specialist to advise on appropriate management throughout their pregnancy.

CANCER SURGERY

As patients undergoing cancer surgery have a high risk of developing both VTE and bleeding, they require special consideration. Due to their illness, they have prolonged immobility and may have further stasis from neoplastic compression of veins. Furthermore, tumor invasion, chemotherapy and vascular access catheters affect vessel wall integrity, and procoagulant changes occur in the coagulation cascade. The risk of developing VTE is two to three times that of benign surgery and may remain high despite thromboprophylaxis. Various therapies have been shown to be efficacious including LMWH, UFH fixed and adjusted doses, dextran, oral anticoagulants, IPC and GCS. In an overview of general surgery, the results of patients with cancer were as follows: low-dose heparin reduced the RR of developing DVT by 53% and PE by 58%; the respective figures for dextran were 46% and 57%. IPC reduced the risk of DVT by 39%, there were too few data to analyze the effect on PE.[1] Orgaran has been used in a trial investigating VTE in 513 patients with malignancy and was compared to low-dose UFH 5,000 units twice daily. There was no difference in bleeding complications and a nonsignificant trend towards less VTE in the Orgaran group, 10.4% versus 14.9%.[30(II)] In general an anticoagulant and a mechanical method, for instance LMWH and GCS should be used for these patients.

METHODS OF PREVENTING DEEP-VEIN THROMBOSIS

Thromboprophylaxis can be directed towards the three components of Virchow's triad, namely blood flow, factors within the blood itself and the vascular endothelium. Some methods act on all three, resulting in a reduction of venous stasis, prevention of the hypercoaguable state induced by tissue trauma and other factors, and protection of the endothelium. Whichever method is used, thromboprophylaxis should probably be initiated prior to induction of anesthesia, as it has been demonstrated that the thrombotic process commences intraoperatively.[31] The ideal thromboprophylactic agent would prevent all DVT's, be free from side-effects, be applicable to all surgical specialities and be simple to apply or administer. No such agent exists. The selection of a particular thromboprophylactic method therefore depends on the type of surgery, the overall risk category into which the patient falls and the preference of the responsible clinician. For example, it may not be appropriate to treat with anticoagulants, patients at very high risk of bleeding or at risk of complications secondary to bleeding, or to use mechanical devices on patients who have peripheral ischemia. For all patients it is important to reduce tissue trauma, shorten the anesthetic time and promote early postoperative mobilization.

MECHANICAL METHODS

Graduated Compression Stockings

Graduated compression stockings are a simple, safe and moderately effective form of thromboprophylaxis. It is by no means clear how GCS achieve a thromboprophylactic effect. It has been shown that they increase the velocity of venous blood flow[32–34] and this may reduce the activation of coagulation systems associated with stasis. It has also been proposed that anesthesia causes venous dilatation and that in unsupported veins this may cause microtears in the endothelium. GCS may prevent this dilatation and therefore prevent exposure of procoagulant subendothelial collagen to circulating coagulation factors.[35]

GCS are recommended in low-risk patients and as an adjunct in those with medium and high risk. The only major contraindication is peripheral vascular disease. The majority of studies in patients undergoing general abdominal and gynecological procedures have shown a reduction in the incidence of DVT. A comprehensive meta-analysis concluded that, in studies using sound methods, there was a highly significant risk reduction of 68% in patients at moderate risk of postoperative thromboembolism.[36] However, there is no conclusive evidence that GCS are effective in reducing the incidence of fatal and nonfatal PE. It is not known whether wearing GCS following discharge from hospital is efficacious.

Intermittent Pneumatic Compression

Intermittent pneumatic compression devices currently in use are more comfortable to wear, less bulky and have been designed to allow greater knee movement than earlier ones. IPC influences all three components of Virchow's triad.[35,37,38] Studies comparing IPC with control, pharmacological agents and combined methods of prophylaxis have been performed in general abdominal, gynecological and urological procedures. IPC is effective in malignant disease,[39(II)] and after urological surgery.[40(I)] However, prospective, randomized, double-blind trials have had insufficient power to show that IPC reduces the incidence of postoperative PE. The optimal duration of IPC application has not been firmly established. However, several studies have shown that commencing IPC in the postoperative period is not so effective as commencing prior to surgery and maintaining it throughout the intraoperative and postoperative periods, until the patient is mobile without requiring aid. Combined use of IPC with GCS may also be more effective than either IPC or GCS alone.[41(I)] There are few contraindications for using IPC, however, care should be taken in patients with heart failure, significant leg edema and for those patients with suspected DVT, since compression of the leg may promote embolization of the thrombus.

PHARMACOLOGICAL METHODS

Dextran

Dextran is a high molecular-weight glucose polymer formed by enzymatic degradation of saccharose. The molecular weight of the most commonly used `Dextrans' in clinical practice are 40,000 and 70,000. Dextran is principally excreted renally at a rate proportional to its molecular weight and it exerts an antithrombotic effect by reducing red cell aggregation, providing a protective coating over the vascular endothelium and erythrocytes, reducing platelet aggregation and by a specific inhibitory effect on Von Willebrand factor. There is also evidence that Dextran may facilitate endogenous thrombolysis and reduce venous stasis by expanding plasma volume. A meta-analysis in general surgical patients showed a significant, 57% reduction in the odds of developing DVT.[1] Clinical trials in general abdominal, urological and gynecological surgery comparing Dextran with other anticoagulants have shown it to be less effective than low-dose unfractionated heparin, low-molecular-weight heparin and warfarin in reducing postoperative DVT. Dextran does however, seem to be effective in reducing extension of DVT beyond the calf and may reduce the incidence of PE.

Dextran used in combination with either GCS[42(I)] or IPC[43(I)] has been shown to be more effective than Dextran alone. The use of Dextran is limited, possibly due to its side-effects, including fluid overload, allergic reactions and anaphylaxis. There is a risk of bleeding and wound oozing comparable to that observed with low-dose heparin. Dextran must also be administered by intravenous infusion and the optimal dosage regimen has not been established.

Aspirin and Other Anti-Platelet Agents

Antiplatelet agents inhibit cyclo-oxygenase, a key enzyme involved in the formation of Thromboxane A_2. Thromboxane A_2 is synthesized and released by platelets in response to various stimuli, such as adenosine diphosphate, thrombin and collagen. By inhibiting the formation of Thromboxane A_2, antiplatelet agents are able to reduce platelet aggregation and inhibit interaction with the vascular endothelium. A large number of clinical trials have investigated the possible thromboprophylactic effect of antiplatelet agents. Many of these have been small or poorly designed studies and the few high quality studies which have been performed have shown conflicting results. However, there are potential advantages of using aspirin and other antiplatelet agents. The drugs are cheap, active when given orally, and are well tolerated when given at doses which effectively inhibit platelets.

Antiplatelet agents have been recommended following a meta-analysis.[44] The results obtained with these drugs showed a risk reduction of 25% for DVT, when compared to control groups. However, this figure is poor when compared with the result of a similar study with heparin which showed a risk reduction of 58%.[45] The comparison of the results for PE showed similar efficacy. Furthermore, the meta-analysis included studies which were clinically and statistically heterogeneous, causing any interpretation to be open to question.[46] Antiplatelet agents used with anticoagulant thromboprophylaxis result in increased bleeding.[47(I)]

Oral Anticoagulants

Oral anticoagulants antagonize the effects of vitamin K, resulting in low levels of vitamin K-dependent coagulation factors II, VII, IX and X. Warfarin is sometimes used in very high-risk patients and may be given in low to moderate doses aiming to increase mildly, the international normalized ratio (INR). It is efficacious in general surgery and has resulted in a risk reduction of 59%,[4] but is associated with a high risk of bleeding complications if not monitored carefully. Patients at very high risk may have undetected DVT prior to surgery and prophylactic oral anticoagulant therapy has the advantage of treating them as well.[48]

Unfractionated Heparin

Heparin, a heterogeneous mixture of sulphated acidic mucopolysaccharides, binds to antithrombin III inducing a structural change which increases the antithrombin catalytic activity (anti-factor IIa) several thousandfold and inhibits activated factors IX, X and XII. At higher concentrations, heparin is able to inhibit thrombin by activating heparin co-factor II; and results in the release of the natural anticoagulant tissue factor pathway inhibitor (TFPI). In addition, heparin inhibits the interactions of coagulant factors on the platelet surface. Low-dose UFH has been used as a thromboprophylactic agent for over 20 years and in many centers has been standard therapy. Used in doses of 5,000 units two or three times daily, it is an effective prophylaxis.[49](I) In a meta-analysis of 62 randomized, placebo-controlled trials in general surgical and urological procedures, the incidence of DVT was reduced by at least two-thirds.[45] UFH also reduces the incidence of PE and fatal PE.[49] However, this benefit is offset by a small but significant increase in minor bleeding complications, especially wound hematomas. The above-mentioned meta-analysis showed there was no difference in the incidence of fatal bleeds, but there was a 2% increase in the incidence of minor bleeding events. In addition to bleeding, standard heparin has other side-effects including thrombocytopenia, pain and bruising, which may occur at the injection site. It has to be administered either two or three times daily, starting the day before surgery and continuing usually until the patient is mobile.

Low Molecular-Weight Heparin

Low-molecular-weight heparins are derived by depolymerization of heparin by either chemical or enzymatic degradation. Conventional unfractionated heparin molecules have molecular weights ranging from 5,000–30,000 daltons, whereas LMWH molecules range from 2,000–8,000 daltons. Several laboratory studies have shown that LMWH produces less bleeding than unfractionated heparin while retaining an equivalent antithrombotic effect.[50,51] This has been explained by the fact that LMWHs have a more specific effect on activated factor X (factor Xa) than on factor II (thrombin). However, the exact mechanism is far from clear. Several meta-analyses have investigated the relative safety and efficacy of LMWH compared to UFH. One meta-analysis has compared UFH with LMWH in general surgical trials with weak and strong methodology.[52] In studies with weak methodology, risk reductions of 33% and 63% were seen for DVT and PE respectively; yet, no overall difference in efficacy and safety was seen in studies with strong methodology. This study was performed before the publication of two large multicenter trials which reinforced the findings of the earlier laboratory studies.

The first was a double-blind multicenter trial in which patients undergoing major abdominal surgery were randomized to receive either LMWH once daily or UFH twice daily.[47] The study included 3,809 patients and found LMWH to have a thromboprophylactic effect equivalent to that of UFH. However, less bleeding occurred in the LMWH group as evidenced by a reduction in the incidence of wound hematoma (1.4% vs 2.7% p = 0.007), severe bleeding (1% vs 1.9% p = 0.02) and in the number of patients requiring reoperation for bleeding (1% vs 1.7% p = 0.05). There was no significant difference between the two groups in the overall incidence of major bleeding events (3.6% vs 4.8% relative risk 0.77 CI 0.56–1.04 p = 0.10). There was also less minor bleeding at the injection sites. The other large multicenter trial produced similar findings with respect to the frequency of wound hematomas and injection site complications.[53] The endpoints of these studies were assessed uniformly and were different from those in the meta-analysis which did not investigate wound hematomas.[52]

ANESTHESIA AND THROMBOEMBOLISM

Lumbar epidural anesthesia results in higher-flow velocity in the femoral vein than general anesthesia (GA).[54] The same is not true for thoracic epidural anesthesia.[55] The incidence of postoperative DVT may be lower in those undergoing lumbar epidurals. In open prostatectomy, epidural anesthesia was compared to GA and less DVT occurred in those having epidurals.[56] Studies comparing the incidence of DVT following general anesthesia, or thoracic extradural anaesthesia in general abdominal surgery have not shown significant differences.[57,58] A randomized study of patients undergoing elective abdominal surgery compared morphine for analgesia and low-dose heparin with epidural analgesia with no prophylactic antithrombotic treatment.[59] The incidence of deep venous thrombosis (I^{125}-fibrinogen scan) was 32% after general anesthesia and low-dose heparin and 34% after epidural analgesia with no prophylactic antithrombotic treatment (P<0.9).

Regional anesthesia combined with UFH or LMWH raises another issue. Spinal hematoma is a recognized complication of epidural and spinal anesthesia and there are obvious concerns regarding the safety of combining these invasive techniques with anticoagulant thromboprophylactic agents. However, intraspinal hemorrhages may occur spontaneously or in conjunction with coexisting pathology, such as bleeding disorders, spinal neoplasia and vascular abnormalities lying in close proximity to the spinal cord. They are well documented in association with therapeutic anticoagulation. The complications of regional anesthesia have been investigated in three studies with a total of 164,701 patients. There were no reported cases of spinal hematomas. A review of surgical patients in clinical trials using heparin thromboprophylaxis where the type of anesthesia was defined showed no intraspinal hematomas in 9,013 patients receiving LMWH in combination with epidural or spinal anesthesia.[60] There is one case report of a spinal hematoma in a patient receiving prophylactic unfractionated heparin in combination with epidural anesthesia, and two case reports of spinal bleeding in patients receiving LMWH prophylaxis. However, only one of these patients had epidural catheterization. This data suggests that there is little or no increased risk associated with a combination of regional anesthesia and heparin thromboprophylaxis. In patients undergoing major surgery, particularly those at high risk of thromboembolic disease, the risks of DVT and fatal PE far outweigh the risks of spinal hemorrhage. They concluded from their review of the literature that the combination of heparin with epidural or spinal anesthesia is safe, provided normal safety precautions are respected.

THE FUTURE OF THROMBOPROPHYLAXIS

Our understanding of the cellular and molecular biology of thrombosis has advanced considerably over the last few years. This, together with a greater awareness of the magnitude of the problem of thromboembolic disease and the more widespread use of thromboprophylactic agents should lead to a reduction in the mortality from postoperative PE. There should also be a reduction in the number of patients with the chronic sequelae of DVT and PE. At present, however, all the thromboprophylactic agents currently in use have potential side effects or limitations in their application. In addition, the incidence of thromboembolic disease remains above 18% for those at highest risk despite thromboprophylactic measures. Further, large clinical trials are required to evaluate low-molecular-weight heparins in different types of surgery and to compare them against and in addition to mechanical methods of prophylaxis and antiplatelet agents. The results of studies on newer agents, such as ultra low-molecular-weight heparins, highly specific thrombin inhibitors, specific anti-Xa inhibitors, antibodies to the fib-

rinogen platelet receptor, the cytoadhesin, glycoprotein IIb/IIIa and other integrins such as the "LeuCAMs" are awaited with interest.

SUMMARY

A range of therapies is available to prevent DVT and PE, which are major causes of morbidity and mortality in patients undergoing general surgery. Anticoagulant prophylaxis and mechanical methods both reduce the incidence of postoperative venous thromboembolism but only the former has been shown to reduce mortality from PE.[45] Thromboprophylactic agents which have been shown to reduce the incidence of DVT and PE should be used in all patients at moderate or high risk of thromboembolism. The choice of a suitable agent depends upon the type of surgery and other risk factors associated with each patient. So far, the evidence from clinical trials does not demonstrate a clear advantage of any one particular agent in preventing thromboembolism. However, a combination of a pharmacological agent with GCS has been shown to be efficacious and should probably be given to both moderate and high-risk patients. IPC is an effective alternative, particularly in those patients for whom anticoagulants are contraindicated. Further large clinical trials and evaluation of more specific antithrombotic agents are under way.

REFERENCES

1. Clagett GP, Reisch JS. Prevention of venous thromboembolism in general surgical patients. Ann Surg 1988;208: 227–240.
2. Bergqvist D. Postoperative thromboembolism: frequency, etiology, prophylaxis. Springer-Verlag, Berlin Heidelberg New York 1983.
3. Kakkar VV, Adams PC. Preventive and therapeutic approach to venous thromboembolism. Can death from pulmonary embolism be prevented? J Am Coll Cardiol 1986;8:146B-158B.
4. Clagett GP, Anderson FA, Levine MN, Salzman E, Brownell Wheeler H. Prevention of venous thromboembolism. Chest 1992;102(4):391S-407S.
5. Mentges B, Buess G, Manncke K, Becker, et al. Minimal invasive surgery of the colon and rectum. MINIMAL INVASIVE CHIRURGIE DES KOLON UND REKTUM. Zentralblatt fur Chirurgie 1993;118:12,746–753.
6. Pitcher DE, Curet MJ, Martin DT, Castillo RR, Gerstenberger PD, et al. Successful management of severe gastroesophageal reflux disease with laparoscopic Nissen fundoplication. Am J Surg 1994;168(6):547–543.
7. Vannucchi PL, Ridolfi B, Biliotti G, et al. Evaluation of prothrombin F1 + 2 fragment after videolaparoscopic surgery. Thromb Res 1994; 75:2,219–222.
(II)8. Cade JF, Clegg EA, Westlake GW. Prophylaxis of venous thrombosis after major thoracic surgery. Austrian and New Zealand J of Surg 1983;53(4):301–304.
9. Kaiser D, Hau H, Strey, M. Prevention of venous thromboembolism during and after surgery of lung cancer. PERI- UND POSTOPERATIVE THROMBOSEPROPHYLAXE BEIM BRONCHIALKARZINOM. Praxis und Klinik der Pneumologie 1981;35(1 Spec):918–921.

10. Malone KM. Coronary artery bypass grafting. In Goldhaber SZ (ed.): Prevention of Venous Thromboembolism 1993;18:439–444.

11. Pogson GW, Reed W, Weinstein GS 1985. Prevention of deep vein thrombosis. Mo Med 1985;82(3)133–136.

12. Reis SE, Polak JF, Hirsch DR, et al. Frequency of deep venous thrombosis in asymptomatic patients with coronary bypass grafts. Am Heart J 1991;122:478–482.

13. Rao G, Zikria EA, Miller WH, Samadani SR, Ford WB. Incidence and prevention of pulmonary embolism after coronary artery surgery. Vasc Surg 1975;9:37–45.

14. Sharma GVRK, Josa M, Khuri SF. Pulmonary embolism is an important sequel of coronary bypass surgery. Circulation 1990;82:II-508(abstract).

15. Antila LE, Markulla H and Iisaly E. Ten years experience of geriatric aspects of surgery of patients with benign prostatic hypertrophy. Acta Chir Scand 1966;357(Suppl):95.

(II)16. Hansberry KL, Thompson IM, Bauman J, Deppe S, Rodriguez FR. A prospective comparison of thromboembolic stockings, external sequential pneumatic compression stockings and heparin sodium/dihydroergotamine mesylate for the prevention of thromboembolic complications in urological surgery. J Urol 1991;1456(6):1205–1208.

17. Brunkwall J, Bergqvist D, Bergentz SE, et al. Deep venous thrombosis in patients undergoing renal transplantation—effects of cyclosporine A. Transplantation Proceedings 1987;19:1II-1814.

18. Allen RDM, Michie CA, Murie JA, Morris PJ. Deep venous thrombosis after renal transplantation. Surg Gynecol and Obstet 1987; 164(2):137–142.

19. Combined report on Regular Dialysis and Transplantation in Europe. European Dialysis and Transplant Association. London: Pitman, 1983.

20. Jeffcoate TNA, Tindall VR. Venous thrombosis and embolism in obstetrics and gynaecology. Aust NZ J Obstet Gynaecol 1965;5:119–130.

21. The Report of the National Confidential Enquiry Into Perioperative Deaths 1990. London: 35–43 Lincoln's Inn Fields, London, 1992.

22. Genton E, Turpie A. Venous thromboembolism associated with gynecologic surgery. Clin Obstet Gynecol 1980;23:209–241.

(III)23. Bonnar J, Walsh H. Prevention of thrombosis after pelvic surgery by British dextran70. Lancet 1972;1:614–616.

(I)24. Clarke-Pearson DL, Synan I, Hinshaw W, Coleman RE, Creasman WT. Prevention of postoperative venous thromboembolism by external pneumatic calf compression in patients with gynecologic malignancy. Obstet Gynecol 1984d;63:92–97.

(I)25. Taberner DA, Poller L, Burslem RW, et al. Oral anticoagulants controlled by the British Comparative Thromboplastin versus low-dose heparin in prophylaxis of deep vein thrombosis. Br Med J 1978;1:272–274.

(II)26. UrlepSalinovic V, Jelatancev B, Gorisek B. Low doses of heparin and heparin dihydergot in postoperative thromboprophylaxis in gynaecological patients. Thrombosis and Haemostasis 1994;72(1):16–20.

(I)27. Kakkar VV, Murray WJG. Efficacy and safety of low molecular weight heparin (CY216) in preventing postoperative venous thromboembolism: a co-operative study. Br J Surg 1985;72:786–791.

28. Briel RC. Low dose heparin prophylaxis and postoperative wound haematoma. Int Surg 1983;68:241–243.

29. Vessey MP, Mant D, Smith A, et al. Oral contraceptives and venous thromboembolism: findings in a large prospective study. Br Med J 1986; 292:526.

(II)30. Gallus A, Cade J, Ockelford P, Hepburn S, Maas M, et al. (ANZ-Organon Investigators' Group). Orgaran (Org 10172) or heparin for preventing venous thromboembolism after elective surgery for malignant disease? A double-blind, randomised multicentre comparison. Thrombsois and Haemostasis 1993;70(4):562–567.

31. Kakkar VV, Howe CT, Flanc C, et al. Natural history of postoperative deep-vein thrombosis. Lancet 1969;230–233.

32. Meyerowitz BR, Nelson R. Measurement of the velocity of blood in lower limb veins with and without compression surgery. Surgery 1964;56:481–486.

33. Sigel B, Edelstein AL, Felix WR. Compression of the deep venous system of the lower leg during inactive recumbency. Arch Surg 1973;106:38–43.

34. Lawrence D, Kakkar VV. Graduated, static, external compression of the lower limb: a physiological assessment. Br J Surg 1980;67:119–121.

35. Comerota AJ, Stewart GJ, Alburger PD, et al. Operative venodilation: A previously unsuspected factor in the cause of postoperative deep vein thrombosis. Surgery 1988;106:301–309.

36. Wells PS, Lensing AWA, Hirsh J. Graduated compression stockings in the prevention of postoperative venous thromboembolism. A meta-analysis. Arch Intern Med 1994;154:67–72.

37. Blackshear VW, Precott C, LePain F, et al. Influence of sequential pneumatic compression on postoperative venous function. J Vasc Surg 1987;5:432–436.

38. Summaria L, Caprini J, McMillan R. Relationship between postsurgical fibrinolytic parameters and deep vein thrombosis in surgical patients treated with compression devices. Am Surg 1988;54:156–160.

(II)39. Butson ARC. Intermittent pneumatic calf compression for prevention of deep vein thrombosis in general abdominal surgery. Am J Surg 1981;142:525–527.

(I)40. Salzman EW, Ploetz J, Bettmann M, et al. Intraoperative external pneumatic calf compression to afford long-term prophylaxis against deep vein thrombosis in urological patients. Surgery 1980;87:239–242.

(I)41. Nicolaides AN, Miles C, Hoare M, et al. Intermittent sequential pneumatic compression of the legs and thromboembolism-deterrent stockings in the prevention of postoperative deep venous thrombosis. Surgery 1983;94:21–25.

(I)42. Bergqvist D, Lindblad B. The thromboprophylactic effect of graded elastic compression stockings in combination with dextran 70. Arch Surg 1984;119:1329–1331.

(I)43. Smith RC, Elton RA, Orr JD. Dextran and intermittent pneumatic compression in prevention of postoperative deep vein thrombosis. Multi-unit trial. Br Med J 1978;1:952–954.

44. Antiplatelet Trialists' Collaboration. Collaborative overview of randomised trials of antiplatelet therapy III. Reduction in venous thrombosis and pulmonary embolism by antiplatelet prophylaxis among surgical and medical patients. Br Med J 1994;308:235–246.

45. Collins R, Scrimgeour A, Yusel S, et al. Reduction in fatal pulmonary and venous thrombosis by perioperative administration of subcutaneous heparin. Overview of randomised trials of general or orthopaedic and urological surgery. New England J Med 1988;318:1162–1173.

46. Cohen AT, Skinner JA, Kakkar VV. Antiplatelet treatment for thromboprophylaxis: a step forward or backwards. Br Med J 1994;309:1213–1217.

(I)47. Kakkar VV, Cohen AT, Edmondson RA, et al. Low molecular weight versus standard heparin for the prevention of venous thrombo-embolism after major abdominal surgery. Lancet 1993;341:259–265.

48. Hirsh J, Dalen JE, Deykin D, Poller L. Oral anticoagulants: mechanisms of action, clinical effectiveness, and optimal therapeutic range. Chest 1992;102(Suppl):312S-326S.

(I)49. Kakkar VV, Corrigan TP, Fossard DP. Prevention of fatal postoperative pulmonary embolism by low doses of heparin: an International Trial. Lancet 1975;ii:45–51.

50. Carter CJ, Kelton JG, Hirsh J, Cerskus AL, Santos AV, et al. The relationship between the haemorrhagic and antithrombotic properties of low molecular weight heparins and heparin. Blood 1982;59:1239.

51. Esquivel CO, Bergqvist D, Bjork C-G, Nilsson B. Comparison between commercial heparin, low molecular weight heparin and pentosan polysulphate on haemostasis and platelets in vivo. Thromb Res 1982;28:389.

52. Nurmohamed MT, Rosendaal FR, Buller HR, et al. Low molecular weight heparin versus standard heparin in general and orthopaedic surgery: a meta-analysis. Lancet 1992;340:152–156.

53. Boneu B. An international multicentre study: Clivarin(R) in the prevention of venous thromboembolism in patients undergoing general surgery. Report of the International Clivarin(R) Assessment Group. Blood Coagulation and Fibrinolysis 1993;4(Suppl 1):S21-S22.

54. Polkolainen E, Hendolin H. Effects of lumbar epidural analgesia and general anaesthesia on flow velocity in the femoral vein and postoperative deep vein thrombosis. Acta Chir Scand 1983;149:361–364.

55. Otton PE, Wilson EJ. The cardiocirculatory effects of upper thoracic epidural analgesia. Can Anaesth Soc J 1966;13:541–549.

56. Hendolin H, Mattila MAK, Poikolainen E. The effect of lumbar epidural analgesia on the development of deep vein thrombosis of the legs after open prostatectomy. Acta Chir Scand 1981;147:425–429.

57. Hendolin H, Tuppurainen T, Lahtinen J. Thoracic epidural analgesia and deep vein thrombosis in cholecystectomized patients. Acta Chir Scand 1982;148:405–409.

58. Mellbring G, Dahlgren S, Reiz S, et al. Thromboembolic complications after major abdominal surgery. Effect of thoracic epidural analgesia. Acta Chir Scand 1983;149:263–268.

59. Hjortso NC, Neumann P, Frosig F, et al. A controlled study on the effect of epidural analgesia with local anaesthetics and morphine on morbidity after abdominal surgery. Acta Anaesth Scand 1985;29(8):790–796.

60. Bergqvist D, Lindblad B, Matzsch T. Low molecular weight heparin for thromboprophylaxis and epidural/spinal anaesthesia—Is there a risk? Acta Anaesth Scand 1992;36:605–609.

6

Orthopedic Surgery

Lars C. Borris, Michael R. Lassen

INTRODUCTION

Major orthopedic operations on the lower extremities, in particular major joint replacements, are main indications for routine use of general thromboprophylaxis due to a very high risk of postoperative thromboembolic complications. The aim is to prevent fatal pulmonary emboli (PE), and thereby decrease the total mortality, and to ultimately avoid the development of deep venous insufficiency with formation of leg oedema and chronic ulceration.

THROMBOEMBOLIC COMPLICATIONS AFTER MAJOR ORTHOPEDIC OPERATIONS

Total Hip Replacement

Deep-vein thrombosis. Thromboembolism in patients undergoing total hip replacement (THR) has been extensively studied since the operation became a standard procedure. One of the first prospective, controlled studies reported an incidence of deep-vein thrombosis (DVT) of 34% in untreated patients;[1(III)] however, it was based on the clinical diagnosis of DVT, which is unreliable for diagnostic purposes due to a very low sensitivity and specificity. The most reliable method for diagnosing postoperative DVT in patients undergoing THR is bilateral ascending phlebography, though this technique is not completely free of methodological problems.[2] Based on phlebographic diagnosis, the incidence of DVT five to 14 days after THR in patients without pharmacological prophylaxis is about 50% (Table 1).[3(III),4(I),5(I),6(III),7(I),8(I),9(I),10(I)] The proportion of patients who develop the classical symptoms of DVT just after operation, however, is much lower; nevertheless, most PE arise from asymptomatic DVT.[11,12] The reason why symptoms very seldom develop in the early postoperative period is that, at this stage most of the thrombi are small (less than 1 cm in diameter),

nonoccluding, and confined exclusively to the veins of the calf.[13,14] A considerable proportion (10% to 20%) of the thrombi formed during surgery are located in the proximal veins, with a typical location at the level of the lesser trochanter (Figure 1). This reason is probably due to direct damage to the deep veins during operation when the joint is dislocated.[15(IV)] Thus, theoretically, thrombus formation may start during operation, but the time interval elapsing from the operation until full development of thrombosis and the length of the risk period are largely unknown. In a previous study using the radio-fibrinogen uptake-test (RFUT), the peak onset of all DVT was on the fourth postoperative day; the risk of proximal-vein thrombosis disappeared after day 11, but the risk of calf-vein thrombosis persisted to day 17, with a second peak on day 13.[16] Although all thrombi were phlebographically confirmed in this study, it has been shown that RFUT may overlook proximal thrombi after THR;[17] furthermore, some of the calf-vein thrombi may extend into the proximal veins after diagnosis, so these data just give an idea of the length of the risk period. Based on these data, it is common practice in some countries to prolong the period of prophylaxis after THR up to three months.

The relationship between DVT and later development of deep venous insufficiency of the lower extremities is not known in detail. The symptoms of venous insufficiency, i.e. varicose veins, ache, pain, ankle or leg oedema, skin irritation, pigmentation, and ulceration, are produced by venous hypertension, which is the result of obstruction, reflux, or a combination of both.[18] It is well known that the end result of a DVT may be obliteration of the vein due to incomplete recanalization and destruction or malfunction of the valves, which in itself predisposes to development of venous hypertension. It is estimated that venous insufficiency may develop in 50% or more of patients about five years after a DVT.

Pulmonary embolism. Only few studies have systematically used screening for PE in untreated patients

From *Venous Thromboembolism: An Evidence-Based Atlas* edited by Russell Hull, Gary Raskob, Graham Pineo © 1996, Futura Publishing Co., Armonk, NY.

Table 1
Incidence of DVT Diagnosed by Bilateral Phlebography After
Total Hip Replacement in Patients Having No
Pharmacological Prophylaxis

Year	Author	N	Day*	DVT %
1971	(3) Evarts	56	10–12	54
1977	(4) Harris	51	7–10	45
1978	(5) Moskovitz	32	10	39
1981	(6) Ishak	41	10–14	54
1983	(7) Gallus	47	7	53
1986	(8) Turpie	50	10	42
1988	(9) Beisaw	74	5	52
1991	(10) Lassen	97	8–10	45

N = number of patients; * postoperative day of phlebography

undergoing THR. In two studies of patients operated under general or epidural anesthesia, the overall frequency of PE, diagnosed by mandatory perfusion lung scanning 14 days after THR, was 9/30 (30%) and 13/60 (22%), respectively.[19(III),20(III)] Less than half of the patients developed clinical symptoms and no fatal PE were observed. The clinical importance of asymptomatic PE is not known. Fatal PE after THR were reported in 1% to 3% of patients in larger studies.[21(III),22(V)] It is commonly accepted that PE originates from thrombi localized in the deep veins of the lower extremities. However, embolization may occur from any thrombus irrespective of the localization in the deep veins,[23,24] although there is no consensus on this matter.

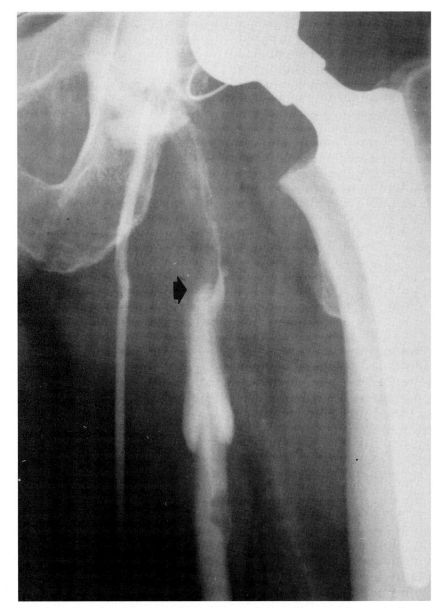

Figure 1. Phlebographic examination 10 days after a total hip replacement. A thrombus is seen in the common femoral vein at the level of the lesser trochanter (arrow).

Table 2
Incidence of DVT Diagnosed by Phlebography After Elective Knee Surgery (mostly total knee replacement) in Patients Having No Pharmacological Prophylaxis

Year	Author	N	Day*	DVT %
1973	(26) Cohen	35	7–14	57
1976	(27) McKenna	30	?	53
1984	(28) Stulberg	49	?	84
1988	(29) Lynch	150	7	41
1989	(30) Stringer	55	10	65
1990	(31) Nielsen	29	10	41

N = number of patients; * postoperative day of phlebography

Total Knee Replacement

Deep-vein thrombosis and pulmonary embolism. The incidence of phlebographically-verified DVT in unprotected patients after elective knee operations is about 60% (Table 2).[25,26(V),27(V),28(IV),29(II),30,31(I)] The incidence of PE in patients undergoing knee surgery is about 7%; the fatality rate is largely unknown.[26(V),28(IV)]

Other Orthopedic Procedures

Documentation of thromboembolic risk is less extensive after other elective orthopedic procedures, but high incidences of DVT have been reported following knee synovectomies, osteotomies, arthrotomies, and lower leg amputations.[26(V),30(V),32]

RISK FACTORS FOR DEVELOPMENT OF THROMBOEMBOLIC COMPLICATIONS AFTER MAJOR ORTHOPEDIC OPERATIONS

In general, both hip and knee arthroplasties must be considered a risk factor in themselves so that all patients subjected to these operations must receive an effective prophylaxis. Additional individual risk factors for development of thromboembolic complications after orthopedic surgery are comparable with the risk factors known in other surgical specialities. The most important are: age (over 40 years), duration of operation (over 30 minutes), obesity, previous thromboembolism, varicose veins, and known malignancy. Furthermore, in knee surgery the use of a thigh tourniquet without exsanguination of the limb may also contribute to an increased thrombosis risk although there is no firm evidence.[26(V),33]

PROPHYLAXIS OF POSTOPERATIVE THROMBOEMBOLISM AFTER MAJOR ORTHOPEDIC OPERATIONS

To reduce the risk of fatal PE after operation, it is important to prevent the development of DVT. Since the late 1960s a very large number of clinical studies have been conducted in orthopedic surgery to evaluate different prophylactic regimens. The quality of these studies is very variable due to differences in design, methodology, and statistical power; as a consequence, direct comparisons between regimens are not possible.

Total Hip Replacement

The regimens evaluated are shown in Table 3. It is not possible to review every study in detail, but for each regimen characteristic results on efficacy and safety will be presented based on selected well-designed clinical studies.

Oral Anticoagulation

One of the most used regimens in the United States has been oral anticoagulation with warfarin. Although many studies have been published with warfarin prophylaxis, only very few meet the modern demands of a proper design. The originally proposed warfarin regimen was to start at a dose of 10 mg on the evening before op-

Table 3
Prophylactic Regimens Evaluated in Patients Undergoing Total Hip Replacement

Regimen	Administration Scheme
Oral anticoagulation	adjusted-dose, low-dose, fixed mini-dose, two-step therapy
Aspirin	orally; 0.3–1.2 g o.d. or high-dose 1.5 g b.i.d.
Dextran 70	intravenous infusion; 500 ml × 4–5 (see text)
Heparin	5000 IU × 2 or 3 daily
Heparin/DHE	5000 IU × 2 daily + 0.5 mg DHE
Low molecular weight heparin	Drug dependent
Graded compression stockings	Applied before operation and worn until mobilization
Intermittent pneumatic compression	Used during and after operation, may be combined with graded compression stockings
Foot pump	Used during and after operation
Regional anesthesia	Spinal or epidural

eration and 5 mg on the night after operation, followed by a daily dose sufficient to keep the prothrombin time at one and a half to two times its control value (adjusted-dose regimen). It has not been possible to find a proper placebo-controlled study with the regimen, but it was evaluated against dextran, aspirin, and unfractionated heparin 5000 IU twice daily started two hours before operation in a randomized study of 187 patients. No fatal PE occurred, but the incidence of DVT was significantly lower in the warfarin group (31%) than in the heparin group (55%) (p<0.01), but warfarin was as effective as each of the two other regimens. Most bleeding complications were observed in the warfarin group.[34(I)] The biggest problem with the use of warfarin is the risk of bleeding, with 1% fatal bleeding. This risk can be reduced by the use of two different dosage regimens: two-step warfarin therapy[35(I)] and low-dose warfarin,[36(II)] without loss of efficacy. The so-called fixed mini-dose warfarin regimen (1 mg daily from the night before surgery) has been advocated by some, but this regimen was less effective compared with adjusted-dose but caused fewer bleeding complications.[37(I)]

The laboratory monitoring that is needed to follow warfarin treatment is cumbersome and expensive, making it less suitable for routine use.

Aspirin

The antiplatelet action of aspirin has been thought to prevent the formation of venous thrombosis. Clinical studies have shown conflicting results. Aspirin is not effective in women,[38(II)] and currently it has no place in the prevention of venous thromboembolism after THR.

Dextran

The effect of dextran, a glucose polymer, is to prevent venous stasis by hemodilution (colloid osmotic effect) and flow improvement. It is this that gives dextran its antithrombotic activity, which has been studied since 1962.[39(III)] Furthermore, dextran probably changes the ultrastructure of fibrin, thereby increasing the lyzability of thrombi formed in the presence of dextran.[40] Two sizes of dextran have been studied in clinical studies, dextran 40 with a mean molecular weight of 40,000, and dextran 70 with a mean molecular weight of 70,000. Dextran 70 is administered by intravenous infusion of 500 ml during induction of anesthesia, repeated four to six hours later on the day of operation, and on days one, three, and five after operation. Dextran has been less preferred partly due to fear of serious allergic reactions, which are very rare when hapten is used, and partly due to fear of bleeding complications, which have been compared in frequency with those of oral anticoagulants.[41]

A retrospective study showed that dextran 70 protected against fatal PE in a mixed surgical population,[42(IV)] and in another study it was comparable in effe-

cacy with low-dose heparin, 5000 IU t.i.d., with respect to the number of deaths due to autopsy-verified PE after orthopedic surgery.[43(II)]

In a controlled study of 106 patients undergoing mixed elective hip surgery, the incidence of postoperative DVT confirmed by phlebography 10 to 12 days after operation, was significantly reduced by two different regimens of dextran 40.[3] Compared with other prophylactic methods, dextran 70 has been equally effective in reducing the incidence of DVT after THR.[44(I),45(I)] Dextran is not suitable in the elderly because of a tendency to volume overloading, for which reason it cannot be recommended as a standard regimen in patients undergoing THR.

Low-Dose Heparin

One of the most used drugs for prophylaxis in Europe has been subcutaneous low-dose unfractionated heparin (5000 IU b.i.d. or t.i.d.) starting two hours before surgery and continued for eight consecutive days, including the day of operation. The antithrombotic action of heparin is not known in detail but the final outcome is potentiation of the natural inhibition of antithrombin III on the activated coagulation factors XIIa, XIa, Xa, IXa, and IIa (thrombin), inhibition of Xa and IIa being the most important. In some reports low-dose heparin was not effective in preventing DVT after THR,[46(V),47(II)] while a definite antithrombotic efficacy was reported by others.[48(I),49(II)] A large number of clinical studies have been performed with heparin, but no study alone has been large enough to be able to show a reduction of fatal PE and even more important of total mortality, the ultimate aim of prevention. However, in a meta-analysis including more than 70 randomized studies in general and orthopedic surgery, low-dose heparin caused a highly significant reduction in the number of deaths due to PE (from 55 in the control patients to 19 in the heparin group), as well as a significant reduction in total mortality.[50] To optimize heparin prophylaxis, it has been tried to adjust the dosage in order to keep the activated partial thromboplastin time within the high-normal range. The antithrombotic efficacy in THR of this regimen has been compared with fixed low-dose heparin (3500 IU t.i.d.) in a study that included 79 patients.[51(I)] The adjusted dosage regimen reduced the incidence of phlebographic DVT significantly from 39% to 13% without increasing the risk of bleeding. This regimen has the disadvantage of needing repeated laboratory monitoring, thus adding to the expense and making it less simple for routine use than the fixed-dose regimen.

Based on the observation that plasma antithrombin III (AT III) concentration declines after THR and the assumption that this may predispose to postoperative DVT, it has been tried to combine fixed low-dose heparin (5,000 IU b.i.d.) and intravenous injections of AT III.[52(I)] However, the combination has never gained any significant usage due to the considerable cost of AT III prepara-

Table 4
Commercially Available LMW Heparins

Trade Name	Generic Name	Manufacturer
Dihydergot-Sandoparin (S)	?	Sandoz AG (Germany)
Fragmin (F)	dalteparin	Kabi Pharmacia AB (Sweden)
Fraxiparine (FX)	nadroparin	Sanofi Pharma (France)
Clexane (lovenox) (K)	enoxaparin	Rhône-Poulenc Rorer (France)
Logiparin (L)	tinzaparin	Novo Nordisk A/S (Denmark)

tions and to the fact that virus transmission cannot be totally ruled out.

Low-Dose Heparin Plus Dihydroergotamine

Another approach to improve the efficacy of fixed low-dose subcutaneous heparin has been combination with 0.5 mg dihydroergotamine (DHE), an ergot alkaloid that was thought selectively to increase the tone of the deep veins and thereby prevent venous stasis. In a study in THR patients, heparin/DHE (5000 IU + 0.5 mg DHE t.i.d.) was more antithrombotic than low-dose heparin alone.[53(I)] In a more recent study, however, the synergistic effect between heparin and DHE was not confirmed.[54(II)] A very large number of clinical studies have been carried out with the combination (heparin/DHE) in elective and emergency hip surgery, comparing the effi-

cacy and safety with other regimens: placebo,[55(I)] dextran 70,[44(I)] and adjusted-dose heparin.[56(II)] However, treatment with DHE may result in severe side-effects due to circulatory disturbances that are often irreversible, especially in patients with arterial insufficiency and trauma.[57] Due to this, combination with DHE has now almost been abolished in orthopedic surgery.

Low-Molecular-Weight Heparin

Low-molecular-weight heparin is a further development of unfractionated heparin. Several different compounds are being manufactured, all with different in vitro and in vivo activities (Table 4).[58] Many studies have been conducted with the different LMW heparins in patients under going THR (Table 5).[8(I),45(I),55(I),59(I),60(II),61(II),62(I),63(I),64(I),65(I),66(I),67(I),68(I)] Most LMW heparins are administered subcutaneously 12 or 2 hours before operation and continued once daily after operation until full mobilization. One LMW heparin (enoxaparin), however, has also been evaluated in a postoperative regimen, in which the first injection is delayed until 12–24 hours after operation and then continued daily at a higher dosage (30 mg b.i.d.) than that used in the preoperative regimen (40 mg o.d.). The postoperative regimen was significantly more effective than placebo and equally safe in one study,[8] and in another study it was comparable in efficacy with a postoperative regimen of unfractionated heparin (7,500 IU b.i.d.) but caused less bleeding.[65] Most LMW heparin studies are included in three meta-analyses.[69–71] Based on these analyses, the following conclusions can be drawn on the use of LMW heparin prophylaxis in patients un-

Table 5
Studies with LMW Heparins Versus Various Controls in Total Hip Replacement

Ref.	Year	Test	Dosage/Day	Control Drug	Dosage/Day	Diagnostic Method(s)
8	1986	K	60 mg	Placebo	—	RFUT/Phleb.
45	1988	F	5000 XaI	Dextran 70	500 ml +	RFUT/Phleb.
55*	1988	S	3000 XaI	Placebo	—	Pla./Phleb.
55*	1988	S	3000 XaI	DHE/Heparin	10000 IU	Pla./Phleb.
59	1988	K	40 mg	Heparin	15000 IU	Bilat. phleb.
60	1989	F	5000 XaI	Heparin	APTT adj.	RFUT/Phleb.
61	1989	S	3000 XaI	DHE/Heparin	10000 IU	RFUT/Phleb. PVLS
10	1991	L	50 XaI/kg	Placebo	—	Bilat. phleb.
62	1991	F	5000 XaI	Placebo	—	RFUT/Phleb.
63	1991	K	40 mg	Dextran 70	500 ml +	Bilat. phleb.
64	1991	L	50 XaI/kg	Dextran 70	500 ml +	RFUT/phleb.
65	1991	K	60 mg	Heparin	15000 IU	RFUT/IPG/Phleb.
66	1991	F	5000 XaI	Heparin	15000 IU	Bilat. phleb.
67	1991	FX	41–62 XaI/kg**	Heparin	APTT adj.	Bilat. phleb.
68	1992	FX	48 mg	Heparin	15000 IU	Bilat. phleb.

Ref. = reference number. Test = the low molecular weight heparin tested. RFUT/Phleb. = ^{125}I-labeled fibrinogen uptake test and unilateral phlebography of positive tests. XaI = factor Xa inhibitory units. DHE = dihydroergotamine. Pla./Phleb. = ^{99m}Tc-plasmin scanning and unilateral phlebography of positive tests. + = 500 ml dextran 70 given two times on the day of operation and 500 ml on the first and third postoperative day. Bilat. Phleb. = bilateral phlebography. APTT adj. = heparin dosage adjusted according to the activated partial thromboplastin time. PVLS = perfusion/ventilation lung scan of all patients. * = 3-armed design: LMW heparin/DHE, Heparin/DHE and Placebo. ** 41 XaI/kg/day for the first three days, then 62 XaI/kg/day from day 4 to day 10. K, S, L, F, FX see Table 4.

dergoing THR: LMW heparin prophylaxis is more antithrombotic than and as safe as placebo, low-dose unfractionated heparin, and dextran 70; it is also as effective and safe as low-dose unfractionated heparin plus DHE. LMW heparin has still not been tested in a large enough study to prove its efficacy against fatal PE and its ability to reduce total mortality. Before deciding to use a certain LMW heparin, it is important to make a critical evaluation of the clinical documentation of the particular compound. At a recent European consensus conference, it was concluded that LMW heparin is currently the most effective antithrombotic for use in THR patients.[72]

Another heparin derivative with antithrombotic potential, a heparinoid, has recently been evaluated in patients undergoing THR in two well-designed comparative studies.[73(I),74(I)] In both of these the compound had an acceptable antithrombotic efficacy and safety.

Mechanical Prophylactic Methods

The antithrombotic action of the mechanical methods is primarily elimination of venous stasis, and an additional effect of pneumatic compression is enhancement of fibrinolysis.[75] The mechanism by which the latter is achieved is poorly understood, but a local release of plasminogen activators has been suggested.[76(I)] Relatively few studies have evaluated the thromboprophylactic efficacy and safety of mechanical prophylaxis in THR patients.

Graded compression stockings alone are considered inadequate prophylaxis in these patients. The efficacy of IPC has been evaluated in a number of studies using phlebographic end-point,[7(III),36(II),77(I)] of which two included an untreated control group.[7(III),77(I)] In the first study, IPC with calf compression protected against calf DVT but did not reduce the incidence of proximal DVT;[7(III)] in the other, IPC with compression of both calf and thigh significantly reduced the incidence of DVT, from 49 % to 24 %.[77(I)] To be effective, the IPC device must be used on both legs from arrival in the recovery room until at least 14 days after operation. Lack of efficacy of the method may be due to low patient compliance or improper use.[78] The device may be combined with graded compression stockings, but it is not known whether this adds to the efficacy. A venous foot pump, tested in 84 patients, reduced the incidence of DVT significantly, from 40% to 5%.[79(I)] In general, mechanical methods should be considered when there are contraindications to pharmacological prophylaxis.

A combination of pharmacological and mechanical methods is used in some countries, but it has been studied only sporadically.[80,81(III)]

Influence of Anesthesia

The role of regional anesthesia (spinal or epidural) as prophylaxis against postoperative DVT after THR has been studied a number of times.[19,20,82(III),83] In all these studies regional anesthesia reduced the incidence of DVT more than general anesthesia in patients having no other specific thromboprophylaxis, but the reduction was only significant in two studies.[20,82] A significant reduction of asymptomatic PE, scintigraphically diagnosed, was also shown.[20] The antithrombotic action of regional anesthesia is due to increased blood flow in the calf veins, reduced tendency for coagulation, and improved fibrinolytic function.[84,85] Blood loss under regional anesthesia was significantly less than in patients operated under general anesthesia in a number of studies.[20,82,86] There was no additional thromboprophylactic effect of epidural anesthesia over general anesthesia in patients on dextran 70 thromboprophylaxis.[87] It seems from this last-named study that the type of anesthesia used in THR may play a minor role as long as an effective thromboprophylaxis is used.

Some countries prohibit the use of any kind of anticoagulation together with regional (spinal/epidural) anesthesia, even low-dose unfractionated heparin and LMW heparin, due to fear of bleeding complications. Based on an extensive review of the world literature, it was concluded that there is no contraindication to the combined use of subcutaneous unfractionated heparin and regional anesthesia.[88]

Total Knee Replacement

The prophylactic regimens evaluated in total knee replacement (TKR) are shown in Table 6 based on a number of studies,[89(I),90(I),91(I),92(II),93(I),94(I),95(I)] of which only a few were controlled.

Pulsatile elastic stockings significantly reduced the incidence of both proximal and calf DVT in a controlled study that included patients undergoing various elective knee operations with the use of a tourniquet.[89(I)] The DVT frequency was significantly reduced by the use of IPC with compression of both calf and thigh.[90(I)] Continuous passive motion was not protective.[92(II)] Prophylaxis with the combination of AT III and low-dose heparin has also been evaluated in TKR patients.[93(I)] LMW heparin has only been evaluated in one study to date in knee surgery.[94(I)] The study, which was randomized and double-blind, compared the antithrombotic efficacy and safety of postoperative enoxaparin (30 mg b.i.d., continued for 14 days) with placebo in 131 patients undergoing TKR or tibial osteotomy. The incidence of postoperative DVT diagnosed by phlebography was significantly reduced from 65% in the placebo group to 19% in the heparin group without an increase in bleeding. No deaths occurred during the study.

A significant reduction in phlebographic DVT was obtained with epidural anesthesia used during operation and continued for three days after operation, compared with general anesthesia, in two well-designed controlled studies in which patients received no other specific prophylaxis.[30,95(I)]

Table 6
Prophylactic Regimens Evaluated in Patients Undergoing Total Knee Replacement

Regimen	Administration Scheme
Aspirin	orally; (1.3 g t.i.d.)
Low molecular weight heparin	drug dependent
Pulsatile elastic stockings	Started postop. and continued for 17 days
Intermittent calf and thigh compression	Started during operation on the non-operated leg Started postop. on the operated leg
Continuous passive motion	Started postop.
Regional anesthesia	Continuous epidural blockade during op. and continued for 3 days postop.

Future Perspectives

An important question for the future is whether it will be possible to improve the efficacy of the existing prophylactic modalities. One way would be to prolong the period of administration after operation in order to prevent late development of thrombi.

How to protect patients with prolonged immobilization in plaster casts against thromboembolic complications is a new challenge for future research.

Some of the newer drugs with known antithrombotic potency, e.g. thrombin inhibitors, may be more antithrombotic and/or safe than the existing pharmacological methods.

CONCLUSION

Effective thromboprophylaxis must be used in all patients undergoing total hip or knee replacement, and in patients having other major operations on the lower extremities in regional or general anesthesia. Prophylaxis must be started preoperatively and continued in the postoperative period until full mobilization (at least 7 days). LMW heparin is currently the most potent and reasonably safe prophylactic to use in this kind of surgery. When there are contraindications to LMW heparin, prophylaxis with intermittent pneumatic compression of thigh and calf must be considered. We would suggest that patients who are immobilized for longer periods must receive oral anticoagulation (INR = 2.5). In general, when a particular prophylactic strategy is considered in a patient, it must always be based on an individual risk/benefit assessment.

REFERENCES

(III)1. Harris WH, Salzman EW, DeSanctis RW. The prevention of thromboembolic disease by prophylactic anticoagulation. A controlled study in elective hip surgery. J Bone Joint Surg 1967;49-A:81–89.

2. Borris LC, Lassen MR. Venography in deep venous thrombosis: postoperative screening of patients in prophylaxis studies. Haemostasis 1993;23(Suppl 1):80–84.

(III)3. Evarts CM, Feil EJ. Prevention of thromboembolic disease after elective surgery of the hip. J Bone Joint Surg 1971; 53–A:1271–1280.

(I)4. Harris WH, Salzman EW, Athanasoulis CA, Waltman AC, DeSanctis RW. Aspirin prophylaxis of venous thromboembolism after total hip replacement. N Engl J Med 1977;297:1246–1249.

(I)5. Moskovitz PA, Ellenberg SS, Feffer HL, et al. Low-dose heparin for prevention of venous thromboembolism in total hip arthroplasty and surgical repair of hip fractures. J Bone Joint Surg 1978;68-A:1065–1070.

(III)6. Ishak MA, Morley KD. Deep venous thrombosis after total hip arthroplasty: a prospective controlled study to determine the prophylactic effect of graded pressure stockings. Br J Surg 1981;68:429–432.

(I)7. Gallus A, Raman K, Darby T. Venous thrombosis after elective hip replacement—the influence of preventive intermittent calf compression and of surgical technique. Br J Surg 1983;70:17–19.

(I)8. Turpie AGG, Levine MN, Hirsh J, et al. A randomized-controlled trial of a low-molecular-weight heparin (Enoxaparin) to prevent deep-vein thrombosis in patients undergoing elective hip surgery. N Engl J Med 1986;315:925–927.

(I)9. Beisaw NE, Comerota AJ, Groth HE, et al. Dihydroergotamine/heparin in the prevention of deep-vein thrombosis after total hip replacement. A controlled, prospective, randomized multicenter trial. J Bone Joint Surg 1988;70-A:2–10.

(I)10. Lassen MR, Borris LC, Christiansen HM, et al. Prevention of thromboembolism in 190 hip arthroplasties. Comparison of LMW heparin and placebo. Acta Orthop Scand 1991;62:33–38.

11. Murphy M, Dalrymple G, Rivarola C. Silent pulmonary embolism in the elderly surgical patient. Geriatrics 1972;27:87–92.

12. Sheppard H, Henson J, Ward DJ, et al. A clinico-pathologic study of fatal pulmonary embolism in a specialist orthopaedic hospital. Arch Trauma Surg 1981;99:65–71.

13. Borris LC, Christiansen HM, Lassen MR, Olsen AD, Schott P. Comparison of real-time B-mode ultrasonography and bilateral ascending phlebography for detection of postoperative deep vein thrombosis following elective hip surgery. Thromb Haemostas 1989;61: 363–365.

14. Kälebo P, Anthmyr B-A, Eriksson BI, Zachrisson BE. Phlebogra phic findings in venous thrombosis following total hip replacement. Acta Radiol 1990;31:259–263.

(IV)15. Planès A, Vochelle N, Fagola M. Total hip replacement and deep vein thrombosis. A venographic and necropsy study. J Bone Joint Surg 1990;72-B:9–13.

16. Sikorski JM, Hampson WG, Staddon GE. The natural history and aetiology of deep vein thrombosis after total hip replacement. J Bone Joint Surg 1981;63-B:171–177.

17. Harris WH, Athanasoulis C, Waltman AC, Salzman EW. Cuff-impedance phlebography and 125I fibrinogen scanning versus roentgenographic phlebography for diagnosis of thrombophlebitis following hip surgery. J Bone Joint Surg 1976;58-A:939–944.
18. Browse NL, Burnand KG. The cause of venous ulceration. Lancet 1982;ii:243.
(III)19. Modig J, Hjelmstedt Å, Sahlstedt B, Maripuu E. Comparative influences of epidural and general anaesthesia on deep venous thrombosis and pulmonary embolism after total hip replacement. Acta Chir Scand 1981;147:125–130.
(III)20. Modig J, Borg T, Karlström G, Maripuu E, Sahlstedt B. Thromboembolism after total hip replacement: role of epidural and general anesthesia. Anesth Analg 1983;62:174–180.
(III)21. Coventry MB, Nolan DR, Beckenbaugh RD. "Delayed" prophylactic anticoagulation: a study of results and complications in 2,012 total hip arthroplasties. J Bone Joint Surg 1973;55–A:1487–1492.
(V)22. Johnson R, Green JR, Charnley J. Pulmonary embolism and its prophylaxis following the Charnley total hip replacement. Clin Orthop 1977;127:123–132.
23. Havig Ö. Deep vein thrombosis and pulmonary embolism. An autopsy study with multiple regression analysis of possible risk factors. Acta Chir Scand 1977;478(Suppl):42–47.
24. Giachino A. Relationship between deep-vein thrombosis in the calf and fatal pulmonary embolism. Can J Surg 1988;31:129–130.
25. Lotke PA, Ecker ML, Alavi A, Berkowitz H. Indications for the treatment of deep venous thrombosis following total knee replacement. J Bone Joint Surg 1984;66-A:202–208.
(V)26. Cohen SH, Ehrlich GE, Kauffman MS, Cope C. Thrombophlebitis following knee surgery. J Bone Joint Surg 1973;55-A:106–112.
(V)27. McKenna R, Bachmann F, Kaushal SP, Galante JO. Thromboembolic disease in patients undergoing total knee replacement. J Bone Joint Surg 1976;58-A:928–932.
(IV)28. Stulberg BN, Insall JN, Williams GW, Ghelman B. Deep-vein thrombosis following total knee replacement. J Bone Joint Surg 1984;66-A:194–201.
(II)29. Lynch AF, Bourne RB, Rorabeck CH, Rankin RN, Donald A. Deep vein thrombosis and continuous passive motion after total knee arthroplasty. J Bone Joint Surg 1988;70-A:11–14.
30. Stringer MD, Steadmen CA, Hedges AR, Thomas EM, Morley TR, et al. Deep vein thrombosis after elective knee surgery. An incidence study in 312 patients. J Bone Joint Surg 1989;71-B:492–497.
(I)31. Nielsen PT, Jørgensen LN, Albrecht-Beste E, Leffers AM, Rasmussen LS. Lower thrombosis risk with epidural blockade in knee arthroplasty. Acta Orthop Scand 1990;61:29–31.
32. Harper DR, Dhall DP, Woodruff WH. Prophylaxis in iliofemoral venous thrombosis. The major amputee as a clinical research model. Br J Surg 1973;60:831.
33. Sharrock NE, Hargett MJ, Urquhart B, et al. Factors affecting deep vein thrombosis rate following total knee arthroplasty under epidural anesthesia. J Arthroplasty 1993;8:133–139.
(I)34 Harris WH, Salzman EW, Athanasoulis C, Waltman AC, Baum S, et al. Comparison of warfarin, low-molecular-weight dextran, aspirin, and subcutaneous heparin in prevention of venous thromboembolism following total hip replacement. J Bone Joint Surg 1974; 56-A:1552–1562.
(I)35. Francis CW, Marder VJ, Evarts CM, Yaukoolbodi S. Two-step warfarin therapy. JAMA 1983;249:374–378.
(II)36. Paiement G, Wessinger SJ, Waltman AC, Harris WH. Low-dose warfarin versus external pneumatic compression for prophylaxis against venous thromboembolism following total hip replacement. J Arthroplasty 1987;2:23–26.
(I)37. Feller JA, Parkin JD, Phillips GW, Hannon PJ, Hennessy O, et al. Prophylaxis against venous thrombosis after total hip arthroplasty. Aust N Z J Surg 1992;62:606–610.
(II)38. Harris WH, Athanasoulis CA, Waltman AC, Salzman EW. High and low-dose aspirin prophylaxis against venous thromboembolic disease in total hip replacement. J Bone Joint Surg 1982;64-A:63–66.
(III)39. Koekenberg LJL. Experimental use of macrodex as a prophylaxis against postoperative thromboembolism. Bull Soc Int Chir 1962;21:501–512.
40. Åberg M, Bergentz SE, Hedner U. The effect of dextran on the lysability of ex vivo thrombi. Ann Surg 1975;181:342–345.
41. Salzman EW, Davies GC. Prophylaxis of venous thromboembolism: Analysis of cost-effectiveness. Ann Surg 1980;191:207–218.
(IV)42. Ljungström K-G. Dextran prophylaxis of fatal pulmonary embolism. World J Surg 1983;7:767–772.
(II)43. Gruber UF, Salden T, Brokop T, et al. Incidence of fatal pulmonary embolism after prophylaxis with dextran 70 and low-dose heparin: an international multicentre study. BMJ 1980;280:69–72.
(I)44. Fredin HO, Rosberg B, Arborelius Jr M, Nylander G. On thromboembolism after total hip replacement in epidural analgesia: a controlled study of dextran 70 and low-dose heparin combined with dihydroergotamine. Br J Surg 1984;71: 58–60.
(I)45. Eriksson BI, Zachrisson BE, Teger-Nilsson AC, Risberg B. Thrombosis prophylaxis with low molecular weight heparin in total hip replacement. Br J Surg 1988;75:1053–1057.
(V)46. Evarts CM, Alfidi RJ. Thromboembolism after hip reconstruction: failure of low doses of heparin in prevention. JAMA 1973;225:515–516.
(II)47. Hampson WGJ, Lucas HK, Harris FC, et al. Failure of low-dose heparin to prevent deep-vein thrombosis after hip-replacement arthroplasty. Lancet 1974;ii:795–797.
(I)48. Morris GK, Henry APJ, Preston BJ. Prevention of deep-vein thrombosis by low-dose heparin in patients undergoing total hip replacement. Lancet 1974;ii:797–798.
(II)49. Sagar S, Stamatakis JD, Higgins AF, et al. Efficacy of low-dose heparin in prevention of extensive deep-vein thrombosis in patients undergoing total-hip replacement. Lancet 1976;i:1151–1154.
50. Collins R, Scrimgeour A, Yusuf S, Peto R. Reduction fatal pulmonary embolism and venous thrombosis by perioperative administration of subcutaneous heparin. N Engl J Med 1988;318:1162–1173.
(I)51. Leyvraz PF, Richard J, Bachmann F, et al. Adjusted versus fixed-dose subcutaneous heparin in the prevention of deep-vein thrombosis after total hip replacement. N Engl J Med 1983;309:954–958.
(I)52. Francis CW, Pellegrini VD, Marder VJ, et al. Antithrombin III/low dose heparin in comparison with dextran 40 in prevention of venous thrombosis following total hip arthroplasty. J Bone Joint Surg 1989;71-A:327–335.
(I)53. Kakkar VV, Stamatakis JD, Bentley PG, Lawrence D, de

Haas H, et al. Prophylaxis for postoperative deep-vein thrombosis: synergistic effect of heparin and dihydroergotamine. JAMA 1979;241:38–42.

(II)54. Gallus A, Cade JF, Mills KW, Murphy W. Apparent lack of synergism between heparin and dihydroergotamine in prevention of deep vein thrombosis after elective hip replacement: a randomized double-blind trial reported in conjunction with an overview of previous results. Thromb Haemost 1992;68:238–244.

(I)55. Lassen MR, Borris LC, Christiansen HM, et al. Heparin/dihydoergotamine for venous thrombosis prophylaxis: comparison of low-dose heparin and low molecular weight heparin in hip surgery. Br J Surg 1988; 75:686–689.

(II)56. Leyvraz P, Bachmann F, Vuilleumier B, Berthet S, Bohnet J, et al. Adjusted subcutaneous heparin versus heparin plus dihydroergotamine in prevention of deep vein thrombosis after total hip arthroplasty. J Arthroplasty 1988;3:81–86.

57. Mattson E, Ohlin A, Balkfors B, Fredin HO, Nilsson P, et al. Lower-limb vasospasm and renal failure during postoperative thromboprophylaxis. Eur J Surg 1991; 157:289–292.

58. Fareed J, Walenga JM, Hoppensteadt D, Huan X, Racanelli A. Comparative study on the in vitro and in vivo activities of seven low molecular weight heparins. Haemostasis 1988;18:3–15.

(I)59. Planes A, Vochelle N, Mazas F, Zucman J, Landais A, et al. Prevention of postoperative venous thrombosis: a randomized trial comparing unfractionated heparin with low molecular weight heparin in patients undergoing total hip replacement. Thromb Haemostas 1988; 60:407–410.

(II)60. Dechavanne M, Ville D, Berruyer M, Trepo F, Dalery F, et al. Randomized trial of a low-molecular-weight heparin (Kabi 2165) versus adjusted-dose subcutaneous standard heparin in the prophylaxis of deep-vein thrombosis after elective hip surgery. Haemostasis 1989;19:5–12.

(II)61. Reilmann H, Bosch U, Creutzig H, Oetting G, Fuchs I, et al. Thromboseprophylaxe mit der niedermolekularem Heparin plus Dihydroergotamin bei Operation an unteren Extremität. Perfusion 1989;234:230–234.

(I)62. Tørholm C, Broeng L, Jørgensen PS, Bjerregaard P, Josephsen L, et al. Thromboprophylaxis by low-molecular-weight heparin in elective hip surgery. J Bone Joint Surg 1991;73-B:434–438.

(I)63. Borris LC, Hauch O, Jørgensen LN, Lassen MR, Wille-Jørgensen P, et al. Low-molecular-weight heparin (Enoxaparin) vs Dextran 70. The prevention of postoperative deep vein thrombosis after total hip replacement. Arch Intern Med 1991;151:1621–1624.

(I)64. Mätzsch T, Bergqvist D, Fredin H, Hedner U, Lindhagen A, et al. Comparison of the thromboprophylactic effect of low molecular weight heparin versus dextran in total hip replacement. Thromb Haemorrh Disorders 1991;3:25–29.

(I)65. Levine MN, Hirsh J, Gent M, Turpie AG, Leclerc J, et al. Prevention of deep vein thrombosis after elective hip surgery. A randomized trial comparing low molecular weight heparin with stan dard unfractionated heparin. Ann Intern Med 1991;114:545–551.

(I)66. Eriksson BI, Kälebo P, Anthmyr A, Wadenvik H, Tengborn L, et al. Prevention of deep vein thrombosis and pulmonary embolism after total hip replacement. Comparison of a low molecular weight heparin and unfractionated heparin. J Bone Joint Surg 1991;73-A:484–493.

(I)67. Leyvraz PF, Bachmann F, Hoek J, Büller HR, Postel M, et al. Prevention of deep vein thrombosis after hip replacement: ran domised comparison between unfractionated heparin and low molecular weight heparin. BMJ 1991;303:543–548.

(I)68. The German Hip Arthroplasty Trial (GHAT) Group. Prevention of deep vein thrombosis with low molecular-weight heparin in patients undergoing total hip replacement. A randomized trial. Arch Orthop Trauma Surg 1992;111:110–120.

69. Lassen MR, Borris LC, Christiansen HM, et al. Clinical trials with low molecular weight heparins in the prevention of postoperative thromboembolic complications: a meta-analysis. Semin Thromb Hemost 1991; 17(Suppl 3):284–290.

70. Nurmohamed MT, Rosendaal FR, Büller H, et al. Low-molecular-weight heparin versus standard heparin in general and orthopaedic surgery: a meta analysis. Lancet 1992;340:152–156.

71. Leizorovicz A, Haugh MC, Chapuis FR, Samama MM, Boissel JP. Low molecular weight heparin in prevention of perioperative thrombosis. BMJ 1992;305:913–920.

72. European Consensus Statement. Prevention of venous thromboembolism. Int Angiol 1992;11:151–159.

(I)73. Hoek J, Nurmohamed MT, Hamelynck KJ, et al. Prevention of deep-vein thrombosis following total hip replacement by a low-molecular-weight heparinoid. Thromb Haemost 1992;67:28–32.

(I)74. Leyvraz P, Bachmann F, Bohnet J, et al. Thromboembolic prophylaxis in total hip replacement: a comparison between the low molecular weight heparinoid Lomoparan and heparin-dihydroer gotamine. Br J Surg 1992;79:911–914.

75. Tarnay TJ, Rohn PR, Davidson AG, Stevenson MM, Byars EF, et al. Pneumatic calf compression, fibrinolysis, and the prevention of deep venous thrombosis. Surgery 1980;84:489–496.

(I)76. Knight MT, Dawson R. Effect of intermittent compression of the arms on deep venous thrombosis in the legs. Lancet 1976; ii:1265–1268.

(I)77. Hull RD, Raskob GE, Gent M, et al. Effectiveness of intermittent pneumatic compression for preventing deep vein thrombosis after total hip replacement. JAMA 1990;263:2313–2317.

78. Comerota AJ, Katz ML, White JV. Why does prophylaxis with external pneumatic compression for deep vein thrombosis fail? Am J Surg 1992;164:265–268.

(I)79. Fordyce MJF, Ling RSM. A venous foot pump reduces thrombosis after total hip replacement. J Bone Joint Surg 1992;74-B:45–49.

80. Wille-Jørgensen P, Bjerg-Nielsen A, Christensen SW, et al. Graded compression stockings with and without heparin-dihydroer gotamine in the prevention of deep venous thrombosis following elective hip alloplasty. Phlebology 1986;1:51–56.

(III)81. Bradley JG, Krugener GH, Jager HJ. The effectiveness of intermittent plantar venous compression in prevention of deep venous thrombosis after total hip arthroplasty. J Arthroplasty 1993;8:57–61.

(III)82. Thorburn J, Louden JR, Vallance R. Spinal and general anaesthesia in total hip replacement: frequency of deep vein thrombosis. Br J Anaesth 1980;52:1117–1121.

83. Pedersen J, Jakobsen BW, Egeberg BB. Thromboembolic complications after total hip replacement. Ugeskr Léger 1987;149: 1463–1466.

84. Modig J, Malmberg P, Karlström G. Effect of epidural versus general anaesthesia on calf blood flow. Acta Anaesth Scand 1980;24:305–309.

85. Modig J. Influence of regional anesthesia, local anesthetics, and sympathicomimetics on the pathophysiology of deep vein thrombosis. Acta Chir Scand 1988; 550(Suppl):119–27.

86. Chin SP, Abou-Madi MN, Eurin B, Witvoët J, Montagne J. Blood loss in total hip replacement: extradural v. phenoperidine analgesia. Br J Anaesth 1982;54:491–495.

87. Fredin H, Rosberg B. Anaesthetic techniques and thromboembolism in total hip arthroplasty. Eur J Anaesthesiol 1986;3: 273–281.

88. Wille-Jørgensen P, Jørgensen LN, Rasmussen LS. Lumbar regional anaesthesia and prophylactic anticoagulant therapy. Is the combination safe? Anaesthesia 1991;46:623–627.

(I)89. Hull R, Delmore TJ, Hirsh J, et al. Effectiveness of intermittent pulsatile elastic stockings for the prevention of calf and thigh vein thrombosis in patients undergoing elective knee surgery. Thromb Res 1979;16:37–45.

(I)90. McKenna R, Galante J, Bachmann F, Wallace DL, Kaushal SP, et al. Prevention of venous thromboembolism after total knee replacement by high-dose aspirin or intermittent calf and thigh compression. BMJ 1980;280:514–517.

(I)91. Haas SB, Insall JN, Scuderi GR, Windsor RE, Ghelman B. Pneumatic sequential-compression boots compared with aspirin prophylaxis of deep-vein thrombosis after total knee arthroplasty. J Bone Joint Surg 1990;72-A:27–31.

(II)92. Lynch AF, Bourne RB, Rorabeck CH, Rankin RN, Donald A. Deep-vein thrombosis and continuous passive motion after total knee arthroplasty. J Bone Joint Surg 1988;70-A:11–14.

(I)93. Stulberg BN, Francis CW, Pellegrini VD, et al. Antithrombin III/low-dose heparin in the prevention of deep-vein thrombosis after total knee arthroplasty. A preliminary report. Clin Orthop 1989;248:152–157.

(I)94. Leclerc JR, Geerts WH, Desjardins L et al. Prevention of deep vein thrombosis after major knee surgery—a randomized, double-blind trial comparing a low molecular weight heparin fragment (enoxaparin) to placebo. Thromb Haemost 1992;67: 417–423.

(I)95. Jørgensen LN, Rasmussen LS, Nielsen PT, Leffers A, Albrecht-Beste E. Antithrombotic efficacy of continuous extradural analgesia after knee replacement. Br J Anaesth 1991;66:8–12.

7

Neurosurgery and Stroke Patients

Alexander G.G. Turpie

INTRODUCTION

Venous thromboembolism is a common complication in patients with acute stroke, in neurosurgical patients and in patients with spinal cord trauma. Venous thrombosis occurs more frequently in patients with lower limb paresis or paralysis. In addition systemic risk factors such as age and medical complications such as chest or urinary tract infections may be added to the local risk factor of venous stasis and increase the risk. Activation of hemostasis which follows brain damage may also contribute to the occurrence of venous thromboembolism in such patients. Clinical recognition of venous thrombosis in stroke and neurosurgical patients is difficult since paralyzed limbs are often edematous without associated thrombosis, while in other patients at risk, thrombosis can occur without any clinical signs. Although antithrombotic prophylaxis with low-dose-heparin or low-molecular-weight heparin is widely accepted for other medium or high-risk medical and surgical patients, there is still reluctance among physicians to use antithrombotic therapy in stroke and neurosurgical patients because of the fear of bleeding into the central nervous system.

The risk of venous thrombosis in stroke and neurosurgical patients has been defined at a number of consensus conferences. The first was in 1986 at the National Institute of Health in Washington.[1] Patients with stroke, neurosurgical patients with lower limb paralysis and paraplegic patients were identified as being in the high-risk category, and neurosurgical patients including patients with brain tumor, subarachnoid hemorrhage and head trauma in the moderate risk category. Since 1986, three additional consensus statements have also defined the risk of venous thromboembolism in such patients using similar classifications.[2-4]

Stroke

Venous thromboembolism is a common complication in patients with acute thrombotic stroke. The estimates of the frequency of deep-vein thrombosis (DVT) in untreated patients ranges from 20% to 75%.[5-7(I)] The wide range of the frequencies reported in the various studies depends on the methods used to detect DVT and, importantly, on the degree of lower-limb paralysis. Most of the thrombi occur in the paralysed limbs in which the frequency ranges from 60% to 75%.[5] Of these thrombi, 25% occur in the proximal segment and present a high risk for pulmonary embolism (PE). Indeed, PE is the third most common cause of death in stroke patients and occurs in 1% to 2% of patients who do not receive prophylaxis.[8] A number of methods of preventing DVT have been shown to be safe and effective in high-risk medical patients. These include low-dose heparin, low-molecular-weight-heparin and graduated compression stockings. Of these, low-dose subcutaneous heparin has been the most extensively evaluated.[9] Three small randomized trials of low-dose heparin prophylaxis in patients with acute stroke have been reported.[10(I),11(I),12] In two studies, low-dose heparin was given subcutaneously in doses of 5,000 units every eight hours. In the first study,[10(I)] low-dose heparin reduced the frequency of DVT from 12 of 16 patients (75%) to two of 16 patients (13%), and in the second study[11(I)] from 117 of 161 patients (73%) to 32 of 144 patients (22%) in the placebo and heparin-treated groups, respectively. In the third study,[12] a combination of low-dose heparin 5,000 units with 0.5 mg dihydroergotamine (DHE) subcutaneous every 12 hours was used. In this study, the frequency of DVT was reduced from 33 of 41 patients (56%) in the placebo-treated group to seven of 40 patients (18%) in the combined heparin/DHE group. Despite the fact that all three studies showed a significant reduction in DVT with treatment, low-dose heparin has not been widely adopted in stroke patients because of concern about the risk of intracranial haemorrhage or haemorrhage transformation of the brain infarct.

Because of the superior pharmacological and pharmacokinetic properties of low-molecular-weight heparin and heparinoids over standard heparin, these agents have

From *Venous Thromboembolism: An Evidence-Based Atlas* edited by Russell Hull, Gary Raskob, Graham Pineo © 1996, Futura Publishing Co., Armonk, NY.

been evaluated in stroke patients particularly since animal experiments have shown that their use is less likely to be associated with bleeding.[14,16(II)]

There have been two studies using the low-molecular-weight heparin (Fragmin) for the prevention of DVT in patients with thrombotic stroke.[15(I),16(II)] The results of these studies were inconsistent. The first study[15] compared low-molecular-weight heparin in a dose of 2,500 anti-factor Xa units twice a day with placebo and demonstrated a reduction in the rate of venous thrombosis from 15 of 30 patients (50%) to 6 of 27 patients (22%). In the second study,[16] low-molecular-weight heparin was given in a dose of 50–65 anti-factor Xa units/kg/body weight once daily (equivalent to 3500–4550 antifactor Xa units daily). In contrast to the first study, there was no difference in the frequency of DVT between the two groups which occurred in 15 of 42 (36%) of the Fragmin-treated patients compared with 17 of 50 (34%) of the placebo-treated patients.

The low-molecular-weight heparinoid, Orgaran which is a nonheparin glycosaminoglycan and distinct from heparin,[17(I)] has been shown to be effective in preventing venous thrombosis without significant bleeding risk in high-risk surgical patients including those undergoing elective joint replacement and fractured hip surgery. Orgaran has also been evaluated for the prevention of DVT in patients with acute ischemic stroke in two studies by Turpie et al.[7(I),18(I)] In the first study,[7] which was double-blind and placebo controlled, 50 patients received Orgaran in a loading dose of 1,000 anti-Xa units intravenously followed by 750 anti-Xa units subcutaneously 12-hourly, and 25 received placebo. Treatment was started within 7 days of stroke onset and continued for 14 days or until discharge from hospital, if earlier. The patients were screened for deep-vein thrombosis using [125]Iodine-labelled fibrinogen leg scanning and impedance plethysmography and the diagnosis of deep vein thrombosis was confirmed by venography which occurred in two of 50 (4%) in the Orgaran group and seven of 25 (28%) in the placebo group (p = 0.005). Proximal DVT occurred in four of the placebo group and none in the Orgaran-treated group. There was one major hemorrhage in the Orgaran-treated group and one minor hemorrhage in the placebo group. Plasma anticoagulant activity measured as anti-factor Xa units/ml (mean ± SED) gradually rose from 0.18 to ± 0.001 and 0.06 ± 0.001, six and 12 hours after injection on the first day to 0.24 ± 0.02 and 0.12 ± 0.01 after 11 days treatment. Thus, the results of the placebo controlled trial demonstrated that Orgaran was effective in the prevention of deep-vein thrombosis in stroke patients without causing significant bleeding. In this study, computerized tomographic (CT) scans of the brain were not repeated after treatment; hence, the rates of hemorrhagic conversion of the infarcts were not determined. In the second study,[18] Orgaran was compared with unfractionated heparin in the prevention of DVT in a double-blind randomized trial in acute stroke patients. In this study, 87 patients who had lower-limb paralysis were randomized to receive Orgaran (45 patients) in a dose of 750 anti-factor Xa units subcutaneously 12-hourly or unfractionated heparin (42 patients) in a dose of 5,000 units subcutaneously 12-hourly. Prophylaxis was started, on average, within 5 days of the onset of the stroke and continued for 14 days. Venous thrombosis surveillance was carried out with [125]Iodine-labelled fibrinogen leg scanning and impedance plethysmography and the diagnosis of DVT confirmed by ascending venography. Venous thrombosis occurred in 4 of 45 (8.9%) of the Orgaran group and 13 of 42 (31%) in the unfractionated heparin group (p = 0.01). Proximal-vein thrombosis occurred in one of the Orgaran-treated group (2.2%) and five of the heparin-treated group (11.9%) respectively (p = 0.08). There were no clinically significant hemorrhagic complications in either group. In this study, the CT scan was repeated at the end of the treatment period. The frequency of hemorrhagic conversion of the infarct was 9.3% in the Orgaran-treated group and 5.6% in the heparin-treated group with no difference in the incidence between the two treatment groups (p>0.10). The results of this study demonstrated that Orgaran was more effective than conventional low-dose subcutaneous heparin in the prevention of DVT in patients with acute stroke. A second study comparing Orgaran with heparin has recently been completed by Dumas et al,[19] comparing 1250 anti-factor Xa units Orgaran given once daily with low-dose heparin 5,000 units 12-hourly. In this study, DVT occurred in 13 of 89 (15%) Orgaran-treated patients and 17 of 70 (18%), heparin-treated patients (p = 0.71). Hemorrhagic transformation of the infarct occurred in two patients in each group. The results of the prophylaxis studies with Orgaran demonstrate low rates of proximal and total venous thrombosis with significantly greater efficacy of Orgaran over standard low-dose heparin without excess bleeding when given twice daily.

The major limitation of the prophylaxis studies in ischemic stroke is the small sample size in each, and although the efficacy of the regimens for the prevention of DVT has been established, their safety remains a question. Additional data on the safety of anticoagulants will be available from the large scale treatment trials in stroke that are underway.[20] Preliminary data indicates that even when administered in therapeutic doses, the low molecular weight heparinoid, Orgaran, is not associated with excess bleeding in patients with ischemic stroke.

Neurosurgery

Deep-vein thrombosis and PE are common causes of morbidity and mortality in neurosurgical patients in whom DVT has been objectively diagnosed by ^{125}I-labelled fibrinogen leg scanning and impedance plethysmography (IPG). DVT has been reported to occur in 20% to 30%[21(I),22(I),23(I),24(II)] and fatal PE approximately 1%.[25,26]

A number of methods for preventing venous thrombosis following neurosurgery are available. Anticoagulant prophylaxis with low-dose heparin is effective in general surgical patients, but its use in neurosurgical patients is problematic because of the potential for serious bleeding. However, there have been few reports on the use of low-dose heparin prophylaxis in neurosurgical patients. Powers and Edwards in a review of the low-dose heparin studies,[27] concluded, from limited data, that low-dose heparin was indicated in all patients undergoing elective neurosurgical procedures and that the regimen was efficacious and safe. However, the studies were too small to exclude an increased risk of clinically important bleeding, including intracranial bleeding, in the heparin group. Therefore, low-dose heparin is not widely used in these patients. The physical methods, including graduated compression stockings or intermittent pneumatic compression (IPC) devices are potentially attractive in this patient group since the hemostatic mechanism is not inhibited, hence the risk of bleeding which may result in serious complications, is low.[9] The use of intermittent pneumatic compression devices has been shown to be, an effective method of prophylaxis in both general surgical patients and neurosurgical patients.[21–23,28(I)] Five studies of thrombosis prophylaxis in neurosurgery have been performed using a variety of pneumatic compression devices.[21–23,28,29(II)] Despite its demonstrated efficacy, pneumatic compression is not widely used for the prevention of DVT in neurosurgical patients, possibly because of the perception that it is inconvenient to both patients and nursing staff. Graduated compression stockings which are much easier to use, are also effective in the prevention of DVT in general surgical patients.[9,30] In a study in neurosurgical patients, graduated compression stockings alone were as effective as graduated compression stockings plus IPC for the prevention of venous thrombosis in neurosurgical patients.[28] The main attraction of physical methods of prophylaxis in neurosurgical patients is that they are effective and are free of the potential for hemorrhagic side-effects.

Spinal Cord Trauma

In patients with spinal cord injuries, venous thrombosis has been reported to occur in 15% to 60% depending upon the severity of the injury, the presence of lower limb paralysis, and the presence of other associated risk factors.[31–33] The reported incidence of fatal PE has ranged from 2% to 16% of patients within two to three months of spinal cord injury.[33]

Because of the evidence for its efficacy and safety in general surgical and medical patients, low-dose heparin has been proposed as a method of preventing DVT in spinal cord injured patients. There have been several reports on the use of low-dose heparin in spinal cord injury patients, but these studies were not randomized and involved only small numbers of patients.[34(V),35(V),36(V)] In one study using retrospective controls, there was a highly significant reduction in the frequency of DVT in spinal cord-injured patients using objective tests to diagnose DVT.[36(V)] In one controlled trial[37(III)] involving 32 patients with spinal cord injury, the frequency of venous thrombosis was unexpectedly low in both the control and heparinized groups, but in this study, only impedance plethysmography was used to detect venous thromboembolism, which would be insensitive to calf-vein thrombi and nonoccluding proximal thrombi. In none of the studies was there a significant increase in bleeding reported. A recent study[38(I)] compared fixed-dose versus adjusted-dose heparin in 58 patients with complete motor paralysis. One-half the patients were randomized to receive 5,000 U of heparin twice daily, while the remainder received sufficient heparin (on average 14,300 U q12h) to prolong their activated partial thromboplastin times to 1.5 times the normal control value. Nine patients received the fixed dose but only two received the adjusted dose developed venous thrombosis ($p<0.05$). However, bleeding necessitating withdrawal of prophylaxis occurred in seven patients treated with the higher dose and none receiving the low-dose regimen ($p<0.02$). The majority of the reports indicate that venous thrombosis is most common during the period of flaccidity, and most authors recommend the use of low-dose heparin or other prophylaxis for the first three months following injury.

Low-molecular-weight heparin, Logiparin, was compared with standard low-dose heparin for the prevention of DVT in spinal cord injured patients.[39(I)] Twenty-one patients were randomized to standard heparin and 20 to low-molecular-weight heparin. Five patients in the standard heparin group had thrombotic events, including two patients with fatal pulmonary embolism; two other patients had bleeding severe enough to necessitate withdrawing the heparin. The cumulative event rate in the heparin group was 34.7% (95% CI, 13.7% to 55.2%) and none in the patients treated with low-molecular-weight heparin (CI, 0% to 14%); the difference between the two groups was significant ($p = 0.006$). The results of this small study suggest that LMWH may be safe and effective in the prevention of thromboembolism in patients with spinal cord injury, and is superior to standard heparin when given in doses of 5,000 units three times per day. However, more extensive experience with low molecular weight heparin in spinal cord injured patients is required before it can be recommended for routine use.

REFERENCES

1. National Institutes of Health Consensus Development Conference Statement. Prevention of venous thrombosis and pulmonary embolism. JAMA 1986; 256(6):744–749.
2. Thromboembolic Risk Factors (THRIFT) Consensus Group. Risk of and prophylaxis for venous thromboembolism in hospital patients. Br Med J 1992; 305(6853):567–574.
3. European Consensus Statement. Prevention of venous thromboembolism. Int Ang 1992;11(3):151–159.

4. Clagett GP, Anderson FA, Levine MN, Salzman EW, Wheeler HB. Prevention of venous thromboembolism. Chest 1992;102(Suppl 4): 391S-407S.

5. Warlow C, Ogston D, Douglas AS. Venous thrombosis following strokes. Lancet 1972;1:1305–1306.

6. McCarthy ST, Robertson D, Turner JJ, Hawkey CJ. Low-dose heparin as a prophylaxis against deep vein thrombosis after acute stroke. Lancet 1977;2:800–801.

(I)7. Turpie AGG, Levine MN, Hirsh J, et al. Double-blind randomised trial of Org 10172 low-molecular-weight heparinoid in prevention of deep vein thrombosis in thrombotic stroke. Lancet 1987;1:523–525.

8. Brown M, Glassenberg M. Mortality factors in patients with acute stroke. JAMA 1973;224:1493–1495.

9. Turpie AGG, Leclerc J. Prophylaxis of venous thromboembolism. In: Leclerc J, ed. Venous Thromboembolic Disorders, 1990;303–345.

(I)10. McCarthy ST, Robertson D, Turner JJ, Hawkey CJ. Low-dose heparin as a prophylaxis against deep vein thrombosis after acute stroke. Lancet 1977;2:800–801.

(I)11. McCarthy ST, Turner J. Low-dose subcutaneous heparin in the prevention of deep vein thrombosis and pulmonary emboli following acute stroke. Age and Aging 1986;15:84–88.

12. Czechanowski B, Heinrich F. Prophylaxe venoser Thrombosen bei frischem ischamischem zerebrovaskularem Indult—Doppelblind studie mit Heparin-Dihydrogot. Dtsch Med Wochenschr 1981;106: 1254–1260.

(V)13. Hirsh J, Levine MN. Low molecular weight heparin. Blood 1992;79(1)1–17.

(II)14. Cade JF, Buchanan MR, Boneu B, Ockelford P, Carter CJ, et al. A comparison of the antithrombotic and haemorrhagic effects of low molecular weight heparin fractions: The influence of the method of preparation. Thromb Res 1984;35:613.

(I)15. Prins MH, Gelsema R, Sing AK, et al. Prophylaxis of deep venous thrombosis with a low-molecular weight heparin (Kabi 2165/Fragmin) in stroke patients. Haemostas 1989;19:245–250.

(II)16. Sandset PM, Dahl T, Stiris M, et al. A double-blind and randomized placebo-controlled trial of low molecular weight heparin once daily to prevent deep vein thrombosis in acute ischemic stroke. Semin Thromb and Hemost 1990;16:25–33.

(I)17. Bergqvist D, Kettunen K, Fredin H, Faunø P, Soumalainen O, et al. Thromboprophylaxis in hip fracture patients—a prospective randomised comparative study between Org 10172 and dextran 70. Surgery 1991;109:617.

(I)18. Turpie AGG, Gent M, Cote R, Levine MN, Ginsberg JS, et al. A low-molecular weight heparinoid compared with unfractionated heparin in the prevention of deep vein thrombosis in patients with acute ischemic stroke. Ann Int Med 1992;117(5):353–357.

19. Dumas R, Woinitas F, Kutnowski M, Nikolic I, Berberich R, et al. Safety and efficacy of ORG 10172 in preventing deep venous thrombosis in patients with acute ischaemic stroke: a multicentre, double-blind, randomised study comparing ORG 10172, 1250 anti-Xa units subcutaneously once daily with low-dose heparin twice daily. Submitted for publication.

20. Massey EW, Biller J, Davis JN, Adams HP Jr, Marler JR, et al. Large-dose infusions of heparinoid ORG 10172 in ischemic stroke. Stroke 1990;21(9):1289–1292.

(I)21. Turpie AGG, Gallus AS, Beattie WS, et al. Prevention of venous thrombosis in patients with intracranial disease by intermittent pneumatic compression of the calf. Neurology 1977;5:435–438.

(I)22. Skillman JJ, Collins EC, Coe NP, et al. Prevention of deep vein thrombosis in neurosurgical patients: A controlled randomized trial of external pneumatic compression boots. Surgery 1978;83:354–358.

(I)23. Turpie AGG, Delmore T, Hirsh J, et al. Prevention of venous thrombosis by intermittent sequential calf compression in patients with intracranial disease. Thromb Res 1979;15:611–616.

(II)24. Turpie AGG, Gent M, Doyle DJ et al. An evaluation of suloctidil in the prevention of deep vein thrombosis in neurosurgical patients. Thromb Res 1985;39:173–181.

25. Sigel B, Ipsen J, Felix WR. The epidemiology of lower extremity deep venous thrombosis in surgical patients. Ann Surg 1974;179:278–290.

26. Watson N. Anticoagulant therapy in the treatment of venous thrombosis and pulmonary embolism in acute spinal injury. Paraplegia 1974;12:197–201.

27. Powers SK, Edwards MSB. Prophylaxis of thromboembolism in the neurological patient: A review. Neurosurgery 1982;10:509–513.

(I)28. Turpie AGG, Hirsh J, Gent M, Julian D, Johnson J. Prevention of deep vein thrombosis in potential neurosurgical patients: A randomized trial comparing graduated compression stockings alone or graduated compression stockings plus intermittent pneumatic compression with control. Arch Intern Med 1979;149: 679–681.

(II)29. Green D, Rossi EC, Yao JST, Flinn WR, Spies SM. Deep vein thrombosis in spinal cord injury: Effect of prophylaxis with calf compression, aspirin and dipyridamole. Paraplegia 1982; 20:227–234.

30. Colditz GA, Tuden RL, Oster G. Rates of venous thrombosis after general surgery: Combined results of randomized clinical trials. Lancet 1986;2:143–146.

31. Hull RD. Venous thromboembolism in spinal cord injury patients. Chest 1992;102(6):658S-663S.

32. Weingarden SI. Deep venous thrombosis in spinal cord injury. Overview of the problem. Chest 1992; 102(6):636S-639S.

33. Turpie AGG. Thrombosis prevention and treatment in spinal cord injured patients. In: Bloch RF, Basbaum M, eds. Spinal Cord Rehabilitation. Williams and Wilkins, 1986:212–240.

(V)34. Rocha Casas E, Sanchez MP, Arias CR, et al. Prophylaxis of venous thrombosis and pulmonary embolism in patients with acute traumatic spinal cord lesions. Paraplegia 1976;14:178.

(V)35. Rocha Casas E, Sanchez MP, Arias CR, et al. Prophylaxis of venous thrombosis and pulmonary embolism in patients with acute traumatic spinal cord lesions. Paraplegia 1977;15:209.

(V)36. Silver JR. The prophylactic use of anticoagulant therapy in the prevention of pulmonary emboli in one hundred consecutive spinal injury patients. Paraplegia 1974;12: 88.

(III)37. Frisbie JH, Sasahara AA. Low dose heparin prophylaxis for deep venous thrombosis in acute spinal cord injury patients: A controlled study. Paraplegia 1981;19:141.

(I)38. Green D, Lee MY, Ito VY, et al. Fixed vs adjusted-dose heparin in the prophylaxis of thromboembolism in spinal cord injury. JAMA 1988;260:1255–1258.

(I)39. Green D, Lee MY, Lim AC, et al. Prevention of thromboembolism after spinal cord injury using low-molecular-weight heparin. Ann Intern Med 1990;113:571–574.

8

Medical Patients

Alexander S. Gallus

INTRODUCTION

There is such a vast amount of published information about venous thrombosis (VT) prevention in surgical patients, that it becomes very tempting to simply extrapolate from this vast body of knowledge directly to medical patients.

There are, after all, obvious similarities: acute medical catastrophes and major surgery both induce an immediate increase in the risk of venous thromboembolism (VTE), a risk which resolves with full functional recovery.

The problems posed by medical illnesses are, however, sufficiently distinct to warrant separate consideration.

First, in almost all surgical evaluations of VT prophylaxis the preventive method was initiated before the thrombogenic stimulus of surgical trauma—and this is clearly not possible in medical emergencies where prophylaxis must wait until some time after the event when small VT may already have been laid down. Second, it is now possible to draw firm conclusions about the impact of at least some prophylactic methods on the incidence of major pulmonary embolism (PE) after elective general surgery, but this is not true for medical patients, where most VT prevention trials have been quite small and limited to measuring an effect on asymptomatic VT. Lastly, there is the additional challenge of chronic medical illnesses where, since hospital admissions are brief interludes in the long-term progression of chronic disability, there may be a need for prolonged prophylaxis.

IMPORTANCE OF VENOUS THROMBOEMBOLISM IN MEDICAL PATIENTS

In autopsy studies, there is more fatal PE in medical than surgical admissions (Tables 1 and 2).[1-6] For instance, in an extensive Swedish series made especially credible by its very high autopsy rate, there was fatal PE in 0.27% of general surgical and 0.42% of orthopaedic surgery admissions, compared with 0.43% of admissions to an infectious diseases unit, 0.58% for internal medicine, and 1.13% in oncology.[3]

From another perspective, medical conditions also predominate as predisposing events in people presenting with VT.[7,8]

The most important question concerns the impact of fatal PE on underlying prognosis, which circumscribes the likely clinical gain from preventing fatal PE.

Although two early autopsy studies suggested the underlying pathology was relatively benign in 25% to 55% of deaths from PE, and these were therefore labelled as potentially 'preventable',[4,9] it is not known if this remains true for medical patients today. In one more recent Danish series, at least, there was a severe and probably terminal underlying disease in 168 of 178 medical patients with fatal, autopsy confirmed, PE;[5] clear evidence that disease prognosis must be a major determinant when selecting patients for VT prophylaxis.

RISK FACTORS IN MEDICAL PATIENTS

Most of these are familiar, since they include previous VTE, increasing age beyond 40 years, obesity (>20% overweight)[10,11], prolonged bed rest, motor paralysis, chronic disabling cerebrovascular disease, myocardial infarction, uncontrolled heart failure,[10] severe infection, trauma, and cancer.[10,12,13] Recently, the use of multi-agent cancer chemotherapy was defined as an additional risk factor.[14,15]

Present formulations of estrogen containing oral contraceptives probably remain mildly thrombogenic,[16] but there is no good evidence that postmenopausal estrogen replacement increases VTE risk.[17]

There a small number of truly 'hypercoagulable' states due to inherited deficiency of one of the physiological anticoagulants: antithrombin III, protein C or protein S, and a few disorders like Behçet's disease and the pri-

From *Venous Thromboembolism: An Evidence-Based Atlas* edited by Russell Hull, Gary Raskob, Graham Pineo © 1996, Futura Publishing Co., Armonk, NY.

Table 1

Reference	Non-operated Patients	Surgical Patients
Hermann et al, 1961	0.49%	0.09%
Dismuke & Wagner, 1986	0.18%	0.05%
Lindblad et al, 1991	0.47%	0.24%

Mortality from PE, estimated from autopsy studies of medical and surgical admission to University general hospitals in the USA and in Sweden. The autopsy rate varied from 50% to 77%.

mary antiphospholipid syndrome where VTE and artery thrombosis form part of the natural history.[18,19]

Large-scale surveys suggest that most patients admitted to hospital have more than one risk factor for VTE,[20] as do most patients who go on to develop VTE.[8]

A number of ^{125}I-fibrinogen leg-scan-based studies, mostly dating from the 1970s, measured VT rates after various acute medical illnesses and looked at the influence of clinical risk factors (Table 3).

Venous thrombosis after myocardial infarction develops most often in older people and when there is heart failure, shock, cardiac arrest, another significant arrhythmia, or continuing chest pain.[21–24] The risk is further increased by transfemoral pacemaker insertion[25] but cigarette smoking may, oddly enough, protect from VT.[26(I)-28]

The risk is especially great when there is a disabling stroke or spinal injury: 25% of people with hemiplegia admitted to a rehabilitation unit have developed symptomatic VT[29] while routine venography finds VT in 40%[30] and leg scanning becomes abnormal in about 50% of paralyzed legs.[31]

Leg scanning also found VT in 13% of bedridden medical inpatients: 20% when there was pneumonia or heart disease and 4% in others,[32] while among inpatients with lung disease confined to bed for longer than three days the VT rate was 26%.[33(III)]

Little is known about the incidence and clinical importance of VTE among chronically debilitated elderly people. Consecutive autopsies from a nursing home showed some degree of PE in 34% of deaths and major PE in 27%, none of them clinically predictable.[34]

Table 2

Reference	Fatal PE	Non Operated (%)	Surgical (%)
Nielsen et al, 1981	220	183 (83%)	37 (17%)
Hauch et al, 1990	74	58 (78%)	16 (22%)
Sperry et al, 1990	78	45 (59%)	31 (41%)

Proportion of all fatal PE found in medical as opposed to surgical patients at autopsy.

Table 3

Condition	Diagnosis	VT	PE	Reference
Myocardial Infarction	leg scan	37%		Maurer et al, 1971
	leg scan	27%		Simmons et al, 1973
	leg scan	29%		Marks and Emerson, 1974
	leg scan	17%		Cristal et al, 1976
Stroke	venography	31%		Cope et al, 1973
	leg scan	53%		Warlow et al, 1976
	clinical/ autopsy		9%	Warlow et al, 1976
Medical	leg scan	13%		Kierkegaard et al, 1987

Selected medical conditions with their associated VT or PE rates determined by leg scanning, routine venography, or at autopsy.

SOME LIMITATIONS OF VENOUS THROMBOSIS PREVENTION TRIALS IN MEDICAL PATIENTS

One severe drawback of most VT prevention trials in medical patients is their small size: few have enrolled enough subjects to indicate an effect on the incidence of extensive VT or major PE.

Most have relied, instead, on convenient tests like ^{125}I-fibrinogen leg scanning to screen for a high-frequency substitute end-point, asymptomatic calf VT, an approach with at least two major limitations: since the evaluations of leg scanning largely failed to meet present-day methodological criteria there is some doubt about its accuracy,[35] and it remains uncertain if prophylactic regimens that prevent small calf VT will also, of necessity, prevent PE.

Leg-scan-based trials do, however, provide a basis for going on to much larger studies which use a clinically more important end-point like PE, but these must, in turn, meet the challenge of diagnostic uncertainty.

Thus, in a recent overview of seven published clinico-pathological correlations, the clinical diagnosis of PE had a very low sensitivity of 11% to 49% but a higher specificity of 89% to 99% for a subsequent finding of PE at autopsy, while the accuracy of a positive clinical diagnosis was 25% to 88% compared with 87% to 99.7% for a negative diagnosis.[36] It is then hardly surprising that PE is perhaps the most frequently misdiagnosed condition relative to its actual presence at autopsy.[37]

One reason is that, typically, only 30% of fatal PE causes the clinical stereotype of sudden death, while 70% result in a gradual deterioration easily mistaken for progressive heart or respiratory failure.[12]

PREVENTING VENOUS THROMBOSIS IN MEDICAL PATIENTS

Logic suggests there should be two clearly distinct clinical settings for VT prevention in medical illnesses:

1. Myocardial infarction or a mild stroke, pneumonia, or other acute problems in previously well people where the thrombogenic stimulus happens at a clearly defined time, there is a full or near-complete functional recovery, and effective preventive therapy during the hospital admission should make a significant impact.
2. Chronically disabling heart, lung, or other major diseases where there is a long-term risk of VTE so that prophylaxis limited to hospital admissions may well have a limited impact and long-term prophylaxis may be more appropriate.

EVIDENCE CONCERNING PREVENTIVE METHODS

Clinical trials have focused on myocardial infarction, on stroke and other neurological disabilities, and on general medical unit admissions.

The preventive methods evaluated have mostly been pharmacological (low doses of unfractionated heparin or low-molecular-weight heparins (LMWHs) given subcutaneously, and oral anticoagulants), although physical measures like graded pressure elastic stockings and intermittent leg compression have also been tested where anticoagulants are thought to be contraindicated.

MYOCARDIAL INFARCTION AND OTHER HEART DISEASES

Myocardial Infarction

The major finding in several early clinical trials was that a moderate level of oral anticoagulant effect, corresponding to an INR of 1.5 to 2.5, prevents symptoms of VT, PE, and systemic embolism after myocardial infarction,[38,39] but failed to resolve if this can also prevent further coronary artery occlusion.

From subsequent leg-scan studies, it appears that unfractionated heparin can prevent VT after myocardial infarction (MI) regardless of whether it is given by intravenous (iv) infusion in therapeutic doses, as continuous iv heparin followed by warfarin, or in low doses given subcutaneously (sc) (5,000 iu, injected two or three times a day),[26,40(I),41(I),42(I),43(I),44(I)] although 7,500 units (U) of heparin given sc twice daily was ineffective in one report (Table 4).[45(II)]

Is Venous Thrombosis Prevention the Only Aim of Anticoagulant Therapy After Myocardial Infarction?

How much heparin is given after myocardial infarction (MI) and by which route depends on the intent of therapy.

To prevent mural thrombus formation and a subsequent embolic stroke, 5,000 u heparin, given sc 12 hourly, is not enough, and the minimum appropriate heparin dose is probably 12,500 iu, given sc twice-daily.[46(I)] To prevent coronary artery reocclusion following thrombolytic therapy, the required dose may well be higher again.[47]

If, on the other hand, the sole purpose is to prevent VTE after an uncomplicated MI, then 5,000 iu heparin, given sc eight or 12 hourly, appears to be safe and effective.

Heart Failure and Cardiac Pacemaker Insertion

Preventing venous and systemic thromboembolism in congestive heart failure was the focus of several early oral anticoagulant trials.

At that time, a high proportion of people with severe and intractable congestive heart failure developed thrombophlebitis, PE and arterial embolism, and several comparisons suggested that long-term dicumarol therapy substantially prevents these complications.[48(II),49(II),50(II)]

Whether these findings remain relevant is uncertain: the extent of heart failure was extreme by today's stan-

Table 4

Heparin Regimen	VT (Active)	VT (Control)	% Risk Reduction	Reference
continuous iv.	0/24 (0%)	7/24 (29%)	100%	Handley et al, 1972
continuous iv, then warfarin.	3/46 (7%)	10/46 (22%)	72% [92 to −3%]	Wray et al, 1973
continuous iv.	4/35 (11%)	11/37 (30%)	66% [89 to −7%]	Pitt et al, 1980
500 u iv 12 hourly.	5/36 (14%)		57% [85 to −23%]	
7,500 u bid sc.	6/26 (23%)	7/24 (29%)	19% [73 to −140%]	Handley, 1972
5,000 u tid sc.	1/38 (3%)	9/40 (23%)	90% [17 to 99%]	Gallus et al, 1973
5,000 u bid.	2/63 (3%)	11/64 (17%)	83% [23 to 96%]	Warlow et al, 1973
low dose heparin.	2/37 (5%)	14/41 (34%)	87% [41 to 97%]	Emerson & Marks, 1977

The effect of various unfractionated heparin regimens on the VT rate after MI, as observed in leg scan based randomised trials (continuous iv = therapeutic doses of intravenous heparin; bid and tid sc = subcutaneous heparin given two or three times daily. The figures in square brackets are 95% confidence intervals for the observed risk reduction, where negative risk reduction reflects an increase in risk).

dards,[48] the diagnosis of VT and PE was based on clinical criteria alone, and case-allocation to treatment or control groups was suboptimal.

Nevertheless, in a recent report, there was a dramatic decrease in pulmonary or arterial embolism after the start of oral anticoagulant therapy, in people with dilated cardiomyopathy, which stood in sharp contrast to a high risk of recurrence when anticoagulants were stopped.[51(V)]

There are reports that low-dose heparin fails to prevent VT after pacemaker insertion.[52]

STROKE AND OTHER NEUROLOGICAL DISORDERS

Disabling stroke is followed by a high risk of developing VT, especially in the paralyzed leg, but most clinicians remain reluctant to use even low doses of anticoagulants to prevent VTE, because they fear to provoke intracranial bleeding.

A number of pilot studies have been done, however (Table 5), and are the subject of a recent overview.[53]

Venous thrombosis rates can be substantially reduced after stroke by low doses of unfractionated sc heparin, by LMWHs, or by heparinoids, although the latter may be superior: in a double-blind comparison, a low-molecular-weight heparinoid (Org 10172, or Lomoparan) gave significantly better results than standard low-dose heparin (5,000 u sc 12 hourly), without causing excess bleeding.[54(I)]

Computed tomography scanning has been used to show that anticoagulant prophylaxis does not increase the risk of subclinical infarct-related intracranial bleeding,[53,54] although the trials done to date have been too small to rule out a small to moderate effect.

Dextran 40 had no demonstrable effect on VT after cerebral infarction in a further small comparison (Table 5),[55(II)] while a randomized pilot study of low-dose-heparin in patients with intracerebral bleeding failed to alter the VT rate shown by blood pool scanning or the incidence of PE found at routine perfusion lung scanning.[56(II)]

In a sequence of trials from the McMaster University group,[57(I),58(I),59(I)] both intermittent leg compression and graded pressure compression stockings, prevented VT in patients admitted to hospital with a variety of intracranial pathologies, generally thought to contraindicate anticoagulant prophylaxis (stroke, subarachnoid haemorrhage, brain tumour and head injury, with or without surgery) and it is of some interest that a combination of graded pressure elastic stockings with intermittent leg compression (calf and thigh) was no more effective than the use of stockings alone (Table 6).[59]

GENERAL MEDICAL UNIT ADMISSIONS

Randomized trials suggest that both low-dose heparin (5,000 iu 8 hourly or 12 hourly sc) and a low-molecular-weight (LMW) heparin given sc once a day, can prevent asymptomatic calf VT in medical inpatients with heart failure or chest infection,[60] after admission to a medical ward or coronary care unit,[61] or following admission to a general medical unit when aged over 65 years (Table 7).[62(I)]

A direct comparison between low-dose standard heparin (5,000 u sc 8 hourly) and a LMW heparin (from Sandoz) given once daily sc, revealed identical VT rates in general medical inpatients expected to stay in bed for longer than 7 days, as measured by clinical examination, doppler ultrasound examination and impedance plethysmography.[63(I)]

Similarly, in a double-blind randomized study of medical inpatients aged over 65 years reported in abstract by the "Geriatric Enoxaparin Study Group", there was leg-scan evidence of VT in 9/207 patients (4.4%) given 20 mg/d of a LMW heparin, Enoxaparin, compared with 10/216 (4.6%) in patients given 5,000 u of unfractionated heparin sc twice-daily. In-hospital mortality and the frequency of bleeding were similar.[64]

Other preventive measures were also evaluated to a limited extent in a further leg-scan-based randomized trial where bedridden patients with lung disease were treated with 5,000 u of standard heparin sc 12 hourly (VT

Table 5
Leg Scan or Venogram Based Randomised VT Prevention Trials in Ischemic Stroke. Active Therapy Compared with Untreated Controls

Preventive Method	VT (Active)	VT (Control)	Risk Reduction	Reference
Low dose sc heparin	32/144 (22%)	117/161 (73%)	73% [60 to 82%]	McCarthy & Turner, 1986
Low dose heparin & dihydroergotamine	11/54 (20%)	23/53 (43%)	53% [4 to 77%]	Czechanowski & Heinrich, 1981
LMW Heparin or Heparinoid:				
Lomoparan	2/50 (4%)	7/25 (28%)	86% [31 to 97%]	Turpie et al, 1987
Fragmin	6/30 (20%)	15/30 (50%)	60% [80 to −3%]	Prins et al, 1989
Fragmin	15/52 (29%)	17/51 (33%)	13% [57 to −73%]	Sandset et al, 1990
CY222	0/15	12/15 (80%)	100%	Elias et al, 1990
Dextran 40	13/24 (54%)	13/26 (50%)	−8% [50 to −134%]	Mellbring et al, 1986

Table 6
Physical Methods of VT Prevention Evaluated Using Randomised Trials in Patients with Intracranial Pathology. Results of Fibrinogen Leg Scanning

Preventive Method	VT (Active)	VT (Control)	Risk Reduction	Reference
Intermittent calf compression	1/65 (1.5%)	12/63 (19%)	92% [38 to 99%]	Turpie et al, 1977
	8/103 (8%)	20/96 (21%)	63% [15 to 84%]	Turpie et al, 1979
graded pressure stockings	7/80 (9%)	16/81 (20%)	55% [82 to −9%]	Turpie et al, 1989
stockings + leg compression	7/78 (9%)		54% [81 to −12%]	

= 1/39), graded compression stockings (VT = 0/39), elastic bandages (VT = 4/33), or 0.5 gm aspirin 12 hourly (VT = 2/35); and all were associated with a significantly lower VT rate than that previously observed in an untreated but non-random control group (12/46 = 26%).[33]

The possible impact of VT prophylaxis on mortality in medical inpatients was examined in two more extensive trials.

In one open comparison, low doses of sc heparin appeared to reduce in-hospital mortality from 10.9% in untreated controls to 7.8% (p = 0.025) but the study design was seriously flawed: treatment allocation was based on 'odd' or 'even' medical record numbers, a significant bias led to more exclusions from the heparin group (32%, compared with 25% of controls; p < 0.01), such that only 411 of 669 people eligible for heparin actually received the drug, and it is unclear if the study size was determined in advance.[65(III)]

The preliminary report from a large placebo-controlled, double-blind, multicentre, randomized trial in 2,474 medical admissions aged over 40 years, and with limited mobility found the LMW heparin CY 216 (Fraxiparin) had no effect on 21-day mortality, as this was similar in the CY216 and placebo groups (10.1% and 10.3%), although prophylaxis was accompanied by non-significant trends towards less PE at autopsy and less VTE diagnosed clinically and/or at autopsy.[66]

CONCLUSIONS

Although epidemiologic surveys and autopsy studies show that more VT and PE arise in medical patients than after surgery, there have been few large-scale trials of VT prevention in medical patients.

Recommendations about prophylaxis therefore remain relatively insecure.

Nevertheless, it seems that low-dose sc heparin, LMW heparins, oral anticoagulants, graded pressure elastic stockings and intermittent leg compression are all effective, at least for preventing asymptomatic calf-vein thrombosis detected by ^{125}I-fibrinogen leg scanning.

After MI, the choice lies between low doses of sc heparin if the infarct is limited and uncomplicated, high doses of sc heparin (12,500 u twice-daily) when there is a need to prevent mural thrombosis, and iv heparin when the drug is given to maintain coronary artery patency.

For paralysis due to stroke or spinal injury, a low-molecular-weight heparin or heparinoid may be the preferred option, although graded pressure stockings or intermittent leg compression are also effective.

In elderly patients with heart failure, chest infection, or general immobility, the only advantage of sc LMW heparins over low doses of unfractionated heparin given sc 8 or 12 hourly, appears to be the convenience of once daily injection.

A recommendation for VT prevention in all hospital patients, medical or surgical, with more than one risk factor for VTE[67,68] has major cost implications,[20] and it is hard to see physicians moving away from selective prophylaxis until they see more extensive and broadly based studies of cost-effectiveness and safety in medical patients, based on large trials which measure the effects of various preventive measures on clinically significant disease (extensive VT, PE, fatal PE and overall mortality).

Table 7

Preventive Regimen	VT (Active)	VT (Control)	Risk Reduction	Reference
Standard Heparin:				
5,000 u 8 hrly sc	2/50 (4%)	13/50 (26%)	85% [32 to 97%]	Belch et al, 1981
5,000 u 12 hrly sc	2%	10%		Cade 1981
LMW heparin:				
Enoxaparin, 60 mg sc daily	4/132 (3%)	12/131 (9%)	67% [89 to −3%]	Dahan et al, 1986

Randomised leg scan based VT prevention trials where active therapy (standard heparin or low molecular weight [LMW] heparin) was compared with no treatment in general medical patients.

REFERENCES

1. Dismuke SE, Wagner EH. Pulmonary embolism as a cause of death. The changing mortality in hospitalized patients. JAMA 1986;255:2039–2042.

2. Hermann RE, Davis JH, Holden WD. Pulmonary ernbolism. A clinical and pathological study with emphasis on the effect of prophylactic therapy with anticoagulants. Am J Surg 1961;102:19–28.

3. Lindblad B, Sternby NH, Bergqvist D. Incidence of venous thromboembolism verified by autopsy over 30 years. Brit Med J 1991;302:709–711.

4. Hauch 0, Jorgensen LN, Khattar SC, et al. Fatal pulmonary embolism associated with surgery. An autopsy study. Acta Chir Scand 1990;156:747–749.

5. Nielsen HK, Bechgaard P, Nielsen PF, Husted SE, Geday E. 178 fatal cases of pulmonary embolism in a medical department. Acta Med Scand 1981;209: 351–355.

6. Sperry KL, Key CR, Anderson RE. Toward a population-based assessment of death due to pulmonary embolism in New Mexico. Hum Pathol 1990;21:159–165.

7. Nordstrom M, Lindblad B, Bergqvist D, Kjellstrom T. A prospective study of the incidence of deep-vein thrombosis within a defined urban population. J Intern Med 1992;232:155–160.

8. Anderson FA, Wheeler HB, Goldberg RJ, et al. A population-based perspective of the hospital incidence and case-fatality rates of deep vein thrombosis and pulmonary embolism. Arch Intern Med 1991;151:933–938.

9. Morrell MT, Dunnill MS. The post-mortem incidence of pulmonary embolisn in a hospital population. Brit J Surg 1968;55:347–352.

10. Coon WW. Risk factors in pulmonary embolism. Surg Gyne Obstet 1976;143:385–390.

11. Goldhaber Z, Savage DD, Garrison RJ, et al. Risk factors for pulmonary embolism. The Framingham Study. Am J Med 1983;74:1023–1028.

12. Havig O. Deep vein thrombosis and pulmonary embolism. Acta Chir Scand 1977; (Supplement) 478:1–120.

13. Anderson FA, Wheeler HB, Goldberg RJ, Hosmer DW, Forcier A, et al. Physician practice in the prevention of venous thromboembolism. Ann Intern Med 1991;115: 591–595.

14. Clarke CS, Otridge BW, Carney DN. Thromboembolism. A complication of weekly chemotherapy in the treatment of Non-Hodgkin's lymphoma. Cancer 1990;66:2027–2030.

15. Levine MN, Gent M, Hirsh J, et al. The thrombogenic effect of anti-cancer drug therapy in women with stage II breast cancer. N Engl J Med 1988;318:404–407.

16. Quinn DA, Thompson BT, Terrin ML, et al. A prospective investigation of pulmonary embolism in women and men. JAMA 1992; 268:1689–1696.

17. Devor M, Barrett-Connor E, Renvall M, Feigal D, Rarnsdell J. Estrogen replacement therapy and the risk of venous thrombosis. Am J Med 1992;92:275–282.

18. Wechsler B, Piette JC, Conard J, Du LTH, Bletry 0, et al. Les thromboses veineuses profondes dans la maladie de Behcet. Presse Med 1987;16:661–664.

19. Hughes GRV. The antiphospholipid syndrome: ten years on. Lancet 1993;342:341–344.

20. Anderson FA, Wheeler HB, Goldberg RJ, Hosmer DW. The prevalence of risk factors for venous thromboembolism among hospital patients. Arch Intern Med 1992; 152:1660–1664.

21. Cristal N, Stern J, Ronen M, Silverman C, Ho W, et al. Identifying patients at risk for thromboembolism. Use of 125I- labeled fibrinogen in patients with acute myocardial infarction. JAMA 1976;236:2755–2757.

22. Hayes MJ, Morris GK, Hampton JR. Lack of effect of bed rest and cigarette smoking on development of deep venous thrombosis after myocardial infarction. Brit Heart J 1976;38:981–983.

23. Maurer BJ, Wray R, Shillingford JP. Frequency of venous thrombosis after myocardial infarction. Lancet 1971;2:1385–1387.

24. Simmons AV, Sheppard MA, Cox AF. Deep venous thrombosis after myocardial infarction. Brit Heart J 1973;35:623–625.

25. Pandian NG, Kosowsky BD, Gurewich V. Transfemoral temporary pacing and deep vein thrombosis. Amer Heart J 1980;100:847–851.

(I)26. Emerson PA, Marks P. Preventing thromboembolism after myocardial infarction:effect of low dose heparin or smoking. Brit Med J 1977;1:18–20.

27. Handley AJ, Teather D. Influence of smoking on deep vein thrombosis after myocardial infarction. Brit Med J 1974;3:230–231.

28. Marks P, Emerson PA. Increased incidence of deep vein thrombosis after myocardial infarction in non-smokers. Brit Med J 1974;3:232–234.

29. Rentsch HP. Thromboembolische Komplikationen nach akuter Hemiplegien. Schweiz med Wschr 1987;117: 1853–1855.

30. Cope C, Reyes TM, Skversky NJ. Phlebographic analysis of the incidence of thrombosis in hemiplegia. Radiol 1973;109:581–584.

31. Warlow C, Ogston D, Douglas AS. Deep venous thrombosis of the legs after strokes. Brit Med J 1976;1: 1178–1183.

32. Kierkegaard A, Norgren L, Olsson C-G, Castenfors J, Persson G, et al. Incidence of deep vein thrombosis in bed-ridden non-surgical patients. Acta Med Scand 1987;222:409–414.

(III)33. Ibarra-Perez C, Lau-Cortes E, Colmenore-Zubiate S, et al. Prevalence and prevention of deep venous thrombosis of the lower extremities in high-risk pulmonary patients. Angiology 1988;39:505–513.

34. Gold G, Pervez N, Kropsky B, Neufeld R, Schwartz I, et al. Pulmonary embolism in the nursing home population: high frequency of autopsy in fernale residents. Arch Gerontol Geriatr 1992;14:117–122.

35. Lensing AWA, Hirsh J. 125I-fibrinogen leg scanning: reassessment of its role for the diagnosis of venous thrombosis in post-operative patients. Thrombos Haemostas 1993;69:2–7.

36. Anderson RE, Hill RB, Key CR. The sensitivity and specificity of clinical diagnosis during five decades. Toward an understanding of necessary fallibility. JAMA 1989;261:1610–1617.

37. Rao MG, Rangwala AF. Diagnostic yield from 231 autopsies in a community hospital. Am J Clin Pathol 1990; 93:486–490.

38. Hirsh J, Dalen JE, Deykin D, Poller L. Oral anticoagulants. Mechanism of action, clinical effectiveness, and optimal therapeutic range. Chest 1992;102 (Supplement):312S–326S.

39. Clagett CP, Anderson FA, Levine MN, Salzman EW, Wheeler HB. Prevention of venous thromboembolism. Chest 1992;102 (Supplement):391S–407S.

(I)40. Warlow C, Beattie AG, Terry G, Ogston D, Kenmure ACF, et al. A double-blind trial of low doses of subcutaneous heparin in the prevention of deep-vein thrombosis after myocardial infarction. Lancet 1973;1:934–936.

(I)41. Wray R, Maurer B, Shillingford J. Prophylactic anticoagulant therapy in the prevention of calf-vein thrombosis after myocardial infarction. N Engl J Med 1973;288: 815–817.

(I)42. Gallus AS, Hirsh J, Tuttle RJ, et al. Small subcutaneous doses of heparin in prevention of venous thrombosis. N Engl J Med 1973;288:545–551.

(I)43. Handley AJ, Emerson PA, Fleming PR. Heparin in the prevention of deep vein thrombosis after myocardial infarction. Brit Med J 1972;2:436–438.

(I)44. Pitt A, Anderson ST, Habersberger PG, Rosengarten DS. Low dose heparin in the prevention of deep vein thrombosis in patients with acute myocardial infarction. Amer Heart J 1980; 99:574–578.

(II)45. Handley AJ. Low-dose heparin after myocardial infarction. Lancet 1972;2:623–624.

(I)46. Turpie AGG, Robinson JG, Doyle DJ, et al. Comparison with high-dose with low-dose subcutaneous heparin to prevent left ventricular mural thrombosis in patients with acute transmural anterior myocardial infarction. N Engl J Med 1989; 320:352–357.

47. Eisenberg PR. Role of heparin in coronary thrombolysis. Chest 1992;101 (Supplement):131S-139S.

(III)48. Harvey WP, Finch CA. Dicumarol prophylaxis of thromboembolic disease in congestive heart failure. N Engl J Med 1950; 242:208–211.

(III)49. Anderson GM, Hull E. The effect of dicumarol upon the mortality and incidence of thromboembolic complications in congestive heart failure. Amer Heart J 1950;39: 697–702.

(III)50. Griffith GC, Stagnell R, Levinson DC, Moore FJ, Ware AG. A study of the beneficial effects of anticoagulant therapy in congestive heart failure. Ann Intern Med 1952;37:867–887.

(V)51. Kyrle PA, Korninger C, Gossinger H, et al. Prevention of arterial and pulmonary embolism by oral anticoagulants in patients with dilated cardiomyopathy. Thrombos Haemostas 1985;54:521–523.

52. Munch U, Mombelli G. Unwirksamkeit der Low-dose-Heparin-Prophylaxe bei Schrittmachereinbau. Schweiz med Wschr 1980;110:1125–1128.

53. Sandercock PAG, van den Belt AGM, Lindle RI, Slattery J. Antithrombotic therapy in acute ischemic stroke: an overview of the completed randomised trials. J Neurol Neurosurg Psychiatry 1993;56:17–25.

(I)54. Turpie AGG, Gent M, Cote R, et al. A low-molecular-weight heparinoid compared with unfractionated heparin in the prevention of deep vein thrombosis in patients with acute ischemic stroke. A randomized, double-blind study. Ann Intern Med 1992;117:353–357.

(II)55. Mellbring G, Strand T, Eriksson S. Venous thromboembolism after cerebral infarction and the prophylactic effect of Dextran 40. Acta Med Scand 1986;220:425–429.

(II)56. Dickmann U, Voth E, Schicha H, Henze T, Prange H, et al. Heparin therapy, deep-vein thrombosis and pulmonary embolism after intracerebral hemorrhage. Klin Wochenschr 1988;66:1182–1183.

(I)57. Turpie AGG, Gallus AS, Beattie WS, Hirsh J. Prevention of venous thrombosis in patients with intracranial disease by intermittent pneumatic compression of the calf. Neurology 1977;27:435–438.

(I)58. Turpie AGG, Delmore T, Hirsh J, et al. Prevention of venous thrombosis by intermittent sequential calf compression in patients with intracranial disease. Thrombos Res 1979;15:611–616.

(I)59. Turpie AGG, Hirsh J, Gent M, Johnson J. Prevention of deep vein thrombosis in potential neurosurgical patients. A randomized trial comparing graduated compression stockings alone or graduated compression stockings plus intermittent pneumatic compression with control. Arch Intern Med 1989;149:679–681.

60. Belch JJ, Lowe GD0, Ward AG, Forbes CD, Prentice CRM. Prevention of deep vein thrombosis in medical patients by low-dose heparin. Scot Med J 1981;26: 115–117.

61. Cade JF. High risk of the critically ill for venous thromboembolism. Crit Care Med 1982;10:448–450.

(I)62. Dahan R, Houlbert D, Caulin C, et al. Prevention of deep vein thrombosis in elderly medical in-patients by a low-molecular weight heparin: a randomized double-blind trial. Haemostasis 1986;16:159–164.

(I)63. Harenberg J, Kallenbach B, Martin U, et al. Randomized controlled study of heparin and low molecular weight heparin for prevention of deep-vein thrombosis in medical patients. Thrombos Res 1990;59:639–650.

64. Mottier D. Prophylaxis of deep vein thrombosis in medical geriatric patients. Thrombos Haemostas 1993; 69(Supplement):1115.

(III)65. Halkin H, Goldberg J, Modan M, Modan B. Reduction of mortality in general medical in-patients by low-dose heparin prophylaxis. Ann Intern Med 1982;96: 561–565.

66. Caulin C. The influence of CY 216 administration on hospital mortality of general medical in-patients. International collaborative double-blind study: methods and preliminary results. In: Breddin K, Fareed J, Samama M, eds. Fraxiparine. First international symposium. Analytical and structural data, pharmacology clinical trials. Stuttgart—New York: Schattauer, 1989: 147–152.

67. Lowe GD0, Greer IA, Dewar EP, et al. Risk of and prophylaxis for venous thromboembolism in hospital patients. Brit Med J 1992;305:567–574.

68. Nicolaides AN, Arcelus J, Belcaro G, et al. Prevention of venous thromboembolism. European consensus statement. Internat Angiol 1992;11:151–159.

9

Trauma

Michael Rud Lassen, Lars C. Borris

INTRODUCTION

Trauma is still a leading cause of death and morbidity in patients under the age of 40 years. Although some of these deaths are directly correlated with injury of vital organs, many patients die from pulmonary embolism (PE) and even more develop sequelae of deep-vein thrombosis (DVT), such as cor pulmonale, venous insufficiency, or chronic ulceration of the lower leg.

Trauma induces activation of the coagulation cascade, through the extrinsic pathway, due to liberation of tissue thromboplastin from soft tissue injury and fractures of the bones.[1] Hemostatic activation with subsequent increased fibrin formation is a basic defense mechanism against exsanguination after tissue trauma. Fibrin formation in the vascular system continues if it is not counteracted by natural anticoagulant mechanisms. Clinically, there may be signs and symptoms of microvascular thrombosis, DVT, and possible pulmonary embulus.

Patients with fracture of a long bone, and especially those with multiple trauma, are at high risk of developing thromboembolic complications.[2,3] Patients with spinal cord and/or head injury have similar risks. The present chapter is concerned only with orthopedic injuries (fractures); head and spinal cord injuries are covered in chapters 8 and 11, respectively.

One of the first studies on DVT after fracture of the long bones in the lower extremity, reported a 10% incidence.[4] Hjemstedt and Bergvall,[5(V)] in a later phlebographic study, showed an incidence of 45% DVT in two series. More recently, Geerts et al, investigated 443 traumatized patients in Canada, 349 of whom had an evaluable venogram; the overall incidence of 70% DVT in patients with fractures of the lower extremities.[6(III)] Incidence for special anatomical regions are shown in Table 1 and 2. These figures are consistent with the findings in another study of 39 multiple trauma patients who were confined to bed for 10 days or longer, showing venographically diagnosed DVT in 67% of the patients with fractures.[7(V)]

Clinical experience has provided evidence that plaster cast immobilization of the lower extremities is frequently associated with DVT. Immobilization, however, should not be considered as the sole pathogenic factor, since swelling, compression, and the type of trauma itself may also significantly influence the probability of thrombus formation. Kujath et al, reported an incidence of 18% DVT in patients with less intensive trauma of the lower legs who were treated by plaster casts.[8(I)] The thrombotic risk depended on the trauma, since only 12% of the patients with ligamental tears developed DVT, compared with 26% of the patients with fractures of the legs.

Multivariate analysis was done in the same Canadian database;[6] age, operation, transfusion, femoral and/or tibial fracture, and spinal injury were significant risk factors for the development of thromboembolic complications. Surprisingly, the Injury Severity Score (ISS) was not a risk factor for DVT. Many patients develop deep venous insufficiency after trauma of the lower extremities, due to silent DVT induced by the trauma itself or due to immobilization. In a study of 170 patients with fractures of the lower extremities, 23% developed symptoms suggestive of venous insufficiency seven to 12 years later, and development of ulcers was a common complication.[9]

In the absence of prophylaxis, 50% to 70% of patients develop DVT following fracture of the hip. In Scandinavia, the mortality rate is very high in these patients during the first months after the fracture.[10,11] An autopsy study showed PE in 46% and DVT in 83% of the patients who died after femoral neck fracture.[12] Both the trauma itself and the surgical treatment are responsible for development of DVT in traumatized patients. The preoperative incidence of DVT is 9% to 15% in patients with hip fracture.[12,13(V),14(III)]

From *Venous Thromboembolism: An Evidence-Based Atlas* edited by Russell Hull, Gary Raskob, Graham Pineo © 1996, Futura Publishing Co., Armonk, NY.

Table 1
Incidence of DVT Following Different Major Injuries

	Face/Chest/ Abdomen	Head	Spine	Lower Limb Orthopedic/ Pelvic
	n = 129	n = 91	n = 66	n = 183
DVT	65 (50%)	49 (54%)	41 (62%)	126 (69%)
Proximal DVT	19 (15%)	17 (19%)	18 (27%)	43 (23%)

DVT: Deep-Vein Thrombosis. By courtesy, William H. Geerts.

PREVENTION OF THROMBOEMBOLISM IN TRAUMATIZED PATIENTS

Prevention of thromboembolism in multiple traumatized patients has not been investigated to the same extent as in hip fracture patients; the recommendations given in this chapter are therefore mostly based on hip fracture studies, but the methods may be used in other types of trauma patients as well.

Oral Anticoagulants

The first published study using oral anticoagulation was the classic one by Sevitt and Gallagher (1959), including 300 elderly patients with hip fracture.[15(II)] The total mortality was reduced by 40%; of the patients who died in the treatment group, 8% died of PE, compared with 26% in the control group (no prophylaxis). These findings have been confirmed in other studies and by compilation of the results, a significant reduction of both mortality and incidence of thromboembolic complications is seen.[16(II),17(II),18(III),19(III),20(I),21(I)] Prophylactic treatment with oral anticoagulation must start before surgery, to be sufficiently protective.[22]

Oral anticoagulation in trauma patients, has been less used outside North America because of the risk of bleeding, and the need for laboratory monitoring.

Dextrans

After the introduction of dextran as a plasma expander, it became obvious that it also possessed an ability

Table 2
Occurrence of DVT in Patients with Fractures of the Lower Extremity

Type of Fracture	Incidence of DVT
Pelvic	62%
Femoral	78%
Tibial	83%
Ankle	67%

DVT: Deep-Vein Thrombosis.

to prevent thrombus formation.[23(III)] Seven placebo-controlled studies have been conducted in hip fracture patients, and dextran reduced the incidence of thromboembolic complications in five of them.[24(III),25(I),26(I),27(I),28(II),29(III),30(I)] Dextran had no antithrombotic effect in the two others.[28,29] Overall, dextran seems to have the same efficacy as oral anticoagulation, but without the need for laboratory monitoring. In one study, dextran caused less bleeding than oral anticoagulation.[31(III)] In combination with dihydroergotamine (DHE), a potent venoconstrictor, dextran decreased the incidence of DVT ten-times more than dextran alone;[32(I)] however, this result was not confirmed in two later studies.[33(II),34(II)] Furthermore, DHE is no longer recommended in traumatized patients because of severe adverse effects (vasospasm resulting in amputation of limbs and death).[35] Dextran is easy to administer, but there is a risk of allergic reactions, which, however, can be prevented by hapten inhibition. Due to the risk of fluid overload, dextran is not the ideal method of prophylaxis in elderly patients with cardiac disease.

Standard Heparin

Low-Dose Heparin (5000 IU × 2 or 3 times daily)

Low-dose heparin has been popular because it is very easy to administer and requires no monitoring. Many comparative studies in hip fracture patients have reported a significantly higher efficacy of low-dose heparin compared with no prophylaxis,[30(I),36(I),37(I),38(II),39(III),40(I),41(I)] even though no difference was found between low-dose heparin and placebo in four other studies.[42(III),43(I),44(II),45(III)] A meta-analysis[46] published in 1988 confirmed that low-dose heparin was more effective than no prophylaxis in the prevention of DVT; however, no significant influence on total mortality and incidence of fatal PE was demonstrated. In one study, low-dose heparin was less effective than warfarin;[47(III)] the methodology used, however, was weak. Low-dose heparin has been administered two and three times daily, but no comparison between the two regimens has been performed. A previous review showed that twice daily low-dose heparin was as effective as three times daily and caused fewer bleeding complications.[48]

Adjusted-Dose Heparin

The more cumbersome adjusted-dose heparin regimen in hip fracture patients was as effective as fixed low-dose heparin.[49(I)] The regimen is therefore not attractive, because of the need for daily measurement of activated partial thromboplastin time (APTT) for adjustment of the heparin dosage.

Low-Dose Heparin Combined with Dihydroergotamine

A combination of low-dose heparin and DHE has shown conflicting results in patients with hip fractures.

One study showed no difference between the combination and a placebo group,[50(II)] whereas others reported that it was as effective as dextran 70.[51(I),52(II)] The combination seems to have the same efficacy as dextran on total mortality and fatal PE,[53(II)] however, the use of the combination has almost stopped because of the adverse effects.[54]

Low-Molecular-Weight Heparin and Other New Compounds

Low-Molecular-Weight Heparin

Low-molecular-weight (LMW) heparin is a highly effective drug, manufactured from unfractionated standard heparin. Several different compounds are available. Currently, LMW heparin is the drug of choice for prevention of postoperative DVT in elective hip surgery (see chapter 6), but the documentation is not so extensive in trauma patients.

LMW heparin is more effective than placebo in hip fracture patients.[55(I),50(II)] In an uncontrolled study using LMW heparin (Enoxaparin 2 times 20 mg or 1 times 40 mg) a very low incidence of DVT (14%) was found.[56(V)] The results were conflicting in five studies that compared LMW heparin with low-dose heparin,[50,57,58,59(I),60(III)] but LMW heparin seems to be significantly more effective than Dextran 70. A recent study of 226 hip fracture patients reported DVT incidences of 15.5% on LMW heparin and 32.6% on Dextran 70,[61(I)] but there was no difference in total mortality. Further studies are needed, especially with respect to reduction in total mortality, such as has been demonstrated with the use of oral anticoagulants.[15]

LMW heparin has the advantage that only one daily subcutaneous injection is sufficient to prevent thrombosis. This opens the possibility of treating outpatients immobilized in plaster casts. In a study of 200 patients wearing plaster casts due to fractures or ligament injuries of the lower extremities, randomized to either injections of LMW heparin once daily or no prophylaxis, 5% of the patients in the LMW heparin group and 18% in the untreated group, developed DVT diagnosed by Ultrasonography with venographic verification.[8] Whether this regimen is possible for outpatients who have to administer one injection daily by themselves, is not yet solved, but no serious difficulties have so far been reported.

Low-Molecular-Weight Heparinoid

Low-molecular-weight heparinoid is, like heparin, a mixture of glycosaminglycans that are extracted from porcine intestinal mucosa. It consists mostly of heparan sulphate and dermatan sulphate.

Two studies have been performed with this compound. In a Scandinavian study of hip fracture patients, LMW heparinoid was significantly more effective than Dextran 70 in the prevention of postoperative DVT.[62(I)]

Warfarin is still used frequently in the United States, and a study was performed to compare the efficacy and safety of the heparinoid and warfarin in hip fracture patients. The treatment group the patients received heparionoid for the first seven days and then warfarin alone for 7 days; the control group received only warfarin for 14 days. Prophylaxis started before operation in both groups. In the heparinoid group, 7% of the patients developed verified DVT, compared with 21% in the control group.[63(I)]

No data are available for patients with multiple trauma.

Dermatan Sulphate

Thromboprophylaxis with dermatan sulphate, which was evaluated in a placebo-controlled study, showed a highly significant efficacy and safety profile.[64(I)] However, only limited data on the compound have been published so far. Further studies are required, especially in comparison with other effective regimens.

Mechanical Methods

In multiple trauma patients, particularly those with fractures of the lower limb, the use of mechanical devices (compression stockings or intermittent pneumatic compression boots) is not possible, though, they may be used in hip fracture patients. There is no clear evidence of the benefit of mechanical methods in hip fracture patients, but in neurosurgery, head injury, and spinal cord injury these methods are well documented and they are currently preferred if the bleeding risk is substantial (see chapters 8 and 11).

Anesthesia

There is a difference of opinion as to the choice of regional versus general anesthesia for surgery in traumatized patients, especially in hip fracture patients. If no other prophylactic method is used, regional anesthesia seems to give a better antithrombotic effect.[65] If an effective pharmacological method is used, however, studies in elective hip surgery have shown that there is no additional effect of regional anesthesia. A recent meta-analysis on the subject identified 13 randomized studies which showed a clearly beneficial effect of regional versus general anesthesia with regard to the incidences of DVT.[66] On the other hand, the analysis did not demonstrate any effect on mortality or bleeding complications. Currently, no conclusions can be made with respect to differences in mortality between the two techniques during the surgical repair of hip fractures.

Surgery

Multiple traumatized patients have been treated for many years by immediate life-saving surgery, while treatment of soft tissue damage and fractures was delayed. It has become increasingly apparent during the last 10 years, that early stabilization of musculoskeletal injuries in association with blunt trauma has decreased systemic complications, including thromboembolism.[67] The introduction of medullary rods has improved the options of stabilization of even very comminuted fractures of the long bones, thus allowing early mobilization of the patients, compared with the previous long-term bed confinement with traction (so-called horizontal crucifixion). Furthermore, the incidence of fracture complications appears not to increase after early operative fracture fixation, compared with conservative fracture management or late fracture fixation.[68]

Conclusion

New epidemiologic research has shown that patients suffering multiple trauma have a high risk of thromboembolic complications. However, very little information is available on prevention of thromboembolism in this group of patients. This might be because the group is very heterogeneous and difficult to study. The treatment of these patients is a multidisciplinary effort involving different medical specialities. Patients suffering multiple injuries are often young and healthy, in contrast to patients with hip fracture. In the latter group, several methods have been studied to prevent complications. They include oral anticoagulants, dextrans, low-dose unfractionated heparin, LMW heparin, LMW heparinoids, and dermatan sulphate. LMW heparin or LMW heparinoid are the methods of choice in the European countries because they are easy to administer, do not require laboratory monitoring, and are clinically safe.

The documentation for the use of thromboprophylaxis in multiple trauma patients is not sufficient, but LMW heparin has been shown to be safe in hip fracture patients and especially in spinal cord injuries,[69(I)] for which reason it seems appropriate also to use the drug in traumatized patients; however, more data are required. In patients immobilized in plaster casts due to minor fractures or ligamental tears, it seems reasonable to use LWM heparin in the prevention of thromboembolism as long as the plaster cast is worn. When thromboprophylaxis is used in fracture patients, administration must start as soon after the trauma as possible.

Studies on total mortality are urgently needed with the modern prophylactic methods to reach the ultimate aim in the prevention of thromboembolic complications; the avoidance of death.

REFERENCES

1. Sørensen JV, Rahr HB, Jensen HP, Borris LC, Lassen MR, et al. Markers of coagulation and fibrinolysis after fractures of the lower extremities. Thromb Res 1992;65:479–486.

2. European Consensus Statement. Prevention of venous thromboembolism. Int Angiol 1992;11:151–159.

3. National Institutes of Health Consensus Development Conference Statement: Prevention of venous thrombosis and pulmonary embolism. JAMA 1986;256:744–749.

4. Bauer G. Thrombosis following leg injuries. Acta Chir Scand 1944;90:229–248.

(V)5. Hjemstedt Å, Bergvall U. Incidence of thrombosis in patients with tibial fractures. A phlebographic study. Acta Chir Scand 1968;134:209–218.

(III)6. Geerts WH, Code KI, Jay RM, et al. A prospective study of venous thromboembolism after major trauma. N Engl J Med 1994;331:1601–1606.

(V)7. Kudsk KA, Fabian TC, Baum S, Gold RE, Mangiante E, et al. Silent deep vein thrombosis in immobilized multi-trauma patients. Am J Surg 1989;158:515–519.

(I)8. Kujath P, Spannagel U, Habscheid W, Schindler G, Weckbach A. Thromboseprophylaxe bei ambulanten patienten mit verletzungen der unteren Extremität. Dtch Med Wschr 1992;117:6–10.

9. Schiøttz-Christensen B, Juul N, Borris LC, Lassen MR. Incidence of venous insufficiency following fractures of the long bones of the lower extremities. Thromb Haemostas 1991;65:1357.

10. Jensen JS, Tøndevold E. Mortality after hip fractures. Acta Orthop Scand 1979;50:161–167.

11. Dahl E. Mortality and life expectancy after hip fractures. Acta Orthop Scand 1980;51:163–170.

12. Freeark RJ, Boswick J, Fardin R. Posttraumatic venous thrombosis. Arch Surg 1967;95:567–575.

(V)13. Stevens J, Fardin R, Freeark RJ. Lower extremity thrombophlebitis in patients with femoral neck fracture. J Trauma 1968;8:527–532.

(III)14. Roberts TS, Nelsson CL, Barnes CL, Ferris EJ, Holder JC, et al. The preoperative prevalence and postoperative incidence of thromboembolism in patients with hip fractures treated with dextran prophylaxis. Clin Orthop 1990;255:198–203.

(III)15. Sevitt S, Gallagher NG. Prevention of venous thrombosis and pulmonary embolism in injured patients: Atrial of anticoagulant prophylaxis with phenindione in middle-aged and elderly patients with fractured necks of femur. Lancet 1959;ii:981–989.

(II)16. Borgström S, Greitz T, van der Linden W, Molin J, Rudics I. Anticoagulant prophylaxis of venous thrombosis in patients with fractured neck of the femur—a controlled clinical trial using venous phlebography. Acta Chir Scand 1965;129:500–508.

(II)17. Eskeland G, Solheim K, Skjörten F. Anticoagulant prophylaxis, thromboembolism and mortality in elderly patients with hip fractures. A controlled clinical trial. Acta Chir Scand 1966;131:16–29.

(III)18. Salzman EW, Harris WH, DeSanctis RW. Anticoagulation for prevention of thromboembolism following fractures of the hip. N Engl J Med 1966;275:122–130.

(III)19. Hamilton HW, Crawford JS, Gardiner JH, Wiley AM. Venous thrombosis in patients with fracture of the upper end of the femur—a phlebographic study of the effect of prophylactic anticoagulation. J Bone Joint Surg 1970;52-B:268–289.

(I)20. Morris GK, Mitchell JRA. Warfarin sodium in prevention of deep venous thrombosis and pulmonary embolism in patients with fractured neck of the femur. Lancet 1976;ii:869–872.

(I)21. Powers PJ, Gent M, Jay RM, et al. A randomized trial of less intense postoperative warfarin or aspirin therapy in the prevention of venous thromboembolism after surgery for fractured hip. Arch Intern Med 1989;149: 771–774.

22. Myhre HO, Storen EJ, Auensen CA. Pre- or post-operative start of anticoagulant prophylaxis in patients with fractured hips? J Oslo City Hosp 1973;23:15–23.

(III)23. Koekenberg LJL. Experimental use of macrodex as a prophylaxis against postoperative thrombembolism. Bull Soc Int Chir 1962;21:501–512.

(III)24. Ahlberg Å, Nylander G, Robertson , Cronberg S, Nilsson IM. Dextran in prophylaxis of thrombosis in fractures of the hip. Acta Chir Scand 1968; 387(Suppl):83–85.

(I)25. Johnsson SR, Bygdeman S, Eliasson R. Effect of dextran on postoperative thrombosis. Acta Chir Scand 1968; 387(Suppl):80–82.

(I)26. Myhre HO, Holen A. Dextran or warfarin in the prophylaxis of venous thrombosis. Nord Med 1969;82: 1534–1538.

(I)27. Stadil F. Prophylaxis of postoperative venous thrombosis with Dextran-70. Ugeskr Laeger 1970;132:1817–1820.

(II)28. Daniel WJ, Moore AR, Flanc C. Prophylaxis of deep vein thrombosis (DVT) with dextran 70 in patients with a fractured neck of the femur. Aust NZ J Surg 1972;41: 289.

(III)29. Darke SG. Ilio-femoral venous thrombosis after operation on the hip—a controlled trial using dextran 70. J Bone Joint Surg 1972;54-B:615–620.

(I)30. Bergqvist D, Efsing HO, Hallböök T, Hedlund T. Thromboembolism after elective and post-traumatic hip surgery—a controlled prophylactic trial with dextran 70 and low-dose heparin. Acta Chir Scand 1979; 145:213–218.

(III)31. Bergqvist E, Bergqvist D, Bronge A, Dahlgren S, Lindqvist B. An evaluation of early thrombosis prophylaxis following fractures of the femoral neck. Acta Chir Scand 1972;138:689–693.

(I)32. Bergqvist D, Lindblad B, Ljungström K-G, Persson NH, Hallböök T. Does dihydroergotamine potentiate the thromboprophylactic effect of Dextran 70? A controlled prospective study in general and hip surgery. Br J Surg 1984;71:516–521.

(II)33. Fredin H, Lindblad B, Jaroszewski H, Bergqvist D. Prevention of thrombosis after hip fracture surgery. Acta Chir Scand 1985;151:681–684.

(II)34. Rørbœk-Madsen M, Jakobsen BW, Pedersen J, Sørensen B. Dihydroergotamine and the thromboprophylactic effect of dextran 70 in emergency hip surgery. Br J Surg 1988;75:364–365.

35. Mattsson E, Öhlin A, Balkfors B, Fredin HO, Nilsson P, et al. Lower limb vasospasm and renal failure during postoperative thromboprophylaxis. Case report. Eur J Surg 1991;157:289–292.

(I)36. Gallus AS, Hirsh J, Tuttle RJ, et al. Small subcutaneous doses of heparin in prevention of venous thrombosis. New Engl J Med 1973;288:545–551.

(I)37. Galasko CSB, Edwards DH, Fearn CBD'A, Barber HM. The value of low dosage heparin for the prophylaxis of thromboembolism in patients with transcervical and intertrochanteric femoral fractures. Acta Orthop Scand 1976;47:276–282.

(II)38. Morris GK, Mischell JRA. Preventing venous thromboembolism in elderly patients with hip fractures: studies of low-dose heparin, dipyridamol, aspirin and flurbiprofen. Br Med J 1977;1:535–537.

(III)39. Xabregas A, Gray L, Ham JM. Heparin prophylaxis of deep vein thrombosis in patients with a fractured neck of the femur. Med J Aust 1978;1:620–622.

(I)40. Rogers PH, Walsh PN, Marder VJ, et al. Controlled trial of low-dose heparin and Sulfinpyrazone to prevent venous thromboembolism after operation on the hip. J Bone Joint Surg 1978;60-A:758–762.

(I)41. Lahnborg G. Effect of low-dose heparin and dihydroergotamine on frequency of postoperative deep-vein thrombosis in patients undergoing post-traumatic surgery. Acta Chir Scand 1980;146:319–322.

(III)42. Checketts RG, Bradley JG. Low-dose heparin in femoral neck fractures. Injury 1974;6:42–44.

(I)43. Moskovitz PA, Ellenberg SS, Feffer Hl, et al. Low-dose heparin for prevention of venous thromboembolism in total hip replacement and surgical repair of hip fractures. J Bone Joint Surg 1978;60-A:1065–1070.

(II)44. Svend-Hansen H, Bremerskov V, Gotrik J, Ostri P. Low-dose heparin in proximal femoral fractures—failure to prevent deep-vein thrombosis. Acta Orthop Scand 1981;52:77–80.

(III)45. Montrey JS, Kistner RL, Kong AYT, et al. Thromboembolism following hip fracture. J Trauma 1985;25: 534–537.

46. Collins R, Scrimgeour A, Yusuf S, Peto R. Reduction in fatal pulmonary embolism and venous thrombosis by perioperative administration of subcutaneous heparin—overview of results of randomized trials in general, orthopedic, and urologic surgery. N Engl J Med 1988;318:1162–1173.

(III)47. Alho A, Strangeland L, Rottingen J, Wiing JN. Prophylaxis of venous thromboembolism by aspirin, warfarin and heparin with hip fractures—a prospective clinical study with cost-benefit analysis. Ann Chir Gyn 1984;73:225–228.

48. Bergqvist D. Prophylaxis of postoperative thromboembolic complications with low-dose heparin. An analysis of different administration intervals. Acta Chir Scand 1979;145:7–14.

(I)49. Taberner DA, Poller L, Thomson JM, Lemon G, Weighill FJ. Randomized study of adjusted versus fixed low dose heparin prophylaxis of deep vein thrombosis in hip surgery. Br J Surg 1989;76:933–935.

(II)50. Lassen MR, Borris LC, Christiansen HM, et al. Prevention of thromboembolism in hip fracture surgery. Comparison of low-dose heparin and low-molecular-weight heparin combined with dihydroergotamine. Arch Orthop Traum Surg 1989;108:10–13.

(I)51. Bergqvist D, Efsing EF, Hallböök T, Lindblad B. Prevention of postoperative thromboembolic complications—a prospective comparison between Dextran 70, dihydroergotamine heparin and a sulphated polysaccharide. Acta Chir Scand 1980;146:559–568.

(II)52. Fredin HO, Nillius SA, Bergqvist D. Prophylaxis of deep vein thrombosis in patients with fracture of the femoral neck. Acta Orthop Scand 1982;53:413–417.

(II)53. Gruber UF. Prevention of fatal pulmonary embolism in patients with fractures of the neck of the femur. Surg Gyn Obst 1985;161:37–42.

54. Borris LC, Lassen MR, Christiansen HM, Møller-Larsen F, Knudsen VE, et al. Circulatory insufficiency during thrombosis prophylaxis with heparin/dihydroergotamine. Effect or side-effect? Ugeskr Laeger 1988;150: 1682–1683.

(I)55. Jørgensen PS, Knudsen JB, Broeng L, et al. The thromboprophylactic effect of a low molecular weight heparin (Fragmin®) in hip fracture surgery. A placebo controlled study. Clin Orthop 1992;278:95–100.

(V)56. Barsotti J, Dabo B, Andreu J, et al. Étude comparative de deux posologie d'heparine de faible masse moléculaire PK 10 169 dans la prévention des accidents thromboemboliques au cours du traitment de 103 fractures du col du fémur. J Mal Vasc 1987;12:96–98.

57. Breyer HG, Al-Therib J, Bacher P, Werner B. Thrombosis prophylaxis with low molecular weight heparin in trauma surgery. Thromb Res 1986;(Suppl VI):84.

58. Korninger C, Schlag G, Poigenfürst J, et al. Randomized trial of low molecular weight heparin (LMWH) versus low dose heparin/acenocoumarin (H/AC) in patients with hip fracture—thromboprophylactic effect and bleeding complications. Thromb Haemostas 1989;62: 187.

(I)59. Monreal M, Lafoz E, Navarro A, et al. A prospective double-blind trial of a low molecular weight heparin once daily compared with conventional low-dose heparin three times daily to prevent pulmonary embolism and venous thrombosis in patients with hip fracture. J Trauma 1989;29:873–875.

(III)60. Pini M, Tagliaferri A, Manotti C, Lasagni F, Rinaldi E, et al. Low molecular weight heparin (Alfa LMWH) compared with unfractionated heparin in prevention of deep-vein thrombosis after hip fractures. Int Angiol 1989;8:134–139.

(I)61. Oertli D, Hess P, Durig M, et al. Prevention of deep vein thrombosis in patients with hip fractures: Low molecular weight heparin versus dextran. World J Surg 1992; 16:980–984.

(I)62. Bergqvist D, Kettunen K, Fredin H, et al. Thromboprophylaxis in patients with hip fractures: a prospective, randomized, comparative study between Org 10172 and dextran 70. Surgery 1991;109:617–622.

(I)63. Gerhart TN, Yett HS, Robertson LK, Lee MA, Smith M, et al. Low-molecular-weight heparinoid compared with warfarin for prophylaxis of deep-vein thrombosis in patients who are operated on for fracture of the hip. J Bone Joint Surg 1991;73-A:494–502.

(I)64. Agnelli G, Casmi B, DiFilippo P, et al. A randomised, double-blind, placebo-controlled trial of dermatan sulphate for prevention of deep vein thrombosis in hip fracture. Thromb Haemost 1992;67:203–208.

65. Prins MH, Hirsh J. A comparison of general anesthesia and regional anesthesia as a risk factor for deep vein thrombosis following hip surgery: a critical review. Thromb Haemost 1990;64:497–500.

66. Sorenson RM, Pace NL. Anesthetic technic during surgical repair of femoral neck fractures. A meta-analysis. Anesthesiology 1992;77:1095–1104.

67. Bone LB. Musculoskeletal management in the multiple injured patient. In: Borris LC, Lassen MR, Bergqvist D, Eds. The Traumatized Patient—with Special Reference to Systemic Complications. Aalborg: The Venous Thrombosis Group 1992:26–29.

68. Ejstrud P, Sorensen JVS. Early osteosynthesis of fractures of the lower extremities in patients with multiple trauma. Ugeskr Laeger 1993;155:1202–1206.

(I)69. Green D, Lee MY, Lim AC, et al. Prevention of thromboembolism after spinal cord injury using low molecular weight heparin. Ann Intern Med 1990;113: 571–574.

10

Prevention of Venous Thromboembolism in Spinal Cord Injury

David Green

INTRODUCTION

Spinal cord injury is a major traumatic event which is associated not only with a risk of paralysis but also with a high incidence of thrombosis. In 16.3% of patients there are signs and symptoms of thromboembolism, and laboratory evidence of deep-vein thrombosis (DVT) in anywhere from 47% to 100%.[1] In past years, massive pulmonary embolism (PE) was the cause of death in one-third of patients[2], and occurred with an overall frequency of 3%.[3] More recently, 61 of 854 deaths in spinal cord injured patients were attributed to PE, giving a standardized mortality ratio of 46.9.[4] Thus, it is apparent that modern methods of thromboprophylaxis have not eliminated this complication, although some progress has been made. In this chapter, the risk factors for thromboembolism in spinal cord injury will be reviewed, and various methods of prophylaxis discussed.

RISK FACTORS FOR THROMBOSIS IN SPINAL CORD INJURY

Patients with spinal cord injury are generally subjected to two major traumas: the injury per se and the surgical procedures necessary for spine stabilization. These two stresses are usually separated by only a few days, providing little opportunity for antithrombotic homeostatic mechanisms to come into play. Thus, the increased levels of clotting factors and platelets stimulated by the initial injury persist for several weeks,[5,6] and antithrombin III levels are probably depressed as well. In addition, fibrinolysis is depressed,[7] probably secondary to an increase in plasminogen activator inhibitor-1.[8]

In addition to these effects on clotting factors, platelets, and fibrinolysis, there are also important alterations in blood vessels and blood flow that predispose to thrombosis. Extrinsic presssure on immobilized or para-

lyzed limbs may result in injury to fragile venous structures providing a nidus for thrombus propagation.[9] There are also fluid shifts from intravascular to extravascular spaces as a result of immobilization and the hypoalbuminemia characteristic of the postoperative period. The resultant hyperviscosity is aggravated by the hyperfibrinogenemia that accompanies stress and trauma.

Lastly, there are patient characteristics that predispose to thrombosis. Obesity is an established risk factor for PE,[10] and this is also true in spinal cord injured patients.[11] Furthermore, in spinal cord injury the location and severity of the lesion predict risk. In a recent survey, it was reported that pulmonary emboli were more common in patients with quadraplegia than paraplegia and complete than incomplete motor paralysis.[4] A delay in the development of spasticity may also predispose to thrombosis[12], perhaps by prolonging the period of venous stasis. There are also data indicating that patients undergoing repeated surgical procedures are at greater risk of having DVT, and that thrombi occur more frequently when there is a delay in initiating thromboprophylaxis.[13(V)] In summary, multiple risk factors coalesce in the spinal cord patient to promote thrombosis (Table 1).

METHODS OF PROPHYLAXIS

Methods that are customarily used to prevent DVT in medical or surgical patients are either inappropriate, dangerous, or ineffectual in the spinal cord injured patient. For example, early ambulation, which is very effective in postoperative subjects, is obviously impossible in paralyzed persons. The use of standard anticoagulants, such as heparin and warfarin, carries a risk of spinal hematoma or bleeding from other injuries sustained at the time of the spine trauma. When anticoagulants are given in low dose, so as to preclude bleeding, they are usually ineffectual

From *Venous Thromboembolism: An Evidence-Based Atlas* edited by Russell Hull, Gary Raskob, Graham Pineo © 1996, Futura Publishing Co., Armonk, NY.

Table 1
Risk Factors for Thrombosis in Spinal Cord Injury

Patient Characteristics
   Obesity
   Complete motor paralysis
   High level of injury
   Absence of spasticity
   Concurrent infections
Hypercoagulability
   Hyperviscosity due to fluid shifts and hyperfibrinogenemia
   Increased platelet aggregability
   Increased factor VIII and von Willebrand factor
   Decreased antithrombin III
   Impaired fibrinolysis due to increase in plasminogen activator
     inhibitor-1.
Management Issues
   Delay in instituting thromboprophylaxis
   Extrinsic pressure on immobile limbs
   Repeated surgical procedures
   Delays in mobilization

(see below). Therefore, only a few modalities of thromboprophylaxis have been attempted in this population.

To assess the baseline incidence of thrombosis in spinal cord injury, we conducted a study in the early 1980s. This investigation reported that positive radiofibrinogen tests developed in 78% of patients, and the presence of thrombosis was confirmed in all instances by venography.[14(II)] Thrombi were detected as early as 4 days after injury, and the peak incidence occurred on days 7 to 10. We then instituted prophylaxis with calf compression leggings.

Compression Leggings

The rationale underlying the use of compression devices is that the rhythmic squeezing of muscle groups will improve venous emptying. It is also possible that they may stimulate vascular endothelium to release tissue plasminogen activator, thereby enhancing fibrinolysis. Leggings have been used effectively in patients having neurosurgery, and orthopedic, urologic, and gynecologic surgery.[15] In the spinal cord injured patient, we found that calf compression leggings decreased the frequency of DVT from 78% to 40%.[14] However, when the leggings were removed at day 30, in order to give patients more freedom to participate in rehabilitation therapies, several subjects developed venous thrombosis. It was concluded that compression leggings are partially effective in thromboprophylaxis and may be used early after spinal cord injury, but should probably be combined with other measures to provide better long-term protection.

Anticoagulant Therapy

Unfractionated Heparin. Low-dose heparin has been the standard thromboprophylactic agent in general surgery patients for many years. In spinal cord injured subjects, 5000 U of heparin given every 12 hours was compared with no specific prophylaxis in 17 and 15 patients respectively.[16(III)] Only one patient in each group was reported to have thrombosis, as detected by impedance plethysmography. This low frequency of thrombosis may have been due to the fact that patients with incomplete injuries were entered into the trial, and that impedance plethysmography does not detect distal thrombi. In contrast, Merli et al,[17(I)] used the fibrinogen uptake test and venography to confirm the presence of thrombosis, and all patients with negative uptake tests had bilateral ascending venography at the end of the trial (4 weeks). Eight of 17 patients receiving no specific prophylaxis, and 8 of 16 given heparin, 5000 U every eight hours, had evidence of thrombosis (p = not significant). In a retrospective study, Kulkarni et al,[13] reviewed the results of low-dose heparin (5000 U every eight hours) given to 97 consecutive patients for 12 weeks. Clinical evidence of thromboembolism was found in 26 patients (17 deep-vein thrombosis and 9 pulmonary emboli). These studies suggest that low-dose heparin is not a very effective antithrombotic agent in these patients.

To determine whether higher doses of heparin would be more effective, we conducted a trial comparing low-dose heparin (5000 U every 12 hours) with doses of heparin adjusted to prolong the activated partial thromboplastin time (APTT) into the upper normal range.[18(I)] In the spinal cord injured patients, doses averaging 13,200 U administered every 12 hours were required to maintain the APTT at one and one-half times control values. One third of patients receiving low-dose heparin had thrombosis as compared to only 7% treated with the adjusted-dose regimen (p<0.05). However, the adjusted-dose heparin was difficult to implement; laboratory tests had to be performed regularly, and doses adjusted often. More importantly, seven of 29 subjects treated with this regimen had bleeding sufficiently severe as to require withdrawal of the heparin. These problems with unfractionated heparin led us to study the use of low-molecular-weight heparin in the spinal cord injured.

Low-Molecular-Weight Heparin. Low-molecular-weight heparins are heparin fragments that retain the ability to potentiate antithrombin III's inhibition of activated factor X, but do not bind to thrombin.[19] They have been shown to be effective in patients undergoing general surgery and orthopedic surgery, and in some trials bleeding has been less than when unfractionated heparin was given.[20] They would therefore appear to be promising agents for thromboprophylaxis in the spinal cord injured.

In a randomized trial, we assigned patients with complete motor paralysis to either unfractionated heparin, 5000 U every eight hours or LMWH, 3500 U once daily.[21(I)] Subjects were excluded if they had concomitant head injuries, hemothorax, long bone fractures, or cardiovascular instability. Patients were begun on prophylaxis within 72 hours of injury, and were followed with clinical examinations, venous ultrasound testing, and venography when the other measures suggested possible thrombosis. After 41 patients had been entered, the trial was stopped because seven patients in the unfractionated heparin group had either thromboembolism or bleeding, whereas no events had occurred in those receiving LMWH (p = 0.006). All subsequent patients were assigned to treatment with LMWH.

Since the completion of that trial, LMWH has been the principal thromboprophylactic agent in more than 60 patients.[22] Treatment has been given for eight weeks. During that interval, DVT has occurred in six subjects and fatal PE in one. Only one patient has had bleeding, and this was in the immediate postoperative period. In comparison with all our previous trials using unfractionated heparin, the frequency of thromboembolism has been less (10% vs 20%, p = 0.15), and bleeding significantly reduced (1% vs 11%, p = 0.04). In view of the very low risk of bleeding with the currently used doses of LMWH (3500 U daily), it is possible that the dose could be safely increased to improve efficacy. For example, 75 U/kg has been given for prophylaxis in patients undergoing hip surgery with a relatively low incidence of bleeding.[23]

Oral Anticoagulants. Oral anticoagulation with warfarin has not been popular in patients with spinal cord injury for a number of reasons: 1) there is a delay in the onset of its action; 2) it is difficult to maintain adequate prophylaxis in patients requiring frequent invasive procedures such as tracheostomy, spinal fusion, and central line placement; 3) many patients have poor nutritional status and are receiving antibiotic therapy, which increase sensitivity to warfarin. In a trial performed 20 years ago, Silver[24(V)] demonstrated good efficacy but frequent bleeding. In this trial, the intensity of treatment was higher than that currently recommended. It is possible that warfarin therapy could be used to advantage in the weeks or months after injury, if the International Normalized Ratio (INR) were maintained in the presently recommended range of two to three.

Combined Modalities for Prophylaxis

In the studies described above using anticoagulants, more than half the spinal cord injured patients screened were excluded because of concerns about bleeding. Therefore, investigators have sought to combine modalities that do not cause bleeding, such as leg compression boots, with doses of heparin that are associated with a low risk of bleeding. In one study, only one of 21 patients treated with a combination of external pneumatic compression boots, graduated elastic hose, and heparin, 5000 U every 12 hours, had thrombosis as detected by the radiofibrinogen uptake test and confirmed by venography.[25(IV)] In another study, the investigators showed that

administering electrical stimulation of the calf muscles combined with heparin, 5000 U every eight hours, decreased the thrombosis rate from 50% with heparin alone to 7% with the combined therapy.[26] Combinations of LMWH and leggings may also improve efficacy, but have not yet been reported.

Vena Caval Filters

Superficially, it would appear that the problem of PE in spinal cord injury could be forestalled by early placement of an inferior vena caval filter. However, while such filters are generally effective,[26,27] they have a number of drawbacks including propagation of ileofemoral thrombi into the vena cava, malpositioning or migration of the filter, and the need for venography and technical expertise in filter placement.[28] Their use should be restricted to patients who are intolerant of anticoagulants because of active bleeding or coagulopathy.

SUMMARY

In early 1992 a consensus conference was held on the subject of DVT in spinal cord injury, and the proceedings published later that year in *Chest*.[29] The conference participants recommended that all spinal cord injury patients with motor paralysis should receive thromboprophylaxis.[30] It was suggested that mechanical compression devices should be applied for the first 10 to 14 days after injury. Anticoagulants could be given beginning 72 hours after injury to augment the antithrombotic effect of the compression leggings, and continued until there was a return of motor function, or for at least 8 to 12 weeks. Suggested anticoagulants included unfractionated heparin in doses of 5000 U every 12 hours or warfarin in doses to achieve an INR of two to three. However, when the compression devices were discontinued, the dose of heparin would need to be increased to prolong the aPTT to the high normal range. Alternatively, LMWH could be administered in doses of 50 to 75 U/kg. Vena caval filters were recommended for those patients who could not be fitted with compression hose because of lower extremity fractures, and in those in whom anticoagulants were contraindicated because of sites of active bleeding, thrombocytopenia or other coagulopathy, renal or hepatic failure, or the need for multiple surgical procedures.

REFERENCES

1. Weingarden SI. Deep vein thrombosis in spinal cord injury: overview of the problem. Chest 1992;102(Suppl):636S-639S.
2. Tribe CR. Causes of death in early and late stages of paraplegia. Paraplegia 1963;1:19–47.
3. Walsh JJ, Tribe CR. Phlebo-thrombosis and pulmonary embolism in paraplegia. Paraplegia 1965;3:209–213.

4. DeVivo MJ, Black KJ, Stover SL. Causes of death during the first 12 years after spinal cord injury. Arch Phys Med Rehabil 1993;74:248–254.

5. Rossi EC, Green D, Rosen JS, et al. Sequential changes in factor VIII and platelets preceding deep vein thrombosis in patients with spinal cord injury. Br J Haematol 1980;45:143–151.

6. Myllynen P, Kammonen M, Rokkanen P, et al. The blood FVIII:Ag/F.VIII:C ratio is an early indicator of deep vein thrombosis during post-traumatic immobilization. J Trauma 1987;27:287–280.

7. Katz RT, Green D, Sullivan T, Yarkony G. Functional electric stimulation to enhance systemic fibrinolytic activity in spinal cord injury patients. Arch Phys Med Rehabil 1987;68:423–426.

8. Petaja J, Myllynen P, Rokkanen P, et al. Fibrinolysis and spinal injury: relationship to post-traumatic deep vein thrombosis. Acta Chir Scand 1989;155:241–246.

9. Mammen EF. Pathogenesis of venous thrombosis. Chest 1992 (Suppl);102:640S–644S.

10. Goldhabver SZ, Savage DD, Garrison RJ, et al. Risk factors for pulmonary embolism: the Framingham study. Am J Med 1983;74:1023–1028.

11. Green D, Twardowski P, Wei R, Rademaker AW. Fatal pulmonary embolism in spinal cord injury. Chest 1994;105:853–855.

12. Waring WP, Kaunas RS. Acute spinal cord injury and the incidence of clinically occurring thromboembolic disease. Paraplegia 1991;29:8–16.

(V)13. Kulkarni JR, Burt AA, Tromans AT, Constable PDL. Prophylactic low dose heparin anticoagulant therapy in patients with spinal cord injury: a retrospective study. Paraplegia 1992;30:169–172.

(II)14. Green D, Rossi EC, Yao JST, et al. Deep vein thrombosis in spinal cord injury : effect of prophylaxis with calf compression, aspirin, and dipyridamole. Paraplegia 1982;20:227–234.

15. Caprini JA, Arcelus JI, Traverso CI, et al. Low molecular weight heparins and external pneumatic compression as options for venous thromboembolism prophylaxis: a surgeon's perspective. Sem Thromb Hemostas 1991;17:356–366.

(III)16. Frisbee JH, Sasahara AA. Low dose heparin prophylaxis for deep venous thrombosis in acute spinal cord injury patients: a controlled study. Paraplegia 1981;19:343–345.

(I)17. Merli GJ, Herbison GJ, DiTunno JF, et al. Deep vein thrombosis: prophylaxis in acute spinal cord injured patients. Arch Phys Med Rehabil 1988;260:1255–1258.

(I)18. Green D, Lee MY, Ito VY, et al. Fixed-vs adjusted-dose heparin in the prophylaxis of thromboembolism in spinal cord injury. JAMA 1988;260:1255–1258.

19. Hirsh J, Levine MN. Low molecular weight heparin. Blood 1992;79:1–17.

20. Green D, Hirsh J, Heit J, Prins M, Davidson B, Lensing AWA. Low molecular weight heparin: a critical; analysis of clinical trials. Pharmacol Reviews. 1994;46:89–109.

(I)21. Green D, Lee MY, Lim AC, et al. Prevention of thromboembolism after spinal cord injury using low-molecular weight heparin. Ann Intern Med 1990;113: 571–574.

22. Green D, Chen D, Chmiel JS, et al. Prevention of thromboembolism in spinal cord injury: role of low molecular weight heparin. Arch Phy Med Rehabil. 1994;75:290–292.

(I)23. Hull RD, Raskob G, Pineo G, et al. A comparison of subcutaneous low-molecular-weight heparin with warfarin sodium for prophylaxis against deep-vein thrombosis after hip or knee implantation. N Engl J Med 1993;329:1370–1376.

(V)24. Silver JR. The prophylactic use of anticoagulant therapy in the prevention of pulmonary embolism in 100 consecutive spinal cord injury patients. Paraplegia 1974;12: 188–196.

(IV)25. Merli GJ, Crabbe S, Doyle L, et al. Mechanical plus pharmacological prophylaxis for deep vein thrombosis in acute spinal cord injury. Paraplegia 1992;30:558–562.

26. Jarrell B, Posuniak E, Roberts J, et al. A new method of management using the Kim-Ray Greenfield filter for deep venous thrombosis and pulmonary embolism in spinal cord injury. Surg Gynecol Obstet 1983;157: 316–320.

27. Merli GJ. Management of deep vein thrombosis in spinal cord injury. Chest 1992;102(Suppl):652S–657S.

28. Balshi J, Cantelmo N, Menzoian J. Complications of caval interruption by Greenfield filter in quadriplegics. J Vasc Surg 1989;9:558–562.

29. Green D, (ed.). Deep vein thrombosis in spinal cord injury. Chest 1992;102(Suppl):633S–663S.

30. Green D, Hull RD, Mammen EF, Merli GJ, Weingarden SI, et al. JST. Deep vein thrombosis in spinal cord injury: summary and recommendations. Chest 1992;102 (Suppl):633S–635S.

SECTION III

Diagnosis of Venous Thrombosis

11

Clinical Features of Deep Venous Thrombosis

Russell D. Hull, Graham F. Pineo

INTRODUCTION

The clinical diagnosis of venous thrombosis is inaccurate, because the clinical findings are both insensitive and nonspecific.[1-6] The sensitivity of clinical diagnosis is low because many potentially dangerous venous thrombi are clinically silent, because they are nonobstructive and not associated with inflammation of the vessel wall or of the perivascular tissues. The specificity of clinical diagnosis is low, because the symptoms or signs of venous thrombosis can all be caused by nonthrombotic disorders.

The differential diagnosis in patients who present with clinically suspected venous thrombosis includes ruptured Baker's cyst, cellulitis, muscle tear, muscle cramp, hematoma, external compression, heart failure, and the postphlebitic syndrome. In some patients, the cause of pain, tenderness, and even swelling remains uncertain and is presumed to be due to inflammation of other soft tissues of the leg. Because of its nonspecificity, it is unacceptable to use clinical diagnosis to make management decisions in patients suspected of venous thrombosis.

CLINICAL DIAGNOSIS

The approach to patients who present or are referred with a possible clinical diagnosis of deep-vein thrombosis (DVT) can be considered in three categories. The first and largest group is patients whose clinical manifestations are compatible with, but not diagnostic of, venous thrombosis. These patients should be investigated by accurate objective tests. In the second group, a diagnosis of venous thrombosis can be excluded by careful history and examination, either because the clinical features clearly indicate the presence of another disorder (e.g., arthritis, nerve compression, cellulitis), or the features are totally inconsistent with a diagnosis of DVT. The third, and least common group, is patients who present with phlegmasia cerulea dolens whose clinical features are so characteristic of venous thrombosis that a diagnosis can be confidently made on clinical grounds.

Although careful documentation of symptoms and signs in patients with clinically suspected DVT is not helpful for diagnosing DVT in the majority of patients, it is of value for identifying the underlying disorders which mimic venous thrombosis, once such a diagnosis has been excluded by obtaining a negative result with an objective test (e.g., in patients with clinically suspected muscle strain or tear or ruptured Baker's cyst, it may be impossible to exclude venous thrombosis unless an objective test is performed). (Table 1)

The unreliability of clinical diagnosis has been demonstrated by numerous studies comparing clinical findings with the results of objective testing[1-10,86]. We have now evaluated over 1,000 patients with clinically suspected venous thrombosis by venography at our institution. Approximately 70% of all patients investigated did not have venous thrombosis and 30% did have deep venous thrombosis. The prevalence of venous thrombosis was lower (only 20%) in patients who were nonhospitalized at the time of presentation. Of those patients who did have venous thrombosis, 90% were in the proximal venous segments and only 10% confined to the deep calf veins. The most common clinical symptoms were pain, tenderness, and swelling. Pain occurred in 50% of the patients with thrombosis, but was not a useful differentiating symptom because it also occurred in 50% of patients who did not have thrombosis. Other clinical features including night cramps, redness, or cyanosis and dilated veins were relatively uncommon and occurred with approximately equal frequency in patients with and without thrombosis. Of interest were the findings that some patients with calf-vein thrombosis had pain and tenderness which extended above the knee.

From *Venous Thromboembolism: An Evidence-Based Atlas* edited by Russell Hull, Gary Raskob, Graham Pineo © 1996, Futura Publishing Co., Armonk, NY.

Evaluation of Symptoms and Signs of Venous Thrombosis

Pain and Tenderness

The severity of these clinical features bears no relationship to the size or extent of thrombosis. Pain and tenderness associated with calf-vein thrombosis are usually localized to the calf, but may extend along the anterior and medial aspects of the thigh and into the groin. Patients with proximal-vein thrombosis may have pain which is localized to the calf or to thigh or buttock. Patients with proximal-vein thrombosis may also have more diffuse pain and tenderness of the calf and thigh.

The pain of venous thrombosis is not characteristic. It may be an ache or a cramp—sharp, dull, severe, or mild.

A number of techniques have been used for eliciting tenderness. The most reliable is to examine the patient in the horizontal position with the knees slightly flexed. The site of maximum pain and tenderness should be determined by careful palpation after the rest of the leg has been carefully examined. Examination should be systematic and include palpation over the posterior tibial veins, the peroneal, popliteal, superficial femoral, common femoral, and iliac veins. Pain and tenderness located away from these regions suggest that these features are not due to venous thrombosis.

The course of pain and tenderness is highly variable. It frequently improves with bed rest and particularly with elevation of the leg, but may recur when the patient becomes mobile and may be falsely attributed to recurrence of venous thrombosis. The pain often disappears after treatment with heparin, but this improvement may be due to the effect of concomitant bed rest.

Swelling

Swelling is due to edema which may be caused either by obstruction of large proximal veins or by inflammation

Table 1
The Alternative Diagnosis in 87 Consecutive
Patients with Clinically Suspected Venous
Thrombosis and Negative Venograms*

Diagnosis	Patients (%)
Muscle strain	24
Direct twisting injury to leg	10
Leg swelling in paralyzed limb	9
Lymphangitis, lymphatic obstruction	7
Venous reflux	7
Muscle tear	6
Baker's cyst	5
Cellulitis	3
Internal abnormality of knee	2
Unknown	26

* The diagnosis was made once venous thrombosis had been excluded by the finding of a negative venogram.

of perivascular tissues. The swelling may be marked and associated with obvious pitting edema, or it may be mild and only detected as increased tissue turgor of calf muscles, which can be appreciated by carefully palpating the relaxed calf. When swelling is due to obstruction of a large proximal vein, it usually occurs distal to the site of obstruction and may be painless, while swelling due to inflammation is usually localized to the site of thrombosis and is associated with pain and tenderness.

Swelling usually subsides when the leg is elevated, however, it frequently recurs during early ambulation and may persist for weeks or months or never entirely subside, particularly in patients with iliofemoral-vein thrombosis.

Homan's Sign

Discomfort in the upper calf on forced dorsiflexion of the foot (Homan's sign) is a time-honored sign of venous thrombosis. It is both insensitive and nonspecific, being present in less than one third of the symptomatic patients with objectively documented DVT and in more than 50% of symptomatic patients who do not have venous thrombosis.

Venous Distension and Prominence of Subcutaneous Vessels

Venous dilatation is a relatively uncommon and nonspecific manifestation of acute venous thrombosis. Prominence of superficial veins was recorded in 17% of symptomatic patients studied with venographically proven thrombosis and in approximately 20% of patients without thrombosis.

When venous distension occurs, it is often a feature of major vein obstruction and usually disappears when the leg is elevated and when new collateral channels form. The distended veins are tense when the affected leg is dependent, and empty slowly as the leg is elevated. Collateral vessels become evident within a few days of major vein obstruction, and appear as prominent, superficial vessels in the region of the groin, anterior abdominal wall, and around the knee. With time, these collateral vessels become tortuous and varicose. Abnormal collaterals over the anterior abdominal wall can be identified because the flow in them is from below upward, whereas veins normally present in the lower part of the anterior abdominal wall drain downward into the proximal portion of the long saphenous vein in the groin.

Discoloration

In patients with venous thrombosis, the leg may be pale, cyanosed, or a reddish-purple color. Marked pallor is an uncommon sign which may occur in the early stages of acute iliofemoral-vein thrombosis; it is thought to be caused by arterial spasm. Cyanosis is caused by impaired venous return and stagnant anoxia and occurs in patients with obstructive iliofemoral-vein thrombosis. Although cyanosis usually subsides over a period of days, it may recur or become more marked, particularly in the calf and ankle, during mobilization and may persist for weeks, months, or even years. Rarely, the leg may be diffusely red, hot, and inflamed due to marked perivascular inflammation, and when this occurs it may be difficult to differentiate from cellulitis.

Phlegmasia Alba Dolens

This is a term used to describe the "milk" leg or white leg caused by iliofemoral-vein thrombosis with associated arterial spasm. The pulses may be weak or absent and the leg is cold. There may be relatively little swelling in the early stages, but as the spasm wears off, the leg becomes swollen and takes on a mottled blue appearance.

Phlegmasia Cerulea Dolens

This is the term used to describe the marked swelling and cyanosis which occurs with obstructive iliofemoral-vein thrombosis. The cyanosis is caused by extensive venous obstruction which, in its most severe form, not only involves most of the deep veins of the leg including the iliofemoral, superficial femoral, and popliteal veins, but also the long saphenous veins and the venous tributaries that drain into the deep venous system. The obstruction to flow caused by venous occlusion and severe edema may impair arterial inflow and so produce marked tissue ischemia. The leg is very painful, swollen, cyanosed, and frequently covered with multiple petechial hemorrhages. The patient may be hypotensive due to marked pooling of blood in the affected leg and there may be a mild thrombocytopenia due probably to platelet consumption. These features usually gradually subside when the patient is treated with heparin and confined to bed with the leg elevated. Occasionally, however, the cyanosis may progress to venous gangrene, and rarely the affected leg may require amputation unless the obstruction is rapidly removed by thrombectomy.

Palpable Cord

When a vessel which is easily palpable becomes thrombosed, it may be felt as an obvious cord.

The palpable cord of superficial phlebitis is readily distinguished from that found in DVT by its immediate subcutaneous location and/or by its anatomical site.

This is an uncommon sign and it may be difficult to differentiate a venous cord from edema or hemorrhage of the calf muscle.

Differential Diagnosis of Symptoms and Signs of Venous Thrombosis

Careful clinical documentation and follow-up often uncover one of the following alternative diagnoses in approximately 70% of patients with clinically suspected venous thrombosis who have negative findings by objective tests.[86]

In many of these, the clinical diagnosis of the alternative condition only becomes obvious on follow-up after venous thrombosis has been excluded by objective testing.

Differential Diagnosis of Pain and/or Tenderness

(a) Muscle Strain or Trauma: Muscle ache may occur when the leg muscles have been subjected to unusual types or amounts of activity. Pain usually occurs in the calf, but may also involve the thigh. There may be tenderness which at times can be quite severe. There is usually no swelling, but occasionally after very marked muscle exertion the leg muscles may feel tense, heavy, and turgid and may be associated with some calf and ankle swelling.

(b) Muscle Tear: Fibers of the gastrocnemius or plantaris muscle may be torn as a result of sudden contraction of calf muscles during plantar flexion. Typically, the muscle tear occurs when the foot is suddenly flexed against resistance, for example, when the individual begins to run. There is a sudden severe pain in the back of the leg which may simulate a direct blow to the calf muscles. Examination reveals local tenderness and it may be possible to palpate the localized swelling caused by hematoma. If there is a complete muscle tear or muscle avulsion at its attachment to the tendon, or tendon rupture, it may be possible to palpate the gap produced by the tear.

After a number of days, a bruise may appear either in the posterior aspect of the medial malleolus or in the anteromedial part of the leg, but his is not invariable. Pain and tenderness may continue for a number of days or even weeks and may be very severe, particularly during any activity involving plantar flexion.

(c) Direct Muscle or Leg Trauma: Direct muscle trauma sustained during a vigorous sporting activity or during an accident may produce delayed pain and swelling due to hematoma formation and inflammation. This can present considerable diagnostic difficulty, since venous thrombosis is a well-recognized complication of leg trauma.

(d) Spontaneous Muscle Hematoma: Occasionally, patients who are being treated with anticoagulants develop pain and swelling of the leg without obvious trauma or following mild trauma. It may be difficult to decide if these symptoms are caused by hemorrhage or recurrent venous thrombosis.

(e) Arterial Insufficiency: Arterial insufficiency is not usually confused with venous thrombosis because the clinical features of the two conditions are sufficiently distinctive.

(f) Neurogenic Pain: Compression of the sciatic nerve or lateral cutaneous nerve of the thigh produces leg pain which is easily differentiated from venous thrombosis.

(g) Ruptured Baker's Cyst: When a Baker's cyst or popliteal cyst ruptures, the fluid contents track down the tissue planes between the calf muscle and produce an inflammatory response to pain, tenderness, heat, and swelling, which may simulate the clinical features of acute venous thrombosis. In most cases, there is a history of arthritis of the knee or of traumatic or operative injury to the knee. Occasionally, this condition may occur without a past history of knee trauma or arthritis or there may be intermittent pain or swelling in the region of the popliteal fossa months or years preceding the acute episode. On examination of the knee, there may be evidence of arthritis or previous surgery or trauma and there may be a fullness of popliteal fossa on the affected side. The diagnosis can be readily established by arthrography, but since venous thrombosis and ruptured Baker's cyst may occur in the same patient, it may be necessary to specifically exclude venous thrombosis before attributing the acute clinical features to a ruptured Baker's cyst.

(h) Arthritis of the Knee or Ankle Joint or Achilles Tendonitis: Deep pain and swelling produced by arthritis of the knee or ankle or by inflammation of Achilles tendon may be occasionally confused with venous thrombosis.

(i) Inflammation of Other Tissues in the Legs: Cellulitis, lymphangitis, vasculitis, myositis, and panniculitis may produce pain and tenderness of the leg. These conditions can usually be differentiated from venous thrombosis on clinical grounds alone when they are fully developed, but they may occasionally be confused with venous thrombosis in their early stages or if they are atypical.

(j) Varicose Veins: Patients with varicose veins frequently have pain and tenderness in the calf when they have been standing for a period of time. Occasionally, an obvious superficial varicose vein becomes inflamed and thrombosed and the pain is more severe. When these clinical features occur in association with more diffuse pain in the calf or with edema of the leg, it may be difficult to exclude an associated DVT without performing objective diagnostic tests.

(k) Pregnancy and Patients Taking the Oral Contraceptive Pill: Pain and tenderness in the leg may occur in pregnancy or in individuals taking an estrogen-containing oral contraceptive pill. Occasionally, the pain and tenderness in pregnant patients are associated with quite marked swelling of the calf or thigh which may be unilateral. In many cases, these symptoms and signs are not due to venous thrombosis. The cause of pain and tenderness is uncertain, but may be due to venous dilation caused by estrogens, to inflammation of the vein wall without associated thrombosis, or to muscle cramps. Unilateral leg swelling occurring in pregnancy may also be caused by compression of the iliac vein by the enlarged uterus.

Differential Diagnosis of Leg Swelling With or Without Associated Pain and Tenderness

A number of conditions other than venous thrombosis can produce edema or swelling of the leg with or without associated pain and tenderness.

Compression Of the Iliac Vein

External compression of the iliac vein by tumor, hematoma, or abscess may be impossible to differentiate from acute iliofemoral-vein thrombosis on clinical grounds alone. The noninvasive tests such as plethysmography and Doppler ultrasound are frequently positive, and even a venogram may be misinterpreted as being positive (falsely) if either a cutoff or abnormal collaterals are accepted as evidence of deep venous thrombosis. Definitive differentiation between acute venous thrombosis and external compression can be made when the venogram shows either a characteristic smooth symmetrical indentation characteristic of the external compression, or an intraluminal filling defect characteristic of acute thrombosis.

Compression of the left common iliac vein by the right common iliac artery may produce chronic swelling which is usually painless, or it may produce acute exacerbations of swelling which last for hours or days and then either completely or only partly subside.[11] The leg swelling which may be intermittent is thought to be due to impaired venous return which occurs as a result of fibrosis and narrowing of the left common iliac vein where it is crossed by the iliac artery.

The Postphlebitic Syndrome

Typically, patients with the postphlebitic syndrome have long-standing symptoms of swelling associated with an ache in the calf which occurs on standing or leg exercise. Some of these patients present with repeated episodes of more severe swelling and pain which may be associated with calf tenderness, and, in these, it may be difficult to exclude a complicating acute venous thrombosis as the cause of the symptoms.[12] The majority of episodes of acute pain, tenderness, and swelling which occur in patients with the postphlebitic syndrome are not caused by acute venous thrombosis and do not require anticoagulant treatment. These acute exacerbations are probably caused by progressive venous dilatation which produces further valvular incompetence and so results in a sudden increase in venous pressure in the calf veins.

Leg Immobilization

Swelling may occur in patients who have their leg immobilized in a plaster cast for a number of weeks or months or who have limb paralysis either because of stroke, paralytic poliomyelitis, or spinal cord injury. Not all of the episodes of swelling are caused by venous thrombosis, although it is well recognized that thrombosis frequently complicates leg immobilization. The mechanism of swelling is uncertain, but may be due to alterations in venous tone or capillary permeability.

Leg Inflammation

Inflammatory conditions of the leg such as cellulitis, panniculitis, erythema nodosum, and severe myositis may cause diffuse swelling, but these can usually be differentiated from venous thrombosis because of other associated characteristic features.

Lymphedema

Leg swelling is a characteristic feature of impaired lymphatic drainage. In its most severe form, lymphedema is nonpitting and brawny, but milder forms of lymphedema may be pitting. When lymphedema occurs as a result of a congenital defect in the lymphatic channels, it is rarely difficult to differentiate from venous thrombosis, but when it is acquired as a result of trauma to the lymphatic vessels which may occur after hip surgery, leg fracture, or from compression of major lymphatic channels by leg plaster—it may be impossible to distinguish it from edema caused by venous obstruction without performing objective tests.

Lipedema

This condition occurs in females often becoming obvious in adult life. The leg swelling is due to accumulation of subcutaneous fat and is, therefore, chronic and not associated with pitting or signs of inflammation. It is readily distinguished from edema caused by venous thrombosis by examination of the leg.

Self-Induced Edema

Occasionally, factitious syndromes may simulate venous thrombosis. Pain, tenderness, and swelling may be produced by self-inflicted injury to the legs, by application of a venous tourniquet, or by other bizarre mechanisms.

REFERENCES

1. Hull R, Raskob G, Leclerc J, Jay R, Hirsh J. The diagnosis of clinically suspected venous thrombosis. Clin Chest Med 1984;5:439.
2. Haeger K. Problems of acute deep venous thrombosis. I. The interpretation of signs and symptoms. Angiology 1969;20:219.
3. Kakkar VV, Howe CT, Flanc C, Clarke MB. Natural history of postoperative deep vein thrombosis. Lancet 1969;2:230.
4. Johnston KW, Kakkar VV. Plethysmographic diagnosis of deep vein thrombosis. Surg Gynecol Obstet 1974;139:41–44.
5. McLachlin J, Richard T, Paterson JC. An evaluation of clinical signs in the diagnosis of venous thrombosis. Arch Surg 1962;85;738.
6. Nicolaides AN, Kakkar VV, Field ES, Renney JTG. The origin of deep vein thrombosis: a venographic study. Br J Radiol 1971;44:653.
7. Barnes RW, Collicott PE, Mozersky DJ, Sumner DS, Strandness DE. Non-invasive quantitation of maximum venous outflow in acute thrombophlebitis. Surgery 1972;72:971–979.
8. Hull R, Hirsh J, Sackett DL, et al. Clinical validity of a negative venogram in patients with clinically suspected venous thrombosis. Circulation 1981;64:622–625.
9. Lensing AWA, Hirsh J, Buller HR. Diagnosis of venous thrombosis. In: Colman RW, Hirsh J, Marder VJ, Salzman EW, eds. Hemostasis and thrombosis: basic principles and clinical practice. Third edition. Philadelphia: JB Lippincott Co., 1994:1297-1321.
10. Wells PS, Hirsh J, Anderson DR, et al. Accuracy of clinical assessment of deep-vein thrombosis. Lancet 1995;345:1326-1330.
11. Verhaeghe R. Iliac vein compression as an anatomical cause of thrombophilia: Cockett's syndrome revisited. Thrombosis and Haemostasis 1995;74(6):1398-1401.
12. Hull R, Carter C, Jay R, et al. The diagnosis of acute recurrent deep-vein thrombosis: A clinical challenge. Circulation 1983;67:901-906.

12

The Diagnosis of Venous Thromboembolism: An Overview

Edwin J.R. van Beek and Jan W. ten Cate

INTRODUCTION

Pulmonary embolism (PE) is one of the most feared complications in hospitalized patients. Deep-vein thrombosis (DVT) and PE have been shown to be closely linked by both postmortem and radiographic studies.[1,2] Later studies demonstrated that half or more of all patients with DVT developed, often clinically silent, pulmonary emboli,[3(I)] while DVT can be venographically detected in 70% to 80% of patients with proven PE.[4] Hence, the term venous thromboembolism (VTE) is currently used for both DVT and PE to acknowledge the fact that we are dealing with one clinico-pathological entity.[5(I)]

Although exact figures are not available, estimates of the incidence of VTE may be calculated from official statistics derived from death certificates. Using these data, Lilienfeld et al, estimated that, in the period of 1980 to 1984, the death rate in the United States for white males and females was four and three per 100,000 respectively, whereas these rates were seven and five per 100,000 for nonwhite males and females respectively.[6] However, the interpretation of these data is often difficult because many diagnoses on death certificates rely solely on clinical diagnosis, which is unreliable in VTE. Furthermore, only one cause of death is allowed which leaves contributing PE often unmentioned. For these reasons, data derived from death certificates must be classified as unreliable.

An alternative source for incidence estimates are discharge diagnosis and case-notes of patients who were diagnosed as having PE. Morrell et al, analyzed 853 patients using a special screening method, while a 97% postmortem rate was obtained in their hospitals.[7] An incidence of 4 to 20 per 1000 inpatients, depending on the age and surgical background of the patient, was reported. Similarly, using discharge diagnoses, a recent study found declining numbers of patients who were dis-

charged with the diagnosis PE (80 per 100,000 in 1979 to 50 per 100,000 in 1984).[8] These data are retrospective, and consequently the diagnostic process may be incomplete. Furthermore, the population studied consists of inpatients who are often more prone to thromboembolism due to operations or underlying illness. Therefore, extrapolation to the general population is not possible.

Many postmortem studies have been performed.[2,9–15] However, the findings vary greatly due to differences in autopsy rates, patient selection, and the techniques used to detect PE. Large macroscopic emboli are unlikely to be missed at postmortem examination, but the rate of PE will rise considerably if microscopic techniques are used. An incidence of pulmonary emboli as low as 12% and as high as 64% have been reported.[9,11] Furthermore, PE is often unrelated or merely contributing to the death of the patient, and there are no clear criteria to distinguish fatal from nonfatal PE in these studies.

A limited number of studies have evaluated the incidence of VTE following discharge from hospital. Incidence varies with types of patients studied (i.e., surgical or nonsurgical, underlying disorders, etc.), and ranges from 7.8% (45% developed after discharge) to 30% (70% developed after discharge).[16–18] A recent, retrospective study evaluated the incidence of symptomatic PE in 19161 operated and 9792 nonoperated patients.[19] The incidence was 0.31% while patients were hospitalized, while a further 0.10% developed after discharge. The incidence was significantly higher in operated patients than in conservatively treated patients (0.42% versus 0.10% respectively).

Few studies have ascertained the incidence of VTE in the general population. This is mainly due to the difficulty of obtaining objective diagnostic tests in the out-of-hospital setting. Gjöres used a questionnaire and case-notes to obtain an incidence of 2.5% for clinically suspected DVT in 15980 persons.[21] In a longitudinal

From *Venous Thromboembolism: An Evidence-Based Atlas* edited by Russell Hull, Gary Raskob, Graham Pineo © 1996, Futura Publishing Co., Armonk, NY.

study which prospectively assessed an 11-year period, it was estimated that there was an overall annual incidence of 0.24 and 1.22 per 1000 inhabitants for PE and DVT, respectively.[21] Kierkegaard was the first to use objective diagnostic tests (phlebography) in the diagnosis of DVT in a community study, and found an incidence of one per 1000 inhabitants per year.[22] More recently, in a community-wide study in which case-notes in 16 short-stay hospitals were assessed, an average overall incidence of DVT alone of 0.48 per 1000 was found, while this was 0.23 per 1000 for PE with or without deep venous thrombosis.[23] From a questionnaire among physicians in the Netherlands, an annual incidence of 2.6 patients with clinically suspected PE per 1000 inhabitants was calculated, which supports the previous studies.[24]

The validity of incidence estimates of VTE can be disputed in many instances. However, the annual incidence for DVT and PE in the general population of the western world may be estimated at 1 and 0.5 per 1000 respectively.

Having established that VTE is one clinical entity, and that it is a frequent clinical problem with considerable mortality, why is it important to correctly identify patients with the disease from those without? Firstly, only 30% of all patients with clinical symptoms suggesting VTE will have their diagnosis objectively demonstrated. Secondly, one aims to prevent mortality and morbidity associated with PE. Treating VTE with anticoagulants reduces the risk of fatal outcome approximately fifteen-fold, which makes the prevention and detection of VTE essential.[6-7] Thirdly, anticoagulants are related to considerable morbidity and mortality.[25] Hence, justification for putting a patient at risk of bleeding complications is required, both from a legal and an ethical point of view. Finally, correct identification of patients who do not require anticoagulant therapy results in considerable costs-savings.[26]

This chapter gives an overview of the diagnostic methods for the detection of deep venous thrombosis. Furthermore, it will discuss the role that various techniques for the diagnosis of DVT may play in the diagnostic management of VTE.

DIAGNOSTIC METHODS FOR DEEP VENOUS THROMBOSIS

Several diagnostic techniques are available for the detection of deep venous thrombosis. However, only a limited number of diagnostic modalities may be of interest for the purpose of diagnosing VTE. These are: contrast venography, impedance plethysmography, compression B-mode ultrasonography and Doppler ultrasonography.

One has to distinguish several patient categories to allow proper interpretation and evaluation of results to take place. Firstly, patients may show signs and symptoms of DVT. Secondly, patients may be asymptomatic for venous thrombosis (as will often be the case in post-operative patients). Finally, patients with a previous DVT may show recurrence of signs and symptoms. The use of tests for DVT for a large part depends on the patient category involved. We will summarize the clinical results of several studies which evaluated the diagnostic tests in the respective patient categories.

CONTRAST VENOGRAPHY

Contrast venography is generally regarded as the gold standard for the diagnosis of DVT.[27,28] Ascending venography is employed to visualize the deep venous system from the calf veins up to the common iliac veins by injecting radio-opaque contrast medium into a dorsal foot vein. Visualization may be improved by using sufficient quantities of contrast medium, by obtaining antero-posterior and oblique views and by tilting of the table with the patient in a semierect position. Either separate films of the calf, knee, thigh and pelvic region or single whole-leg films may be used.[28,29] Deep venous thrombosis is diagnosed if intraluminal filling defects or persistent nonfilling of segments of the deep venous system is seen in at least two projections.

Unfortunately, a 4% to 12% inadequacy rate has been reported for venography.[30,31(I),32(I)] Furthermore, interobserver variability varies from 2% to 10%.[29,33] Finally, due to its invasive nature and the use of contrast media, venography cannot be performed in patients with renal failure, a history of a reaction to contrast media, or patients who are generally in poor condition. Contrast venography may be used in both symptomatic and asymptomatic patients, as well as in patients with recurrent signs of DVT.

Hull et al, performed the only management study of venography in 160 patients with clinically suspected deep venous thrombosis.[34(I)] In this study, anticoagulants were withheld in patients with normal venograms. In the 3-month follow-up period, two of those patients (1.3%) developed DVT, and no patient died or developed clinically overt PE. Although the study showed the relative safety of withholding anticoagulants in patients with normal venograms, the 95% confidence interval of the deep venous thrombosis rate is 0.15% to 4.44%. Furthermore, venography took place in a specialized center, and inadequacy rates were probably lower than one would expect in less experienced centers. This may imply that the gold standard, contrast venography, is not necessarily fail-proof in the correct identification of patients with deep venous thrombosis in less equipped or less specialized centers.

IMPEDANCE PLETHYSMOGRAPHY

Impedance plethysmography (IPG) is a noninvasive technique which reflects volume changes of the leg which are produced by inflating and deflating an air cuff.

Impedance plethysmography has been extensively evaluated and several venography controlled studies have shown high accuracy for the detection of proximal venous thrombosis.[35(II),36(I),37(I)]

In a Canadian study by Hull and colleagues, 922 patients with suspected deep venous thrombosis were studied using IPG as the initial test.[35(I)] In 834 patients a normal IPG was found, and 645 patients were subsequently randomized for either serial IPG (317 patients) or a combination of IPG and legscanning (328 patients). Anticoagulants were withheld in all patients with persistent normal test results, while abnormal test results were confirmed by venography. During the one-year follow-up period, only one of 634 patients (0.16%) with initial normal IPG findings developed PE. In 90 of 95 patients with initially abnormal IPG results, venography confirmed DVT (positive predictive value 95%).

Two studies by Huisman et al, showed the safety of serial IPG in the management of symptomatic outpatients with suspected DVT.[32(I),36(I)] In one study, 426 consecutive outpatients underwent serial IPG testing (days 1, 2, 5, and 10).[32(I)] In 289 patients IPG remained normal, and anticoagulants were withheld. During follow-up only one patient (0.3%) developed PE. In the remaining 137 patients, IPG results were abnormal on day 1 (117; 85%), day 2 (12; 9%), day 5 (6; 4%) and day 10 (2; 2%), respectively. Venography was obtained in 130 patients, and was adequate for interpretation in 123(95%). Confirmation of deep venous thrombosis was obtained in 113 patients (92%). To evaluate the accuracy of IPG outside specialized centers, a study was carried out in a community hospital.[36(I)] The study comprised 243 patients, and showed similar results with a positive predictive value of 90%, and only one of 131 patients (0.8%) with repeated normal test results returned with deep venous thrombosis during a 6-month follow-up period.

Finally, Heijboer et al, performed two studies comparing IPG and B-mode compression ultrasonography in 801 outpatients with clinically suspected deep venous thrombosis and in 83 patients who developed clinically suspected DVT while hospitalized.[37(I),38(I)] The results of IPG confirmed those of previous studies in outpatients, while IPG was found to be equally useful for inpatients.

Unfortunately, two problems arise. Firstly, the technique is insensitive for distal vein thrombosis (i.e., isolated calf-vein thrombi) and nonoccluding thrombi. Furthermore, false-positive results may be obtained in patients with poor venous outflow (i.e., congestive heart failure, severe dyspnea, tumor compression in the pelvis region) or with arterial insufficiency of the legs. Finally, even with this noninvasive technique, 2% to 3% of patients are unable to undergo IPG.[35(I)]

More recently, some doubt has been cast on the reliability of IPG. A computerized version (CIPG) proved unsafe in a management study, while another recent study showed a sensitivity of only 66%.[39(I),40] Possible explana-

tions of these discrepancies with previous studies are changes in the performing of the IPG or the use of different (less sensitive) equipment. This is a good example of the necessity to prospectively validate any new equipment both with venography as the reference method and in a management study.

In conclusion, IPG must be considered an effective tool for the detection of DVT in symptomatic in- and outpatients. However, in asymptomatic patients the sensitivity of IPG proved insufficient for proper identification of patients with or without postoperative thrombosis.[41(I),42(I),43] In patients with recurrent symptoms suggestive for deep venous thrombosis, an abnormal IPG test may only be used to confirm the diagnosis if a normal base-line IPG is available.[44(I)]

B-MODE ULTRASONOGRAPHY

Real-time B-mode ultrasonography is a noninvasive direct imaging technique, which gives a two-dimensional image of the blood vessels by transforming reflected ultrasound signals. Compression of the veins of the leg is the most accurate method for the detection of DVT: noncompressibility is the criterium for the presence of DVT.[45,46(I)] The technique has several advantages over IPG: raised venous pressure does not influence ultrasonography and it is easier to perform in severely ill patients. Ultrasonography has a high sensitivity and specificity for proximal-vein thrombi, but is insensitive for isolated calf-vein thrombi. The addition of (color coded) Doppler images may improve the diagnostic accuracy for small veins[47], but studies to evaluate this possible improvement are not yet completed.

Lensing and associates performed B-mode ultrasonography and contrast venography in a prospective study in 220 outpatients with clinically suspected DVT.[46(I)] Ultrasonography proved to be highly sensitive for proximal-vein thrombosis (66/66; 100%) and at the same time highly specific (only one false-positive test; specificity 99%). Furthermore, interobserver agreement was 100% in this study. However, only four out of 11 isolated calf vein thrombi could be detected by ultrasonography for a sensitivity of 36%.

In the studies by Heijboer, compression B-mode ultrasonography proved to be highly accurate for the diagnosis of proximal-vein thrombosis in both inpatients (sensitivity 96%, specificity 83%) and outpatients (positive predictive value 94%).[37(I),38(I)] Furthermore, one of these studies randomly compared serial IPG with serial B-mode ultrasonography in the management of outpatients with suspected deep venous thrombosis, using venography as the reference method.[37(I)] The IPG group consisted of 494 patients, while the ultrasonography group contained 491 patients. Anticoagulants were withheld in patients with serially normal test results and patients were followed for 6 months. The positive predictive value of compression ultrasonography proved significantly better than IPG (94% versus 83%). During the 6-month follow-up period, the incidence of VTE was 1.5% and 2.2% for ultrasonography and IPG, respectively.

In conclusion, real-time B-mode compression ultrasonography is highly accurate for the detection of symptomatic proximal-vein thrombosis, and is probably better than IPG. Furthermore, it is less operator-dependent and more widely available. In patients with recurrent symptoms, the use of an abnormal ultrasound result is limited to patients with a previous normal baseline test. Finally, ultrasonography is not sufficiently sensitive to use as a screening test in asymptomatic patients.

DOPPLER ULTRASONOGRAPHY

Doppler ultrasonography is based on the transformation of bloodflow into sound. The technique was first introduced by Strandness et al, in 1972.[48] The test can be rapidly performed, the equipment is portable and simple to use. The problem with this technique was its lack of uniformity and standardization.

A recent study determined objective diagnostic criteria in 110 patients, and subsequently evaluated the technique in a further 155 patients with clinically suspected DVT.[49(1)] Venography was used as the reference method. For proximal-vein thrombosis a sensitivity and specificity of 91% and 99%, respectively, were obtained.

Unfortunately, at present, no management studies have been performed with this technique.

ROLE OF DEEP-VEIN THROMBOSIS TESTS IN THE DIAGNOSTIC MANAGEMENT OF PATIENTS WITH SUSPECTED VENOUS THROMBOEMBOLISM

Only a limited number of studies have been performed in which tests for deep venous thrombosis have been used to assess the potential utility for the diagnosis of PE. Even fewer studies have been performed in which tests for DVT were part of the management of patients with clinically suspected PE.

In a study by Moser and LeMoine the embolic risk was assessed for different locations of venous thrombi in the legs.[50] Abnormal lung scans were found in eight of 15 patients (53%) with proximal DVT, while no patients with isolated calf-vein thrombi showed perfusion lung scan defects. These findings were confirmed in a subsequent study by Huisman and colleagues.[3] Thus, patients with proven proximal deep venous thrombosis often have asymptomatic PE. However, the question we need to address is how many patients with proven PE have asymptomatic deep venous thrombosis?

Hull and associates performed a study in 139 patients with suspected PE and an abnormal perfusion lung scan.[5(1)] Pulmonary angiography could be obtained in 88 of 107 patients (82%) with perfusion defects and normal chest radiography. Contrast venography and IPG was performed in 74 and 85 of these 88 patients, respectively. The venography results showed DVT in 29 of 41 patients (71%) with angiographically proven PE, while 21 of 37 patients (57%) had both an abnormal IPG result and PE as shown by angiography. Thus, 70% of patients with proven PE may have deep venous thrombosis confirmed by contrast venography. This could imply that venography may be used as an alternative to pulmonary angiography in a substantial proportion of patients with nondiagnostic lung scan results. This would mean less expensive equipment and expertise needed, reduction of invasiveness to the patients, and reduction of angiography associated mortality and morbidity. On the other hand, in 30% of patients with proven PE venography was unable to show deep venous thrombi in the legs. This may be due to the fact that the thrombus has completely migrated to the lungs, or that the location of thrombosis is outside the legs (i.e., in the pelvic veins or arm-vein thrombosis, which makes up 1% to 2% of the total number of venous thrombosis and gives rise to PE in 30%[51]).

In another study, 169 patients with clinically suspected PE were managed according to lung scan and contrast venography results.[4] In 44 patients a normal perfusion lung scan was obtained, and anticoagulants were withheld. In the 125 patients with abnormal lung scan findings, bilateral venography was performed: in 63 (50%) patients deep venous thrombosis was diagnosed (93% of high probability lung scans and 30% of nondiagnostic lung scans). Of these patients with confirmed DVT, only 21 (33%) thrombi were limited to the calf veins, while only 18 (28%) were symptomatic for DVT. Patients with DVT were treated with anticoagulants, while anticoagulant therapy was withheld in the remaining 62 patients with abnormal lung scans and normal venograms. On follow-up recurrent venous thromboembolism was diagnosed in 2.3%, 6.4% and 1.6% of patients with normal lung scan results, abnormal and normal venograms, respectively. At first glance, this study would indicate that venography adequately identifies patients at risk for recurrent venous thromboembolic complications, and therefore pulmonary angiography could be replaced by contrast venography. However, the outcome of the study population shows an alarming mortality rate of 12.9% (95% confidence interval: 5.7% to 23.9%) in the patient group with abnormal lung scan and normal venography results. Although no symptomatic PE was seen, it cannot be ruled out that thromboembolism played a major role in this relatively high mortality rate.

Noninvasive tests for deep venous thrombosis in patients with symptoms suggesting PE have been evaluated in a limited number of studies. Impedance plethysmography was evaluated in a large prospective management study of 874 patients with clinically suspected PE.[52(I)] Deep-vein thrombosis was detected in only 19%, 8% and 1% of patients with a high probability, nondiagnostic and normal lung scan result, respectively. This is considerably less than the prevalence of DVT as shown by contrast venography studies,[4(I),5(I),50] but in agreement with the low yields of IPG in patients with asymptomatic DVT.[41(I), 42(I), 43(I)] The main aim of this study was to evaluate the possible use of serial IPG to replace pulmonary angiography in patients with nondiagnostic lung scan results. Therefore, 371 patients with nonhigh probability lung scan results were managed with serial IPG up to 2 weeks. Deep-vein thrombosis was detected in nine (2%) and these patients received anticoagulant therapy. In the remaining 362 patients anticoagulants were withheld, and within 3 months, 10 (2.7%) returned with symptomatic and objectively documented VTE. No fatal complications were noted, suggesting the safety of this management strategy with serial IPG as an alternative to pulmonary angiography. However, since this is the only study of its kind, the results of this study require confirmation.

In another study, Glew and others compared the results of lung scintigraphy with IPG in 125 patients.[53] However, the IPG equipment used was self-designed and not properly evaluated and validated with the use of contrast venography. This could explain the high number of patients with normal lung scan results and abnormal IPG findings (22%) when compared to the study by Hull, et al.[52(I)] Furthermore, IPG results may be false-positive in patients with symptoms suggesting PE, such as severe dyspnea.

In a retrospective study by Schiff et al, records of 50 patients were collected who underwent pulmonary angiography and noninvasive thrombosis tests (either Doppler ultrasonography or IPG).[54] Both tests were positive (10 patients), negative (18 patients), or showed conflicting results (six angiography normal with abnormal thrombosis test, 16 angiography abnormal and noninvasive test normal). This study shows a sensitivity of only 38% and a specificity of 74%, which compares unfavorably with the study by Hull, et al.[52(I)]

Doppler ultrasonography was evaluated in 79 patients with pulmonary angiography proven PE.[55] In 61 patients, Doppler ultrasonography did not detect DVT, yielding a sensitivity of only 23%. This finding could partly be explained by the fact that Doppler ultrasonography is insensitive to distal-vein thrombi.

In conclusion, only two management studies for suspected PE have been performed in which diagnostic tests for DVT (contrast venography or IPG) were used.[5,52] All other reported studies have been either small, retrospective, or of poor quality in study design. Thus, the efficacy and safety of tests for deep venous thrombosis in the diagnostic and therapeutic management of patients with clinically suspected PE remains to be proven, and further prospective management trials are urgently required.

FUTURE DIRECTIONS FOR NONINVASIVE SCREENING TESTS IN THE DIAGNOSIS OF VENOUS THROMBOEMBOLISM

What we have discussed so far leaves us to conclude that only limited studies have investigated the potential use of noninvasive (DVT) tests, for the diagnosis of PE. However, one would also have to conclude that promising findings have been described, and several techniques are currently undergoing clinical testing. The main points of interest are noninvasive DVT tests (especially ultrasonography could be of value due to the wide availability and ease with which the test may be performed) and blood tests for D-dimer.

Ultrasonography was discussed previously, and seems more accurate in symptomatic DVT patients than IPG.[37(I)] The ease with which it can be performed, even in severely ill patients, and the lack of false positive results in severely dyspneic patients make it especially promising for the diagnosis of symptomatic PE. One could thus use this test as a positive identifier for the presence of PE. Of course, normal ultrasonography findings are unable to exclude thromboembolism. The addition of color coded Doppler ultrasonography may be of use, but clinical experience is lacking. Furthermore, one recent report found that this technique was insensitive for asymptomatic proximal-vein thrombi.[56(I)] The exact place of ultrasonography in the diagnostic work-up for PE is a further point of interest. A recent cost-effectiveness analysis, which used data derived from the literature, found that ultrasonography as a first screening test in patients with clinically suspected PE would be highly cost-effective.[26] However, clinical implementation of such a strategy may be difficult. Furthermore, no studies have been performed assessing the possible role of compression B-mode ultrasonography in patients with clinically suspected PE. Thus, the practical value of B-mode ultrasonography remains to be determined.

The use of blood tests for VTE has been attempted for many years. However, Bounameaux and colleagues recently pointed out that D-dimer may be of value for the exclusion of PE.[57] In 170 patients with clinically suspected PE, lung scanning was performed, and this was followed by pulmonary angiography if a nondiagnostic lung scan result was obtained. Using a cut-off value of 500 μg/l, a sensitivity and specificity of 98% and 39%, respectively, were found. A major disadvantage in the study was, that the complete population was studied, which could only be useful if the blood test can be performed before lung scintigraphy is carried out. Due to the fact that the ELISA technique that is used takes 3 hours to perform, and is unavailable 24 hours a day, the main attraction of D-dimer would probably be the exclusion of emboli in patients with nondiagnostic lung scan results.

Using the same D-dimer assay in 130 patients with

clinically suspected PE, Demers et al, showed a sensitivity and specificity of 96% and 52%, respectively.[58] However, a cut-off level of 300 μg/l was used compared to 500 μg/l as found by Bounameaux, et al. Furthermore, pulmonary angiography was often replaced by serial IPG in patients with nondiagnostic lung scan results, and in 40% of all patients no definite diagnosis was made.

The disadvantage of D-dimer is that ELISA techniques are required to obtain reasonably reliable results. These are time-consuming and impractical for use in individual patients. Furthermore, high coefficients of variation have been found for various D-dimer assays when applied to patients with clinically suspected PE.[59] Faster techniques, such as latex methods, are too insensitive for use as a screening test for PE. Thus, the need for a fast, individual, easy to perform, and reliable D-dimer test remains.

In conclusion, several new options are currently underinvestigation as an alternative for pulmonary angiography. However, at this moment, none have been adequately investigated in management studies to allow them to replace angiography. Thus, it would be unsafe to conclude that noninvasive tests are validated and may be used as an alternative to lung scintigraphy and/or pulmonary angiography in patients with clinically suspected PE.

REFERENCES

1. Havig O. Deep vein thrombosis and pulmonary embolism. Acta Chir Scand 1977;478(Suppl):42–47.
2. Sevitt S, Gallagher N. Venous thrombosis and pulmonary embolism. A clinico-pathological study in injured and burned patients. Br J Surg 1961;48:475–489.
(I)3. Huisman MV, Büller HR, ten Cate JW, et al. Unexpected high prevalence of silent pulmonary embolism in patients with deep venous thrombosis. Chest 1989;95:498–502.
4. Kruit WHJ, de Boer AC, Sing AK, van Roon F. The significance of venography in the management of patients with clinically suspected pulmonary embolism. J Intern Med 1991;230:333–339.
(I)5. Hull RD, Hirsh J, Carter CJ, et al. Pulmonary angiography, ventilation lung scanning, and venography for clinically suspected pulmonary embolism with abnormal perfusion lung scan. Ann Intern Med 1983;98:891–899.
6. Lilienfeld DE, Chan E, Ehland J, Godbold JH, Landrigam PJ, et al. Mortality from pulmonary embolism in the United States: 1962 to 1984. Chest 1990;98:1067–1072.
7. Morrell MT, Truelove SC, Barr A. Pulmonary embolism. Br Med J 1963;2:830–835.
8. Lilienfeld DE, Godbold JH, Burke GL, Sprafko JM, Pham DL, et al. Hospitalization and case fatality for pulmonary embolism in the twin cities: 1979 to 1984. Am Heart J 1990;120:392–395.
9. Morrell MT, Dunnill MS. The post-mortem incidence of pulmonary embolism in a hospital population. Br J Surg 1968;55:347–352.
10. Dismuke SE, Wagner EH. Pulmonary embolism as a cause of death. The changing mortality in hospitalized patients. JAMA 1986;255:2039–2042.
11. Freiman DG, Suyemoto J, Wessler S. Frequency of pulmonary thromboembolism in man. N Engl J Med 1965;272:1278–1280.
12. Goldhaber SZ, Hennekens CH, Evans DA, Newton EC, Godleski JJ. Factors associated with correct antemortem diagnosis of major pulmonary embolism. Am J Med 1982;73:822–826.
13. Dismuke SE, Wagner EH. Pulmonary embolism as a cause of death. The changing mortality in hospitalized patients. JAMA 1986;255:2039–2042.
14. Svendsen E, Karwinski B. Prevalence of pulmonary embolism at necropsy in patients with cancer. J Clin Pathol 1989;42:805–809.
15. Karwinski B, Svendsen E. Comparison of clinical and postmortem diagnosis of pulmonary embolism. J Clin Pathol 1989;42:135–139.
16. Clarke-Pearson DL, Jelovsek FR, Creasman WT. Thromboembolism complicating surgery for cervical and uterine malignancy: incidence, risk factors and prophylaxis. Obstet Gynecol 1983;61:87–94.
17. Clarke-Pearson DL, Synan IS, Coleman RE, Hinshaw W, Creasman WT. The natural history of postoperative venous thromboemboli in gynecologic oncology: a prospective study of 382 patients. Am J Obstet Gynecol 1984;148:1051–1054.
18. Scurr JH, Coleridge-Smith PD, Hasty JH. Deep venous thrombosis: a continuing problem. Br Med J 1988;297:28.
19. Huber O, Bounameaux H, Borst F, Rohner A. Postoperative pulmonary embolism after hospital discharge. An underestimated risk. Arch Surg 1992;127:310–313.
20. Gjöres JE. The incidence of venous thrombosis and its sequelae in certain districts of Sweden. Acta Chir Scand 1956;206(Suppl):1–88.
21. Coon WW, Willis PW III, Keller JB. Venous thromboembolism and other venous disease in the Tecumseh community health study. Circulation 1973;48:839–846.
22. Kierkegaard A. Incidence of acute deep venous thrombosis in two districts. A phlebographic study. Acta Chir Scand 1980;146:267–269.
23. Anderson FA, Wheeler HB, Goldberg RJ. A population-based perspective of the hospital incidence and case-fatality rates of deep vein thrombosis and pulmonary embolism. The Worcester DVT study. Arch Intern Med 1991;151:933–938.
24. Van Beek EJR, Büller HR, Van Everdingen JJE, Zwijnenburg A, ten Cate JW. Diagnostic management of suspected pulmonary embolism in the Netherlands: results from a questionnaire. Thromb Haemostas 1991;65:1171.(Abstract).
25. Levine MN, Hirsh J, Landefeld S, Raskob G. Hemorrhagic complications of anticoagulant treatment. Chest 1992;102:352S–363S.
26. Oudkerk M, van Beek EJR, van Putten WLJ, Büller HR. Cost-effectiveness analysis of various strategies in the diagnostic management of pulmonary embolism. Arch Intern Med 1993;153:947–954.
27. Bauer G. A venographic study of thromboembolic problems. Acta Chir Scand 1940;61(Suppl):1–75.
28. Rabinov K, Paulin S. Roentgen diagnosis of venous thrombosis in the leg. Arch Surg 1972;104:134–144.
29. Lensing AWA, Büller HR, Prandoni P, et al. Contrast venography, the gold standard for the diagnosis of deep vein thrombosis: improvement in observer agreement. Thromb Haemostas 1992;67:8–12.
30. Lensing AWA, Prandoni P. Distribution of venous thrombi in symptomatic patients. Thromb Haemostas 1991;65:1176.(Abstract).

(I)31. Hull RD, van Aken WG, Hirsh J, et al. Impedance plethysmography using the occlusive cuff technique in the diagnosis of venous thrombosis. Circulation 1976;53:696–700.

(I)32. Huisman MV, Büller HR, ten Cate JW, Vreeken J. Serial impedance plethysmography for suspected deep venous thrombosis in outpatients. The Amsterdam General Practitioner Study. N Engl J Med 1986;314:823–828.

33. MacLachlan MSF, Thomson JG, Taylor DW, Kelly ME, Sackett DL. Observer variation in the interpretation of lower limbs venograms. Am J Radiol 1979;132:227–229.

(I)34. Hull RD, Hirsh J, Sackett DL, et al. Clinical validity of a negative venogram in patients with clinically suspected venous thrombosis. Circulation 1981;64:622–625.

(I)35. Hull RD, Hirsh J, Carter CJ, et al. Diagnostic efficacy of impedance plethysmography for clinically suspected deep-vein thrombosis: a randomized trial. Ann Intern Med 1985;102:21–26.

(I)36. Huisman MV, Büller HR, ten Cate JW, Heijermans HSF, van der Laan J, et. al. Management of clinically suspected acute venous thrombosis in outpatients with serial impedence plethysmography in a community hospital setting. Arch Intern Med 1989;149:511–513.

(I)37. Heijboer H, Büller HR, Lensing AWA, Turpie AG, Colly LP, et al. A randomized comparison of the clinical utility of real-time compression ultrasonography versus impedance plethysmography in the diagnosis of deep-vein thrombosis in symptomatic outpatients. N Engl J Med. 1993;329:1365–1369.

(I)38. Heijboer H, Cogo A, Büller HR, Prandoni P, ten Cate JW. Detection of deep vein thrombosis with impedance plethysmography and real-time compression ultrasonography in hospitalized patients. Arch Intern Med 1992;152:1901–1903.

(I)39. Prandoni P, Lensing AWA, Büller HR, et al. Failure of computerized impedance plethysmography in the diagnostic management of patients with clinically suspected deep-vein thrombosis. Thromb Haemostas 1991;65:35–39.

40. Andersen DR, Lensing AWA, Wells PS, Levine MN, Weitz JI, et al. Limitations of impedance plethysmography in the diagnosis of clinically suspected deep-vein thrombosis. Ann Intern Med 1993;118:25–30.

(I)41. Paiement G, Wessinger SJ, Waltman AC, Harris WH. Surveillance of deep vein thrombosis in asymptomatic total hip replacement patients. Am J Surg 1988;155:400–404.

(I)42. Cruickshank MK, Levine MN, Hirsh J, et al. An evaluation of impedance plethysmography and ^{125}I-fibrinogen leg scanning in patients following hip surgery. Thromb Haemostas 1989;62:830–834.

43. Agnelli G, Cosmi B, Ranucci V, et al. Impedance plethysmography in the diagnosis of asymptomatic deep vein thrombosis in hip surgery. Arch Intern Med 1991;151:2167–2171.

(I)44. Hull RD, Carter CJ, Jay R, et al. The diagnosis of acute recurrent deep-vein thrombosis: a diagnostic challenge. Circulation 1983;67:901–905.

45. Cronan JJ, Dorfman GS, Scola FH, Schepps B, Alexander J. Deep venous thrombosis: US assessment using vein compressibility. Radiology 1987;162:191–194.

(I)46. Lensing AWA, Prandoni P, Brandjes DPM, et al. Accurate detection of deep-vein thrombosis by real-time B-mode ultrasonography. N Engl J Med 1989;320:342–345.

47. White RH, McGahan JP, Dasenbach MM, Hartling RP. Diagnosis of deep vein thrombosis using duplex ultrasound. Ann Intern Med 1989;111:297–304.

48. Strandness DE Jr, Sumner DS. Ultrasonic velocity detector in the diagnosis of thrombophlebitis. Arch Surg 1972;104:180–183.

(I)49. Lensing AWA, Levi MM, Büller HR, et al. Diagnosis of deep-vein thrombosis using an objective Doppler method. Ann Intern Med 1990;113:9–13.

50. Moser KM, LeMoine JR. Is embolic risk conditioned by location of deep venous thrombosis? Ann Intern Med 1981;94:439–444.

51. Harley DP, White RA, Nelson RJ, Mehringer CM. Pulmonary embolism secondary to venous thrombosis of the arm. Am J Surg 1984;147:221–224.

(I)52. Hull RD, Raskob GE, Coates G, Panju AA, Gill GJ. A new noninvasive management strategy for patients with suspected pulmonary embolism. Arch Intern Med 1989;149:2549–2555.

53. Glew D, Cooper T, Mitchelmore AE, et al. Impedance plethysmography and thromboembolic disease. Br J Radiol 1992;65:306–308.

54. Schiff MJ, Feinberg AW, Naidich JB. Noninvasive venous examinations as a screening test for pulmonary embolism. Arch Intern Med 1987;147:505–507.

55. Cheely R, McCartney WH, Perry JR, et al. The role of noninvasive tests versus pulmonary angiography in the diagnosis of pulmonary embolism. Am J Med 1981;70:17–22.

(I)56. Davidson BL, Elliott CG, Lensing AWA, et al. Low accuracy of color Doppler ultrasound in the detection of proximal leg vein thrombosis in asymptomatic high-risk patients. Ann Intern Med 1992;117:735–738.

57. Bounameaux H, Cirafici P, de Moerloose P, et al. Measurement of D-dimer in plasma as diagnostic aid in suspected pulmonary embolism. Lancet 1991;337:196–200.

58. Demers C, Ginsberg JS, Johnston M, Brill-Edwards P, Panju A. D-dimer and thrombin-antithrombin III complexes in patients with clinically suspected pulmonary embolism. Thromb Haemostas 1992;67:408–412.

59. Van Beek EJR, van den Ende A, Berckmans RJ, et al. A comparative analysis of D-dimer assays in patients with clinically suspected pulmonary embolism. Thromb Haemostas 1993;70:408–413.

13

Contrast Venography

Brian G. Birdwell

INTRODUCTION

Venography is accepted as the standard of accuracy for diagnosing deep-vein thrombosis (DVT).[1,2(I)] Impedance plethysmography (IPG) and compression ultrasound have also proven accurate for DVT diagnosis in symptomatic patients. These noninvasive tests are less morbid, less expensive and easier to perform than venography, and have largely replaced it as the initial test for patients with suspected DVT. What, then, is the role of venography today? For diagnosis and management of venous thromboembolic disease, the venogram remains indispensable in four major areas.

Determining Operating Characteristics for Noninvasive Tests

It is not safe to assume that published operating characteristics for noninvasive tests apply to every clinical setting. Each noninvasive laboratory should determine positive and negative predictive value for the tests they use to diagnose DVT, and anytime test procedures are changed significantly. This is accomplished by blinded comparison of noninvasive test results with venographic findings.

Clinical Management of Patients with Abnormal Noninvasive Tests

Diagnoses of DVT made via noninvasive testing should be confirmed by venography, for three important reasons: (1) False-positive test results lead to unnecessary treatment and inaccurate labeling of patients. (2) Venography is the only objective test currently available which is accurate for calf DVT. Since IPG detects up to 20% of patients with thrombi limited to the calf,[3(I)] and compression ultrasound abnormalities in the distal popliteal fossa can be difficult to localize anatomically, venography is key in identification of patients with proximal versus calf DVT. This distinction can directly impact treatment: studies suggest that calf DVT (if treated) may require less long-term treatment, e.g. 6 weeks versus three to 6 months for proximal DVT.[3,4] Venography can define the extent and precise location of thrombus in patients with abnormal noninvasive tests. This baseline information is often pivotal in the assessment of future symptomatic episodes in patients with a history of DVT (see *Recurrence*).

Case-Finding in Asymptomatic High-Risk Patients

Some patients—notably those who undergo major hip and knee surgery—are at significant risk for DVT, and thrombosis in many of these patients is clinically silent. Impedance plethysmography and duplex Doppler ultrasound are insensitive to 20% to 60% of these clots,[5(I),6(I)] whereas venography is both sensitive and specific. Noninvasive tests may be useful in the clinical management of such patients, but in clinical trials, often the important endpoint is the presence or absence of thrombus. Only venography can reliably assess this endpoint in asymptomatic patients.

Research and Development of New Diagnostic Methods

The gold standard for a test of DVT diagnosis is the outcome for patients managed according to the results of the test. But a new test should be proven accurate before an outcome study is undertaken, and accuracy is defined by comparison of the test's results with the results of the venogram.

From *Venous Thromboembolism: An Evidence-Based Atlas* edited by Russell Hull, Gary Raskob, Graham Pineo © 1996, Futura Publishing Co., Armonk, NY.

Less common indications for venography include investigation of venous malformations, discerning extrinsic compression by mass lesions (e.g., in the pelvis), assessing the site and extent of traumatic vein injury, and reconstructive surgery of lower extremity veins. Upper extremity phlebography is also a useful procedure, but axillosubclavian vein thrombosis constitutes a distinct entity and is not considered here. In this chapter, the term venography comprises contrast venography only. Contrast venography and nuclear venography are not the same test. Studies purporting to assess accuracy of nuclear venography are methodologically limited,[7] and no prospective clinical management studies have been performed with nuclear venography.

Thus, for the reasons listed above venography remains an important diagnostic tool in clinical care and research. The following sections detail lower extremity venous anatomy, technical issues and pitfalls encountered in the performance and interpretation of venography, and application of venographic results in patient management.

NORMAL ANATOMY OF THE VENOUS SYSTEM OF THE LOWER EXTREMITIES

Accurate interpretation of venograms requires knowledge of normal and variant anatomy of the venous system of the legs and pelvis. Venous drainage of the lower extremities is accomplished via three systems: the deep system, which carries approximately 85% of the blood to the central circulation; the superficial system, which comprises the visible and often palpable leg veins familiar to patients and clinicians; and the perforator (communicating) venous system, small but important veins which connect the superficial and deep systems.

Deep System

In the lower leg the deep system consists of the deep plantar veins of the foot, and six paired veins in the calf which run parallel to corresponding named arteries (posterial tibial, peroneal, anterior tibial). In the upper third of the calf the six paired veins converge to form three veins. The soleal vein plexus and the gastrocnemius vein plexus drain into the posterior tibial and peroneal veins, respectively, which then converge to form the tibio-peroneal trunk in the distal popliteal fossa. The popliteal vein is formed by the convergence of the anterior tibial vein and tibio-peroneal trunk. At the level of the obturator canal in the distal thigh the popliteal vein becomes the superficial femoral vein (still very much a "deep vein"). In the upper thigh, the deep femoral vein, which drains the muscles of the thigh, joins the superficial femoral vein to form the common femoral vein. Above the inguinal ligament this vein is called the external iliac which when joined by the internal iliac becomes the common iliac vein. The right

and left common iliac veins converge to form the inferior vena cava.

Superficial System

Lying within the subcutaneous tissues, the superficial veins of the leg are familiar to clinicians and patients. "Cording" is one manifestation of thrombus in a superficial vein, varicose veins are dilated superficial veins, and many other normal superficial veins may be visible and/or palpable. The superficial system consists of two major veins and their small tributaries: the greater (long) saphenous vein, and the lesser (short) saphenous vein. The greater saphenous vein is formed by the confluence of veins from the medial sole of the foot and the medial marginal vein, courses upward anterior to the medial malleolus and along the anteromedial surface of the leg and thigh, finally emptying into the common femoral vein just distal to the inguinal ligament. It receives many tributaries throughout its course, most notably the posterior arch veins in the calf. The lesser saphenous vein, which begins at the outer border of the foot behind the lateral malleolus, drains the lateral aspect of the heel and calf. It ascends along the lateral border of the Achilles tendon on the deep fascia until it reaches the middle third of the calf. There it lies within the fascial layer covering the gastrocnemius muscle and runs along the middle of the back of the calf. Typically it empties into the popliteal vein in the popliteal fossa, but it may join the greater saphenous vein in the calf, the popliteal vein high in the popliteal fossa, or join the femoral vein in the upper thigh.

The Communicating Veins

Blood from the superficial system flows into the deep system via the communicating veins. The communicating veins normally feature one-way valves which prevent the refluxing of blood from the deep system back into the superficial system. (Such pathological reflux is the cause of the postphlebitic syndrome.) The largest communicating veins are the terminal portions of the greater and lesser saphenous veins; they drain into the femoral and popliteal veins, respectively. Communicating veins are particularly numerous in the lower leg, some of which have been a target of surgical ligation in the face of recalcitrant post-phlebitic ulceration.

TECHNICAL ISSUES AND PITFALLS IN THE PERFORMANCE AND INTERPRETATION OF VENOGRAPHY

The following points are common to all accepted approaches to the performance of venography and interpretation of venograms. (Three published venographic techniques are extensively utilized, and these are discussed in section IV.)

Performing the Venogram

Position. Venographic dye is heavier than blood. When injected into a dorsal foot vein, the dye displaces the blood as it ascends in the leg. Therefore the ideal position for performing venography would be with the patient erect. This would assure that all patent vessels of the deep venous system would fill with contrast dye, and achieve maximum mixing of blood with contrast. Unfortunately this position is technically difficult and not well tolerated by patients. Tilting the examination table 40° downward will usually promote sufficient filling of the deep leg veins.

Weightbearing. Contraction of the calf muscles (as occurs with weightbearing) often results in incomplete filling of the deep leg veins. This is obviated by having the patient support body weight on the other leg.

Injection site. Contrast media must be injected into a vein on the distal half of the foot, else the deep calf veins may be bypassed. Some also inject contrast against the venous flow, i.e., pointing the needle toward the toes, to facilitate deep calf-vein filling.[8]

Adequately visualizing IVC and proximal veins. With routine venography the inferior vena cava is usually not visualized, and other proximal veins are often poorly opacified. Filling of the inferior vena cava, iliac and upper common femoral vein is enhanced by compressing the calf, having the patient extend the foot against resistance, and/or removing tourniquets (if used). If some veins are still not seen, direct injection via a femoral vein puncture may be necessary.

Tourniquets. The use of tourniquets is controversial, and no objective data are available to resolve the issue. Advocates of their use contend that: (1) deep-vein filling is enhanced by placing a tourniquet just above the ankle, with its pressure adjusted during injection to preserve deep-vein filling but minimize flow into the superficial system; (2) restricting the filling of the superficial system facilitates the visualization of deep veins in patients with large superficial veins or extensive varicosities; and (3) a second tourniquet above the knee may further improve deep-vein filling by delaying the emptying of contrast from the deep calf veins. Those discouraging use of tourniquets contend that contrast injected into a superficial foot vein of patients in a near-upright position will readily and necessarily enter the deep veins as well; and that the tourniquet may actually prevent complete filling of the deep system.

Criteria for Diagnosis of Deep-vein Thrombosis

The venographic diagnosis of DVT is based on specific radiographic characteristics:

1. An intraluminal filling defect (ILFD), consistent in its appearance in all films. (Exam must include ≥ 2 views). This is the only direct and unequivocal radiographic sign of the presence of thrombus.
2. Abrupt termination of the opaque contrast column, seen at a constant site (≥ 2 views) in a vein segment. This may be seen either above or below the thrombotic obstruction.
3. Nonfilling of deep veins above the knee, when proper venographic technique is employed. This finding may be artifactual, even with meticulous attention to technique.

Age of Thrombus, by Venographic Criteria

An ILFD may persist indefinitely, so not even an ILFD can be assumed to represent new thrombosis in a patient with prior venous thromboembolic episodes. A previous venogram is required for comparison, to assess whether the finding is new or old. Conversely, findings which would seem to connote an old thrombus are unreliable. "Well-developed" collaterals are seen acutely with occlusive thrombi;[9] other putatively old findings such as recanalized flow through thrombus or narrowed, torturous veins can mask the presence of new thrombus.[9–11(I)]

Technical Issues and Pitfalls in Interpretation

Flow defects. Flow defects result when contrast-opacified blood mixes with the non-opacified blood. On still radiographs these lucent areas can mimic a true ILFD. Measures employed to avoid flow defects include: (1) viewing the veins during injection under fluoroscopy, which may reveal the ephemeral nature of the lucency; (2) positioning the patient at least 40° from the horizontal, thereby promoting filling and opacification of deep veins; (3) use of the Valsalva maneuver, which may be helpful when flow from the deep femoral vein and/or internal iliac vein has produced a flow defect in the common femoral vein or the common iliac vein, respectively. Though thrombus involving the deep femoral or internal iliac veins is rarely a clinical issue, positive identification of these veins using Valsalva should be attempted in this situation.

Lack of filling. When a vein fails to fill adequately with contrast, the lucent area may be ascribed to thrombus or regarded as normal because no filling defect is outlined. Common examples include missing a nonobstructive thrombus in the common femoral region when the flow into the external and common iliac veins appears adequate but filling of the common femoral vein is inadequate; misdiagnosing a thrombus in the common femoral or iliac veins due to inadequate opacification.

SPECIFIC VENOGRAPHIC METHODS

These three published methods are the most widely employed techniques for contrast venography. Rabinov and Paulin is fully described; for the other methods, only details which differ from Rabinov and Paulin are listed.

Method of Rabinov and Paulin[9]

• Tilting (movable) table, image intensifier, fluoroscopy, and spot film with fine focus are strongly recommended.

• To facilitate nonweightbearing, a box is placed under the opposite foot, allowing the injected leg to remain relaxed and be properly positioned.

• No tourniquet is used.

• Venipuncture using a No. 21 scalp vein needle.

• Contrast of moderate concentration and density (280 to 300 mg of iodine per ml.); 75 to 125 ml injected over 1½ to three minutes.

• To facilitate contrast filling of the area of the upper common femoral and external iliac veins, the patients flexes the foot against the hand of the examiner, utilizing the calf pump to propel contrast material upward.

• Fluoroscopic monitoring is carried out during the injection; each segment of the venous system is screened fluoroscopically and documented by films with legs at various degrees of rotation.

• Multiple spot films are taken over the entire extremity; a small focus tube and automatic phototimer are used.

• Radiographs are taken after the injection and spot films: AP stereoscopic views and a single lateral view.

Method of Lea-Thomas[10]

(1) No special radiographic equipment is required; (2) tourniquets are used, one above the ankle and another above the knee; (3) strong recommendation for non-ionic contrast, generally 50 ml. per leg, although up to 200 ml. for bilateral leg and vena cava exams regarded as safe.

Long-Leg Method[11]

(1) Use of tourniquet in patients with obvious venous insufficiency; (2) injection of greater volume of contrast (150 ml.); (3) use of long-leg films instead of spot films, i.e., the entire venous system of the leg is outlined in a single film.

Comments on these Methods

With proper technique ascending contrast venography outlines the entire deep venous system of the lower extremities and pelvis, and because of this it became and remains the reference standard for diagnosis of DVT. Rabinov and Paulin's methodology is widely employed, with differences in the use of tourniquets, and type and amount of contrast being important variations. The long-leg method represents an attempt to contend with interobserver variation in the interpretation of venograms and the frequency of technically inadequate venograms. In this study[13] comparing the long-leg method with the method of Rabinov and Paulin, interobserver variation in interpretation was significantly decreased and technically inadequate venograms occurred much less frequently with the long-leg method. However, the study design was limited due to the comparisons being made between venograms performed using the long-leg method in one hospital while the Rabinov-Paulin method was performed on different patients by different teams in a different outpatient center. The differences in interobserver variation and technically adequate venograms detected in the study could have been due to variables other than the different venographic methods employed, e.g., differences in patients studied, experience and expertise of operators, etc. The issue of interobserver variability therefore remains unresolved.

SIDE EFFECTS OF VENOGRAPHY

Generalized/Systemic Reactions

The contrast media used for venography and many other radiographic studies can cause a wide range of idiosyncratic and systemic reactions, rarely of great clinical consequence.

• Minor reactions such as mild urticaria, nausea, sneezing, pruritis, etc., occur in about 8% of cases, and they usually require no treatment.[8]

• Anaphylactic reactions require immediate—sometimes lifesaving—treatment. The mortality rate from intravenous injection of iodinated contrast media is approximately one in 40,000 but may be lower when low osmolality media are employed.[12] These reactions are unpredictable, and a history of uneventful exposure to iodinated contrast is no assurance that it will not happen in the future.

• Cardiac dysrhythmias and/or arrest may occur in patients with pulmonary hypertension who undergo venography. Contrast media induces significant vasodilatation, which can critically reduce cardiac output in these patients; prophylactic administration of plasma expanders or a vasoconstrictor may lower the risk.

• Renal complications from use of contrast media are uncommon (probably <5%) among patients without renal insufficiency, diabetes or congestive heart failure.[14] Even among "high-risk" patients, the risk is surprisingly small: in a controlled prospective study of 34 patients with renal insufficiency and diabetes given contrast dye, about 9% had a short-lived drop in creatinine clearance, and none required dialysis.[15] Use of nonionic dye does not appear to further decrease this modest risk of nephrotoxicity.[16]

Local Reactions

• Pain at the injection site is the most common side effect of venography, due primarily to the osmolality of the contrast. Severe pain should alert the venographer to the possibility of extravasation of contrast into the tissues.

• Thrombosis: hyperosmolar solutions like contrast media injure vein endothelium, theoretically promoting thrombosis. Prospective clinical trial data suggests that this occurs in 1% to 2% of cases.[2] No documentation exists linking pulmonary embolism (PE) to venography.

• Extravasation into surrounding tissues manifests a spectrum of severity from minor pain to extensive chemical cellulitis, necrosis and even gangrene. The injection site must be closely observed for swelling throughout the examination with fluoroscopic screening if extravasation is suspected. Significant extravasation merits stopping the exam, injection of physiological saline to dilute the contrast media, and gentle massage to promote quick dispersion.

CONTRAST MEDIA

The most serious complications associated with injection of contrast are anaphylactic reactions, which are idiosyncratic responses to iodine. Iodine imparts the quality of radiopacity and is thus present in all contrast media, including low osmolality preparations. Nothing presently can be done to obviate these reactions, although severity is believed to be mitigated by pretreatment in high-risk patients. Local reactions are by and large the product of the osmolality of the contrast medium employed. Standard contrast media have an osmolality of 1.5 osmols/kg, compared to 0.3 osmols/kg of plasma. Reduction of the osmolality is approached in several ways.

Dilution

This approach is limited because the iodine content of the media decreases in direct proportion to the dilution and the resulting venographic images may not be adequate for accurate diagnosis.

Nonionic Solution

By making the iodine molecule nondissociable in solution, the osmolality of "nonionic" contrast media may be lowered to approximately 0.5 osmols/kg while maintaining fully adequate iodine content. M. Lea Thomas reports that use of the nonionic media produces painless injection, virtual elimination of thrombosis from endothelial damage due to contrast, and no tissue necrosis with accidental extravasation.[12] However, this product currently costs about 20 times as much as conventional media.

Increased Molecular Weight

If the molecule, an iodinated benzoic acid derivative, is forged into a dimer, the molecular weight is increased, preserving the total iodine content but lowering the os-

molality of the medium. This product is similar to the nonionic media in cost and osmolality.

CLINICAL VALIDITY OF A NEGATIVE VENOGRAM

When a properly performed venogram is diagnostic of thrombus, no other evidence should reasonably dissuade the clinician that thrombus is not present. However, what is the meaning of a normal venogram in a patient with clinical findings highly suspicious for DVT? Can a negative venogram dictate management of asymptomatic patients at high risk for DVT?

Symptomatic Patients

As recently as 1980, some authorities insisted that no reasonable clinician would fail to anticoagulate a patient with classic clinical features of DVT, even in the face of a negative venogram.[17] Since the majority of patients with suspected DVT will have a negative venogram, the question is critical: is it safe to withhold anticoagulants from patients with clinical presentation suspicious for DVT but a normal venogram? This issue was addressed in a landmark study wherein 160 consecutive symptomatic patients with negative venograms had anticoagulants withheld, then were carefully followed to determine the frequency of subsequent DVT or PE.[2] Only two of the 160 patients returned with symptoms suspicious for DVT and both were found to have DVT on repeat venogram. Both occurred within 5 days of the original venogram, suggesting that the venogram itself probably induced the thrombosis. No patient had a PE. Only 1.3% of patients with suspected DVT but negative venography had recurrent thromboembolic events. These data established the safety of withholding anticoagulation from patients with negative venograms.

Case-Finding Among Patients at High Risk

As noted above, patients who have recently undergone hip and knee surgery comprise a group at high risk for proximal DVT, but screening has proven difficult because the sensitivity of noninvasive tests is unacceptably low in asymptomatic patients. An approach to management might include screening with venography, rather than waiting for the patient to progress to either leg symptoms or PE. However, it remains to be shown in prospective clinical trials whether, and when, a negative venogram connotes a good outcome in asymptomatic patients, with known high risk of venous thromboembolic disease.

SUMMARY

Venography continues to play a pivotal role in patient care and research. Thoughtful attention to the utilization, performance and interpretation of this test is vital for proper management of patients and the continued growth of our knowledge and capacities in venous thromboembolic disease.

REFERENCES

1. Cranley JJ, Canos AJ, Sull WJ. The diagnosis of deep venous thrombosis: fallibility of clinical symptoms and signs. Arch Surg 1976;111:34–36.

(I)2. Hull R, Hirsh J, Sackett DL, et al. Clinical validity of a negative venogram in patients with clinically suspected venous thrombosis. Circulation 1981;64:622–625.

(I)3. Hull R, Delmore T, Genton E, et al. Warfarin sodium versus low-dose heparin in the long-term treatment of venous thrombosis. N Engl J Med 1979;301:855–858.

(I)4. Hull R, Hirsh J, Carter CJ, et al. Diagnostic efficacy of impedance plethysmography for clinically suspected deep-vein thrombosis: a randomized trial. Ann Intern Med 1985;102:21–28.

(I)5. Ginsberg JS, Caco CC, Brill-Edwards PA, et al. Venous thrombosis in patients who have undergone major hip or knee surgery: detection with compression ultrasound and impedance plethysmography. Radiology 1991;181:651–654.

(I)6. Davidson BL, Elliott CG, Lensing AWA. Low accuracy of color Doppler ultrasound in the detection of proximal leg vein thrombosis in asymptomatic high-risk patients. Ann Intern Med 1992;117:735–738.

7. Gomes AS, Webber MM, Buffkin D. Contrast venography vs. radionuclide venography: a study of discrepancies and their possible significance. Radiology 1982;142:719–728.

8. Thomas ML. Phlebography of the Lower Limb. Edinburgh, Churchill-Livingstone, 1982, p.28.

9. Rabinov K, Paulin S. Roentgen diagnosis of venous thrombosis in the leg. Arch Surg 1972;104:134–144.

10. Harris WH, Waltmen AC, Athanasoulis C, et al. The accuracy of the *in vivo* diagnosis of deep vein thrombosis in patients with prior venous thrombembolic diesase or severe varicose veins. Thromb Res 1981;21:137–145.

(I)11. Hull R, Carter C, Jay R, et al. The diagnosis of acute recurrent deep-vein thrombosis: A diagnostic challenge. Circulation 1983;67:901–906.

12. Thomas ML. Techniques of phlebography: a review. Eur J Radiol 1990;11:125–130.

13. Lensing AWA, Büller HR, Prandoni P, et al. Contrast venography, the gold standard for the diagnosis of deep-vein thrombosis: improvement in observer agreement. Thromb Hemost 1992;67:8–12.

14. Brezis M, Epstein FH. A closer look at radiocontrast-induced nephropathy. N Engl J Med 1989;320:179–181.

(I)15. Parfrey PS, Griffiths SM, Barrett BJ, et al. Contrast material-induced renal failure in patients with diabetes mellitus, renal insufficiency, or both. A prospective controlled study. N Engl J Med 1989;320:143–149.

(I)16. Schwab SJ, Hlatky MA, Pieper KS, et al. Contrast nephrotoxicity: a randomized controlled trial of a nonionic and an ionic radiographic contrast agent. N Engl J Med 1989;320:149–153.

17. Fitzer PM. Contrast venography: a "golden oldie". Virginia Medical 1980;107:210–214.

14

Impedance Plethysmography

Gary E. Raskob, Graham F. Pineo, Russell D. Hull

INTRODUCTION

Plethysmography is a noninvasive method for measuring changes in blood volume in the leg. Three plethysmographic techniques have been applied to the diagnosis of venous thrombosis. These are: impedance plethysmography (IPG), strain-gauge plethysmography, and air-cuff plethysmography or phleborrheography. The difference between these techniques is the method by which they record the changes in blood volume which occur with venous filling or emptying of the leg. Impedance plethysmography measures changes in electrical resistance (impedance) of the limb. Strain-gauge plethysmography measures changes in the circumference of the limb. Phleborrheography measures changes in pressure transmitted from the leg to an air-filled cuff. Impedance plethysmography has been the most thoroughly evaluated technique.

Impedance plethysmography has been extensively evaluated by clinical trials using two different approaches: (1) studies evaluating the diagnostic accuracy of IPG by comparison to ascending contrast venography, the diagnostic reference standard,[1,2,3(I),4(I),5(I),6,7(I)12(I)–14] and (2) studies evaluating the clinical outcome of patients with symptoms or signs suggesting venous thromboembolism (VTE) in whom the decision to administer or withhold anticoagulant therapy is based on the results of IPG testing.[15(I),16(I),17(I),18(I),19(I)] The cumulative data from the diagnostic accuracy studies indicate that IPG is a sensitive and specific test for thrombosis of the popliteal, femoral and iliac veins (proximal-veins) in symptomatic patients.[1,2,3(I),4(I),5(I),6,7(I)12(I)–14] The results from the clinical outcome studies are consistent and establish unequivocally that serial testing with IPG is a safe and cost-effective approach for managing patients with clinically suspected venous thrombosis.[15–20] Impedance plethysmography has also been extensively evaluated in patients with suspected pulmonary embolism (PE), by both ac-

curacy and clinical outcome studies,[21(I),22(I),23(I)] (see chapter 24). Impedance plethysmography is also a useful test in patients with suspected acute recurrent venous thrombosis.[24(I)]

In 1993 and 1994, two accuracy studies[25,26(IV)] were reported by the same investigators which have created potential confusion about the clinical value of IPG in patients with suspected venous thrombosis. These two studies did not evaluate clinical outcome, but confined the assessment of IPG to a comparison of a single evaluation with that of venography. These studies[25,26] reported considerably lower sensitivity (65%) for proximal-vein thrombosis than had been reported by more than 12 previous accuracy studies by different groups of investigators (sensitivity range 87% to 100%, see Table 1).[1–14] The results of these accuracy studies[25,26] can be explained based on the knowledge of the natural history of venous thrombosis and the operating characteristics of IPG, and these findings will be discussed in more detail later in the chapter. The crucial issue is more fundamental: the decision to continue using or to abandon a particular diagnostic technology, such as IPG, should be based on the findings of clinical outcome studies. Indeed, there has been a recent call for clinical outcome studies to replace studies of accuracy as the reference standard for evaluating the clinical application of IPG.[27] It is not appropriate to recommend abandoning an approach such as IPG which has been established by clinical outcome studies to be safe[15–19] and cost-effective,[20] based on the findings of one or two recent studies of accuracy by investigators in one center. Serial testing with IPG is a relatively simple, portable, cost-effective and safe approach for evaluating patients with symptoms or signs suggesting venous thrombosis. This approach should continue to play an important role in the evaluation of patients with suspected VTE for those centers in which the technology is currently available, and for those centers which are considering making this technology available.

Table 1
Sensitivity and Specificity of Occlusive-Cuff Impedance Plethysmography for Proximal-Vein
Thrombosis in Symptomatic Patients

Study	Year	Sensitivity	Specificity
Wheeler and Anderson[1]	1974	98% (88/90)	92% (191/208)
Todd et al[2]	1976	100% (11/11)	100% (11/11)
Hull et al[3]	1976	93% (124/133)	97% (386/397)
Hull et al[4]	1977	98% (59/60)	95% (108/114)
Toy and Schrier[5]	1978	94% (15/16)	100% (9/9)
Flanigan et al[6]	1978	96% (52/54)	95% (93/98)
Hull et al[7]	1978	92% (155/169)	96% (304/317)
Gross and Burney[8]	1979	100% (9/9)	94% (32/34)
Cooperman et al[9]	1979	87% (20/23)	96% (72/75)
Liapis et al[10]	1980	91% (43/47)	90% (219/243)
Foti and Gurewich[11]	1980	90% (19/21)	79% (19/24)
Hull et al[12]	1981	95% (74/78)	98% (157/160)
Clarke-Pearson and Creasman[13]	1981	100% (10/10)	40% (2/5)
Peters et al[14]	1982	92% (36/39)	93% (115/124)
Anderson et al[25]	1993	66% (37/56)	-
Ginsberg et al[26]	1994	65% (26/40)	93% (79/85)

THEORETICAL AND PHYSIOLOGICAL BACKGROUND

Impedance plethysmography is based on the principle that changes in the blood volume of the calf produced by temporary venous occlusion, result in changes in electrical resistance (impedance) which are detected by four skin electrodes placed around the calf.[1,3] A high-frequency current which is imperceptible to the patient is passed through the outer electrodes and the impedance across the field is measured by the two inner electrodes. Proximal venous occlusion produced by the inflation of a pneumatic thigh cuff results in pooling of blood in the calf. Blood is a good conductor of electricity and this pooling results in a decrease in the electrical impedance across the field measured by the electrodes placed around the calf. Using this technique, it is possible to quantitate the capacity of the venous system of the leg to fill and empty in response to temporary occlusion of venous outflow.[1,3,7] The relationship between venous filling and venous emptying in response to temporary venous occlusion is markedly different between patients with normal veins, and those with thrombosis of the popliteal or more proximal deep-veins. When the pneumatic cuff is inflated in a normal limb, the calf begins to fill with blood, at first rapidly and then more slowly as the venous pressure gradient equalizes. If there is obstruction to venous outflow, for example by a thrombus, cuff occlusion produces less venous filling because venous pooling is already present and when the cuff is deflated, the reduction in calf blood volume (venous emptying) occurs much more slowly.

The clinical application of IPG is based on the physiological relationship between venous filling and venous emptying in response to temporary venous occlusion.[7] The sensitivity and specificity of IPG for proximal-vein thrombosis are directly linked to the relationship between venous filling and venous emptying.[7] The relationship between venous filling and venous emptying in patients with and without proximal-vein thrombosis is shown in Figure 1. In patients without proximal-vein thrombosis, a progressive increase in venous filling is accompanied by an increase in venous emptying. If proximal-vein thrombosis is present, however, increased venous filling is not associated with a proportionate increase in venous emptying (because of obstruction to venous outflow by the thrombus). Consequently, the regression lines relating venous filling and venous emptying for patients with and without proximal-vein thrombosis diverge progressively as venous filling increases (see Figure 1). Thus, the accuracy of IPG for proximal-vein thrombosis is enhanced with increased venous filling due to a progressive separation of test results between patients with and without thrombosis.[7] The current technique for performing IPG is designed to ensure that maximum venous filling occurs in each patient, in order to provide maximum separation of test results between patients with and without proximal-vein thrombosis. The maneuvers which are employed to achieve maximal venous filling are: (1) the use of a pneumatic occlusive-cuff to produce temporary occlusion of venous outflow, rather than using maximum respiratory effort or the Valsalva maneuver, which frequently did not produce maximum venous filling, and (2) the use of prolonged cuff occlusion times (120 seconds) and repeated sequential testing. Early studies with IPG documented that venous filling was frequently suboptimal after cuff occlusion for only 45 seconds. Prolonging the period of cuff occlusion from 45 seconds to 120 seconds ensures that maximum venous filling occurs for any single test, since 95% or more of patients reach a plateau of venous filling after cuff occlusion for 120 seconds.[7] Repeated sequential testing produces a further increase in venous filling (capacitance) by stretching the vessel wall,

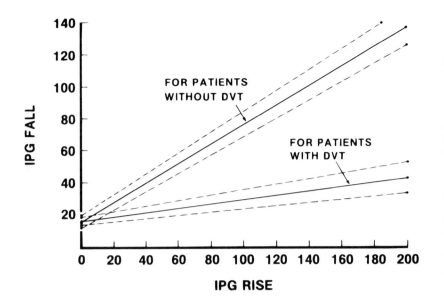

Figure 1. Relationship between venous filling and venous emptying in patients with and without proximal deep-vein thrombosis (DVT). Venous filling (IPG rise) is shown on the horizontal axis and venous emptying (IPG fall) is plotted on the vertical axis. The solid lines are the regression lines indicating the relationship between venous filling and venous emptying in symptomatic patients without proximal DVT and in those with proximal DVT by venography. The dotted lines indicate the 95% confidence interval around these regression lines. As venous filling is increased, there is a progressive separation of the regression lines relating venous filling and venous emptying between the two populations. Thus, the ability to discriminate between patients with proximal DVT and those without proximal DVT using IPG is enhanced as venous filling is increased.

such that greater filling is possible with each successive period of cuff occlusion.[7] This increased venous filling observed with repetitive filling and emptying of the vein is based on the physiological principle known as stress-relaxation of the vessel wall.[7] The technique for performing occlusive-cuff IPG using the sequential testing approach is outlined below.

It should be noted that the comments about the physiological basis and clinical application of IPG discussed so far, apply to one specific IPG machine. This machine has been evaluated in the accuracy studies,[1–14] and the clinical outcome studies[15–19] and the physiological basis for IPG testing applies specifically to this machine.[7] More recently, an alternate IPG device became available[28(I),29(I)] which reported a lower sensitivity for proximal-vein thrombosis[29] and an unacceptably high rate of pulmonary embolism, including fatal pulmonary embolism, on follow-up in patients with serially negative results.[28] The remainder of this chapter focuses on IPG measured using the original technology which has now been extensively validated.

Technique for Performing Occlusive-Cuff Impedance Plethysmography

Occlusive-cuff IPG is performed with the patient supine and with the lower limb elevated about 30° from horizontal, the knee flexed 10° to 20°, and the ankle 8 cm to 15 cm higher than the knee. The hip may be externally rotated provided that the patient is comfortable in this position and that there are no contraindications to this maneuver (e.g., recent hip surgery). External rotation of the hip is optional, however, and the patient should not be forced into this position because it may result in muscle tension with the potential for a false-positive test result.

The electrodes are applied 8 cm to 12 cm apart following the natural contour of the calf and encircling the maximum circumference of the calf without applying excessive tension. If reusable electrodes are used, a thin coating of electroconductive cream is applied to each electrode to guarantee good electrode-to-skin contact. In more recent years, disposable electrodes have been developed and applied which do not require the use of electroconductive cream.

A pneumatic cuff 15 cm wide is applied to the midthigh. Care should be taken to ensure that the cuff is not applied too tightly because this may result in a false-positive test. It should be possible to comfortably slip four fingers under the upper and lower edges of the cuff. The thigh cuff is then inflated to a pressure of 45 mmHg to temporarily occlude venous return. After a predetermined period of time, the cuff is rapidly deflated and the change in electrical impedance (resistance) resulting from alteration in blood volume distal to the cuff is detected by the calf electrodes and recorded on a strip of electrocardiograph paper. Both the total increase in venous capacitance (IPG rise) during cuff inflation and the total venous outflow occurring in the first three seconds of cuff deflation (IPG fall) are plotted on a two-way IPG graph (Figure 2). The graph includes a "discriminant line" which provides optimal separation of the results into normal and abnormal for proximal-vein thrombosis.

The sequential IPG technique is performed using a five-test sequence with the following cuff occlusion times:

Test 1: 45 seconds
Test 2: 45 seconds
Test 3: 120 seconds
Test 4: 45 seconds
Test 5: 120 seconds

The effect of increasing cuff occlusion time and of sequential testing on both venous filling and the accuracy of IPG was evaluated in a prospective study of over 300 patients with clinically suspected venous thrombosis.[7] It was noted that as venous filling increased, there was a corresponding increase in both the sensitivity and specificity of

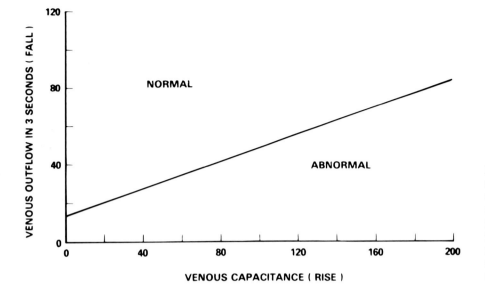

Figure 2. Two-way IPG graph with venous filling or capacitance (IPG rise) indicated on the horizontal axis, and venous outflow or emptying in 3 seconds (IPG fall) on the vertical axis. The solid line is the discriminant line which provides optimal separation of IPG results into normal and abnormal for proximal-vein thrombosis.

the test.[7] Termination of the IPG evaluation after a single 45-second occlusion time was associated with a decline in sensitivity of 10% and a loss of specificity of 20%.

The importance of sequential testing is further illustrated by the analysis of patterns of IPG response in patients with and without proximal-vein thrombosis (demonstrated by venography). Four patterns of IPG response were observed (Figure 3). In 76% of 317 legs that were normal by venography, the initial test in the sequence fell above the discriminant line, as did all subsequent tests (Figure 3A). However, in the remaining 20% of legs that were normal by venography, the initial 45-second test fell below the discriminant line (Figure 3B). When venous filling was improved by prolonged cuff occlusion and by performing sequential tests, the subsequent tests fell above the discriminant line indicating the

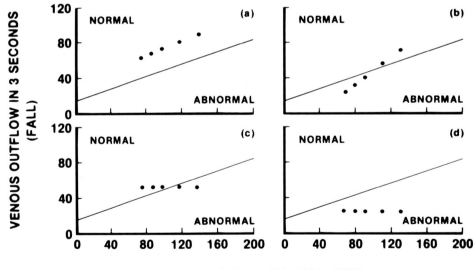

Figure 3. Patterns of IPG response using the five-test sequential testing protocol. **(A)**, shows that in 76% of legs normal be venography, the initial test and all subsequent tests in the five-test sequence fall above the discriminant line. **(B)**, shows that in 20% of legs normal by venography, the initial one or two tests in the sequence fall below the discriminant line, but as venous filling (capacitance) is increased, subsequent tests land above the discriminant line indicating a normal result. Thus, the use of the five-test sequential method produces improved venous filling and an increase in the specificity of IPG of 20% (from 76% to 96%). **(D)**, shows that, in 85% of legs with proximal-vein thrombosis by venography, the initial test and all subsequent tests in the five-test sequence land below the discriminant line. However, in 10% of limbs with proximal-vein thrombosis by venography (Figure **3C**), the initial one or two tests in the sequence land above the discriminant line, but as venous filling is improved, there is not a corresponding increase in venous outflow, and the subsequent tests land below the discriminant line, indicating an abnormal result. Thus, the five-test sequential technique produces an increase in sensitivity of 10% (from 85% to 95%).

absence of proximal-vein thrombosis (Figure 3B). Thus, the improved venous filling obtained by using the sequential IPG technique resulted in an improvement of specificity of 20%.[7]

In 82% of 169 legs with proximal-vein thrombosis by venography, the initial test result and all subsequent test results fell below the discriminant line, indicating the presence of proximal-vein thrombosis (Figure 3D). However, in 10%, the initial tests fell above the discriminant line and would have been falsely read as negative for proximal-vein thrombosis if the test sequence had been terminated (Figure 3C). When venous filling was improved by prolonged cuff occlusion and sequential testing, the subsequent tests fell below the discriminant line because the improved venous filling was not accompanied by a corresponding improvement in venous outflow (Figure 3C). This latter pattern of IPG response is sometimes seen in patients with nonobstructive proximal-vein thrombosis or proximal-vein thrombosis associated with extensive collaterals. Thus, the sequential IPG technique resulted in an improvement in sensitivity for proximal-vein thrombosis of 10% compared to the use of a single 45-second test.[7]

Scoring and Interpreting Impedance Plethysmography Results

The result of each IPG test is recorded on the two-way IPG graph containing the discriminant line and the "stop-line" (Figure 4). Each IPG test is recorded by plotting the total IPG rise during cuff inflation (venous filling or capacitance) on the horizontal axis, and the total IPG fall during the first three seconds of cuff deflation (venous outflow) on the vertical axis. The test result with both the highest rise (greatest venous capacitance) and the greatest fall (venous outflow) is taken as the patient's IPG result.

The IPG result is considered abnormal if the point with both the highest rise and the greatest fall lies on or below the discriminant line.

The two-way IPG graph includes the "stop-line" which allows early termination of sequential IPG testing without loss of accuracy in a significant proportion of patients with normal IPG results. If any point in the five-test sequence is above the "stop-line", the test sequence can be terminated and that point is taken as the patient's test result. Since any test result which falls above the "stop-line" also lands above the "discriminant line", a result which lands above the stop-line is by definition a normal IPG result. The validity of the stop-line was established in a prospective study[30] which demonstrated that when any test in the IPG sequence falls above the stop-line, the sequential IPG technique can be terminated without loss of sensitivity for proximal-vein thrombosis. In over 300 symptomatic legs negative by venography, the use of the "stop-line" provided termination of the sequential technique in 45% of limbs following one test with the 45-second occlusion time, in 59% following the second test in the sequence, and in 80% after the third test of the sequence. If the test result does not fall above the "stop-line", the complete sequential protocol should be carried out. The test is terminated when a result is obtained that either falls above the stop-line, or when the five-test sequence is completed, whichever occurs first.

The "stop-line" was added to provide efficiency in testing and to simplify the technique by avoiding unnecessary sequential tests. It is emphasized that the area between the "stop-line" and the "discriminant line" is not a "grey zone" or region of "borderline" IPG results. If the test result with both the greatest rise and greatest fall in a five-test sequence lands above the discriminant line, this is a normal test result and is not considered "borderline". Thus, there are only three possible interpretations of IPG results when

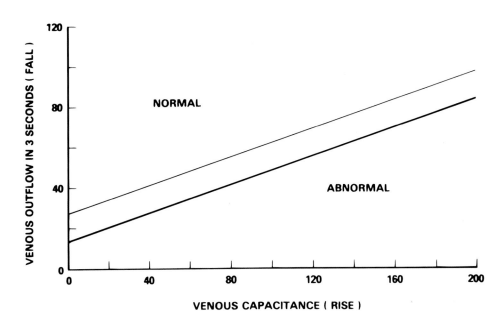

Figure 4. Two-way IPG graph with discriminant line (bold solid line) and stop-line (thin solid line). The discriminant line (bold solid line) defined the test result as normal or abnormal. The IPG result is defined as abnormal if the single test with *both* the greatest venous capacitance (IPG rise) and greatest venous outflow (IPG fall) lands on or below the discriminant line. The stop-line (thin solid line) runs parallel to the discriminant line and provides for early termination of the five-test sequence if the test result lands above this stop-line. This enables the five-test sequential technique to be terminated without loss of accuracy in 45% of normal limbs following one test, in 59% following the second test in the sequence, and in 80% after the third test of the sequence.

the five-test sequential procedure is used. These are: (1) normal because the test with the highest rise and greatest fall lands above the discriminant line, (2) abnormal because the test with the both the highest rise and greatest fall lands on or below the discriminant line, and (3) technically inadequate if the maximum venous filling and outflow (highest rise and fall) do not occur in the same test of the sequence. The most common cause of technically inadequate IPG results is unrecognized muscle tension or contraction of leg muscles which may lead to impairment of venous outflow and a false-positive IPG result. This IPG result is easily recognized by a deterioration in venous outflow despite an increase in venous filling.

CAUSES OF FALSE-POSITIVE OR FALSE-NEGATIVE IMPEDANCE PLETHYSMOGRAPHY RESULTS

Technical Causes

The most serious technical error may be a false-negative IPG result caused by skin movement artifact due to incorrect positioning of the cuff too far distally on the thigh, particularly in patients with obese legs; when the thigh cuff is inflated, the skin over the calf may stretch and cause movement of the electrodes. This skin movement artifact is exaggerated by increased knee flexion. The skin movement artifact is easily identified as a large, fast rise of the IPG tracing in the first two to three seconds after cuff inflation. It is easily distinguished from the normal IPG rise since it is much more abrupt and does not contain an arterial pulse. It is easily corrected by moving the cuff higher up on the thigh and ensuring that the appropriate amount of knee flexion of 10° to 20° is present. All individuals performing IPG should be familiar with the "rapid-rise" tracing and be able to identify this because it could lead to the potential for undetected proximal-vein thrombosis.

The potential technical causes of a false-positive IPG result include the tourniquet effect, incorrect positioning of the leg (hyperextension), or instrumentation problems. The tourniquet effect, resulting in obstruction to venous outflow, may be caused by tight clothing or pressure dressing, or by the thigh cuff or electrodes if they are applied too tightly. Clothing which may potentially produce external constriction and obstruction to venous outflow should be removed during IPG testing. The operator should be able to easily slide four fingers under both the proximal and distal edge of the thigh cuff. The electrodes should be applied with as little tension as necessary to provide adequate skin contact. Hyperextension of the knee may produce a false-positive result due to compression of the popliteal vein by the posterior aspect of the tibia; the leg should be positioned with the knee flexed 10° to 20°. Successful testing with IPG depends on rapid deflation of the cuff, since the venous outflow is measured during the first three seconds. If the thigh cuff does not deflate properly, this may lead to a false-positive result and could be due to either a problem with the cuff or a kink or obstruction in the pneumatic outflow line. Finally, the manufacturers recommendation should be followed for appropriate calibration, quality control checking and instrument maintenance.

Pathophysiological Causes

The most common causes of a false-positive result are: (1) muscle tension (this is the most common cause), (2) increased central venous pressure due to congestive cardiac failure or constrictive pericarditis (this usually produces an abnormal result bilaterally), (3) external venous compression due to pelvic tumors or abscess, (4) venoconstriction due to severe cold or shock which impairs venous filling (this usually produces an abnormal result bilaterally), and (5) arterial insufficiency which impairs venous filling, and is usually associated with clinically evident and severe peripheral ischemia.

Impedance plethysmography may remain abnormal for weeks to months in patients with proximal-vein thrombosis. Therefore, in patients with a previous history of venous thrombosis who present with new symptoms and have a positive IPG, it is difficult to distinguish acute recurrent thrombosis from the postphlebitic syndrome if it has not been documented that the IPG had returned to normal during the interim. The IPG returns to normal in 30% of patients with proximal-vein thrombosis by 3 weeks after the initial episode, in 60% to 70% by 6 months, in about 80% by 6 months, and in 95% by one year.[31,32(I)] This makes the IPG a particularly useful test in patients with suspected recurrent venous thrombosis, particularly when it is documented that the IPG has returned to normal after the initial episode.

The IPG has the potential to be false-negative in patients with a history of previous venous thrombosis if well developed or extensive collaterals have formed. Impedance plethysmography does not detect most thrombi confined to the calf-veins, and may fail to detect small nonocclusive proximal-vein thrombi. These potential limitations are overcome for practical clinical purposes by performing serial testing. The clinical outcome studies have shown that serial testing is effective for identifying clinically important thrombi which may result from either extension of isolated calf-vein thrombosis or evolution of nonocclusive proximal thrombi to become occlusive.

CLINICAL APPLICATION OF IMPEDANCE PLETHYSMOGRAPHY

Results in the Diagnosis of Clinically Suspected Deep-Vein Thrombosis

The studies evaluating the sensitivity and specificity of occlusive-cuff IPG for proximal-vein thrombosis in symptomatic patients are summarized in Table 1. Between 1974 and 1982, studies by several groups reported consistently high sensitivity and specificity of IPG for proximal-vein thrombosis (Table 1). The cumulative sensitivity during this period was 94% and the cumulative specificity was 94%. During the mid-1980s, the focus of studies with IPG shifted to evaluating clinical outcome in patients in whom management decisions were based on the results of IPG testing. The main objective of these outcome studies was to test the safety of withholding anticoagulant therapy in patients with symptoms or signs suggesting deep-vein thrombosis (DVT) in whom repeated testing with IPG over a 10- to 14-day period had remained negative. The results of the five prospective studies[15-19] evaluating clinical outcome in patients managed using serial IPG are summarized in Table 2. The results indicate that if serial testing with IPG remains negative, the risk of clinically important PE is low (less than 1%). Similarly, the rate of symptomatic venous thrombosis on follow-up for 3 to 6 months is also low (1% to 2%). Thus, it is safe to withhold anticoagulant therapy if the results of serial testing with IPG remain negative.

The results of the two most recent accuracy studies[25,26] from the same institution are in striking contrast to the consistent findings of 14 previous studies published between 1974 and 1982 (Table 1). In the study by Ginsberg et al,[26] most of the thrombi which were not detected by IPG extended just into the popliteal vein. It is well documented that a single IPG test may fail to detect such nonocclusive thrombi which barely extend out of the calf-veins. The clinical outcome studies summarized in Table 2 indicate that these thrombi either were detected by serial testing, or if such thrombi were present in patients negative by serial IPG, they did not result in subsequent clinically important VTE. Recent observations[33] suggest that B-mode imaging may be more sensitive to popliteal extension of calf-vein thrombosis than IPG. The large outcome studies, however document equivalent safety in patients with negative results with either serial IPG or B-mode ultrasound imaging.[15,19]

In conclusion, serial testing with IPG is an effective and safe approach for evaluating patients with clinically suspected venous thrombosis. If the IPG at presentation is negative, it is safe to evaluate such patients with serial testing in which the IPG is repeated four to five times over a 10 to 14 day interval. This repeated testing can be performed on an outpatient basis.

A positive IPG result is highly specific for proximal-vein thrombosis in the absence of clinical conditions known to produce false-positive test results (e.g., CHF, severe peripheral arterial disease, etc). In patients with positive IPG results, a bedside examination of the patient is needed to rule out clinical disorders known to produce false-positive findings. In patient subgroups with disorders known to produce false-positive IPG results (for example, those in intensive care who frequently suffer from cardiac failure), the use of serial B-mode imaging would avoid the potentially higher false-positive rates associated with IPG testing in such a population.

Application in Patients with Clinically Suspected Pulmonary Embolism

Impedance plethysmography is sensitive and specific for proximal-vein thrombosis in patients who present with symptoms or signs suggesting PE.[21] Serial testing with IPG in patients with suspected PE who have nondiagnostic lung scans and adequate cardiorespiratory reserve provides a practical noninvasive strategy that: (1) avoids pulmonary angiography, (2) identifies patients with proximal-vein thrombosis who require treatment, and (3) avoids the need for treatment and further investigation in the majority of patients.[23] The role of testing with IPG and other objective tests for venous thrombosis in patients with suspected PE is discussed in more detail in chapter 24.

Table 2
Incidence of Clinically Important Pulmonary Embolism in Patients with Suspected Venous Thrombosis and Negative Results by Serial Impedance Plethysmography Testing: Prospective Studies

Study and Year	No. of Patients with Negative Results	Fatal PE No. of Patients (%)	Symptomatic Non-fatal PE No. of Patients (%)
Hull et al. 1985[15]	311	0	0
Huisman et al. 1986[16]	289	0	0
Huisman et al. 1989[17]	131	0	0
Hull et al. 1990[18]	139	0	0
Heijboer et al. 1993[19]	361	0	2 (0.6%)
Total	1,231	0*	2 (0.2%)

IPG = impedance plethysmography
* 95% confidence intervals: 0/1231, 0% to 0.24% and 2/1231, 0.02% to 0.59%.

REFERENCES

1. Wheeler HB, O'Donnell JA, Anderson F, Benedict KJ. Occlusive impedance phlebography: a diagnostic procedure for venous thrombosis and pulmonary embolism. Prog Cardiovasc Dis 1974;17:199–205.

2. Todd JW, Frisbie JH, Rossier AB, et al. Deep venous thrombosis in acute spinal cord injury: a comparison of ^{125}I fibrinogen leg scanning and venography. Paraplegia 1976;14:50–57.

(I)3. Hull R, van Aken WG, Hirsh J, Gallus AS, Hoicka G, et al. Impedance plethysmography using the occlusive cuff technique in the diagnosis of venous thrombosis. Circulation 1976;53:696–700.

(I)4. Hull R, Hirsh J, Sackett DL, Powers P, Turpie AGG, Walker I. Combined use of leg scanning and impedance plethysmography in suspected venous thrombosis: an alternative to venography. N Engl J of Med 1977;296:1497–1500.

(I)5. Toy PTCY, Schrier SL. Occlusive impedance plethysmography: a noninvasive method of diagnosis of deep vein thrombosis. West J Med 1978;129:89.

6. Flanigan DP, Goodreau JJ, Burnham S, Bergan JJ, Yao JST. Vascular-laboratory diagnosis of clinically suspected acute deep vein thrombosis. Lancet 1978;2(8085):331-334.

(I)7. Hull R, Taylor DW, Hirsh J, Sackett DL, Powers P, et al. Impedance plethysmography: the relationship between venous filling and sensitivity and specificity for proximal vein thrombosis. Circulation 1978;58:898–902.

8. Gross WS, Burney RE. Therapeutic and economic implications of emergency department evaluation for venous thrombosis. J Am Coll Emer Physicians 1979;8:110–113.

9. Cooperman M, Martin EW Jr, Satiani B, et al. Detection of deep venous thrombosis by impedance plethysmography. Am J Surg 1979;137:252–254.

10. Liapis CD, Satiani B, Kuhns M, Evans WE. Value of impedance plethysmography in suspected venous disease of the lower extremity. Angiology 1980;31:522–525.

11. Foti ME, Gurewich V. Fibrin degradation products and impedance plethysmography: measurements in the diagnosis of acute deep vein thrombosis. Arch Intern Med 1980;140:903–906.

(I)12. Hull R, Hirsh J, Sackett DL, Taylor DW, Carter C, et al. Replacement of venography in suspected venous thrombosis by impedance plethysmography and ^{125}I-fibrinogen leg scanning: a less invasive approach. Ann Intern Med 1981;94:12–15.

13. Clarke-Peterson DL, Creasman WT. Diagnosis of deep venous thrombosis in obstetrics and gynecology by impedance phlebography. Obstet Gynecol 1981;58:52–57.

14. Peters SHA, Joncker JJ, de Boer AC, Ottlander GJ. Home-diagnosis of deep venous thrombosis with impedance plethysmography. Thromb and Haemost 1982;48:297–300.

(I)15. Hull RD, Hirsh J, Carter CJ, Jay RM, Ockelford PA, et al. Diagnostic efficacy of impedance plethysmography for clinically suspected deep-vein thrombosis: a randomized trial. Ann Intern Med 1985;102:21–28.

(I)16. Huisman MV, Buller HR, ten Cate JW, Vreeken J. Serial impedance plethysmography for suspected deep venous thrombosis in outpatients. The Amsterdam general practitioner study. N Engl J of Med 1986;314:823–828.

(I)17. Huisman MV, Buller HR, ten Cate JW, Heijermans HSF, van der Laan J, et al. Management of clinically suspected acute venous thrombosis in outpatients with serial impedance plethysmography in a community hospital setting. Arch Intern Med 1989;149:511–513.

(I)18. Hull RD, Raskob GE, Carter CJ. Serial impedance plethysmography in pregnant patients with clinically suspected deep-vein thrombosis: clinical validity of negative findings. Ann Intern Med 1990;112:663–667.

(I)19. Heijboer H, Buller HR, Lensing AWA, Turpie AGG, Colly LP, et al. A comparison of real-time compression ultrasonography with impedance plethysmography for the diagnosis of deep-vein thrombosis in symptomatic outpatients. N Engl J of Med 1993;329:1365–1369.

20. Hull RD, Feldstein W, Pineo GF, Raskob GE. Cost effectiveness of diagnosis of deep vein thrombosis in symptomatic patients. Thromb Haemost 1995;74:189–196.

(I)21. Hull R, Hirsh J, Carter C, Jay R, Dodd P, et al. Pulmonary angiography, ventilation lung scanning, and venography for clinically suspected pulmonary embolism with abnormal perfusion lung scans. Ann Intern Med 1983;98:891–899.

(I)22. Hull R, Raskob G, Coates G, Panju A, Gill G. A new noninvasive management strategy for patients with suspected pulmonary embolism. Arch Intern Med 1989;149:2549–2555.

(I)23. Hull R, Raskob G, Ginsberg J, Panju A, Brill-Edwards P, et al. A noninvasive management strategy for patients with suspected pulmonary embolism. Arch Intern Med 1994;154:289–297.

(I)24. Hull R, Carter C, Jay R, Ockelford P, Hirsh J, et al. The diagnosis of acute recurrent deep-vein thrombosis: a diagnostic challenge. Circulation 1983;67:901–906.

25. Anderson DR, Lensing AWA, Wells PS, Levine MN, Weitz JI, et al. Limitations of impedance plethysmography in the diagnosis of clinically suspected deep-vein thrombosis. Ann Intern Med 1993;118:25–30.

(IV)26. Ginsberg J, Wells P, Hirsh J, Panju A, Patel MA, et al. Reevaluation of the sensitivity of impedance plethysmography for the detection of proximal deep vein thrombosis. Arch Intern Med 1994;154:1930–1933.

27. Akers SM, Bartter T, Pratter MR. Impedance plethysmography: it's the clinical outcome that counts. Chest 1994;106:1317–1318.

(I)28. Prandoni P, Lensing AWA, Buller HR, Carta M, Vigo M, et al. Failure of computerized impedance plethysmography in the diagnostic management of patients with clinically suspected deep-vein thrombosis. Thromb Haemost 1991;65:233–236.

(I)29. Prandoni P, Lensing AWA, Huisman MV, Jonker JJC, Vigo M, et al. A new computerized impedance plethysmograph: accuracy in the detection of proximal deep-vein thrombosis in symptomatic outpatients. Thromb Haemost 1991;65:229–232.

30. Taylor D, Hull R, et al. Simplification of the sequential impedance plethysmography technique without loss of accuracy. Thromb Res 1980;17:561–565.

31. Jay R, Hull R, Carter C, Ockelford P, Buller H, et al. Outcome of abnormal impedance plethysmography results in patients with proximal-vein thrombosis: frequency of return to normal. Thrombosis Research 1984;36:259–263.

(I)32. Huisman M, Buller H, ten Cate JW. Utility of impedance plethysmography in the diagnosis of recurrent deep-vein thrombosis. Arch Intern Med 1988;148:681–683.

33. Kearon C, Hirsh J. Factors influencing the reported sensitivity and specificity of impedance plethysmography for proximal deep vein thrombosis. Thromb Haemost 1994;72:652–658.

15

Diagnosis of Deep-Vein Thrombosis with Ultrasound Imaging in Symptomatic Patients and Asymptomatic High-Risk Patients

Anthonie W.A. Lensing, Bruce L. Davidson, Martin H. Prins, Harry R. Büller

INTRODUCTION

Recent advances in ultrasound instrumentation, including the application of high-resolution real-time equipment, have provided a new noninvasive approach for the diagnosis of venous thrombosis. The following ultrasound techniques are available: conventional gray-scale real-time ultrasonography, duplex ultrasonography, and color-coded Doppler ultrasonography. The gray-scale real-time image is obtained by real-time computation of the reflected signals from an array of ultrasound sources, resulting in two-dimensional images. The reflections are due to boundaries between adjacent structures with different acoustic properties. Duplex ultrasonography is based on the combined use of the gray-scale real-time image and pulsed Doppler technology, permitting simultaneous imaging of anatomic structures and audible or visual characterization of venous and arterial blood flow. Color-coded Doppler ultrasonography is a recent development in which Doppler shift information from moving erythrocytes, is color coded both for velocity and direction, and is superimposed in real-time on the gray-scale image.

Since the introduction of venous ultrasound imaging in 1982,[1] many articles have appeared evaluating its use for the diagnosis of deep-vein thrombosis (DVT) in symptomatic and asymptomatic high-risk patients. The latter group consists of patients at high risk for developing DVT following a major surgical procedure or a prolonged period of immobilization. These studies varied in selection of the ultrasound technique, use of diagnostic criteria, number of patients studied, and compliance with methodologic standards for the proper evaluation of a diagnostic test.

In this chapter, we will provide details of performing and interpreting the imaging techniques, discuss their potential advantages and drawbacks, and review their accuracy for the diagnosis of DVT in symptomatic and asymptomatic patients. In addition, accuracy was calculated separately for studies which minimized the potential for bias and those investigations with such a potential.

ULTRASONOGRAPHY TECHNIQUES

Conventional Gray-Scale Real-Time Ultrasonography

Venous ultrasound imaging is performed with the patient in the supine position, with the head of the bed elevated approximately 30° to ensure adequate venous filling of the legs. The ultrasound probe is placed in the groin to identify the common femoral vein, which is always medial to the common femoral artery. The transducer is then moved distally to visualize the superficial femoral vein throughout its course. For examination of the popliteal vein, the patient is in the prone or the lateral decubitus position, with the knees flexed to prevent spontaneous collapse of the vein. The lumen of a normal vein is free of echoes and, as opposed to arteries, veins have thin walls and are held open primarily by the low venous blood pressure. Therefore, the vein lumen can be easily obliterated by a small amount of extrinsic pressure.

The most accurate and simple ultrasonic criterion for diagnosing venous thrombosis, is noncompressibility of the vascular lumen under gentle probe pressure (compression ultrasound). Vein compressibility is considered present if no residual lumen is observed and indicates the absence of venous thrombosis. The images can be ob-

From *Venous Thromboembolism: An Evidence-Based Atlas* edited by Russell Hull, Gary Raskob, Graham Pineo © 1996, Futura Publishing Co., Armonk, NY.

tained in either the transverse or longitudinal plane. However, vein compressibility is best evaluated in the transverse view because it allows visualization of both the vein and the adjacent artery. With the vein imaged in the longitudinal plane, the vein may slide out of the image plane during compression with the ultrasound probe and so falsely simulate compressibility of the venous segment. The presence of echogenic bands in the vein might be helpful to diagnose venous thrombosis but are often observed in patients in whom contrast venography clearly proves the absence of venous thrombosis. In general, the common femoral and popliteal vein can be visualized most easily due to their superficial location. The superficial femoral vein, especially its segment that passes through the adductor canal, is localized deeper and is often difficult to evaluate. The calf veins can not be evaluated with conventional ultrasound techniques, because they cannot be visualized adequately, due to their small size and insufficient resolution of the ultrasound device.

Duplex Ultrasonography

Patients are examined in an identical way as with conventional compression ultrasound. In addition, blood flow characteristics may be evaluated using the pulsed Doppler capability. Blood flow in normal veins is spontaneous and phasic with respiration, can be augmented by elevating the distal lower extremity or by manual compression distal to the ultrasound transducer, and can be interrupted by performing the Valsalva maneuver. When the phasic pattern is absent, flow is defined as continuous, indicating the presence of venous outflow obstruction especially when there is no or minimal change after the Valsalva maneuver. Absence of spontaneous venous flow may result from complete obstruction of the vein lumen.

A major drawback of the duplex examination is the lack of objective and standardized diagnostic criteria for the Doppler assessment. Sometimes spontaneous flow may not be detected in normal veins due to slow flow in small veins, and augmentation techniques will not always result in a clear venous Doppler signal. Furthermore, continuous flow with no response or poor response to the Valsalva maneuver, can be observed in patients without venous thrombosis. In patients with nonocclusive venous thrombosis the normal finding, i.e., phasic spontaneous flow interrupted by the Valsalva maneuver, may be observed.

The assessment of the calf veins by duplex ultrasound is, as for the conventional gray-scale examination, hampered by the poor visualization of these veins.

Color-Coded Doppler Ultrasonography

The technique of the color-coded Doppler ultrasonography (color Doppler) examination is basically identical with that of compression ultrasound and duplex ultrasonography. In color flow sonography, pulsed Doppler signals are used to produce the images. When a

Doppler shift is recognized, it is assigned a color (e.g., red or blue) according to its forward or reverse direction. Therefore, the technique of color Doppler mapping results in a display of flowing blood as a color overlay to the gray-scale ultrasound image, which has the potential to enhance the ability to identify the veins, even when they are obscured by soft tissue edema or by excessive depth from the transducer. Color Doppler has the potential to visualize the calf veins.

Images in the longitudinal axis are used for the assessment with color Doppler. The interpretation of venous flow whether with color Doppler or duplex ultrasonography, is essentially the same. The criterion for an abnormal color Doppler test is the absence of color in a vein after augmentation or a focal intraluminal filling defect.

As with the duplex examination, "venous flow" is Doppler wave information detected as a Doppler shift, rather than true flow measured in volume per unit of time. Therefore, Doppler-detected flow may be absent in normal veins due to slow flow and augmentation does not always result in a clear color image. The color Doppler examination might be falsely interpreted as normal in patients with nonocclusive thrombosis due to persistent venous flow (and, therefore, normal color coding of venous flow) around the thrombus.

EVALUATION OF STUDY METHODOLOGY

We critically reviewed all articles published in the English literature that evaluated the accuracy of ultrasound imaging techniques for the diagnosis of proximal or distal calf-vein thrombosis in symptomatic patients or asymptomatic high-risk patients. All reports were reviewed to determine whether they truly evaluated accuracy and whether they included the essential design features required for the evaluation of a diagnostic test[2]; these criteria are listed in Table 1. These methodological criteria were considered to be mandatory since their absence from the study design may introduce biases which invalidate the results of the studies. The design features are: (1) explicitly defined criteria for a normal and abnormal test result. In addition, the criteria for the interpretation of the reference method (venography) to which the outcomes were compared needed to be specified; (2) an

Table 1
Essential Design Features for the Evaluation of a Diagnostic Tests for Venous Thrombosis

1) Establishment of a priori objective criteria for a normal and abnormal test results.
2) Independent comparison with the gold standard for venous thrombosis, i.e., contrast venography, by investigators blinded to clinical and prior test information.
3) Inclusion of consecutive patients and prospective analysis.

independent and blind assessment of the ultrasound and venography results by observers who had no knowledge of the other test result; and (3) the inclusion of consecutive patients who were studied prospectively.

The interpretation of ultrasound tests and venography have subjective elements so that failure to define the criteria used for a normal and abnormal test result, and failure to ensure that the results of each test are interpreted independently and without knowledge of the other test result, introduces a number of biases which could invalidate the findings.[3-5] Failure to include consecutive patients or a retrospective analysis of results, can lead to the exclusion of patients in certain risk categories and so produce false estimates of accuracy. A study was considered to have included consecutive patients if this was explicitly mentioned in the article or if the exclusion criteria were described in sufficient detail to allow this judgment to be made.

Reports which met these criteria were classified as level 1 studies (potential for bias minimized), while reports which did not include all three criteria were classified as level 2 studies (potential for bias). The indices of diagnostic accuracy were calculated as follows: sensitivity was assessed by dividing the number of patients with an abnormal ultrasound result and venographically proven venous thrombosis, by the total number of patients with venographically proven venous thrombosis; specificity was assessed by dividing the number of patients with a normal ultrasound result and a normal venogram, by the total number of patients with normal venograms; the positive predictive value was determined by dividing the number of patients with a venogram-confirmed abnormal ultrasound result, by the total number of patients with an abnormal ultrasound result.

DIAGNOSIS OF SYMPTOMATIC DEEP-VEIN THROMBOSIS

A total of 46 reports could be identified that reported on the ultrasonic diagnosis of DVT in symptomatic patients. Eighteen reports were not eligible for the analysis, because they did not truly evaluate accuracy[6-16]; used symptomatic and asymptomatic patients without providing separate results for both groups[17]; used a small number of pregnant patients[18]; reported results obtained in patients with symptomatic DVT or pulmonary embolism (PE) without providing subgroup analysis[19]; provided insufficient data to allow a proper calculation of sensitivity and specificity[20(I),21]; reported results of the combination of upper and lower extremity thrombosis without providing data on the number of patients with proximal thrombosis[22]; or evaluated a selection of patients with isolated calf-vein thrombosis using a biased venographic interpretation.[77] Of the remaining 28 reports, 14 evaluated compression ultrasound, eight used duplex ultrasonography, and six assessed color-coded ultrasonography.

Accuracy for Proximal-Vein Thrombosis

Compression Ultrasound

Of the 14 studies evaluating compression ultrasound, 12 included symptomatic outpatients and two hospitalized patients who became symptomatic for venous thrombosis during their stay in the hospital. The methodology of the outpatients studies was graded as level 1 in eight studies[23,24(I),25-27(I),28-30] and as level 2 in four studies[(31-34); Table 2]. The combined analysis of the level 1 studies demonstrates that compression ultrasound correctly identified proximal-vein thrombosis in 354 of

Table 2
Classification of Study Methodology and Results for Reports Evaluating Gray-Scale Real-Time
Ultrasonography in Patients with Clinically Suspected Deep-Vein Thrombosis

Investigators	Standards Satisfied	Sensitivity for Proximal DVT		Specificity	
		Level 1			
Dauzat et al., 1986	1,2,3	97%	(89/92)	100%	(45/45)
Appelman et al., 1987	1,2,3	92%	(48/52)	97%	(58/60)
Aitken and Godden, 1987	1,2,3	94%	(15/16)	100%	(26/26)
Cronan et al., 1987	1,2,3	93%	(25/27)	100%	(23/23)
Lensing et al., 1989	1,2,3	100%	(66/66)	99%	(142/143)
Monreal et al., 1989	1,2,3	93%	(40/43)	86%	(18/21)
Habscheid et al., 1990	1,2,3	95%	(57/60)	100%	(91/91)
Chance et al., 1991	1,2,3	100%	(14/14)	93%	(56/60)
Total		96%	(354/370)	98%	(459/469)
		Level 2			
Effeney et al., 1984	1	83%	(19/23)	86%	(12/14)
Raghavendra et al., 1984	1	100%	(6/6)	100%	(5/5)
Raghavendra et al., 1986	1	100%	(14/14)	100%	(6/6)
Fletcher et al., 1990	1,3	100%	(14/14)	93%	(28/30)
Total		93%	(53/57)	93%	(51/55)

Sensitivity level 1 versus level 2: p = 0.62, Specificity level 1 versus level 2: p < 0.03.

the 370 patients, for a sensitivity of 96%. Thrombosis was correctly excluded in 459 of the 469 patients with normal venograms, for a specificity of 98%. The results of the four level 2 studies did slightly differ from the results in the level 1 studies; sensitivity and specificity were both 93%. The difference between sensitivity of the level 1 studies versus level 2 studies was not statistically significant (p = 0.62). Therefore, regardless of quality of study design, compression ultrasound of the proximal veins has a consistently high accuracy for the diagnosis of proximal-vein thrombosis in symptomatic patients. Feasibility of the compression ultrasound test was consistently high in all studies. Inconclusive compression ultrasound test results occurred infrequently (less than 1% of patients). Two large studies limited the compression ultrasound evaluation to the common femoral vein and the popliteal vein.[24(I),27(I)] Combining the data, the sensitivity and specificity for proximal-vein thrombosis was 97% and 99%, respectively—these results are fully comparable with the results of studies that evaluated the entire proximal venous system. Both compression ultrasound studies, which evaluated hospitalized patients who became symptomatic for venous thrombosis during hospitalization, had level 1 methodology.[35(I),36(I)] In these patients, the combined sensitivity and specificity for proximal-vein thrombosis were 91% (135/148) and 94% (102/109), respectively. These findings in hospitalized patients are fully comparable with the results obtained in symptomatic outpatients.

Duplex Ultrasonography

Eight studies evaluated the accuracy of duplex ultrasonography for the diagnosis of proximal-vein thrombosis (seven in symptomatic outpatients, one in hospitalized patients who became symptomatic during hospitalization). Of the outpatients studies, four had level 1 methodology,[37,38(I),39,40(I)] and three were classified as level 2

([41–43]; Table 3). In the level 1 studies, the sensitivity was 95% (98/103), and specificity was 93% (134/144). In the studies which used less strict methodology, sensitivity and specificity were 99% and 96%, respectively. The difference between sensitivity of the level 1 studies versus level 2 studies was statistically significant (p = 0.02) in favor of the studies which had a potential for bias. The single duplex ultrasonography study which evaluated hospitalized patients who became symptomatic for venous thrombosis during hospitalization had level 1 methodology.[44(I)] In this study, sensitivity and specificity for proximal-vein thrombosis were 97% and 98%, respectively.

Color Doppler Ultrasonography

The accuracy of color Doppler ultrasonography for the diagnosis of venous thrombosis has thus far been investigated in four methodologically sound studies (level 1; [45–48]; Table 4), whereas two studies had level 2 methodology.[49,80] In the level 1 studies, color Doppler correctly diagnosed proximal-vein thrombosis in 123 of the 127 patients, for a sensitivity of 97%. The presence of proximal-vein thrombosis was correctly excluded in 207 of the 213 patients, for a specificity of 97%.

In both studies with potential for bias, sensitivity and specificity were 99% and 100%, respectively.[49,80]

Accuracy for Isolated Calf-Vein Thrombosis

The assessment of accuracy for isolated calf-vein thrombosis was limited to level 1 studies. Of the eight compression ultrasound studies in which the potential for bias was minimized, only one evaluated the accuracy for isolated calf-vein thrombosis;[29](Table 5). In this study, isolated calf-vein thrombosis was demonstrated by venography in 23 patients and compression ultrasound identified 20 of these (sensitivity, 87%). Of the four duplex ultrasonography studies which had adequate methodol-

Table 3
Classification of Study Methodology and Results for Reports Evaluating Duplex
Ultrasonography in Patients with Clinically Suspected Deep-Vein Thrombosis

Investigators	Standards Satisfied	Sensitivity for Proximal DVT	Specificity
Level 1			
Vogel et al., 1987	1,2,3	95% (19/20)	100% (33/33)
O'Leary et al., 1988	1,2,3	92% (22/24)	96% (25/26)
Mantoni et al., 1989	1,2,3	97% (34/35)	97% (48/50)
Mitchell et al., 1991	1,2,3	96% (23/24)	80% (28/35)
Total		95% (98/103)	93% (134/144)
Level 2			
George et al., 1987	1	92% (22/24)	100% (26/26)
Elias et al., 1987	1,3	100% (241/241)	98% (583/606)
Comerota et al., 1990	1	100% (37/37)	86% (24/28)
Total		99% (300/302)	96% (633/660)

Sensitivity level 1 versus level 2: p < 0.02.
Specificity level 1 versus level 2: p = 0.21.

Table 4
Classification of Study Methodology and Results for Reports Evaluating Color-Coded Doppler
Ultrasonography in Patients with Clinically Suspected Deep-Vein Thrombosis

Investigators	Standards Satisfied	Sensitivity for Proximal DVT	Specificity
		Level 1	
Baxter et al., 1990	1,2,3	92% (11/12)	100% (26/26)
Rose et al., 1990	1,2,3	92% (23/25)	100% (50/50)
Schindler et al., 1990	1,2,3	98% (54/55)	100% (100/100)
Mattos et al., 1992	1,2,3	100% (35/35)	84% (31/37)
Total		97% (123/127)	97% (207/213)
		Level 2	
Belcaro et al., 1992	1,2	100% (90/90)	100% (16/16)
Bradley et al., 1993	1,3	97% (33/34)	100% (50/50)
Total		99% (123/124)	100% (66/66)

ogy, the ability to detect isolated calf-vein thrombosis was addressed in one.[40] In this study, duplex ultrasonography identified two of the five patients with isolated calf-vein thrombosis (sensitivity, 40%). The sensitivity of color Doppler ultrasonography for isolated calf-vein thrombosis was determined in two of the four methodologically sound studies[45,46]; color Doppler correctly identified 24 of the 32 patients with isolated calf-vein thrombosis, for a sensitivity of 75%.

Diagnostic Management of Symptomatic Patients

Compression, duplex, and color Doppler ultrasonography have a high and comparable sensitivity and specificity for the diagnosis of proximal-vein thrombosis in symptomatic patients, but have limitations for the detection of isolated calf-vein thrombosis. The results of this review indicates that for the diagnosis of symptomatic DVT, duplex and color-coded ultrasonography do not offer any advantage over conventional compression ultrasound since use of the former tests does not result in an increased accuracy for proximal-vein thrombosis. Duplex and color Doppler ultrasonography have the disadvantages of being more expensive than compression ultra-

sound, because the devices cost more and the procedures are more time consuming. Moreover, false-positive results are likely to occur more often using duplex and color-coded Doppler because of difficulty evaluating Doppler signals from venous flow in the superficial femoral vein in the adductor canal. Also, the potential for false-negative results, secondary to preserved apparently normal Doppler signals, is higher for duplex and color Doppler assessments than for compression ultrasound, since approximately 10% to 20% of symptomatic patients have nonocclusive proximal-vein thrombosis.

At present, compression ultrasound limited to the assessment of the common femoral vein and the popliteal vein is the test of choice in the evaluation of symptomatic patients.[24,27] An abnormal compression ultrasound test justifies the initiation of anticoagulant treatment since the predictive value of an abnormal test outcome is high (i.e., 98%). Although a normal compression ultrasound result essentially excludes a diagnosis of proximal-vein thrombosis (negative predictive value, 96%), it does not exclude the presence of isolated calf-vein thrombosis.[27] Therefore, patients with a normal test outcome should be retested after five to 7 days to detect the small proportion of patients (approximately 1% of patients with an initial normal ultrasound test) with proximally extending calf-vein thrombosis.[50(II),51–52,53(I),54(II)]

Table 5
Sensitivity for Isolated Calf-Vein Thrombosis for Studies in
Symptomatic Patients which Minimized the Potential for Bias

	Sensitivity	95% Confidence Interval
Gray-Scale Real-Time Ultrasonography		
Habscheid et al., 1990	87% (20/23)	65–92%
Duplex Ultrasonography		
Mitchell et al., 1991	40% (2/5)	13–93%
Color Doppler Ultrasonography		
Baxter et al., 1990	100% (2/2)	23–100%
Rose et al., 1990	73% (22/30)	54–87%
Total	75% (24/32)	56–88%

DIAGNOSIS OF ASYMPTOMATIC DEEP-VEIN THROMBOSIS IN HIGH-RISK PATIENTS

A total of 26 studies (25 in orthopedic surgical patients; one in neurosurgical patients) could be identified that reported on the accuracy of ultrasound imaging techniques for the diagnosis of asymptomatic venous thrombosis in high-risk patients. Of these, seven were excluded from the analysis, since results were reported for both asymptomatic high-risk patients and patients with clinically suspected venous thrombosis,[17,55] or PE.[28] without providing subgroup analyses, two because venography was not performed or was done only in patients with abnormal ultrasound results,[56(I),57(I)] one because results were not specified for proximal-vein thrombosis separately,[58(I)] and one because results were published later in full.[79] Of the remaining 19 reports, 10 evaluated compression ultrasound, six used duplex ultrasonography, and three assessed color-coded ultrasonography.

Results

Compression Ultrasound

Of the 10 compression ultrasound studies, study methodology was graded as level 1 in eight studies,[59(I),60,61(I),62(I),63(I),64(I),65,66] and as level 2 in two studies.[67,68] Compression ultrasound identified 80 of the 129 legs with proximal-vein thrombosis, for a sensitivity of 62%; Table 6. An abnormal ultrasound test was found in 21 of the 769 legs with normal venogram results, for a specificity of 97%. The positive predictive value was 79% (80/101).

The combined results of the level 2 reports suggest that compression ultrasound had a very high sensitivity (94%) for proximal-vein thrombosis and was highly specific (100%). Since no false-positive ultrasound results were observed in these studies the positive predictive value was 100%. Comparison of the sensitivities observed in the level 1 and 2 studies demonstrates a statistically but also clinically important difference in favor of the less rigorously designed studies.

Duplex Ultrasonography

Six studies evaluated the accuracy of duplex ultrasonography for the diagnosis of proximal-vein thrombosis in asymptomatic high-risk patients. Of these, four had level 1 methodology,[69,70(I),71(I),72(I)] and two were classified as level 2 ([73,74]; Table 7). All results were reported in legs and not in patients. In the level 1 studies, the sensitivity was 79% (34/43), and specificity was 97% (473/488). The predictive value of an abnormal test was low (69%; 34/49). In the level 2 studies, sensitivity was 95%, specificity 100%, and positive predictive value was 100%.

Color Doppler Ultrasonography

The accuracy of color Doppler ultrasonography as a screening test for proximal-vein thrombosis has thus far been investigated in three methodologically sound studies[48,66,75(I)]; Table 8). Color Doppler correctly diagnosed proximal-vein thrombosis in only 28 of the 56 legs, for a sensitivity of 50%. The presence of proximal-vein thrombosis was correctly excluded in 528 of the 548 legs, for a specificity of 96%. Proximal-vein thrombosis was demonstrated by venography in only 28 of the 48 legs with an abnormal color Doppler test result, for a positive predictive value of 58%.

Accuracy for Isolated Calf-Vein Thrombosis

The assessment of accuracy for isolated calf-vein thrombosis was limited to level 1 studies.[76] Of the eight compression ultrasound studies in which the potential for bias was minimized, four evaluated the accuracy for isolated calf-vein thrombosis;[62,64–66](Table 9). In these studies, compression ultrasound identified 17 of the 42 isolated calf-vein thromboses, for a sensitivity of 40%. Of the four duplex ultrasonography studies which had adequate methodology, a single study evaluated the accuracy for

Table 6
Classification of Study Methodology and Results for Reports Evaluating Compression Ultrasonography in Asymptomatic High-Risk Patients

Investigators	Standards Satisfied	Sensitivity for Proximal DVT	Specificity	Positive Predictive Value
		Level 1		
Borris et al., 1989	1,2,3	63% (15/24)	91% (29/32)	83% (15/18)
Borris et al., 1990	1,2,3	73% (8/11)	94% (44/47)	73% (8/11)
Agnelli et al., 1992	1,2,3	57% (12/21)	99% (165/166)	92% (12/13)
Ginsberg et al., 1991	1,2,3	52% (11/21)	99% (184/186)	89% (11/13)
Cronan et al., 1991	1,2,3	100% (12/12)	100% (64/64)	100% (12/12)
Tremaine et al., 1992	1,2,3	100% (2/2)	95% (55/58)	40% (2/5)
Jongbloets et al., 1992	1,2,3	38% (5/13)	96% (83/87)	56% (5/9)
Lensing et al., 1994	1,2,3	60% (15/25)	96% (124/129)	75% (15/20)
Total		62% (80/129)	97% (748/769)	79% (80/101)
		Level 2		
Woolson et al., 1990	1	89% (17/19)	100% (133/133)	100% (17/17)
Dorfman et al., 1990	1,3	100% (14/14)	100% (75/75)	100% (14/14)
Total		94% (31/33)	100% (208/208)	100% (31/31)

Sensitivity level 1 versus level 2: $p < 0.001$.
Specificity level 1 versus level 2: $p < 0.04$.
Positive predictive value level 1 versus level 2: $P < 0.02$.

Table 7
Classification of Study Methodology and Results for Reports Evaluating Duplex Ultrasonography in Asymptomatic High-Risk Patients

Investigators	Standards Satisfied	Sensitivity for Proximal DVT	Specificity	Positive Predictive Value
		Level 1		
Froehlich et al., 1989	1,2,3	100% (5/5)	97% (33/34)	83% (5/6)
Barnes et al., 1991	1,2,3	79% (15/19)	98% (283/289)	71% (15/21)
Woolson et al., 1991	1,2,3	67% (10/15)	99% (72/73)	91% (10/11)
Elliott et al., 1993	1,2,3	100% (4/4)	92% (85/92)	36% (4/11)
Total		79% (34/43)	97% (473/488)	69% (34/49)
		Level 2		
Comerota et al., 1990	3	100% (7/7)	100% (29/29)	100% (7/7)
White et al., 1990	3	92% (11/12)	100% (20/20)	100% (11/11)
Total		95% (18/19)	100% (49/49)	100% (18/18)

Sensitivity level 1 versus level 2: $p = 0.24$.
Specificity level 1 versus level 2: $p = 0.43$.
Positive predictive value level 1 versus level 2: $P < 0.02$.

isolated calf-vein thrombosis.[71] In this study, duplex ultrasonography identified 13 of the 23 patients with isolated calf-vein thrombosis (sensitivity, 57%). The sensitivity of color Doppler ultrasonography for isolated calf-vein thrombosis was determined in one of the three methodologically sound studies.[66] In addition, a color Doppler ultrasonography study which minimized the potential for bias was identified which evaluated only patients with isolated calf-vein thrombosis.[78(I)] The combined results of these studies demonstrate that 24 of the 49 patients with isolated calf-vein thrombosis (sensitivity, 49%) were correctly diagnosed.

Conclusions

At present, there is sufficient evidence from well performed studies in patients presenting with clinically suspected DVT, to conclude that all three ultrasonographic diagnostic tests have a very high and fully comparable ability, to confirm or refute proximal-vein thrombosis in these patients. This conclusion appears to be valid both for patients who are referred to the hospital with clinical signs and symptoms, as well as for patients who become symptomatic during their stay in hospital. The confidence

that these results reflect the true accuracy and comparability of the three ultrasound methods is further strengthened by the narrow ranges of accuracy indices for proximal DVT reported by the individual studies.

The accuracy of the various ultrasound techniques for the detection of isolated calf-vein thrombosis has thus far been investigated in a limited number of studies. The sensitivity for isolated calf-vein thrombosis appears to be considerably lower than for proximal-vein thrombosis. Therefore, the clinical utility of these techniques to rule out isolated calf-vein thrombosis is insufficient, making repeated testing necessary to detect patients with proximally extending calf-vein thrombosis. Hence the most cost-effective approach for symptomatic patients is to perform compression ultrasound at the day of referral and repeat the test in patients with normal initial test outcomes after 5 to 7 days.

This analysis clearly illustrates the fact that the excellent accuracy of ultrasonography tests found in symptomatic patients cannot be extrapolated to asymptomatic high-risk patients. In actual fact, the sensitivity for proximal-vein thrombosis of all three ultrasound methods are 30% to 40% lower than the sensitivity in symptomatic patients, whereas the sensitivity for isolated calf-vein

Table 8
Classification of Study Methodology and Results for Reports Evaluating Color Doppler Ultrasonography in Asymptomatic High-Risk Patients

Investigators	Standards Satisfied	Sensitivity for Proximal DVT	Specificity	Positive Predictive Value
		Level 1		
Davidson et al., 1992	1,2,3	38% (8/21)	94% (225/239)	36% (8/22)
Mattos et al., 1992	1,2,3	50% (5/10)	99% (179/180)	83% (5/6)
Lensing et al., 1994	1,2,3	60% (15/25)	96% (124/129)	75% (15/20)
Total		50% (28/56)	96% (528/548)	58% (24/48)

Table 9
Sensitivity for Isolated Calf-Vein Thrombosis for Studies in Asymptomatic High-Risk Patients which Minimized the Potential for Bias

	Sensitivity	95% Confidence Interval
Gray-Scale Real-Time Ultrasonography		
Cronan et al., 1991	0% (0/1)	—
Tremaine et al., 1992	50% (2/4)	12–100%
Jongbloets et al., 1994	38% (5/13)	8–69%
Lensing et al., 1994	42% (10/24)	20–63%
Total	40% (17/42)	24–57%
Duplex Ultrasonography		
Elliott et al., 1993	57% (13/23)	34–79%
Color Doppler Ultrasonography		
Lensing et al., 1994	42% (10/24)	20–63%
Rose et al., 1993	58% (14/24)	37–80%
Total	49% (24/49)	34–64%

thrombosis is approximately 50%. Consequently, all three ultrasound methods analyzed have an insufficient clinical utility to rule in or rule out venous thrombosis in asymptomatic high-risk patients. It is most likely that differences in characteristics of the thrombi account for the different sensitivities of ultrasonography in symptomatic patients compared with asymptomatic high-risk patients. Indeed, in symptomatic patients proximal thrombi are usually large, and occlusive, whereas in asymptomatic high-risk patients proximal thrombi are often small, fresher and nonocclusive.

The separate analyses of studies with and without the potential for bias, showed a disturbing difference in accuracy towards almost ideal sensitivities and specificities in those studies with less stringent methodology. This illustrates that enthusiasm is not a substitute for careful validation of these tests, and it may be particularly troublesome if the introduction and adoption of poorly validated tests is associated with increased risk of morbidity, due to unnecessary anticoagulant therapy and missed venous thrombosis.

The technology of ultrasonography is evolving rapidly as new transducer materials and electronic components become available and new methods of data acquisition, signal processing, and image display will be developed. It is possible that with further refinement in ultrasound technology its resolution will be improved to enable it to detect small nonocclusive thrombi. At present, however, color Doppler and duplex ultrasonography have no advantage in the diagnosis of DVT over the much less expensive conventional real-time compression ultrasound technique.

REFERENCES

1. Talbot SR. Use of real-time imaging in identifying deep venous obstruction: a preliminary report. Bruit 1982;6:41–42.

2. Sackett DL, Haynes RB, Tugwell P. The interpretation of diagnostic data. In: Sackett DL, Haynes RB, Tugwell P (eds.): Clinical Epidemiology. A basic science for clinical medicine. Boston, Toronto, Little, Brown and Company, 1985.

3. McLachlan MSF, Thomson JG, Taylor DW, Kelly ME, Sackett DL. Observer variation in the interpretation of lower limbs venograms. Am J Radiol 1979;132:227–229.

4. Lensing AWA, Büller HR, Prandoni P, et al. Contrast venography, the gold standard for the diagnosis of deep vein thrombosis: improvement in observer agreement. Thromb Haemostas 1991;67:8–12.

5. Lensing AWA, Hirsh J. ^{125}I-fibrinogen leg scanning: reassessment of its role for the diagnosis of venous thrombosis in post-operative patients. Thromb Haemostas 1993;69:2–7.

6. Langsfeld M, Hershey FB, Thorpe L, et al. Duplex B-mode imaging for the diagnosis of deep venous thrombosis. Arch Surg 1987;122:587–591.

7. Rollins DL, Semrow CM, Friedell ML, Calligaro KD, Buchbinder D. Progress in the diagnosis of deep venous thrombosis. J Vasc Surg 1988;7:638–641.

8. Rosner NH, Doris PE. Diagnosis of femeropopliteal venous thrombosis. AJR 1988;150:623–627.

9. Persson AV, Jones C, Zide R, Jewell ER. Use of triplex scanner in diagnosis of deep venous thrombosis. Arch Surg 1989;124:593–596.

10. Fobbe F, Koennecke HC, Bedewi M, Heidt P, Boese-Landgraf J, et al. Diagnostik der tiefen beinvenenthrombose mit der farbkodierten duplexsonographie. Fortschr Roentgenstr 1989;151:569–573.

11. Killewich LA, Bedford GR, Beach KW, et al. Diagnosis of deep venous thrombosis. Circulation 1989;79:810–814.

12. Cavaye D, Kelly AT, Graham JC, Appleberg M, Briggs GM. Duplex ultrasound diagnosis of lower limb venous thrombosis. Aust N Z J Surg 1990;60:283–288.

13. George JE, Berry RE. Noninvasive detection of deep venous thrombosis. Am Surg 1990;56:76–78.

14. Wright DJ, Shepard AD, McPharlin M, Ernst CB. Pitfalls in lower extremity venous duplex scanning. J Vasc Surg 1990;5:675–679.

15. Foley WD, Middleton WD, Lawson TL, Erickson S, Quiroz FA, et al. Color Doppler ultrasound imaging of lower-extremity venous disease. AJR 1991;152:371–376.

16. AbuRahma AF, Kennard W, Robinson PA, et al. The judicial use of venous duplex imaging and strain gauge plethysmography (single or combined) in the diagnosis of acute and chronic deep vein thrombosis. Surg Gynecol Obstet 1992;174:52–58.

17. Mussurakis S, Papaioannou S, Voros D, Vrakatselis T. Compression ultrasonography as a reliable imaging monitor in deep venous thrombosis. Surg Gynecol Obstet 1990;171:233–239.

18. Greer IA, Barry J, Mackon N, Allan PL. Diagnosis of deep venous thrombosis in pregnancy: a new role for diagnostic ultrasound. Br J Obstet Gyn 1990;97:53–57.

19. Ramshorst B, Legemate DA, Verzijlbergen JF, et al. Duplex scanning in the diagnosis of acute deep vein thrombosis of the lower extremity. Eur J Vasc Surg 1991;5:255–260.

(I)20. Irvine AT, Thomas ML. Colour-coded duplex sonography in the diagnosis of deep vein thrombosis: a comparison with phlebography. Phlebography 1991;6:103–109.

21. Lindqvist R. Ultrasound as a complementary diagnostic method in deep vein thrombosis of the leg. Acta Med Scand 1977;201:435–438.

22. Montefusco-von Kleist CM, Bakal C, Sprayregen S, Rhodes BA, Veith FJ. Comparison of duplex ultrasonog-

raphy and ascending contrast venography in the diagnosis of venous thrombosis. Angiology 1993;44:169–175.

23. Dauzat MM, Laroche JP, Charras C, et al. Real-time B-mode ultrasonography for better specificity in the noninvasive diagnosis of deep venous thrombosis. J Ultrasound Med 1986;5:625–630.

(I)24. Appelman PT, de Jong TE, Lampman LE, et al. Deep venous thrombosis of the leg: US findings. Radiology 1987;163:743–746.

25. Aitken AGF, Godden DJ. Real-time ultrasound diagnosis of deep vein thrombosis: a comparison with venography. Clin Radiol 1987;38:309–313.

26. Cronan JJ, Dorfman GS, Scola FH, Schepps B, Alexander J. Deep venous thrombosis: US assessment using vein compressibility. Radiology 1987;162:191–194.

(I)27. Lensing AWA, Prandoni P, Brandjes D, et al. Detection of deep-vein thrombosis by real-time B-mode ultrasonography. N Eng J Med 1989;320:342–345.

28. Monreal M, Montserrat E, Salvador R, et al. Real-time ultrasound for diagnosis of symptomatic venous thrombosis and for screening of patients at risk. Angiology 1989;40:527–532.

29. Habscheid W, Hohmann M, Wilhelm T, et al. Real-time ultrasound in the diagnosis of acute deep venous thrombosis of the lower extremity. Angiology 1990;599–608.

30. Chance JF, Abbitt PL, Tegtmeyer CJ, Powers RD. Real-time ultrasound for the detection of deep venous thrombosis. Ann Emerg Med 1991;20:494–496.

31. Effeney DJ, Friedman MD, Gooding GAW. Iliofemoral venous thrombosis: real-time ultrasound diagnosis, normal criteria, and clinical application. Radiology 1984;150:787–793.

32. Raghavendra BN, Rosen RJ, Lam S, et al. Deep venous thrombosis: detection by high resolution real-time ultrasonography. Radiology 1984;152:789–793.

33. Raghavendra BN, Horii SC, Hilton S, et al. Deep venous thrombosis: detection by probe compression of veins. J Ultrasound Med 1986;5:89–95.

34. Fletcher JP, Kershaw LS, Barker DS, Koutts J, Varnava A. Ultrasound diagnosis of lower limb deep venous thrombosis. Med J Australia 1990;153:453–455.

(I)35. Pedersen OM, Aslaksen A, Vik-Mo H, Bassoe AM. Compression ultrasonography in hospitalized patients with suspected deep venous thrombosis. Arch Intern Med 1991;151:2217–2220.

(I)36. Heijboer H, Cogo A, Büller HR, et al. Detection of deep vein thrombosis with impedance plethysmography and real-time compression ultrasonography in hospitalized patients. Arch Intern Med 1992;152:1901–1903.

37. Vogel P, Laing FC, Jeffrey RB, Wing VW. Deep venous thrombosis of the lower extremity: US evaluation. Radiology 1987;163:747–751.

(I)38. O'Leary DH, Kane RA, Chase BM. A prospective study of the efficacy of B-scan sonography in the detection of deep venous thrombosis in the lower extremities. J Clin Ultrasound 1988;16:1–8.

39. Mantoni M. Diagnosis of deep venous thrombosis by duplex sonography. Acta Radiologica 1989;30:575–579.

(I)40. Mitchell DC, Grasty MS, Stebbings WSL, et al. Comparison of duplex ultrasonography and venography in the diagnosis of deep venous thrombosis. Br J Surg 1991;78:611–613.

41. George JE, Smith MO, Berry RE. Duplex scanning for the detection of deep venous thrombosis of lower extremities in a community hospital. Curr Surg 1987;44:203–206.

(I)42. Elias A, LeCorff G, Bouvier JL, et al. Value of real-time B-mode ultrasound imaging in the diagnosis of deep vein thrombosis of the lower limbs. Int Angiol 1987;6:175–182.

43. Comerota AJ, Katz ML, Greenwald LL, et al. Venous duplex imaging: should it replace hemodynamic tests for deep venous thrombosis. J Vasc Surg 1990;11:53–57.

(I)44. Quintavalla R, Larini P, Miselli A, Mandrioli R, Ugolotti U, et al. Duplex ultrasound diagnosis of symptomatic proximal deep vein thrombosis of lower limbs. Eur J Radiol 1992;15:32–36.

45. Baxter GM, McKechnie S, Duffy P. Colour Doppler ultrasound in deep venous thrombosis: a comparison with venography. Clin Radiol 1990;42:32–36.

46. Rose ST, Zwiebel WJ, Nelson BD, Priest DL, Knighton RA, et al. Symptomatic lower extremity deep venous thrombosis: accuracy, limitations, and role of color duplex flow imaging in diagnosis. Radiology 1990;175:639–644.

47. Schindler JM, Kaiser M, Gerber A, et al. Colour coded duplex sonography in suspected deep vein thrombosis of the leg. Br Med J 1990;301:1369–1370.

48. Mattos MA, Londey GL, Leutz DW, et al. Color-flow duplex scanning for the surveillance and diagnosis of acute deep venous thrombosis. J Vasc Surg 1992;15:366–376.

49. Belcaro GV, Laurora G, Cesarone MR, Errichi BM. Colour duplex scanning and phlebography in deep vein thrombosis. Panminerva Med 1992;34:1–3.

(I)50. Huisman MV, Büller HR, ten Cate JW, Vreeken J. Serial impedance plethysmography for suspected deep venous thrombosis in outpatients. The Amsterdam General Practitioner Study. N Engl J Med 1986;314:823–826.

51. Cronan JJ, Dorfman GS, Grusmark J. Lower-extremity deep venous thrombosis: further experience with and refinements of US assessment. Radiology 1988;168:101–107.

52. Vaccaro JP, Cronan JJ, Dorfman GS. Outcome analysis of patients with normal compression US-examinations. Radiology 1990;175:645–649.

(I)53. Sluzewski M, Koopman MMW, Schuur KH, Vroonhoven TJMV, Ruijs JHJ, et al. Influence of negative ultrasound findings on the management of in- and outpatients with suspected deep-vein thrombosis. Eur J Radiol 1991;13:174–177.

(I)54. Heijboer H, Büller HR, Lensing AWA, et al. A comparison of real-time compression ultrasonography with impedance plethysmography for the diagnosis of deep-vein thrombosis in symptomatic outpatients. N Engl J Med 1993;329:1365–1369.

55. Nix ML, Nelson CL, Harmon BH, Ferris EF, Barnes RW, et al. Duplex venous scanning: image vs Doppler accuracy. J Vasc Tech 1989;13:123–126.

(I)56. Flinn WR, Sandager GP, Cerullo LJ, Havey RJ, Yao JST. Duplex venous scanning for the prospective surveillance of perioperative venous thrombosis. Arch Surg 1989;124:901–905.

(I)57. Kraay MJ, Goldberg VM, Herbener TE. Vascular ultrasonography for deep venous thrombosis after total knee arthroplasty. Clin Orthop 1993;286:18–26.

(I)58. Vanninen R, Manninen H, Soimakallio S, Katila T, Suomalainen O. Asymptomatic deep venous thrombosis in the calf: accuracy and limitations of ultrasonography as a screening test after total knee arthroplasty. Br J Radiol 1993;66:199–202.

(I)59. Borris LC, Christiansen HM, Lassen MR, et al. Comparison of real-time B-mode ultrasonography and bilateral ascending phlebography for detection of postoperative deep vein thrombosis following elective hip surgery. Thromb Haemost 1989;61:363–365.

60. Borris LC, Christiansen HM, Lassen MR, et al. Real-time B-mode ultrasonography in the diagnosis of postoperative deep-vein thrombosis in non-symptomatic high-risk patients. Eur J Vasc Surg 1990;4:473–475.

(I)61. Ginsberg JS, Caco CC, Brill-Edwards P, et al. Venous thrombosis in patients who have undergone major hip or knee surgery: Detection with compression US and impedance plethysmography. Radiology 1991;181:651–654.

(I)62. Cronan JJ, Froehlich JA, Dorfman GS, Image-directed Doppler ultrasound: a screening technique for patients at high risk to develop deep vein thrombosis. JCU 1991;19: 133–138.

(I)63. Agnelli G, Volpato R, Radicchia S, et al. Detection of asymptomatic deep vein thrombosis by real-time B-mode compression ultrasound in hip surgery patients. Thromb Haemostas 1992;68:257–260.

(I)64. Tremaine MD, Choroszy CJ, Gordon GH, Menking SA. Diagnosis of deep vein thrombosis by compression ultrasound in knee arthroplasty patients. J Arthroplasty 1992;7:187–192.

65. Jongbloets LMM, Lensing AWA, Koopman MM, Büller HR, ten Cate JW. Limitations of real-time compression ultrasound for the detection of asymptomatic deep-vein thrombosis in postoperative patients. submitted.

66. Lensing AWA, McGrath F, Doris I, et al. Color Doppler versus real-time ultrasonography in the diagnosis of postoperative asymptomatic deep-vein thrombosis. Submitted.

67. Woolson ST, McCrory DW, Walter JF, et al. B-mode ultrasound scanning in the detection of proximal venous thrombosis after total hip replacement. J Bone Joint Surg 1990;72:983–987.

68. Dorfman GS, Froehlich JA, Cronan JJ, Urbanek PJ, Herndon JH. Lower-extremity venous thrombosis in patients with acute hip fractures. AJR 1990;154:851–855.

69. Froehlich JA, Dorfman GS, Cronan JJ, et al. Compression ultrasonography for the detection of deep venous thrombosis in patients who have a fracture of the hip. J Bone Joint Surg 1989;71:249–253.

(I)70. Barnes CL, Nelson CL, Nix ML, et al. Duplex scanning versus venography as a screening examination in total hip arthroplasty patients. Clin Orthop 1991;271:180–189.

(I)71. Elliott GC, Suchyta M, Rose SC, et al. Duplex ultrasonography for the detection of deep vein thrombi after total hip or knee arthroplasty. Angiology 1993;44:26–33.

(I)72. Woolson ST, Pottorf G. Venous ultrasonography in the detection of proximal vein thrombosis after total knee arthroplasty. Clin Orthop 1991;273:131–135.

73. Comerota AJ, Katz ML, Greenwald LL, et al. Venous duplex imaging: should it replace haemodynamic tests for deep venous thrombosis? J Vasc Surg 1990;11:53–61.

74. White RH, Goulet JA, Bray TJ, et al. Deep-vein thrombosis after fracture of the pelvis: assessment with serial duplex ultrasound screening. J Bone Joint Surg 1990;4: 495–500.

(I)75. Davidson B, Elliott GC, Lensing AWA. Low accuracy of color Doppler ultrasound to detect proximal leg vein thrombosis during screening of asymptomatic high-risk patients. Ann Intern Med 1992;117:735–738.

76. Mussurakis S. Compression US in isolated calf vein thrombosis. Radiology 1991;181:351–35

77. Yucel EK, Fisher JS, Egglin TK, Geller SC, Waltman AC. Isolated calf vein thrombosis: diagnosis with compression ultrasound. Radiology 1991;179:443–446.

(I)78. Rose SC, Zwiebel WJ, Murdock LE, et al. Insensitivity of color Doppler flow imaging for detection of acute calf deep venous thrombosis in asymptomatic postoperative patients. J Vasc Interv Radiol 1993;4:111–117.

79. Barnes RW, Nix ML, Barnes CL, et al. Perioperative asymptomatic venous thrombosis: Role of duplex scanning versus venography. J Vas Surg 1989;9:251–260.

80. Bradley MJ, Spencer PA, Elaxander L, Milner GR. Colour flow mapping in the diagnosis of calf deep vein thrombosis. Clin Radiol 1993;47:399–402.

16

Doppler Ultrasonography

Anthonie W.A. Lensing, Marcel Levi, Harry R. Büller

BACKGROUND

In 1845, Dr. Buys Ballot confirmed Doppler's theory under experimental conditions using a locomotive and two musicians (one blowing a horn and the other perceiving the tone).[1] A century later, blood flow velocity measurement based on the Doppler principle was introduced as a diagnostic test for vascular disease.[2,3]

The Doppler ultrasound flow-velocity detector contains an oscillator that activates a piezoelectric crystal in a hand-held probe, resulting in the generation of an ultrasound beam at a frequency of 2–10 MHz. If this beam is directed percutaneously at an underlying vein, the beam will be reflected by moving red blood cells and is received by a second piezoelectric crystal. The difference in frequency between the incident and reflected ultrasound beam is proportional to the velocity of the blood cells. This difference in frequency (the Doppler shift) is translated into an audible or graphical signal. If blood flow is absent (or too slow to induce a Doppler shift), no signal will be generated. Therefore, the Doppler signals reflect Doppler shift information rather than true flow measurements.

TECHNIQUE

The Doppler ultrasound examination is performed with the patient lying in bed in the semi-upright position with the hip slightly externally rotated. Care should be taken to remove garments that constrict venous outflow because this may interfere with venous return. The common femoral vein is located by initially placing the probe over the common femoral artery, which can be easily identified, and it is then moved medially until the low-pitched sound, typical of venous flow, is heard. The intensity of this low-pitched sound decreases with inspiration and increases with expiration, resulting in a phasic signal. Abdominal compression will result in interruption of venous flow in the leg and when abdominal compression is released, there is an augmented sound as blood flow in the veins suddenly increases. Manual compression of the thigh and calf produces an augmented venous sound due to sudden acceleration of venous flow. Patency of the entire superficial femoral vein can be confirmed by moving the probe distally along this vein and repeating calf and distal thigh compression. However, care must be taken not to confuse the sounds with those produced by the long saphenous vein. Augmentation of flow is also induced by sudden release of thigh compression proximal to the probe. The probe is then placed over the posterior tibial vein, which is located adjacent to the corresponding artery behind the ankle. Augmentation of flow is produced by squeezing the foot and by suddenly releasing proximal calf compression.

Doppler ultrasound is sensitive to thrombi in the popliteal and more proximal veins which completely occlude the vein but is less sensitive to nonocclusive proximal thrombi. The ultrasonic detection of isolated calf-vein thrombosis is cumbersome due to slow venous flow which is often beyond the detection limit of the Doppler equipment and the complicated anatomy of the calf veins.

DIAGNOSTIC CRITERIA

Obstruction to venous outflow may result in an absent venous signal, provided that the thrombus completely occludes the vein. Augmentation of the venous signal, which normally occurs as a result of compression of the limb distal to the probe or to release of compression proximal to the probe, may in case of intravascular thrombus formation be diminished, high-pitched and of short duration, or absent. Maneuvers such as deep breathing, or Valsalva's may also result in increase of venous flow and may produce additional information regarding the patency of veins.

It should be noted however that venous flow may be

interpreted as normal in patients with nonocclusive thrombosis which does not cause hemodynamic changes and in patients with collateral veins. False abnormal results may be found in patients with extrinsic venous compression, or with previous deep-vein thrombosis (DVT), but may also be the result of inexperience of the examiner. The interpretation of Doppler ultrasound results are in part subjective and requires considerable skill and experience to perform reliably.

Recently, a modified Doppler ultrasound method has been evaluated which combines a standardized protocol for the execution of the examination and objective criteria for interpretation of the test result.[4(1)] With this modified technique, manual compression is not used to augment sounds. Instead, a standardized Valsalva maneuver employing a pressure device is used to measure the Valsalva pressure required to abolish the venous Doppler signal. This modified technique is based on the observation that in the horizontal position patients without venous thrombosis have low venous pressures (approximately 5 mm Hg), whereas in patients with proximal-vein thrombosis, venous pressures are much higher as a result of outflow obstruction. Performance of Valsalva's maneuver increases intra-abdominal pressure and, therefore, interrupts venous flow when intra-abdominal pressure equals the venous pressure. The Valsalva pressure and the venous Doppler signal are recorded simultaneously on a strip-chart.

CLINICAL RESULTS

The Doppler ultrasound examination has been compared with venography in several studies. A review of study methodology demonstrated that most studies did not adhere to the essential criteria for the evaluation of a diagnostic test.[5] Thus, the interpretation of venography was often done with knowledge of the results of the Doppler ultrasound examination, resulting in a high potential for bias towards a more optimistic accuracy for the Doppler examination. Furthermore, many studies assessed, selected patients (with a higher pre-test likelihood) rather than a consecutive series of patients. For the present analysis, studies were selected if the essential criteria for the evaluation of a diagnostic test were met.

Nine studies had no or minimal potential for bias and were selected for this review.[6–11,12(1),13,14] (Table 1) A pooled analysis of these studies demonstrate that this technique is sensitive to proximal-vein thrombosis but less sensitive to calf-vein thrombosis. Of the 315 patients with venographically proven proximal-vein thrombosis, 280 had an abnormal Doppler ultrasound result, for a sensitivity of 89%. The Doppler ultrasound result was falsely abnormal in 93 of the 706 patients without evidence of proximal-vein thrombosis on their venograms, for a specificity of 87%. Consequently, the predictive value of an abnormal Doppler ultrasound test is 75%.

Table 1
Sensitivity and Specificity for the Doppler Ultrasound Method for the Detection of Proximal-Vein Thrombosis in Symptomatic Patients

Investigators	Sensitivity		Specificity	
Yao et al., 1972	100%	(33/33)	88%	(15/17)
Holmes et al., 1973	100%	(17/17)	94%	(46/49)
Meadway et al., 1975	85%	(29/34)	72%	(55/76)
Dosick et al., 1978	96%	(50/52)	93%	(100/102)
Flanigan et al., 1978	65%	(35/54)	96%	(94/98)
Sumner and Lambeth, 1979	94%	(34/36)	90%	(35/39)
Hanel et al., 1981	92%	(49/53)	91%	(118/130)
Zielinsky et al., 1983	95%	(20/21)	76%	(117/153)
Turnbull et al., 1990	87%	(13/15)	78%	(33/42)
Total	89%	(280/315)	87%	(613/706)

MODIFIED DOPPLER ULTRASOUND METHOD

Recently, we reported on the development of a standardized protocol to perform the examination, and on the definition of objective criteria for normal and abnormal Doppler ultrasound results. The Doppler method was prospectively validated in a large series of consecutive outpatients with clinically suspected DVT. Contrast venography was used as the reference method.

The Doppler ultrasound test was performed at the level of the popliteal vein with the patient in the prone position, the knees flexed and the feet supported by a pillow (to prevent spontaneous collapse of the vein). The popliteal artery was located and the probe was moved laterally towards the popliteal vein. Manual compression to augment sounds was not used, instead a standardized Valsalva maneuver using a pressure device connected to a disposable mouth-piece was utilized. The pressures (expressed in mm Hg) were simultaneously recorded with the Doppler ultrasound signal.

The Valsalva-Doppler test criteria have been developed in 110 patients with clinically suspected DVT. Criteria for a normal Doppler ultrasound examination include: 1) cyclic spontaneous signal, i.e. the zero-line is intermittently printed; or 2) continuous signal with Valsalva pressure < 6.5 mm Hg to stop venous flow; or 3) absent venous signal with augmentation of venous flow after cessation of the Valsalva maneuver. Criteria for an abnormal Doppler ultrasound result were: either 1) absent venous signal without augmentation of venous flow after cessation of the Valsalva maneuver; or 2) continuous venous flow signals which can not be interrupted at a Valsalva pressure > 6.5 mm Hg.

RESULTS

A total of 155 consecutive outpatients with clinically suspected DVT and interpretable Doppler and venography results were studied. Venography demonstrated proximal-vein thrombosis in 45 patients, isolated calf-vein thrombosis in another three patients, while the remaining 107 patients had normal venograms. An abnormal Doppler test was obtained in 41 of the 45 patients with proximal-vein thrombosis (sensitivity, 91%). A false abnormal Doppler test result was obtained in only one of the 107 patients with completely normal venograms, for a specificity of 99%.

CONCLUSION

Doppler ultrasound flow-meter examination has been extensively evaluated as a noninvasive diagnostic test in patients with clinically suspected DVT. In expert hands, Doppler ultrasound is a sensitive method for detecting proximal-vein thrombosis, but is not reliable in the diagnosis of isolated calf-vein thrombosis. Advantages of this technique are that it can be performed rapidly at the bedside and that it is convenient for patients. Doppler ultrasound is more reliable than plethysmographic methods for detecting proximal-vein thrombosis in patients with raised central venous pressure or arterial insufficiency and can be used in patients who have their legs in plaster or who are in traction. However, the major limitation is that the interpretation of the Doppler signal is subjective, thereby making this test potentially unreliable in the hands of examiners with knowledge less than an expert. The recent modifications of the Doppler method which use objective and reproducible criteria for interpretation of the signal might improve its clinical usefulness. However, studies evaluating the safety of withholding anticoagulant treatment in symptomatic patients, with normal Doppler test results, have not been performed. The value of Doppler ultrasound for the diagnosis of recurrent venous thrombosis and for the screening of post-operative high-risk patients has not been formally studied.

REFERENCES

1. Jonkmans EJ. Doppler research in the nineteenth century—a historical note. Ultrasound Med Biol 1980;6:1–5.
2. Sigel B, Felix WR, Popky GL, Ispen J. Diagnosis of lower limb venous thrombosis by Doppler ultrasound technique. Arch Surg 1972;104:174–179.
3. Strandness DE Jr, Sumner DS. Ultrasonic velocity detector in the diagnosis of thrombophlebitis. Arch Surg 1972;104:180–183.
(I)4. Lensing AWA, Levi MM, Büller HR, et al. An objective Doppler method for the diagnosis of deep-vein thrombosis. Ann Intern Med 1990;113:9–13.
5. Sackett DL, Haynes RB, Tugwell P. The interpretation of diagnostic data. In: Sackett DL, Haynes RB, Tugwell P, eds. Clinical Epidemiology, A Basic Science for Clinical Medicine. Boston, Toronto: Little, Brown and Company, 1983;59–138.
6. Yao ST, Gourmos C, Hobbs JT. Detection of proximal vein thrombosis by Doppler ultrasound flow detection. Lancet 1972;1:1–4.
7. Holmes MCG. Deep venous thrombosis of the lower limbs diagnosed by ultrasound. Med J Aus 1973;1:427–431.
8. Meadway J, Nicolaides AN, Walker CJ, et al. Value of Doppler ultrasound in diagnosis of clinically suspected deep vein thrombosis. Br Med J 1975;4:552–556.
9. Dosick SM, Blakemore WS. The role of Doppler ultrasound in acute deep vein thrombosis. Am J Surg 1978;136:265–270.
10. Flanigan DP, Goodreau JJ, Burnham SJ, et al. Vascular laboratory diagnosis of clinically suspected acute deep vein thrombosis. Lancet 1978;2:331–334.
11. Sumner DS, Lambeth A. Reliability of Doppler ultrasound in the diagnosis of acute venous thrombosis both above and below the knee. Am J Surg 1979;138:205–209.
(I)12. Hanel KC, Abbott WM, Reidy NC, Fuldhino D, Miller A, et al. The role of two noninvasive tests in deep venous thrombosis. Ann Surg 1981;194:725–730.
13. Zielinsky A, Hull R, Carter C, Raskob G, Hirsh J. Doppler ultrasonography in patients with clinically suspected deep vein thrombosis. Thromb Haemostas 1983;50:153.
14. Turnbull T, Dymowski JJ, Zalut TE. A prospective study of hand-held Doppler ultrasonography by emergency physicians in the evaluation of suspected deep vein thrombosis. Ann Emergency Med 1990;19:691–695.

17

Laboratory Tests for the Diagnosis of Venous Thromboembolism

Marie-Helene Horellou, Jacqueline Conard, Meyer M. Samama

INTRODUCTION

It has long been the goal of clinicians and biologists to develop blood tests that can be used to predict thrombosis in the high-risk patient (predictive testing), or to confirm or exclude the diagnosis of thrombosis when this is clinically suspected (diagnostic testing). Sensitive and specific biochemical and immunochemical tests have been developed to detect activation of coagulation and/or fibrinolysis. Thus, circulating activated clotting factors, activation peptides, complexes of activated clotting factors and their inhibitors, and products of degradation of fibrin (resulting from the action of thrombin and plasmin on the fibrinogen), have been investigated in the diagnosis of venous thrombosis.

MARKERS OF THE ACTIVATION OF COAGULATION AND FIBRINOLYSIS

Several groups of tests are available for assessing *in vivo* coagulation (Figure 1): the first measures the plasma concentration of prothrombin fragment 1 + 2 (F_{1+2}), which is released during the conversion of prothrombin to thrombin; the second group includes tests measuring the interaction of thrombin with its substrates (fibrinopeptide A: FPA) and/or *in vivo* inhibitors (complexes thrombin-antithrombin III = TAT). After conversion of the fibrinogen in fibrin by thrombin *in vivo*, the fibrinolytic system is stimulated to lyse the fibrin. There is a subsequent increase in the levels of fibrin degradation products in plasma (D-Dimer). Markers of fibrinolysis such as plasmin-$\alpha_2$antiplasmin-complexes also provide information on in vivo coagulation. Blood cells, including platelets, participate in coagulation by serving as surfaces for assembling clotting factors. Moreover, platelets acti-

vated by thrombin release a variety of granular contents, some of which have been evaluated as markers of increased in vivo coagulation and thrombosis. These molecular markers elaborated by activated platelets have been studied in patients with arterial thrombosis and will not be discussed in this review.

Prothrombin Fragment $_{1+2}$ (F_{1+2})

Prothrombinase, including factor Xa (enzyme) and factor Va (cofactor for factor Xa) bound to procoagulant surfaces (phospholipids), converts prothrombin into equimolar concentrations of thrombin and F_{1+2}. These prothrombin fragments can be detected by immunoassays (ELISA). The concentration of F_{1+2} in normal adult citrated plasma varies between 0.3 and 1.5 nmol/l and increases significantly with age.[1,2,3] Because no specialized anticoagulant appears to be necessary, F_{1+2} can be measured on blood collected into citrate.[4] The half-life of F_{1+2} is 90 minutes. The plasma of patients with deep-vein thrombosis (DVT) shows high levels of F_{1+2}, and heparin therapy causes a rapid reduction of their concentration. Oral anticoagulant treatment suppresses the production of F_{1+2} correlating with the prolongation of the prothrombin time.[32]

Fibrinopeptide A (FPA)

Fibrinopeptide A (FPA), one of the two terminal peptides cleaved from fibrinogen by thrombin, can be identified by immunoassay.[5] The half-life of FPA is very short (3 minutes). The concentration in normal individuals is 1.5 pmol/ml or less. The considerable overlap between the values in patients with and without detectable thrombosis limits the clinical relevance of this assay.

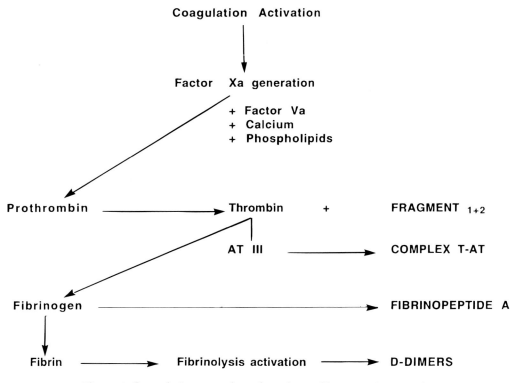

Figure 1. Coagulation cascade and markers of hemostatic activation.

Thrombin-Antithrombin III Complexes (TAT)

Thrombin is rapidly inactivated by antithrombin III, and the endogenous concentrations of TAT reflect the amount of thrombin generated. The concentration of TAT in normal volunteers (measured using commercial ELISA kits) varies between 15 to 32 pmol/l.[1,3] The half-life of TAT, 3 minutes, is as short as that of FPA.

D-Dimer

The blood of patients with active thrombotic and fibrinolytic disorders contains a large spectrum of fibrin or fibrinogen derivatives as a consequence of the separate or combined actions of thrombin, factor XIIIa, and plasmin on fibrinogen.[6] Plasmin digestion of crosslinked fibrin produces the D-Dimer fragment. Because D-Dimer is not found in digests of fibrinogen or non-crosslinked fibrin. the presence in blood of crosslinked fragments, such as D-Dimer, indicate active fibrinolysis. Monoclonal antibodies specific for antigenic determinants on D-Dimer are used in latex agglutination and enzyme immunoassays for the specific measurement of D-Dimer. The lack of cross-reactivity for the monoclonal antibody with fibrinogen allows these assays to be performed in plasma. The minimum detectable amount of D-Dimer in plasma using Latex agglutination is approximately 400 ng/ml and, by ELISA assay, approximately 10 ng/ml. The half-life of D-Dimer is 8 hours.[6]

LABORATORY TESTS FOR THE PREDICTION OF VENOUS THROMBOSIS

Predictive Tests

Preoperative Prediction of Thrombosis: Several risk factors, including preoperative parameters, physical examination, and laboratory tests, have been proposed to predict preoperatively which patient will experience venous thrombosis after a surgical procedure.[8] Several laboratory tests—fibrinolytic variables, especially prolonged clot lysis time, raised serum or plasma levels of fibrin(ogen) degradation products, and increased plasminogen activator inhibitor (PAI 1) levels—can predict postoperative DVT.[8–12] Predictive indices have been proposed.[8] For example, in a prospective study, Clayton et al, investigated 124 patients undergoing gynecologic surgery.[10] The incidence of thrombosis was 16% as assessed by leg scanning followed by venography in all patients with a positive scan. They concluded that, of all the clinical and laboratory data collected preoperatively, the euglobulin clot lysis time (*a*) was the best predictor for postoperative thrombosis. Other variables that added to the prediction power were age (*b*), presence of varicose veins (*c*), FDP levels (*d*), and a high weight/height ratio (*e*). The Clayton risk factor formula is as follows:

$$I = 11.3 + 0.0090a + 0.22d + 0.085b + 0.043e + 2.19c$$

It was calculated that all patients with postoperative thrombosis were correctly identified using an index of −5. It was found that using a cut-off point of −5 for the Clayton index, prophylaxis could be safely withheld in 21% of the total patient group (27 out of 127). However, such predictive indices are not widely used by surgeons because the illness for which surgery is performed also influences the preoperative levels of hematological tests.[13]

Postoperative Prediction of Thrombosis: Increased plasma TAT levels have been observed after surgery, particularly in the first postoperative day[14–16]; lower levels were seen in patients receiving heparin prophylaxis.[14] Significantly higher levels were observed in patients developing DVT (proven by phlebography) compared to patients without DVT, but the predictive power in individual patients to rule-in or rule-out DVT was unsatisfactorily low.[14]

In contrast, Ofosu et al, found higher concentrations of TAT in the plasma of patients who developed postoperative DVT than in plasma of patients who remained DVT-negative.[17] Comparable concentrations of TAT were observed in postunfractionnated and low-molecular-weight heparin plasmas.

A marked increase in D-Dimer levels were also observed after orthopedic surgery[16] or general abdominal surgery.[18] This increase in D-Dimer level had no predictive value for DVT in 11 total knee replacement patients.[16] In general surgery, the most accurate cut-off of D-Dimer (ELISA) for discriminating patients with or without DVT was 3000 ng/ml (as determined by ROC curve analysis); the sensitivity of using a D-Dimer level of more than 3000 ng/ml to indicate the presence of phlebographically documented DVT on the 8th day postoperatively was 89% for a specificity of 48%, with a positive predictive value of 35%.[18]

Prediction of Thrombosis in Thrombophilic Patients: In asymptomatic patients with heterozygous antithrombin III deficiency, it was initially reported that in F_{1+2} levels on heparin therapy were frequently increased compared with those of age-matched unaffected siblings[19]: 3.91 ± 1.13 versus 1.51 ± 0.63 nmol/l. Subsequently, it was shown that the high concentration of the fragment resulted from an in vitro anticoagulant effect resulting from the action of low amounts of heparin in the presence of reduced levels of antithrombin III.[20] A recent study of 26 Antithrombin III-deficiency subjects did not show significant elevation in citrated plasma F_{1+2}[21]: four patients had high F_{1+2} values (15%) and nine had high FPA values (35%). In contrast, in 63 members of a large family with normal levels of Antithrombin III antigen and reduced protease inhibitory activity, the mean level of F_{1+2} in citrated plasma was significantly higher in the deficient adults (0.87 ± 0.26 nmol/l) compared with both the nondeficient adults (0.70 ± 0.21, p. 0.03) and deficient adults receiving warfarin (0.16 ± 0.01). The differences in the mean values of TAT

complexes and FPA between deficient and nondeficient individuals were not statistically significant.[22] Therefore, overall, the present evidence indicates that patients with antithrombin deficiency do not have excessive thrombin generation in the basal state, as measured by the F_{1+2} assay.

In 23 non-anticoagulated patients with an isolated deficiency of protein C, mean levels of F_{1+2} were significantly elevated: 2.54 versus 1.51 ± 0.68 nmol/l, with a minimal fibrinopeptide A increase.[23] Approximately one-third of patients had F_{1+2} levels greater than the upper limit of normal control values; FPA levels were elevated in 20% of patients. In 57 patients with asymptomatic protein C deficiency, Mannucci et al, found a similar frequency of elevated F_{1+2} and FPA, 25% and 18%, respectively. The predictive value for a thrombotic event of an increase of F_{1+2} levels has not been determined.

When oral anticoagulants were used and equivalent levels of intensity of oral anticoagulant were achieved, the mean plasma F_{1+2} level in patients with ATIII deficiency was significantly elevated, compared with the mean level in subjects with protein C deficiency, or in a group of anticoagulated subjects without an inherited thrombotic disorder: 0.714, 0.205, and 0.231 nmol/l, respectively (in three). These immunochemical techniques should be useful in designing optimal therapeutic regimens for suppressing the in vivo generation of thrombin in such individuals. Normalization of markers of coagulation activation have been obtained after infusion of a purified protein C concentrate in two adults with homozygous protein C deficiency.[24]

LABORATORY TESTS FOR THE DIAGNOSIS OF DEEP VENOUS THROMBOSIS

Diagnostic Tests

Clinical diagnosis of DVT is unreliable, and objective testing of the venous system is needed to confirm the diagnosis of DVT before starting anticoagulant treatment. Contrast venography remains the gold standard, but this test has several major limitations: patient discomfort, allergic reactions, limited out-patient availability, and cost. Several noninvasive tests have been developed, such as venous occlusion plethysmography and ultradoppler scanning examinations. Published comparisons with contrast venography show that, in most centers, a sensitivity for the detection of proximal venous thrombosis of approximately 90% can be obtained. In addition to these physical techniques, the usefulness of plasma markers reflecting activation of hemostasis has been evaluated. A rapid blood test that could be done in the emergency room or office and that could exclude clinically significant DVT would greatly simplify patient management. At the present time the most promising results have been obtained with the measurement of D-Dimer.

(1) FPA determination: Nossel et al,[4] was the first to report elevated levels of FPA in the plasmas of patients with thrombosis: the normal level was increased up to thirty-fold. However, FPA assays have poor sensitivity and specificity for the diagnosis of DVT.[25]

(2) D-Dimer determination: Several studies have evaluated D-Dimer in patients with clinically suspected DVT (Table 1) which was confirmed by contrast venography or noninvasive methods. D-Dimer can be measured using an enzyme-linked immunosorbent assay (ELISA) or a latex agglutination assay.[26,27(I),28(I),29(I),30,31(I),32–36] In cumulative results,[37] the performance (sensitivity, specificity, positive and negative values) of the test was calculated with respect to the presence of DVT: D-Dimer ELISA tests have a high sensitivity of 96.8% (95% CI: 95.2–98.4) and a high negative predictive value of 95%, with a low specificity of 35.2% (95% CI: 32.0–38.4). Therefore, the measurement of D-Dimer by the ELISA method in symptomatic patients with clinically suspected DVT allows the diagnosis of DVT to be excluded when it is negative (<500 ng/ml), with a predictive value of 95%. An increased value (>500 ng/ml) could be explained by other conditions (such as septicaemia, malignant and inflammatory diseases, etc), and should be confirmed by other objective tests.

Although the ELISA test is very reliable in excluding the diagnosis of DVT when it is negative, it does not provide a rapid result and cannot be used as a routine screening test. The measurement of plasma D-Dimer using the latex immunoassay method is more practical and suitable for emergencies: in cumulative results, the sensitivity of the latex D-Dimer assay is only 82.9% (CI 95%: 78.4–87.4) with a specificity of 67.9% (CI 95%: 63.7–72.1). This sensitivity of only 82% is not sufficient to allow this type of assay to be used as an exclusion test for DVT. A rapid test with a sensitivity of approximately 185 ng/ml, as shown by a mathematical model (ROC analysis), could exclude the diagnosis of DVT in 62% of patients with a 98% sensitivity.[37]

The combination of a D-Dimer test and a noninvasive test has also been studied for the diagnosis of DVT and/or pulmonary embolism (PE). The diagnostic value of this combination of two noninvasive tests, i.e., computerized impedance plethysmography (IPG) and a latex test for D-Dimer measurement in plasma, was assessed in 112 consecutive patients[38]: one or both tests were positive in 59 of 60 patients with positive venograms (a sensitivity of 98%) and both were negative in 36 of 52 patients with negative venograms (a specificity of 69%). The positive predictive value when both tests were positive was 100%

Table 1

Study	n	n (DVT)	Se %	Sp %	PPV %	NPV %
D-Dimer latex						
• DVT confirmed by venography						
HEATON	57	26	73	69	63	78
OTT	108	39			59	98
BOUNAMEAUX	53	21	76	87	80	85
de BOER	33	21	43	100	100	52
ACHKAR	119	58	80	70	68	80
• DVT confirmed by non invasive methods (Doppler ultrasound, impedance phlethysmography)						
ELIAS	100	45	98	22	50	92
BONEU	116	34	76	58	43	85
LESPRIT	44	22	96	77	81	94
CARTER	190	36	80	84	54	95
D-Dimer ELISA						
• DVT confirmed by venography						
HEATON	57	26	100	47	53	100
ROWBOTHAM	104	45	100	34	54	100
OTT	108	39	97	37	61	98
BOUNAMEAUX	53	21	95	47	54	94
MOSSAZ	112	64	98	6	57	75
HEIJBOER	309	70	100	29		100
ACHKAR	119	58	90	68	68	80
• DVT confirmed by non invasive methods						
Van Bergen	239	60	92	20	28	87
ELIAS	100	45	98	29	53	94
BONEU	116	34	94	51	44	95

Sensitivity (Se), specificity (Sp), Positive (PPV) and Negative (NPV) predictive values of the D-Dimer (ELIAS and Latex assay) for the diagnosis of deep-vein thrombosis.

(39/39) and 97% when both tests were negative (36/37). Combining tests is useful in patients with clinically suspected DVT because of the very high accuracy of concordant test results. Venography should only be performed in patients with discordant test results (36 out of 112 patients). Using the combined approach, the diagnosis of DVT could either be established (positive IPG) or rejected (normal level of D-Dimer) in 42% of 309 referred patients on entry, as opposed to only 19% of patients using serial noninvasive testing alone.[39]

In studies evaluating D-Dimer testing in patients with clinically suspected PE, using a cut-off of 145 to 500 ng/ml for the ELISA assay yielded a sensitivity of 89% to 100% with a specificity ranging between 39% and 81%.[40–43] In patients with inconclusive lung scans (representing about two thirds of all scintigraphic examinations), plasma measurement of D-Dimer by ELISA is a particularly useful diagnostic approach: the diagnosis of PE can be ruled out when the level is less than 500 ng/ml (a cut-off that should be validated for each assay).[44]

(3) Thrombin-Anthithrombin III complexes or Fragment $_{1+2}$: TAT complexes[31,33] and F_{1+2}[33] determinations were less sensitive than D-Dimer assays in the diagnosis of DVT. The relatively longer D-Dimer half-life (compared to TAT and F_{1+2}) and the rapid decrease of TAT and F_{1+2} levels under heparin therapy, can explain the greater accuracy of D-Dimer testing for the diagnosis of DVT. Comparative evaluation of the usefulness of tests for D-Dimer, TAT complexes, and F_{1+2} has been performed for the diagnosis of clinically suspected DVT.[33] The most accurate assay was the D-Dimer ELISA which had both a higher sensitivity (94%) and a higher negative predictive value (95%) than those for TAT complexes (64% and 84%, respectively) and for F_{1+2} (47% and 78%, respectively). In spite of positive and significant correlations between the levels of the three different markers, their association did not improve their overall occuracy for DVT detection.[33]

Because heparin significantly decreases plasma levels of F_{1+2} and TAT complexes in less than three days, it rapidly improves the hypercoagulable state associated with acute venous thrombosis.[45] High levels of D-Dimer persisted during 9 days of heparin therapy[45] and 35 days of oral anticoagulant treatment,[46] suggesting a very long-term fibrinolytic process which occurs independently of thrombin generation. Eight days after the initiation of oral anticoagulant treatment, in spite of a correctly adjusted treatment (INR 2 to 3), increased levels of TAT complexes were associated with subnormal levels of F_{1+2} suggesting the persistence of a hypercoagulable state. After the first month, TAT complexes were normalized while F_{1+2} levels were at least three times lower than those of a young control population.[46] Monitoring the intensity and the duration of oral anticoagulant treatment based on F_{1+2} and TAT complexes levels could be determined by prospective clinical trials.

In summary, highly sensitive immunological assays for quantifying *in vivo* coagulation and/or fibrinolysis, i.e., assays for fragment $_{1+2}$, thrombin-antithrombin III complexes, fibrinopeptide A, and D-Dimer, are avalaible. These tests have been used to confirm or refute the existence of hypercoagulation in patients at high risk or with symptoms of thrombosis. With the exception of D-Dimer ELISA, these markers are of little value for the diagnosis of DVT. When the level of D-Dimer ELISA is normal (<500 ng/ml), the diagnosis of DVT can be ruled out with a risk of error of <5%. The lower sensitivity (80%) of the latex D-Dimer test is not sufficient to allow this type of assay to be used as an exclusion test for DVT. ELISA assay is not a rapid test and is not suitable for immediate clinical decision-making. Attempts should be made to simplify and shorten the time necessary to perform ELISA before the assay can be effectively used in an emergency. A rapid test with a high sensitivity could be a highly economical way to screen out-patients to determine whether they need direct vascular testing for the management of suspected acute venous thrombosis.

Suppression of the *in vivo* coagulation markers by anticogulants in patients with thrombosis, or who are at high risk for developing DVT, has been well documented. Whether or not the decision to reduce the intensity of anticoagulant treatment can be based on the measurement of these markers needs to be determined by prospective clinical trials.

REFERENCES

1. Lau HK, Rosenberg JS, Beeler DL, Rosenberg RD. The isolation and characterization of a specific antibody population directed aginst the prothrombin activation fragments F_2 and F_{1+2}. J Biol Chem 1979;254:8751–8756.
2. Teitel JM, Bauer KA, Lau H, Rosenberg RD. Studies of the prothrombin activation pathway utilizing radioimmuno assays for the F_{1+2} and thrombin-antithrombin III. Blood 1982;59:1086–1097.
3. Bauer KA, Rosenberg RD. The pathophysiology of the prethrombotic state in humans: insights gained from studies using markers of hemostatic system Activation. Blood 1987;70:343–349.
4. Pelzer H, Schwarz A, Stuber W. Determination of human prothrombin activation fragment 1 + 2 in plasma with an antibody against a synthetic peptide. Thrombosis Haemost 1991;65:153–159.
5. Nossel HL, Yudelman I, Canfiel RE, et al. Measurement of fibrinopeptide A in human blood. J Clin Invest 1974;54:43–55.
6. Gaffney PJ. The occurence and clinical relevance of fibrin fragments in blood. Ann NY Acad Sci 1983;408:407–422
7. Francks JJ, Kirsch RE, Kao B, Koppel TM. Fibrinogen and fibrinogen related peptides in cancer. In: Mariani (ed.): Pathophysiology of plasma protein metabolism. Mc Millan, London 1984:265–269
8. Ninet J, Horellou MH, Darjinoff JJ, Caulin C, Leizorovicz A. Assessment of preoperative risk factors. Ann Fr Anesth Reanim 1992;11:252–281.
9. Crandon AJ, Peel KR, Anderson JA. Post operative deep

vein thrombosis identifying high risk patients. Brit Med J 1980;281:343–344.

10. Clayton JK, Anderson JA, McNicol GP. Preoperative prediction of postoperative deep vein thrombosis. Brit Med J 1976;2:910–912.

11. Sue-Ling HM, Johnston D, McMahon MJ. Preoperative identification of patients at high risk of deep venous thrombosis after elective major abdominal surgery. Lancet 1986;l:1173–1176.

12. Paramo JA, Alfaro MJ, Rocha E. Post operative changes in the plasmatic levels of tissue type plasminogen activator and its fast acting inhibitor. Relationship to deep vein thrombosis and influence of prophylaxis. Thromb and Haemost 1985;57:713–716.

13. Lowe GD, McArdle BM, Carter DC, McLarem D, Osborme DH, et al. Prediction and selective prophylaxis of venous thrombosis in elective gastrointestinal surgery. Lancet, 1982;1:409–412.

14. Hoek JA, Nurmohamed MT, ten Cate JW, Büller HR, Knipscheer HC, et al. Thrombin-Antithrombin III complexes in the prediction of deep vein thrombosis following total hip replacement. Thromb Haemost 1989;62:1050–1052.

15. Bogaty-Yver J, Samama M. Thrombin-Antithrombin III complexes for the detection of postoperative hypercoagulable state in surgical patients receiving heparin prophylaxis. Thromb Haemost 1989;61:538. (Letter)

16. De Prost D, Ollivier V, Vie P, Benacerraf F, Duparc K, et al. D Dimer and Thrombin-antithrombin III complex levels uncorrelated with phlebographic findings in 11 total knee replacement patients. Ann Biol Clin 1990;48:235–238.

17. Ofosu FA, Levine M, Craven S, Dewar L, Shawai S, et al. Prophylactically equivalent doses of Enoxaparin and unfractionnated heparin inhibit in vivo coagulation to the same extent. Brit J Haematol 1992;82:400–405.

18. Bounameaux H, Khabiri E, Huber O, Schneider PA, Didier P, et al. Value of liquid chrystal contact thermography and plasma level of D-Dimer for screening of deep venous thrombosis following general abdominal surgery. Thromb Haemost 1992;67:603–606.

19. Bauer KA, Goodman TL, Kass BL, Rosenberg RD.Elevated factor Xa activity in the blood of asymptomatic patients with congenital antithrombin deficiency. J Clin Invest 1985;76:826–836

20. Bauer KA, Barzegar S, Rosenberg RD. Influence of anticoagulants used for blood collection on plasma prothrombin fragment F_{1+2} measurements. Thromb Res 1991;63:617–628.

21. Mannucci PM, Tripodi A, Bottasso B, Baudo F, Finazzi G, et al. Markers of procoagulant imbalance in patients with inherited thrombophilic syndromes. Thromb Haemost l992;67:200–202.

22. Demers C, Ginsberg J, Henderson P, Ofosu F, Weitz J, et al. Measurement of markers of activated coagulation in antithrombin III deficient subjects. Thromb Haemost 1992;67:542–544.

23. Bauer KA, Broekmans AW, Bertina RM, Conard J, Horellou MH, et al. Hemostatic enzyme generation in the blood of patients with hereditary protein C deficiency. Blood 1988;71:1418–1426.

24. Conard JC, Bauer KA, Griffin JH, Schwarz HP, Horellou MH, et al. Normalization of markers of coagulation activation with a purified protein C concentrate in adults with homozygous protein C deficiency. Blood 1993;82:1159–1164.

25. Wojchechoswski J, Olausson M, Korsan-Bengtsen K. Fibrinopeptide A, Beta thromboglobulin and fibrin degradation products as screening test for the diagnosis of deep venous thrombosis. Haemostasis 1983;13:254–261.

26. Rowbotham BJ, Carroll P, Whitaker AN. Measurement of cross linked fibrin derivatives—Use in the diagnosis of venous thrombosis. Thromb Haemost 1987;57:59–61.

(I)27. Heaton DC, Billings JD, Hickton CM. Assessment of D-Dimer assays for the diagnosis of deep vein thrombosis. J Lab Clin Med 1987;110:588–591.

(I)28. Ott P, Astrup L, Hartvin G, Jensen R, Nyeland P, Pedersen B. Assessment of D-Dimer in plasma: diagnostic value in suspected deep venous thrombosis of the leg. Acta Med Scand 1988;224:263–267.

(I)29. Bounameaux H, Schneider PA, Reber G, De Moerloose P, Krahenbuhl B. Measurement of plasma D-Dimer for diagnosis of deep venous thrombosis. Am J Clin Path 1989;91:82–85.

30. Mossaz A, Gandrille S, Vitoux JF, Abdouchel-Baudot N, Aiach M, et al. Valeur des D-Dimeres dans le diagnostic en urgence des thromboses veineuses. Presse Med 1990;19:1055.

(I)31. Van Bergen PFMM, Ear K, Jonker JJC, De Boer AC, De Mart MPM. Is quantitative determination of fibrinogen degradation products and thrombin-antithrombin III complexes useful to diagnose deep venous thrombosis in out-patients. Thromb Haemost 1989;62:1043–1045.

32. Elias A, Aillaud MF, Roul C, Villain PH, Serradimigni A, et al. Assessment of D-Dimer measurement by ELISA or latex methods in deep vein thrombosis diagnosed by ultrasonic duplex scanning. Fibrinolysis 1990;4:237–240.

33. Boneu B, Bes G, Pelzer I, Sie P, Boccalon H. D-Dimers thrombin-antithrombin III complexes and prothrombin Fragments $_{1+2}$ diagnostic value in clinically suspected deep vein thrombosis. Thromb Haemost 1991;65:28–32.

34. De Boer WA, De Haan MA, Huisman JW, Klaassen CHL. D-Dimer latex assay as screening method in suspected deep venous thrombosis of the leg. A clinical study and the review of the literature. Neth J Med 1991;38:65–69.

35. Achkar A, Laaban JP, Horellou MH, Conard J, Rabbat A, et al. Evaluation of repeated measurements of D-Dimers in the diagnosis of venous thromboembolic diseases. Thromb Haemost l993;69:620.(Abstract)

36. Lesprit P, Gepner P, Piette AM, De Tovar G, FIlilole M, et al. Phlebites profondes des membres inférieurs. Intér diagnostic du dosage des D-Dimeres. Press Med 1991;20:1927–1929.

37. Carter CJ, Doyle DL, Dawson N, Fowler A, Devine DV. Investigations into the clinical utility of Latex D-Dimer in the diagnosis of deep venous thrombosis. Thromb Haemost 1993;69:8–11.

38. Pini M, Biazzi A, Pattacini C, Megha A, Tagliaferri A, et al. Combined used of impedance plethysmography and plasma D-Dimer determination in clinically suspected deep venous thrombosis. Thromb Haemost 1991;65:1176.(Abstract)

39. Heijboer H, Ginsberg J, Buller H, Lensing AWA, Colly LP, et al. The use of the D-Dimer test in combination with noninvasive testing versus serial noninvasive testing alone for the diagnosis of deep vein thrombosis. Thromb Haemost 1992;67:510–513.

40. Bounameaux H, Slosman D, De Moerloose P, Reber G. Laboratory diagnosis of pulmonary embolism. Value of increased levels of plasma D-Dimer and thrombin-antithrombin III complexes. Biomed Pharmacother 1989;43:385–388.

41. Bridey F, Philipotteau C, Dreyfus M, Simonneau G.

Plasma D-Dimer and pulmonary embolism. Lancet 1989;1:791–792.

42. Speiser W, Leitha T, Dudczak R, Lechner K. Plasma D-Dimer levels in patients with pulmonary embolism. Lancet 1989;1:792.(Letter).

43 Goldhaber SZ, Vaughan DE, Tumeh SS, Loscalzo J. Utility of crosslinked fibrin degradation products in the diagnosis of pulmonary embolism. Am Heart J 1988;116: 505–508.

44. Bounameaux H, Cirafici P, De Moerloose P, Schneider PA, Slosman D, et al. Measurement of D-Dimer in plasma as diagnostic aid in suspected pulmonary embolism. Lancet 1991;337:196–200.

45. Estivals M, Pelzer H, Sie P, Pichon J, Boccalon H, et al. Prothrombin fragment $_{1+2}$, thrombin-antithrombin III complexes and D-Dimers in acute deep vein thrombosis. Effects of heparin treatment. Brit J Haematol 1991;78:421–424.

46. Elias A, Bonfils S, Daoud-Elias M, Gauthier B, Sie P, et al. Influence of long term oral anticoagulants upon prothrombin fragment $_{1+2}$, thrombin-antithrombin III complex and D-Dimer levels in patients affected by proximal deep vein thrombosis. Thromb Haemost 1993;69:302–305.

18

Cost-Effectiveness of Diagnosis of Deep-Vein Thrombosis in Symptomatic Patients

Russell D. Hull, William Feldstein, Graham F. Pineo, Gary E. Raskob

INTRODUCTION

Since the late 1980's, Doppler ultrasonographic imaging of the lower extremities has become the dominant test for deep-vein thrombosis (DVT). It has, in general, replaced impedance plethysmography (IPG) for noninvasive testing. Clinical trials have indicated that serial negative findings by IPG or Doppler ultrasonography are equivalent.[1–6] The positive predictive value of IPG is slightly less than that of Doppler ultrasonography.[3] Falsely positive IPG results can occur in the presence of congestive cardiac failure, hematoma, and severe vascular disease. However, these can be readily identified if a clinical examination at the bedside is performed.[4,6]

Objective diagnosis of DVT will allow treatment of such patients. If a diagnosis is not confirmed by objective tests, a unnecessary treatment and prolonged hospital stays can then be avoided.[7] It is much more likely that proximal-vein thrombosis, rather than calf-vein thrombosis, will lead to fatal pulmonary embolism (PE).[8,9] The incidence of fatal PE can be markedly reduced if DVT is treated with anticoagulant therapy.[10–12] Another important complication of DVT is the postphlebitic syndrome. However, this important complication is not considered in the cost-effectiveness analysis, because no reliable information is available on its prevalence in treated versus untreated patients with DVT.

Decision-makers try to maximize the health of the population served within the confines of the available resources by applying economic evaluation. Cost-effectiveness analysis is an economic tool that ranks alternative approaches to the same health problem to determine which is "best".[13] In economic terms, the best approach is defined as the approach that: (1) accomplishes the desired health effect at minimum cost (cost minimization), (2) produces the maximal health benefit for a given cost, or (3) provides the maximum effectiveness/cost ratio.

Cost minimization is utilized to apply cost-effectiveness analysis to the diagnosis of DVT.[7] The diagnostic approaches can be ranked from "worst" to "best", the "best" approach being defined as that which accomplishes the desired health effect at minimum cost.

Effectiveness, or health benefit, is defined as the number or proportion of patients with DVT correctly identified by objective testing, or the number or proportion in whom treatment was correctly withheld. The group in which treatment was correctly withheld is important because large-outcome studies have confirmed the safety of withholding or withdrawing anticoagulant therapy in symptomatic patients who have negative sonographic findings or who are negative by serial noninvasive leg testing.[1–3,14,15] The impact of the analysis on the use of objective testing in outpatient care is also examined.

METHODS

Objective Tests for Deep-Vein Thrombosis

Deep-vein thrombosis in symptomatic patients is diagnosed from clinical findings, venography, and one or more noninvasive tests. The best evaluated of the diagnostic tests are ascending contrast venography, IPG, and Doppler ultrasonography with B-mode imaging.[1–6,14,15] A prospective study of approximately 500 patients who, after a first episode of clinically suspected DVT, had been referred to a regional thromboembolism program, provided the data for this cost-effectiveness analysis.[7] Each patient was assessed clinically and then investigated by venography and IPG. Adequate venograms were obtained in 478 of these patients.[7]

At the time the prospective study was performed, Doppler ultrasonography with B-mode imaging, a highly sensitive and specific technique for detecting proximal-vein thrombosis in symptomatic patients,[3,5] was not available. However, like IPG, it is relatively insensitive for identifying calf-vein thrombosis. As a consequence, serial testing is required. Clinical trials comparing serial IPG with Doppler ultrasonography with B-mode imaging have been subsequently completed.[3,5] Serial Doppler ultrasonography is at least as effective as serial IPG, and may be more so because it has a higher positive predictive value.[3,5] Doppler ultrasonography using B-mode imaging is formally evaluated in our study from these direct comparisons against IPG.[3,5]

COST-EFFECTIVENESS

Cost: The cost of each diagnostic alternative has been defined as the direct cost of administering the diagnostic test plus the treatment cost associated with a positive test. The treatment cost consisted of the cost of anticoagulant therapy (including drugs and laboratory tests for monitoring anticoagulant therapy), and "hotel" costs of hospitalization (rooming, laundry, food, etc.). Costs for treating the complications and side effects of the diagnostic tests and of the anticoagulant therapy are not included because these costs were relatively minor.

The findings shown in the Results section are expressed in both 1992 Canadian and American dollars (to the nearest dollar), according to the costs at the urban-based hospital site in Canada and the charges at the urban-based hospital site in the U.S., respectively. Detailed cost items for both countries were determined at the time at which the study was completed ($1.00 Canadian was equivalent to $0.80 U.S.).

Unit Costs At An Urban Teaching Hospital In Canada: Cost data used are based on actual quantities and costs were derived from the operating costs incurred in an urban hospital affiliated with a university medical school. The costs were $542.50 per day for hotel costs, $137 for venography, and $150 and $400 for serial IPG or serial Doppler ultrasonography with B-mode imaging, respectively. The cost of administering intravenous heparin therapy for 6 days was $142.78 per patient: $48.91 for heparin (5,000 Units initial bolus; constant infusion of 30,000 Units for 6 days) and $93.87 for partial thromboplastin time tests (three tests during the first 24 hours and once per day thereafter).

The cost of long-term therapy with warfarin sodium for 3 months was $471.72 per patient: $44.21 for warfarin sodium, $153.51 for prothrombin-time monitoring (five prothrombin-time tests per day for days 2–6, followed by 1 test per week for 12 weeks), and $274.00 for physicians' fees.

Unit Charges At An Urban Teaching Hospital in the United States: This economic analysis was repeated using actual 1992 charges in U.S. dollars at an urban hospital in the midwestern United States. Teaching hospital hotel and diagnostic charges were derived from standard step-down cost accounting and work sampling procedures. The ranking of these estimates of costs (although they differ from true economic costs) is similar to the ranking of costs observed for Canada (for example, this facility's hotel charge was U.S. $575.00 per day compared with CDN $542.50 per day for the facility in Canada). The economic evaluation of each therapeutic approach was the same as that used for Canada (Appendix).

Effectiveness: Three criteria of effectiveness were used. They involved the correct identification of: (1) DVT (thrombosis involving the calf, popliteal, femoral, or iliac veins), (2) thrombosis involving the proximal veins (popliteal, femoral, or iliac veins) with or without calf-vein thrombosis, and (3) the number of patients in whom treatment was correctly withheld.

SENSITIVITY ANALYSIS

Multiple-sensitivity analyses were performed. The variables examined were: (1) the prevalence of DVT, (2) the cost of the hospital bed, (3) the cost of treatment, and (4) the cost of the diagnostic tests used. For prevalence, a range of five to 80 cases of DVT per 100 symptomatic patients with clinically suspected DVT was used. This range exceeds the prevalence of DVT reported in the literature. A range of 40% to 300% was used for the costs of the hospital bed and treatment. A range of 50% to 195%, reflecting regional variations in costs in Canada was used for objective testing. For 7% of patients venograms were inadequate; in these cases, the costs of other objective tests were examined by sensitivity analysis. For the inpatients who had DVT while they were convalescing from some other disorder, the number of extra days in the hospital attributed to the diagnosis of DVT ranged from one to six.

The impact of false-positive results by noninvasive testing was also examined by sensitivity analysis.

RESULTS

The 516 patients with clinically suspected venous thrombosis who were referred to the venous thromboembolism program ranged from 15 to 86 years of age (mean 53 years). The ratio of males to females was 41:55. Two hundred and sixty-eight (52%) were outpatients at the time they were referred to the program; 248 (48%) were inpatients. Of the 248 symptomatic patients who were inpatients at the time of referral, 165 were admitted to the hospital for suspected DVT. The remaining 83 patients (16% of the population studied) had symptoms of DVT during their convalescence from an acute surgical or medical illness, and management based on the clinical diagnosis would have prolonged their hospital stays. For this reason, these patients were included in the analysis.

Ascending venograms were technically adequate in 478 of the 516 patients (93%), and the cost-effectiveness comparison was performed in these patients. In 277 of the

Table 1
Total Costs and Results of the Alternative Strategies to Diagnose Deep-Vein Thrombosis

	No. of Correct Diagnoses	Cost	
		Canadian $	United States $
Clinical Diagnosis	201	$1,590,784	$2,624,220
Inpatient Venography	201	$1,207,707	$2,087,417
Outpatient Venography	201	$ 734,314	$1,450,040
Doppler Ultrasonography	142	$ 618,265	$1,326,180
Combined Doppler and Impedance Plethysmography	142	$ 551,065	$1,124,580
Impedance Plethysmography	142	$ 527,165	$1,052,880

(Used with permission from Hull, et al. Thromb Haemostas 1995;74(1):191)

478 patients (58%) venography was negative. Of the remaining 201 patients, 139 had proximal-vein thrombosis with or without calf-vein thrombosis on venography, and 62 had thrombosis that was limited to the calf.

The Appendix gives a detailed analysis of the cost-effectiveness of clinical diagnosis, venography, and noninvasive testing. Table 1 shows total costs and results of the alternative strategies to diagnose DVT. Table 2 shows total costs of the alternative strategies for each patient correctly managed.

COST-EFFECTIVENESS OF DIAGNOSTIC APPROACHES FOR DEEP-VEIN THROMBOSIS

Clinical Diagnosis: According to the clinical diagnosis alone, 478 symptomatic patients would have received care and treatment in the hospital. Because the venograms were normal in 277 (58%) of these 478 patients with clinically diagnosed DVT, more than half of these patients would have been incorrectly labelled and treated in the hospital on the basis of the clinical diagnosis alone. For a correct diagnosis in 201 patients with DVT the total

Canadian dollar cost in 1992 of diagnosis and treatment in 478 patients would be $1,590,784 ($2,624,220 in the U.S.). The cost per patient with DVT that was correctly identified and treated would be $7,914 ($13,055 in the U.S.), the cost per patient with proximal-vein thrombosis would be $11,444 ($18,879 in the U.S.), and the cost per patient correctly withheld from therapy would be $5,743 ($9,474 in the U.S.).

Venography: The diagnostic reference standard for identifying venous thrombosis and against which noninvasive tests are measured is venography. There are, however, disadvantages to venography. It is invasive and is associated with patient morbidity. It requires admission to the hospital if it is not readily available on an outpatient basis. Costs will be considered on the basis of outpatient and inpatient diagnosis.

Venography As An Outpatient Diagnostic Approach: In 277 of the 478 patients, venography was negative. These 277 patients would have been spared inpatient care and therapy. The cost incurred in this group would be only the cost of venography. The diagnosis of DVT was confirmed in 201 patients. In these patients the costs incurred were for venography, inpatient care, and treat-

Table 2
Total Costs of the Alternative Strategies for Each Patient Correctly Managed

		Cost/Patient Correctly Withheld from Treatment	Cost/Patient with Correct Diagnosis of Proximal Deep-Vein Thrombosis	Cost/Patient with Correct Diagnosis of Deep-Vein Thrombosis
Clinical Diagnosis	CDN $	$5,743	$11,444	$ 7,914
	US $	$9,474	$18,879	$13,055
Inpatient Venography	CDN $	$4,360	$ 8,689	$ 6,008
	US $	$7,536	$15,017	$10,385
Outpatient Venography	CDN $	$2,651	$ 5,283	$ 3,653
	US $	$5,235	$10,432	$ 7,214
Doppler Ultrasonography	CDN $	$1,840	$ 4,684	$ 4,354
	US $	$3,947	$10,047	$ 9,339
Combined Doppler and Impedance Plethysmography	CDN $	$1,640	$ 4,175	$ 3,881
	US $	$3,347	$ 8,520	$ 7,920
Impedance Plethysmography	CDN $	$1,569	$ 3,994	$ 3,712
	US $	$3,134	$ 7,976	$ 7,415

(Used with permission from Hull, et al. Thromb Haemostas 1995;74(1):191)

ment. The total Canadian dollar cost in 1992, for outpatient venography in 478 patients yielding a diagnosis of DVT in 201 patients would be $734,314 ($1,450,040 in the U.S.). The cost per patient with DVT correctly identified and treated would be $3,653 ($7,214 in the U.S.), the cost per patient with proximal DVT would be $5,283 ($10,432 in the U.S.), and the cost per patient correctly withheld from therapy would be $2,651 ($5,235 in the U.S.).

Venography As An Elective Inpatient Diagnostic Approach: If immediate outpatient venography is not available, it may be necessary to admit symptomatic patients to the hospital for elective venography. Patients with clinically suspected DVT subsequently ruled out by elective venography had an average hospital stay of 3 days.

If all 478 symptomatic patients were admitted to the hospital for elective venography, 277 patients would have been hospitalized unnecessarily, incurring the costs of anticoagulant therapy and hospitalization for 3 days.

The total Canadian dollar cost in 1992 of using inpatient venography in 478 patients to yield a diagnosis in 201 patients would be $1,207,707 ($2,087,417 in the U.S.). The cost per patient with DVT correctly identified and treated would be $6,008 ($10,385 in the U.S.), the cost per patient with proximal DVT would be $8,689 ($15,017 in the U.S.), and the cost per patient correctly withheld from therapy would be $4,360 ($7,536 in the U.S.).

Serial Occlusive Cuff Impedance Plethysmography: Impedance plethysmography using the occlusive cuff technique is sensitive and specific for detecting proximal-vein thrombosis but is insensitive for identifying calf thrombi. Impedance plethysmography is an objective diagnostic method that can be carried out in the outpatient clinic, ward, or emergency room.

Impedance plethysmography detected the disease in 132 (95%) of 139 patients with proximal-vein thrombosis and in 10 (16%) of 62 patients with calf-vein thrombosis. Therefore, a correct diagnosis was made in 142 of 201 patients with DVT (71%). Impedance plethysmography was falsely positive in five patients (2%) in whom there was no obvious clinical cause.

The total Canadian dollar cost in 1992 of using IPG in 478 patients for a diagnosis in 142 patients would be $527,165 ($1,052,880 in the U.S.). The cost per patient with DVT correctly identified and treated was $3,712 ($7,415 in the U.S.), the cost per patient with proximal DVT was $3,994 ($7,976 in the U.S.), and the cost per patient correctly withheld from therapy would be $1,569 ($3,134 in the U.S.).

Ultrasonography: B-mode imaging is sensitive and specific for detecting proximal-vein thrombosis but is insensitive for identifying calf thrombi. B-mode imaging is an objective diagnostic method that can be carried out in the outpatient clinic, ward, or emergency room, but in many centers this test is done in a centralized facility.

Ultrasonography would have detected the disease in 132 (95%) of 139 patients with proximal-vein thrombosis and in 10 (16%) of 62 patients with calf-vein thrombosis. Therefore, a correct diagnosis would have been made in 142 of 201 patients with DVT (71%). Ultrasonography would have been falsely positive in two patients.

The total Canadian dollar cost in 1992 of using ultrasonography in 478 patients for a diagnosis in 142 patients would be $618,265 ($1,326,180 in the U.S.). The cost per patient with DVT correctly identified and treated would be $4,354 ($9,339 in the U.S.), the cost per patient with proximal DVT would be $4,684 ($10,047 in the U.S.), and the cost per patient correctly withheld from therapy would be $1,840 ($3,947 in the U.S.).

Initial Negative Doppler Ultrasonography Examination Leading to Serial Impedance Plethysmography: A higher positive predictive value is observed with ultrasonography. Therefore, an efficient approach may be an initial B-mode image evaluation, followed by less costly serial IPG if the initial evaluation was negative.

The total Canadian dollar cost in 1992 of using combined ultrasonography/impedance plethysmography in 478 patients, for a diagnosis in 142 patients would be $551,065 ($1,124,580 in the U.S.). The cost per patient with DVT correctly identified and treated would be $3,881 ($7,920 in the U.S.), the cost per patient with proximal DVT would be $4,175 ($8,520 in the U.S.), and the cost per patient correctly withheld from therapy would be $1,640 ($3,347 in the U.S.).

Sensitivity Analysis: We performed multiple sensitivity analyses using the variables outlined in the Methods section, and this procedure did not alter the findings of this study.

DISCUSSION

Clinical diagnosis, venography, and serial noninvasive testing are the diagnostic approaches to DVT. The clinical diagnosis of DVT is non-specific and insensitive.[4,14] In approximately 50% or more of patients with clinically diagnosed DVT, the results of objective testing are negative.[7] This approach is not cost effective because one of two patients with clinically diagnosed DVT will be inappropriately admitted to the hospital and given anticoagulant therapy. Accurate identification of patients with DVT is accomplished by means of venograph[14] or noninvasive leg testing, using either IPG or Doppler ultrasonography with B-mode imaging.[1-7,15]

Venography is the standard diagnostic reference test against which noninvasive tests are evaluated.[1-7,14] It has disadvantages: it is invasive, it is associated with patient discomfort, and it induces postvenography phlebitis in approximately 1% to 3% of patients. Venography is readily available in many centers on an outpatient basis. This avoids the unnecessary costs associated with inpatient testing.

In ranking the approaches discussed, it is evident that clinical diagnosis is the least cost effective. Noninvasive testing is the most cost effective. Serial IPG is less expensive than venography or Doppler ultrasonography with B-mode imaging. It is also more versatile than venography, and can be carried out in the outpatient clinic, ward, or emergency room. B-mode imaging is carried out in a centralized facility in many centers. Noninvasive testing with serial IPG or B-mode imaging avoids the risk of unnecessary anticoagulant therapy in those patients without proximal-vein thrombosis.[1–3,5,15]

The disadvantage of Serial B-mode imaging is that it costs more than serial IPG, even though it is equally effective in ruling out proximal-vein thrombosis. It has the advantage, however, that a bedside examination of the patient is not required to rule out clinical disorders known to produce false-positive results, unlike IPG which requires such an examination.[3] Therefore, in patients without clinical disorders known to produce a false-positive IPG result, it would make economic sense to use serial IPG in this large patient population. On the other hand, in patient subgroups that frequently suffer from cardiac failure (for example, those in the Intensive Care Unit), the use of serial B-mode imaging would avoid the otherwise high false-positive rates associated with IPG testing in such a patient population.

Recent observations[16] suggest that B-mode imaging may be more sensitive to popliteal extension of calf-vein thrombosis than IPG. However, large-outcome studies have demonstrated equivalent safety in patients with negative outcomes when either serial IPG or ultrasonography was used.[3,15]

Our cost-effectiveness analyses suggest that IPG and B-mode imaging, if used selectively in the appropriate patient populations, would maximize effectiveness but would avoid the excessive cost associated with the routine use of B-mode imaging in all patients. A strategy which would optimize both effectiveness and cost would be an initial Doppler ultrasonography B-mode examination, and if this initial evaluation was negative, mandatory serial testing would be deployed using IPG. The result would be significant cost savings. Our cost-effectiveness analyses suggest that Doppler ultrasonography with B-mode imaging and IPG are complementary rather than competitive.

In patients in whom IPG or B-mode imaging is initially negative, serial testing is mandatory to detect nonocclusive proximal thrombi which subsequently extend, or isolated calf-vein thrombi which propagate proximally.[1–3,5,15,16] Finally, in patients with a negative noninvasive test result (either by IPG or B-mode imaging) in whom the clinical suspicion of DVT remains high, it is likely that a diagnosis of a nonocclusive thrombus could be made earlier by adjunctive ascending venography as an alternative to serial testing.[16]

Serial testing is only feasible on an outpatient basis in patients who can and will return for follow-up. Outpatient ascending venography remains the diagnostic method of choice in outpatients who are unwilling or unable to return for serial follow-up.

Although the actual cost of each component will be dictated by regional differences and will change in the future, the proportion each component contributes to the total cost will remain linked. Thus, ranking of the diagnostic approaches from "worst" to "best" as determined by cost-effectiveness analysis should continue to be relevant. Because inpatient diagnosis is likely to remain a major cost, emphasis should be placed on outpatient diagnosis.

APPENDIX

Cost-effectiveness findings for Canada (shown in the Results section) are expressed in 1992 Canadian dollars, to the nearest dollar using the Canadian dollar cost described in the Methods section. The findings for the United States are expressed in U.S. dollars and are calculated using the U.S. dollar cost described in the Methods section.

CANADIAN COSTS:

Treatment Costing Details

Hotel Cost: $542.50 per day

Intravenous Heparin by Continuous Infusion for 5–6 Days: The 1992 Canadian dollar cost per patient was $142.78. It consisted of $0.61 for a drug bolus ($0.61 × 1), $0.01 for a bolus swab ($0.007 × 1), $0.12 for a bolus syringe with needle ($0.12 × 1), $48.10 for infusion bags with heparin drug ($4.81 × 10); $0.07 for infusion swabs ($0.007 × 10), $92.70 for PTT tests ($10.30 × 9), and $1.17 for PTT blood vials with needles ($0.13 × 9).

Intravenous Heparin by Continuous Infusion for 3 Days: The 1992 Canadian dollar cost per patient was $81.05. It consisted of $0.61 for drug a bolus ($0.61 × 1), $0.01 for a bolus swab ($0.007 × 1), $0.12 for a bolus syringe with needle ($0.12 × 1), $28.86 for infusion bags with heparin drug ($4.81 × 6), $0.04 for infusion swabs ($0.007 × 6), $51.50 for PTT tests ($10.30 × 5), and $0.65 for PTT blood vials with needles ($0.13 × 5).

Long-term Treatment with Warfarin Sodium: Long-term treatment with warfarin sodium ranged between 2 and 15 mg per day. The 1992 Canadian dollar cost per patient for this 12-week warfarin sodium treatment was $471.72 and consisted of $1.92 for the drug while in hospital ($0.32 × 6), a one-time cost of $42.29 for warfarin drug prescription (this includes the cost of 90 5 mg tablets, plus dispensing fee), $151.30 for PT/INR tests ($8.90 × 17), $2.21 for PT/INR blood vials with needles ($0.13 × 17), $100.00 for in-hospital physician fees ($20.00 × 5), and $174.00 for out-patient physician fees ($14.50 × 12).

Clinical Diagnosis

The cost per patient with the clinical diagnosis of DVT would consist of the intrinsic technical cost of $0, a hospital room for 5–6 days (at $542.50 a day) for a cost of $2,713, plus the $615 combined cost of anticoagulant therapy, laboratory testing, and monitoring for 3 months (initial treatment with intravenous heparin costing $143 plus long-term treatment with warfarin sodium costing $472), for an overall cost of $3,328. The cost for 478 patients was 478 × $3,328 = $1,590,784.

Effectiveness: The correct diagnosis and treatment of each patient with DVT is the desired result. Only 201 of the 478 patients had DVT: 139 had proximal DVT and 62 had DVT involving only calf veins.

Cost-Effectiveness: The cost per patient with a correct diagnosis of DVT would be $1,590,784 ÷ 201 = $7,914. The cost per patient with a correct diagnosis of proximal DVT would be $1,590,784 ÷ 139 = $11,444. The cost per patient in whom treatment was correctly withheld would be $1,590,784 ÷ 277 = $5,743.

Ascending Venography for Outpatient Diagnosing

The intrinsic cost of venography at $137 per patient in 478 patients would be $65,486. For 201 patients with DVT the cost of the hospital rooms for 5–6 days per patient (at $542.50 per day) would be $545,213 and the cost of anticoagulant therapy, laboratory tests, and monitoring (at a total of $615 per patient) would be $123,615. The total cost for 478 patients would be $734,314.

Effectiveness: In 201 patients with DVT, venography correctly identified the disease: 139 had proximal DVT and 62 had calf-vein thrombosis.

Cost-Effectiveness: The cost per patient with a correct diagnosis of DVT would be $734,314 ÷ 201 = $3,653. The cost per patient with a correct diagnosis of proximal DVT would be $734,314 ÷ 139 = $5,283. The cost per patient in whom treatment was correctly withheld would be $734,314 ÷ 277 = $2,651.

Ascending Venography for Inpatient Diagnosing

The intrinsic cost of venography at $137 per patient in 478 patients would be $65,486. For 201 patients with DVT the cost of the hospital rooms for 5–6 days per patient (at $542.50 a day) would be $545,213 and the cost of anticoagulant therapy, laboratory tests, and monitoring (at a total of $615 per patient) would be $123,615. Additionally, each of the 277 patients in whom venogra-

phy was subsequently negative would receive 3 days of hospital care (3 × $542.50 = $1,628) and anticoagulant therapy and monitoring ($81) at a cost of $1,709. The cost for 277 patients would be 277 × $1,709 = $473,393. The total cost for the 478 patients would be $1,207,707.

Effectiveness: In 201 patients with DVT, venography correctly identified the disease: 139 had proximal DVT and 62 had calf-vein thrombosis.

Cost-Effectiveness: The cost per patient with a correct diagnosis of DVT would be $1,207,707 ÷ 201 = $6,008. The cost per patient with a correct diagnosis of proximal DVT would be $1,207,707 ÷ 139 = $8,689. The cost per patient in whom treatment was correctly withheld would be $1,207,707 ÷ 277 = $4,360.

Impedance Plethysmography

The intrinsic cost of impedance plethysmography at $30 per test per patient in 478 patients would be $14,340. For the 336 negative patients the cost of serial impedance plethysmography (four tests) would be $120 × 336 = $40,320. For the 142 positive patients the cost of the hospital rooms for 5–6 days per patient (at $542.50 per day) would be $385,175 and anticoagulant therapy, laboratory testing, and monitoring at a cost of $615 per patient would be $87,330. The total cost for the 478 patients would be $527,165.

Effectiveness: In 142 patients, DVT was correctly identified: 132 had proximal DVT and 10 had calf-vein thrombosis.

Cost-Effectiveness: The cost per patient with a correct diagnosis of DVT would be $527,165 ÷ 142 = $3,712. The cost per patient with a correct diagnosis of proximal DVT would be $527,165 ÷ 132 = $3,994. The cost per patient in whom treatment was correctly withheld would be $527,165 ÷ 336 = $1,569.

Ultrasonography

The intrinsic cost of Doppler ultrasonography at $80 per test per patient in 478 patients would be $38,240. For the 336 negative patients the cost of serial ultrasonography (four tests) would be $320 × 336 = $107,520. For the 142 patients in whom ultrasonography was positive, the cost of the hospital rooms for 5–6 days per patient (at $542.50 per day) would be $385,175 and anticoagulant therapy, laboratory testing, and monitoring at a cost of $615 per patient would be $87,330. The total cost for the 478 patients would be $618,265.

Effectiveness: In 142 patients, DVT was correctly identified: 132 had proximal DVT and 10 had calf-vein thrombosis.

Cost-Effectiveness: The cost per patient with a correct diagnosis of DVT would be $618,265 ÷ 142 = $4,354. The cost per patient with a correct diagnosis of proximal DVT would be $618,265 ÷ 132 = $4,684. The cost per patient in whom treatment was correctly withheld would be $618,265 ÷ 336 = $1,840.

Initial Negative Doppler Ultrasonography Examination Leading to Serial Impedance Plethysmography

The intrinsic cost of Doppler ultrasonography at $80 per test per patient in 478 patients would be $38,240. For the 336 negative patients the cost of serial IPG (four tests) would be $120 × 336 = $40,320. For the 142 positive patients the cost of the hospital rooms for 5–6 days per patient (at $542.50 per day) would be $385,175 and anticoagulant therapy, laboratory testing, and monitoring at a cost of $615 per patient would be $87,330. The total cost for the 478 patients would be $551,065.

Effectiveness: In 142 patients, DVT was correctly identified: 132 had proximal DVT and 10 had calf-vein thrombosis.

Cost Effectiveness: The cost per patient with a correct diagnosis of DVT would be $551,065 ÷ 142 = $3,881. The cost per patient with a correct diagnosis of proximal DVT would be $551,065 ÷ 132 = $4,175. The cost per patient in whom treatment was correctly withheld would be $551,065 ÷ 336 = $1,640.

UNITED STATES COSTS:

Treatment Costing Details

Hotel Charge: $575.00 per day

Intravenous Heparin by Continuous Infusion for 5–6 Days: The 1992 U.S. dollar charge per patient was $966.36. It consisted of $0.36 for a drug bolus ($0.36 × 1), $3.00 for a bolus swab ($3.00 × 1), $1.50 for a bolus syringe with needle ($1.50 × 1), $20.00 pharmacy charge for dispensing of the bolus ($20.00 × 1), $396.50 for infusion bags with heparin drug ($39.65 × 10), $30.00 for infusion swabs ($3.00 × 10), $200.00 in pharmacy charges for dispensing the infusion bags ($20.00 × 10), and $315.00 for PTT tests ($35.00 × 9) which includes the cost of blood vials and needles.

Intravenous Heparin by Continuous Infusion for 3 Days: The 1992 U.S. dollar cost per patient was $575.76. It consisted of $0.36 for a drug bolus ($0.36 × 1), $3.00 for a bolus swab ($3.00 × 1), $1.50 for a bolus syringe with needle ($1.50 × 1), $20.00 pharmacy charge for dispensing of the bolus ($20.00 × 1), $237.90 for infusion bags with heparin drug ($39.65 × 6), $18.00 for infusion swabs ($3.00 × 6), $120.00 in pharmacy charges for dispensing the infusion bags ($20.00 × 6), and $175.00 for PTT tests ($35.00 × 5) which includes the cost of blood vials and needles.

Long-term Treatment with Warfarin Sodium: Long-term treatment with warfarin sodium ranged between 2 and 15 mg per day. The 1992 U.S. dollar charge per pa-

tient for this 12-week warfarin sodium treatment was $1,649.40. It consisted of $10.80 for the in-hospital drug ($1.80 × 6), a one-time $79.60 drug prescription charge ($79.60 × 1), $323.00 for PT/INR tests ($19.00 × 17) which includes the cost of blood vials and needles, $600.00 for in-hospital physician fees ($120.00 × 5), and $636.00 for out-patient physician fees ($53.00 × 12).

Clinical Diagnosis

The charge per patient with the clinical diagnosis of DVT would consist of the intrinsic technical cost of $0, a hospital room for 5–6 days (at $575.00 per day) for a cost of $2,875, plus the $2,615 combined cost of anticoagulant therapy, laboratory testing, and monitoring for 3 months (initial treatment with intravenous heparin costing $966 plus long-term treatment with warfarin sodium costing $1,649) for an overall charge of $5,490. The cost for 478 patients would be 478 × $5,490 = $2,624,220.

Effectiveness: The correct diagnosis and treatment of each patient with DVT is the desired result. Only 201 of the 478 patients had DVT: 139 had proximal DVT and 62 had calf-vein thrombosis only.

Cost Effectiveness: The charge per patient with a correct diagnosis of DVT would be $2,624,220 ÷ 201 = $13,055. The charge per patient with a correct diagnosis of proximal DVT would be $2,624,220 ÷ 139 = $18,879. The cost per patient in whom treatment was correctly withheld would be $2,624,220 ÷ 277 = $9,474.

Ascending Venography for Outpatient Diagnosing

The intrinsic cost of venography at $725 per patient in 478 patients would be $346,550. For 201 patients with DVT the cost of the hospital rooms for 5–6 days per patient (at $575 per day) would be $577,875 and the cost of anticoagulant therapy, laboratory tests, and monitoring (at a total of $2,615 per patient) in 201 patients with DVT would be $525,615. The total charge for 478 patients would be $1,450,040.

Effectiveness: In 201 patients with DVT, venography correctly identified the disease; 139 had proximal DVT, and 62 had calf-vein thrombosis.

Cost Effectiveness: The charge per patient with a correct diagnosis of DVT would be $1,450,040 ÷ 201 = $7,214. The charge per patient with a correct diagnosis of proximal DVT would be $1,450,040 ÷ 139 = $10,432. The cost per patient in whom treatment was correctly withheld would be $1,450,040 ÷ 277 = $5,235.

ASCENDING VENOGRAPHY FOR INPATIENT DIAGNOSING

The intrinsic cost of venography at $725 per patient in 478 patients would be $346,550. For 201 patients with

DVT the cost of the hospital rooms for 5–6 days per patient (at $575 a day) would be $577,875 and the cost of anticoagulant therapy, laboratory tests, and monitoring (at a total of $2,615 per patient) in 201 patients with DVT would be $525,615. Additionally, each of the 277 patients in whom venography was subsequently negative would receive 3 days of hospital care (3 × $575 = $1,725) and anticoagulant therapy and monitoring ($576) at a cost of $2,301. The cost for 277 patients would be 277 × $2,301 = $637,377. The total charge for 478 patients would be $2,087,417.

Effectiveness: In 201 patients with DVT, venography correctly identified the disease: 139 had proximal DVT and 62 had calf-vein thrombosis.

Cost-Effectiveness: The charge per patient with a correct diagnosis of DVT would be $2,087,417 ÷ 201 = $10,385. The charge per patient with a correct diagnosis of proximal DVT would be $2,087,417 ÷ 139 = $15,017. The cost per patient in whom treatment was correctly withheld would be $2,087,417 ÷ 277 = $7,536.

IMPEDANCE PLETHYSMOGRAPHY

The intrinsic cost of IPG at $150 per test per patient in 478 patients would be $71,700. For the 336 negative patients the cost of serial IPG (four tests) would be $600 × 336 = $201,600. For the 142 positive patients the cost of the hospital rooms for 5–6 days per patient (at $575 per day) would be $408,250 and anticoagulant therapy, laboratory testing, and monitoring at a cost of $2,615 per patient would be $371,330. The total charge for the 478 patients would be $1,052,880.

Effectiveness: In 142 patients, DVT was correctly identified: 132 had proximal DVT and 10 had calf-vein thrombosis.

Cost-Effectiveness: The charge per patient with a correct diagnosis of DVT would be $1,052,880 ÷ 142 = $7,415. The charge per patient with a correct diagnosis of proximal DVT would be $1,052,880 ÷ 132 = $7,976. The cost per patient in whom treatment was correctly withheld would be $1,052,880 ÷ 336 = $3,134.

Ultrasonography

The intrinsic cost of Doppler ultrasonography at $300 per test per patient in 478 patients would be $143,400. For the 336 negative patients the cost of serial ultrasonography (four tests) would be $1,200 × 336 = $403,200. For the 142 positive patients the cost of the hospital rooms for 5–6 days per patient (at $575 per day) would be $408,250 and anticoagulant therapy, laboratory testing, and monitoring at a cost of $2,615 per patient in 142 patients would be $371,330. The total charge for the 478 patients would be $1,326,180.

Effectiveness: In 142 patients, DVT was correctly identified: 132 had proximal DVT and 10 had calf-vein thrombosis.

Cost-Effectiveness: The charge per patient with a correct diagnosis of DVT would be $1,326,180 ÷ 142 = $9,339. The charge per patient with a correct diagnosis of proximal DVT would be $1,326,180 ÷ 132 = $10,047. The cost per patient in whom treatment was correctly withheld would be $1,326,180 ÷ 336 = $3,947.

Initial Negative Doppler Ultrasonography Examination Leading to Serial Impedance Plethysmography

The intrinsic cost of Doppler ultrasonography at $300 per test per patient in 478 patients would be $143,400. The cost of serial IPG (four tests) in the 336 negative patients would be $600 × 336 = $201,600. The cost of the hospital rooms for 5–6 days per patient (at $575 per day) for the 142 positive patients would be $408,250. The cost of anticoagulant therapy, laboratory testing, and monitoring at a cost of $2,615 per patient in 142 patients would be $371,330. The total charge for the 478 patients would be $1,124,580.

Effectiveness: In 142 patients, DVT was correctly identified: 132 had proximal DVT and 10 had calf-vein thrombosis.

Cost-Effectiveness: The charge per patient with a correct diagnosis of DVT would be $1,124,580 ÷ 142 = $7,920. The charge per patient with a correct diagnosis of proximal DVT would be $1,124,580 ÷ 132 = $8,520. The cost per patient in whom treatment was correctly withheld would be $1,124,580 ÷ 336 = $3,347.

REFERENCES

1. Huisman MV, Buller HR, ten Cate JW, Vreeken J. Serial impedance plethysmography for suspected deep venous thrombosis in outpatients. The Amsterdam General Practitioner Study. N Engl J Med 1986;314:823–828.
2. Huisman MV, Buller HR, ten Cate JW, Heljermans HSF, van der Laan J, et al. Management of clinically suspected acute venous thrombosis in outpatients with serial impedance plethysmography in a community hospital setting. Arch Intern Med 1989;149:511–513.
3. Heijboer H, Buller HR, Lensing AWA, Turpie AGG, Colly LP, et al. A comparison of real-time compression ultrasonography with impedance plethysmography for the diagnosis of DVT in symptomatic outpatients. N Engl J Med 1993;329:1365–1369.
4. Wheeler HB, O'Donnell JA, Anderson FA, Benedict K, Jr. Occlusive impedance phlebography: a diagnostic procedure for venous thrombosis and pulmonary embolism. Prog Cardiovasc Dis 1974;17:199–205.
5. Heijboer H, Cogo A, Buller HR, Prandoni P, ten Cate JW. Detection of DVT with impedance plethysmography and real-time compression ultrasonography in hospitalized patients. Arch Intern Med 1992;152:1901–1903.
6. Hull RD, Van Aken WG, Hirsh J, Gallus AS, Hoicka G, et al. Impedance plethysmography using the occlusive cuff technique in the diagnosis of venous thrombosis. Circulation 1976;53:697–700.
7. Hull RD, Hirsh J, Sackett DL, Stoddart G. Cost effectiveness of clinical diagnosis, venography, and noninvasive

testing in patients with symptomatic DVT. N Engl J Med 1981;304:1561–1567.

8. Kakkar VV, Howe CT, Flanc C, Clarke MB. Natural history of postoperative DVT. Lancet 1969;2:230–232.

9. Moser KM, LeMoine JR. Is embolic risk conditioned by location of deep venous thrombosis? Ann Intern Med 1981;94:439–444.

10. Hull RD, Raskob GE, Hirsh H, Jay RM, Leclerc JR, et al. Continuous intravenous heparin compared with intermittent subcutaneous heparin in the initial treatment of proximal-vein thrombosis. N Engl J Med 1986;315:1109–1114.

11. Hull RD, Delmore T, Genton E, Hirsh J, Gent M, et al. Warfarin sodium versus low-dose heparin in the long-term treatment of venous thrombosis. N Engl J Med 1979;301:855.

12. Brandjes DPM, Heijboer H, Buller HR, De Rijk M, Jagt H, et al. Acenocoumarol and heparin compared with aceno-coumarol alone in the initial treatment of proximal vein thrombosis. N Engl J Med 1992;327:1485–1489.

13. Weinstein MC, Stason WB. Foundations of cost effectiveness analysis for health and medical practices. N Engl J Med 1977;296:716.

14. Hull RD, Hirsh J, Sackett DL, Taylor DW, Carter C, et al. Clinical validity of a negative venogram in patients with clinically suspected venous thrombosis. Circulation 1981;64:622.

15. Hull RD, Hirsh J, Carter CJ, Jay R, Ockelford P, et al. Diagnostic efficacy of impedance plethysmography for clinically suspected deep-vein thrombosis. Ann Intern Med 1985;102:21–28.

16. Kearon C, Hirsh H. Factors influencing the reported sensitivity and specificity of impedance plethysmography for proximal deep-vein thrombosis. Thromb Haemost 1994;72:652–658.

19

The Diagnosis of Recurrent Deep-Vein Thrombosis

Menno V. Huisman, Maria M.W. Beaumont-Koopman

INTRODUCTION

Considerable progress has been made over the last 20 years in the diagnosis and treatment of acute deep-vein thrombosis (DVT) presenting as a first episode. It has been shown in several studies that the clinical diagnosis is nonspecific.[1-3] More objective testing for DVT has become feasible using contrast venography,[4(I),5] and noninvasive techniques such as impedance plethysmography (IPG),[6(I),7(I),8(I)] compression ultrasonography (US)[9(I),10(I)] and Doppler ultrasonography[11] and fibrinogen ^{125}I leg scanning.[6,12] Most studies evaluating these techniques have included patients with a first episode of clinically suspected DVT. In contrast, relatively few studies have been performed in patients with a history of DVT who present with recurrent symptoms.[13(I),14,15(I),16] An accurate diagnosis of recurrent DVT is important because a patient may be labelled as being thrombophilic and be exposed to the risk of the complications of prolonged anticoagulant treatment.

EPIDEMIOLOGY

The incidence of a first episode of proven DVT is estimated to vary from 0.56 to 1.6 per 1000 people each year.[17,18] Figures for recurrent DVT can be derived from treatment studies in patients with proven DVT who have careful long-term follow-up.[19(I),20(I),21(I),22(I),23(I),24(I),25(I)] From these studies an aggregate incidence of recurrent DVT of 7.5% was calculated after the start of anticoagulant treatment.[26] In a recent large randomized trial, patients with DVT and/or pulmonary embolism (PE) were followed over 2 years.[27(I)] Thromboembolic recurrences—mostly recurrent DVT—occurred in 18.1% of patients treated with oral anticoagulation for 6 weeks and in 9.5% of patients who were on oral anticoagulants for 6 months. Importantly, in the 6-week anticoagulation group there was a sharp increase in the recurrence rate immediately after the cessation of the oral anticoagulation therapy, while this was not observed in the 6-month treatment group.[27(I)] In another large follow-up study of 352 patients with treated DVT, the cumulative incidence of recurrent venous thromboembolism was 15% and 22% after one and 2 years respectively.[28] From epidemiological studies it has become clear that several factors can increase the risk of recurrent DVT. These include hereditary inhibitor deficiencies (antithrombin, protein C, protein S, activated protein C resistance), cancer, and previous thromboembolism.[29]

Finally, it is important to realize that the rate of clinically suspected recurrent DVT is three to fivefold higher than the reported recurrence rates, since only 20%–30% of the patients have a recurrence proven by objective tests.[13(I),15(I)]

DIFFERENTIAL DIAGNOSIS

Until recently, most of the patients with a history of venous thrombosis who had recurrent symptoms of leg pain and swelling were considered to have recurrent DVT based on their clinical presentation alone. They then experienced the inconvenience of multiple hospital admissions, long-term anticoagulant therapy—with associated need for laboratory control—and the considerable mental anguish because of fear of a fatal recurrent episode. It is now clear that this approach is inappropriate because in studies it has been shown that the diagnosis of recurrent DVT cannot be established—or, of equal importance, ruled out, by clinical assessment.[13(I),14,15(I),16]

Recurrent leg symptoms following DVT may be caused by acute recurrent DVT, the postthrombotic syndrome or nonthrombotic disorders that may mimic recurrent DVT symptoms such as Baker's cyst, hematoma, muscle strain, sciatic pain, arthralgia or lumbosacral disc

From *Venous Thromboembolism: An Evidence-Based Atlas* edited by Russell Hull, Gary Raskob, Graham Pineo © 1996, Futura Publishing Co., Armonk, NY.

disease. Finally, some patients, out of fear of venous thromboembolic complications, have an exaggerated perception of their symptoms, which is called "thromboneurosis".[14] This latter, poorly recognized diagnosis should be reserved for the patient who has a history of multiple hospital admissions for "recurrent DVT" and may present with leg pain and tenderness; in its most severe form there is such fear for recurrent DVT and/or PE, limb loss, and death that a patient becomes totally incapacitated. It can be prevented by objective testing in every patient with the clinical suspicion of recurrent DVT.

OBJECTIVE DIAGNOSIS OF RECURRENT DVT

Recurrent DVT represents a diagnostic dilemma because the clinical diagnosis is nonspecific and the gold standard for a first episode of DVT, venography, is potentially less useful. This is because it may be difficult to visualize a constant intraluminal filling defect in previously thrombosed veins. Furthermore, venography is difficult to perform in patients who have multiple episodes of clinically suspected recurrence.[14]

IPG, either alone or in combination with ^{125}I fibrinogen leg scanning, and compression ultrasonography have been thoroughly investigated as alternative techniques to venography in patients with the clinical suspicion of recurrent DVT, satisfying the aforementioned criteria of evaluating diagnostic tests.

VENOGRAPHY

The hallmark sign for acute venous thrombosis is an intraluminal filling defect that is constant in shape and projection in two different projections.[30] When present in patients with recurrent DVT it gives firm proof for the presence of fresh thrombi. The interpretation of venograms in patients with recurrent DVT is often difficult because of obliteration of the legs' veins due to previous thrombotic occlusion.

The diagnostic utility of venography was evaluated in a study where IPG was used as a screening test with subsequent venography if the IPG was abnormal.[13] Seventy of 270 patients with clinically suspected recurrent DVT had an abnormal IPG and in 45 (64%) of these patients new intraluminal filling defects could be detected; two patients had normal venograms, whereas venography was indeterminate in 23 (33%) patients. On follow-up with ^{125}I fibrinogen leg scan 10 of these 23 patients had positive scans and were treated for recurrent DVT.

IMPEDANCE PLETHYSMOGRAPHY AND ^{125}I FIBRINOGEN LEG SCANNING

The combination of IPG and ^{125}I leg scanning as a diagnostic method is based on the assumption that they are complementary. IPG has been shown to be sensitive for detecting proximal-vein thrombosis[6(I)], while ^{125}I leg scanning is sensitive for distal thrombosis[6]. In a prospective study involving 270 patients with clinically suspected recurrent DVT the diagnostic utility of this combination was evaluated.[13] At the outset of the study it was decided to withhold anticoagulant treatment in patients with normal IPG and leg-scanning results, irrespective of the clinical findings. IPG was performed on referral. If normal, ^{125}I fibrinogen was injected and the patient scanned one and 3 days later. IPG was also repeated on these days. If the IPG was abnormal, venography was performed (see above) and anticoagulant therapy started in patients with abnormal venograms. When venography was normal, ^{125}I fibrinogen was injected and the patients scanned one and 3 days later. If the scan became positive, patients were treated with anticoagulants. All patients were followed-up long-term at 3 and 12 months.

Of the 270 patients, 181 (67%) had normal IPG and leg scan results and anticoagulant therapy was withheld in these patients. None of them died of PE and three (1.7%) patients returned with documented recurrent DVT. In contrast, 18 of the 89 (20%) patients with abnormal IPG or leg scan results had new episodes of recurrent venous thromboembolism, including four deaths due to PE. This diagnostic approach therefore has high clinical utility. Ninety-five percent of the 270 patients could be managed using this rather complex combination of diagnostic tests. Moreover in 67% of the patients, a decision not to treat again with anticoagulants was possible, and this proved to be safe on long-term follow-up.

IMPEDANCE PLETHYSMOGRAPHY

An alternative approach to combined IPG and leg scanning is the use of serial IPG based on the assumption that serial IPG detects proximally-extending calf DVT, as was demonstrated in two large studies in patients with a first episode of DVT.[7(I),8(I)] For this approach knowledge of the normalization of IPG after a first episode of DVT is important because of the need of a normal base-line result of IPG before the onset of recurrent symptoms. Both this normalization rate and the safety and efficacy of serial IPG has been evaluated in a study in 161 patients with proven DVT.[15(I)] IPG had normalized in 67%, 85%, 92% and 95% of patients after 3, 6, 9 and 12 months respectively. Thirty-five (22%) patients returned with suspected recurrent DVT. Anticoagulant therapy was withheld in 18 (51%) of these patients and in follow-up there was no recurrence of venous thromboembolism. In 13 patients, IPG became again abnormal and venography showed new intraluminal filling defects in 11 of them. In this study it was possible to manage 29 (83%) patients with suspected recurrence with serial IPG alone. These results suggest that it may be impossible to simplify the combined approach of IPG—or another noninvasive method—and leg scanning for recurrent DVT by using serial IPG alone, but larger studies are required to confirm these observations. Furthermore, it recommends that noninvasive tests be repeated routinely in patients at follow-up visits or at least before discharge from the hospital.

COMPRESSION ULTRASONOGRAPHY

Real-time B-mode ultrasonography has great utility in the diagnosis of proximal-vein thrombosis. In several studies the single criterion of noncompressibility in either the popliteal or femoral veins has been shown to be highly specific for the presence of DVT, while compressibility rules out proximal-vein thrombosis.[31(I),32(I)] A few studies have performed serial ultrasound examinations after an acute episode of DVT.[33–37] Applying the criterion of full compressibility of the common femoral and popliteal veins, that is, compression ultrasound (C-US), a normalization of the test was shown in only 21% to 52% after 6 months and 30% to 55% after 12 months.[33–37] These studies suggest that real-time C-US cannot be reused in patients with clinically suspected recurrent DVT.

Recently, studies have demonstrated progressive decreases in thrombus mass after the initial thrombosis.[34,38] Furthermore, in two studies it was shown that the apposition of fresh thrombi to the pre-existing clot follows the anatomical distribution pattern of the first episode, involving the common femoral vein, the popliteal vein, or both.[23(I),39(I)] It is therefore hypothesized that in the presence of a recurrent thrombosis, the residual thrombus mass enlarges, and that the enlargement is measurable by application of the ultrasound procedure to a limited number of fixed points over the upper leg.[26,37] This ultrasound procedure consists of measuring the thickness of the thrombus mass in abnormal venous segments over the saphenofemoral junction—for the femoral vein— and/or in the midpopliteal fossa—for the popliteal vein, as follows.[37] The maximum compressibility of the vein is assessed in the transverse section by pressing on the vein with the transducer probe. A freeze image is obtained and the residual vein diameter—representing the indicator for the thickness of thrombus mass—is measured on line and recorded on the patient's chart.

In the study by Prandoni and colleagues, noncompressibility of previously normalized venous segment and/or enlargement of thrombus thickness of 2 mm or more, were considered as evidence of recurrent proximal DVT.[37] A statistically significant reduction ($p<0.0001$) in thrombus mass was observed in both the femoral and popliteal vein, with a major reduction (62% in the femoral and 50% in the popliteal veins) within the first 3 months. During the study, 29 of the 149 patients developed a clinical recurrence (19.5%), of whom 22 (15%) within one year. Compression Ultrasound had normalized in only six (21%) of the 27 patients with suspected DVT recurrence and reverted to normal in the three patients with proximal DVT recurrence (sensitivity and specificity 100%). In all 10 patients with venographically confirmed

proximal recurrent DVT, the ultrasound test demonstrated noncompressibility of a previously normalized popliteal or common femoral vein and/or an increased vein diameter (2 mm or more), compared with the previous assessment (sensitivity of the combined C-US and thrombus thickness methods 100%; 95% CI 61–100%). In one patient with recurrent calf-vein thrombosis the test was unchanged. In all 18 patients without venographically proven DVT, the US test demonstrated an unchanged or improved residual vein diameter as compared with the previous US test (specificity, 100%; 95% CI 81–100%). In the seven patients in whom thrombus thickness determination confirmed the diagnosis of recurrent DVT, the enlargement was 2 mm in one patient, 3 mm in two patients and more than 4 mm in four patients.

A potential flaw of this method might be the tiny echographic separation between patients with and without recurrent DVT, raising questions of the consistency and reliability of this technique, especially in the hands of untrained operators. In this study an inter-observer variability of 1 mm was accepted, which resulted in a high reproducibility.

In another study the intra- and inter-observer variability of the thrombus thickness determination was determined.[26] The intra-test variability never exceeded 1 mm, while the inter-test variability was one millimeter in 32 patients, 2 mm in three patients, and 4 mm in two patients. Based on these findings, Koopman et al, in contrast to the findings of Prandoni et al,[37] defined three different categories: an unchanged diameter or a decrease in diameter makes recurrent DVT very unlikely, changes up to 4 mm are considered nondiagnostic, whereas an increase in diameter of more than 4 mm is highly suggestive of recurrent DVT. In the nondiagnostic group it was concluded that repeated testing would be appropriate.

Clearly, there is a need for confirmation of the accuracy of the quantitative ultrasound test for recurrent DVT with respect to reproducibility, specificity for recurrent DVT and most importantly, clinical outcome associated with normal tests.

Whether the adjunct of duplex or color Doppler facilities improves the diagnostic accuracy of real-time B-mode US is uncertain, since prospective studies in symptomatic patients are lacking. In a study in asymptomatic high-risk patients, color Doppler had an unacceptably low sensitivity and clinical utility for detection of proximal-vein thrombi.[40(I)]

BLOOD TESTS

Although no rigorous studies have been performed evaluating the accuracy of blood tests measuring breakdown products of cross-linked fibrin, such as Fpa or D-dimer, in patients with suspected recurrent DVT, these tests have shown to have very high negative predictive values and can thus be applied successfully to exclude first episode venous thrombosis.[41(I),42(I),43(I)] The reported sensitivity of an elevated D-dimer level (>300 microgr/l) for the presence of DVT was 100% (95% CI 95–100%) in a recent large prospective study.[44](I) The main disadvantage of this test is its low specificity (29%, 95% CI 23%–34%), thus necessitating repeated testing with a noninvasive test in many patients. In the same study in 309 consecutive patients with clinically suspected DVT, 69 of 249 patients (28%)—all of whom had normal IPG or C-US results on the day of referral—had normal D-dimer levels.[44] They would have been spared the inconvenience of serial testing with IPG of C-US. In total, using a combination of IPG or C-US and D-dimer test, a definitive diagnosis could be made on the day of presentation in 42% of referred patients (60/309 patients; 60 with either abnormal IPG or C-US and 69 patients with a normal D-dimer test). Importantly, in this study a rapid bedside ELISA test was used, opposed to the more laborious tests used in older studies. In the diagnosis of recurrent DVT it is conceivable to select a subset of patients on the basis of a normal D-dimer test, in whom recurrent DVT is highly unlikely. Such a subgroup of patients would be spared the need for serial testing with noninvasive tests. This strategy in combination with noninvasive tests such as IPG or quantitative C-US would be both practical and cost-effective, but follow-up studies have to confirm the safety of such an approach.

MAGNETIC RESONANCE IMAGING

Magnetic resonance imaging (MRI) has, to a limited extent, been evaluated in acute venous thrombosis.[45,46] Its role in the diagnosis of recurrent DVT has not been determined. It is questionable whether this expensive technique warrants further development for the diagnosis of recurrent DVT.

CONCLUSIONS

The diagnosis of recurrent DVT is difficult and requires careful evaluation. The diagnosis cannot be established on the basis of clinical symptoms because of the unacceptably low specificity. The combination of IPG and ^{125}I fibrinogen leg scanning represents an accurate but rather intensive approach. Serial IPG has been evaluated to a limited extent, but this method is not widely available. The combination of C-US and quantitative ultrasound measurement of thrombus thickness, seems to be the most promising technique for the diagnosis of recurrent DVT. Whether this approach can be used either alone as a serial test or in combination with a D-dimer test, should be tested in prospective studies.

REFERENCES

1. Haeger K. Problems of acute deep venous thrombosis: The interpretation of signs and symptoms. Angiology 1969;20:219–223.
2. Barnes RW, Wu KK, Hoak JC. Fallibility of the clinical diagnosis of venous thrombosis. JAMA 1975;234:605–607.
3. Cranley JJ, Canes AJ, Sull WJ. The diagnosis of deep vein thrombosis: Fallibility of clinical symptoms and signs. Arch Surg 1976;111:34–36.
(I)4. Hull RD, Hirsh J, Sackett DL, et al. The clinical validity of a negative venogram. Circulation 1981;64:622–625.
5. Bueller HR, Lensing AWA, Hirsh J, ten Cate JW. Deep vein thrombosis: new noninvasive tests. Thromb Haemost 1991;636:133–137.
(I)6. Hull RD, Hirsh J, Sackett DL, et al. The combined use of leg scanning and impedance plethysmography in suspected venous thrombosis: an alternative to venography. N Engl J Med 1977;296:1497–1500.
(I)7. Hull RD, Hirsh J, Carter C, et al. Diagnostic efficacy of impedance plethysmography for clinically suspected deep vein thrombosis: a randomized trial. Ann Int Med 1995;102:21–28.
(I)8. Huisman MV, Bueller HR, ten Cate JW, et al. Serial impedance plethysmography for suspected deep venous thrombosis in outpatients. The Amsterdam General Practitioner Study. N Engl J Med 1986;314:823–828.
(I)9. Lensing AWA, Prandoni P, Brandjes DPM, et al. Detection of deep vein thrombosis by real time B-mode ultrasonography. N Engl J Med 1989;320:342–345.
(I)10. Heijboer H, Bueller HR, Lensing AWA, et al. A randomized comparison of the clinical utility of real-time compression ultrasonography versus impedance plethysmography in the diagnosis of deep vein thrombosis in symptomatic outpatients. N Engl J Med 1993;
(I)11. Lensing AWA, Levi M, Bueller HR, et al. An objective Doppler method for the diagnosis of deep vein thrombosis. Ann Int Med 1990;113:9–14.
12. Moser KM, Brach BB, Dolan GF. Clinically suspected deep venous thrombosis of the lower extremities: A comparison of venography, impedance plethysmography and radio-labeled fibrinogen. JAMA 1977;237:2195–2198.
(I)13. Hull RD, Carter C, Jay R. The diagnosis of acute recurrent DVT: A diagnostic challenge. Circulation 1983;67:901–906.
14. Leclerc J, Jay R, Hull RD, et al. Recurrent leg symptoms following deep vein thrombosis. A diagnostic challenge. Arch Int Med 1985;145:1867–1869.
(I)15. Huisman MV, Bueller HR, ten Cate JW. Utility of impedance plethysmography in the diagnosis of recurrent deep-vein thrombosis. Arch Int Med 1988;148:681–683.
16. Prandoni P, Cogo A, Bernardi E. A simple ultrasound approach for detection of recurrent proximal-vein thrombosis. Circulation 1993;88:1730–1735.
17. Nordstroem M, Lindblad B, Bergqvist D, Kjellstroem T. A prospective study of the incidence of deep vein thrombosis within a defined urban population. J Int Med 1992;232:155–160.
18. Anderson Jr FA, Wheeler HB, Goldberg RJ, et al. A population-based perspective of the hospital incidence and case-fatality rates of deep vein thrombosis and pulmonary embolism. The Worcester DVT Study. Arch Int Med 1991;151:933–938.
(I)19. Hull RD, Delmore T, Genton E, et al. Warfarin sodium versus low dose heparin in the long-term treatment of venous thrombosis. N Engl J Med 1979;301:855–858.
(I)20. Hull RD, Delmore T, Carter C, et al. Adjusted subcutaneous heparin versus warfarin sodium in the longterm treatment of venous thrombosis. N Engl J Med 1982;306:189–194.
(I)21. Shulman S, Lockner D, Juhlin-Danfelt A. The duration of oral anticoagulant after deep vein thrombosis. Acta Med Scand 1985;217:547–552.

(I)22. Hull RD, Raskob GE, Hirsh J, et al. Continuous intravenous heparin compared with intermittent subcutaneous heparin in the initial treatment of proximal-vein thrombosis. N Engl J Med 1986;1109–1114.

(I)23. Prandoni P, Lensing AWA, Bueller HR, et al. Comparison of subcutaneous low molecular weight heparin with intravenous heparin in proximal deep vein thrombosis. Lancet 1992;339:441–445.

(I)24. Brandjes DPM, Heijboer H, Bueller HR, et al. Acenocoumarol and heparin compared with acenocoumarol alone in the initial treatment of proximal-vein thrombosis. N Engl J Med 1992;327:1485–1489.

(I)25. Hull RD, Raskob GE, Pineo GF, et al. Subcutaneous low molecular weight heparin compared with continuous intravenous heparin in the treatment of proximal vein thrombosis. N Engl J Med 1992;326:975–982.

26. Koopman MMW, Bueller HR, ten Cate JW. Diagnosis of recurrent deep-vein thrombosis. Hemostasis 1995;25:49–57.

(I)27. Shulman S, Rhedin AS, Lindmarker P, et al. A comparison of six weeks with six months of oral anticoagulant therapy after a first episode of venous thromboembolism. N Engl J Med 1995;332:1661–1665.

28. Prandoni P, Lensing AWA, Cogo A, et al. The clinical course of deep-vein thrombosis. Thromb Haem 1995;73:1092. (Abstract)

29. Salzman EW, Hirsh J. The epidemiology, pathogenesis, and natural history of venous thrombosis. In: Hemostasis and Thrombosis: Basic Principles and Clinical Practice. Third Edition. Colman RW, Hirsh J, Marder VJ, et al. (eds.): Philadephia, PA, JB Lippincott Co., 1994, Chapter 65, pp. 1275–1298.

30. Rabinov K, Paulin S. Roentgen diagnosis of venous thrombosis in the leg. Arch Surg 1972;104:134–144.

(I)31. Lensing AWA, Prandoni P, Brandjes DPM, Huisman PM, et al. Detection of deep vein thrombosis by real time B-mode ultrasonography. N Engl J Med 1989;320:342–345.

(I)32. Heijboer H, Lensing AWA, Bueller HR, et al. A comparison of real-time compression ultrasonography with impedance plethysmography for the diagnosis of deep vein thrombosis in symptomatic outpatients. N Engl J Med 1993;329:1365–1369.

33. Cronan JJ, Leen V. Recurrent deep venous thrombosis: limitations of CUS. Radiology 1989;170:739–742.

34. Murphy TP, Cronan JJ. Evolution of deep venous thrombosis: a prospective evaluation with US. Radiology 1990;177:543–548.

35. Mantoni M. Deep venous thrombosis: longitudinal study with duplex US. Radiology 1991;179:271–273.

36. Heijboer H, Jongbloets LMM, Bueller HR, et al. Clinical utility of real-time compression ultrasonography for diagnostic management of patients with recurrent venous thrombosis. Acta Radiol 1992;33:297–300.

37. Prandoni P, Cogo A, Bernardi E, et al. A simple ultrasound approach for detection of recurrent proximal-vein thrombosis. Circulation 1993;88:1730–1735.

38. van Ramshorst B, van Bemmelen PS, Hoeneveld H, et al. Thrombus regression in deep venous thrombosis: quantification of spontaneous thrombolysis with duplex scanning. Circulation 1992;86:414–419.

(I)39. Prandoni P, Lensing AWA, Bueller HR, et al. Deep vein thrombosis and the incidence of subsequent symptomatic cancer. N Engl J Med 1992;327:1128–1133.

(I)40. Davidson BL, Elliott CG, Lensing AWA. Low accuracy of color-Doppler ultrasound in the detection of proximal leg vein thrombosis in asymptomatic high risk patients. Ann Int Med 1992;117:735–738.

(I)41. Heaton DC, Billings JD, Hicton CM. Assessment of D-dimer assays for the diagnosis of deep vein thrombosis. J Lab Clin Med 1987;110:588–591.

(I)42. Ott P, Astrup L, Jansen RH, et al. Assessment of D-dimer in plasma: Diagnostic value in suspected deep venous thrombosis of the leg. Acta Med Scand 1988;224:263–267.

(I)43. Bounameaux H, Schneider PA, Reber G, et al. Measurement of plasma D-dimer for diagnosis of deep venous thrombosis. Am J Clinic Pathol 1989;91:82–85.

(I)44. Heijboer H, Ginsberg JS, Bueller HR, et al. The use of D-dimer test in combination with noninvasive testing alone for the diagnosis of deep vein thrombosis. Thromb Haem 1992;67:510–513.

45. Spritzer CE, Sussman SK, Blinder RA, et al. DVT evaluation with limited flip-angle, gradient refocused MRI: Preliminary experience. Radiology 1988;166:371–375.

46. Erdman WA, Jayson HT, Redman HC, et al. DVT of extremities: Role of MRI in the diagnosis. Radiology 1990;174:425–429.

SECTION IV

Diagnosis of Pulmonary Embolism

20

Overview of the Diagnosis of Pulmonary Embolism

Mark A. Kelley

INTRODUCTION

Pulmonary embolism (PE) is a major international health problem with an annual estimated incidence of over 500,000 cases in the United States alone.[1] Recent reports have confirmed that PE continues to be prevalent among hospitalized patients and remains as a common cause of mortality.[2–4] This situation may actually worsen as the demographics of the disease evolve. In the recent multicenter study, Prospective Investigation of Pulmonary Embolism Diagnosis (PIOPED), malignancy, congestive heart failure and pulmonary diseases were commonly associated with PE.[5] As modern medicine improves patient longevity with these chronic diseases, PE may become an even more common clinical problem.

Because of its lethal potential, PE has been the subject of considerable research over the last 20 years. The most important outcomes of these investigations have been: (1) most pulmonary emboli arise from deep-vein thrombosis (DVT); (2) prophylaxis of DVT is very effective in reducing the incidence of PE; and (3) anticoagulation greatly reduces the mortality of PE. However despite these important observations, prophylaxis for DVT is still not used appropriately in many clinical settings.[6] In addition, PE remains a difficult disorder to diagnose and its therapy, anticoagulation, is too risky to apply without a firm diagnosis.

The diagnosis of PE is a major clinical challenge because PE often accompanies other diseases and overlaps with their clinical presentations. Findings such as chest pain, shortness of breath, and arrhythmias can occur with PE and a variety of other cardiopulmonary disorders. However, once PE is diagnosed, the treatment is highly effective. In the recent PIOPED study, patients with correctly diagnosed and treated PE had only a 2% mortality from this disorder.[5] This contrasts with uncontrolled series which have estimated the fatality rate for undiagnosed PE to be as high as 30%.[7] There are few disorders in clinical medicine where there is such a tremendous premium on correct diagnosis and treatment. Therefore, there has been a long-standing quest to improve the accuracy of diagnosing PE.

During the past three decades, there have been many advances in understanding PE which have led to new clinical approaches and the development of diagnostic technology. However, despite these advances, many unresolved issues remain. This chapter will provide a chronologic view of our understanding of PE. The end of the chapter will summarize our current state of knowledge and serve as a frame of reference for subsequent chapters, which describe more detailed approaches.

1960s—THE DECADE OF DISCOVERY

Pulmonary embolism has been recognized as a clinical condition for centuries. Virchow reported the triad of venous stasis, hypercoagulability and vessel injury leading to PE.[8] Trousseau described migratory thrombophlebitis and fatal PE associated with pancreatic carcinoma. Osler described pulmonary infarction and embolus in the setting of chronic heart disease.

However, while PE was well known clinically, it was not until 1960 that the effective therapy was defined. At that time, a controlled trial in patients with massive PE proved that anticoagulation improved survival.[9] Additional clinical investigation demonstrated that the pulmonary emboli arose from clots in large capacitance vessels of the lower extremities.[10] Particularly at risk were surgical patients who seemed to form clot avidly, even on the operating table.

Simultaneously, radiographic imaging technology was rapidly coming to the forefront. Radioactive isotopes

From *Venous Thromboembolism: An Evidence-Based Atlas* edited by Russell Hull, Gary Raskob, Graham Pineo © 1996, Futura Publishing Co., Armonk, NY.

were used to image the liver, brain, lung, and skeletal system. The technique of vascular catheterization permitted visualization of the vascular anatomy of vital organs.

These imaging techniques were immediately applied to diagnosing PE in several different ways. For those interested in peripheral vascular disease, the radioactive fibrinogen scan documented the formation and evolution of venous clot in the lower extremities. However, this technique failed to detect proximal DVT, the most common cause of PE. This shortcoming led to the development of other noninvasive techniques which were better at documenting proximal venous clot. Studies such as impedance plethysmography (IPG) and Doppler measured the flow characteristics of the venous system before and after occlusion of the venous return. These techniques became standard in some hospitals and were often used in large clinical trials.

At the end of this decade, angiographic imaging techniques became standardized. Advances in technology, such as magnification and selective contrast injections, led to more sophisticated imaging of small vascular abnormalities. In the field of PE, venography could document DVT and pulmonary angiography could detect clots within the central circulation. While pulmonary angiograms were initially primitive, improved techniques allowed imaging of even small clots.

Radionuclide scanning had great appeal because of its noninvasive nature. For diagnosing PE, perfusion scans could define abnormalities in the pulmonary circulation. Such images, coupled with ventilation scans could, in theory, document occlusion of pulmonary blood flow from PE. Enthusiasm for this technology was heightened when imaging improved as rectilinear scanners were replaced by the current gamma cameras.

Thus in the 1960s, the rapid explosion of technology led to a great deal of optimism about improving the accuracy of PE diagnosis. However, during the next decade of the 1970s, this optimism was replaced by skepticism as controversy surrounded these new technologies.

1970s—DECADE OF CONTROVERSY

As PE was increasingly recognized as a preventable and treatable condition, there was an explosive interest in the clinical investigation of this disorder. The National Institutions of Health commissioned historically important multicenter trials on the role of thrombolytic therapy in PE.[11] Using diagnostic technology to document PE, these trials compared heparin therapy alone to heparin and thrombolytic therapy. These trials not only provided information about the efficacy of thrombolytic therapy, but also gave a glimpse of performance characteristics of diagnostic imaging technology. This technology would be considered, by current standards, primitive, since it utilized rectilinear radionuclide scanning and main pulmonary artery and/or right ventricular injections for an-

giography. Since the trials focused on therapy, the implication was that the diagnosis of PE was no longer the challenge it had been in previous decades.

As is well known, the thrombolytic trials were largely inconclusive. While thrombolytic therapy dissolved clot more rapidly than heparin, the studies did not have the statistical power to demonstrate any effect on mortality.

The major importance of these clinical trials is that they demonstrated the complexity of patients presenting with suspected PE. Such patients often presented with overlapping symptoms which could be confused with other cardiopulmonary disorders. Frequently, chest radiographic findings and electrocardiograms were diagnostically nonspecific. Therefore, it appeared that diagnostic imaging techniques were critical for diagnosis and attention began to focus on the accuracy of these techniques.

Meanwhile, nuclear medicine began to proliferate as a discipline even among small community hospitals. Radionuclide imaging techniques were used extensively for such disorders as stroke (before CAT scanning); staging of cancer; and in the evaluation of pulmonary vascular disease, particularly PE. These techniques were noninvasive, provided permanent images and used simple technology. These features made nuclear medicine attractive to clinicians and hospital administrators alike. In contrast, angiography was invasive and technically challenging, thereby confining this technology to tertiary referral centers. In addition, the equipment was expensive and required a substantial volume of patients to sustain clinical activity.

Soon, the lung scan became more widely available than pulmonary angiography. Physicians found the scanning techniques to be easily tolerated by most patients. Radiologists, while often comfortable with such techniques as venography, did not have the same degree of confidence when studying the central circulation. Thus, clinicians found the lung scan to be more appealing to them and their radiology colleagues, and soon this test was accepted as the diagnostic procedure of choice for PE.

In the late 1970s, this concept was boldly challenged. An historically important paper by Robin suggested that the lung scan may be inaccurate and that it had never been proven in comparison with pulmonary angiography.[12] Furthermore, he contended that all the diagnostic technology in PE had never been subjected to appropriate scrutiny.

This challenge stimulated predictable responses from the nuclear medicine and angiography communities. Multiple reports, largely derived from uncontrolled retrospective studies, compared the diagnostic accuracy of lung scanning and angiography.[13–16] These studies, suggested that the lung scan was a good screening test for PE but when abnormal could be associated with varying degrees of diagnostic accuracy. These conclusions remained controversial. In addition, as the field of decision analysis emerged, there were attempts to link elements of clinical history, clinical findings, laboratory data, and imaging studies into algorithms which accurately would diagnose PE. These attempts were plagued by lack of prospective studies which included all patients suspected of PE rather than those who were subselected for pulmonary angiography. Thus, the end of the 1970s was punctuated by a great deal of confusion as to the best diagnostic approach for PE and whether imaging techniques had reliable accuracy.

1980s—THE STORM CLOUDS BEGIN TO CLEAR

In the early 1980s, the National Institutes of Health recognized that PE was a major health problem which remained a great diagnostic challenge. For this reason, the National Institutes of Health sponsored the PIOPED project to compare directly the performance of pulmonary angiography and radionuclide lung scanning in the diagnosis of PE. The study, conducted in six tertiary care referral centers, had a strict prospective study design, as described elsewhere in this volume.[17]

Prospective Investigation of Pulmonary Embolism Diagnosis confirmed a long-held clinical dictum: a normal lung scan or pulmonary angiogram rules out clinically important PE. For the first time, PIOPED investigators prospectively categorized abnormal lung scans and compared them to angiograms. In PIOPED, a high probability lung scan was highly suggestive of PE but had about a 15% error margin. This error was magnified when the patient had previous PE since the abnormal scan could indicate an old clot. An intermediate probability lung scan was associated with approximately a 30% likelihood of PE. For patients with low probability scans, 13% had PE. A lung scan which is neither normal nor abnormal enough to be classified as low probability, had a less than 5% likelihood of being associated with PE.

One of the most significant findings in PIOPED was that among the patients with PE, the majority did not have high probability scans. Of all patients with PE, 40% had high probability scans, 42% intermediate scans, and 18% low or near normal scan findings.

PIOPED is historically important in the diagnosis of PE for several reasons. First, this study was one of the first diagnostic technology assessments ever performed by the National Institutes of Health. Such technology research has now become essential in healthcare economics. Second, PIOPED confirmed what had long been suspected—namely that the radionuclide lung scan is a perfect screening test for PE. Thus a normal lung scan absolutely rules out the diagnosis of PE. The problem is that an abnormal lung scan result is nonspecific and is associated with variable probabilities of PE depending on details of the lung scan image. Finally, and most notably, PIOPED demonstrated that most patients with PE have

"non-diagnostic scans", i.e. neither high probability nor normal. Therefore, with these patients, the lung scan results still leave the clinician guessing as to the correct diagnosis.

As the PIOPED study was being conducted, other research introduced the concept of "thromboembolism."[18] This term describes the condition which begins with thrombus formation in the venous circulation and embolization of this thrombus to the pulmonary circulation, leading to the condition we recognize as PE. Many studies had linked DVT, particularly of the lower extremities with PE. In addition, in patients with DVT, as many as 50% may have asymptomatic PE as documented by lung scan.[19] Investigators at McMaster University had also discovered that at least half of patients with angiographically proven PE had proximal-vein thrombosis detected by either noninvasive or invasive techniques.[20]

Because of this overlap between DVT and PE, it was proposed that a combined approach of noninvasive technology might be useful in diagnosing PE. Specifically it was suggested that if patients had nondiagnostic lung scans (as defined above), they should undergo venous studies of the lower extremities to detect DVT. If this condition were found, patients could then be placed on anticoagulation.

Two major studies used noninvasive technologies to document thromboembolism. In a large study of outpatients suspected of DVT, serial impedance plethysmography successfully detected clinically important proximal DVT.[21] Hull and colleagues extended these observations to patients suspected of PE. In this series, patients with nondiagnostic lung scans underwent serial IPGs to detect proximal DVT either in initial presentation, or in subsequent days to weeks.[22] The results suggested that this combined approach of lung scanning and serial IPGs had a highly acceptable diagnostic accuracy.

1990s—THE ERA OF CLINICAL OUTCOMES

As this decade began, many more facets were known about diagnosing PE. The diagnostic accuracy of both the radionuclide lung scan and pulmonary angiogram were documented by PIOPED.[17] There had been at least two decades of experience with venous imaging by contrast venography and conventional Doppler and IPG (noninvasive techniques). The latter were felt to be 90% to 95% sensitive for the diagnosis of DVT. The nonspecific nature of an abnormal lung scan, meant that, this technology alone was insufficient for diagnostic confidence in most patients suspected of PE. It appeared to be logistically and economically impractical to provide pulmonary angiography to all patients suspected of PE. Therefore the early part of this decade was characterized by a quest for noninvasive approaches which would lead to a correct diagnosis.

As had been traditional in the field for thirty years, novel methods to image clot continued to be reported. For at least 10 years, a variety of studies have examined techniques to provide radiolabeling of the venous clot. For example, the role of radioactive platelets have been studied in imaging clot. Unfortunately, these platelets may not participate in active clot formation or the aggregation may be so slow as to preclude timely diagnosis. Monoclonal antibodies directed against fibrin have also been employed, and while these may accurately detect leg-vein thrombosis, they have not had similar accuracy in the lung. The role of this technology compared to other venous studies has yet to be determined.[23]

An important sidelight of the PIOPED study was to underscore the role of the clinical impression or prior probability assessment of patients suspected of PE. In the PIOPED project, participating clinicians were asked to estimate the probability of PE before any imaging studies were performed. The results demonstrated that when lung scan results supported clinical impression, this combination was highly accurate. Thus, a low clinical suspicion of PE, combined with a low probability lung scan, effectively ruled out the diagnosis. A similar analysis has also shown that the receiver operating curve characteristics of lung scan interpretations, are widely influenced by the prevalence of the disease as reflected by clinical probability estimates.[24] The role of clinical probability estimates has been undervalued in previous studies of diag-

nostic technology and more recent research, particularly in the area of critical care, has suggested that clinical probability estimates may be highly accurate.[25]

Using this information plus that from PIOPED, Kelley et al, suggested a diagnostic algorithm for PE.[26] (Figure 1) In this approach, patients suspected of this diagnosis undergo lung scanning first, as a screening test. In the presence of a nondiagnostic lung scan, IPGs could be employed. An important caveat to this approach is that serial IPGs have not been studied in patients with major cardiopulmonary disease. Therefore, the serial IPG approach combined with lung scanning, needs to have further confirmation. In situations of diagnostic uncertainty, the pulmonary angiogram or empiric heparin remain as alternatives.

This noninvasive approach to thromboembolism has recently been challenged. Prandoni and colleagues applied the serial IPG technique to patients suspected of DVT and found there was 1.3% mortality rate.[27] The doubt was reinforced by reports in which noninvasive studies failed to detect proximal DVT in patients undergoing hip surgery and in screening for thromboembolism.[28–30]

These results have raised the whole question as to whether venous diagnostic imaging should be subjected to more rigorous clinical trials. Currently, IPG is viewed as an excellent screening test which is technically simple and does not depend on operator skill. In contrast,

DIAGNOSTIC ALGORITHM

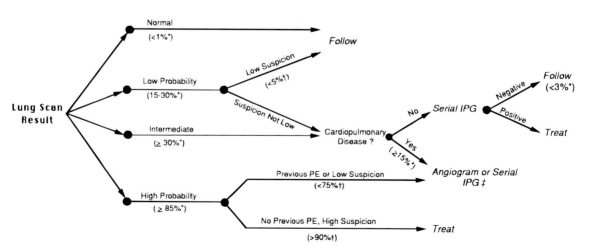

Figure 1. Diagnostic Algorithm A normal scan result effectively rules out pulmonary embolism *(PE)*. A high probability scan supports the diagnosis of PE except in the presence of previous PE or low clinical suspicion. Other scan results were less helpful, except the combination of low probability scan result and low clinical suspicion. A positive impedance plethysmograph *(IPG)* result supports the diagnosis of thromboembolism. A negative result, when done serially, reliably excludes this disorder only in patients with nondiagnostic scans and no cardiopulmonary disease. The likelihood of pulmonary embolism is indicated in parenthesis. * = strongly supported by clinical studies; † = suggested by clinical studies, needs confirmation; ‡ = a serially negative IPG result may not be sufficient to rule out thromboembolism. (Kelley MA, Carson JL, Palevsky HI, Schwartz JS: Diagnosing Pulmonary Embolism: New Facts and Strategies. Ann Int Med 114:304 February, 1991, Figure 1.)

Doppler ultrasound, which may be somewhat more sensitive for calf-vein thrombosis, requires a high degree of operator skill but may be more effective in detecting nonoccluding disease. Thus, in the 1990s controversy has surrounded the more classic venous noninvasive studies.

WHERE WE ARE NOW AND WHERE ARE WE GOING IN DIAGNOSING PULMONARY EMBOLISM?

After nearly three decades of research, we have a better understanding of the approach to the diagnosis of PE but many questions still remain. The diagnostic accuracy of lung scanning and angiography are now well documented and unless there are new breakthroughs in these technologies, these data seem very secure. In addition, as a result of multiple retrospective and several prospective series, it is clear that patients suspected of PE have the prevalence of this disorder of around 25% to 33%. This statistic is important in determining the predictive value and clinical utility of any diagnostic technology. Finally, with the PIOPED study, the outcome of patients with recognized and treated PE has now been clarified. These patients have an overall mortality of approximately 23% after one year, but from PE itself, the mortality is only 2%. The rest is due to underlying diseases such as cardiac conditions, pulmonary problems and malignancy.

From this secure knowledge base, we then move into theories that are suggested by clinical studies but are not yet firm enough to be conclusive. As described above, the noninvasive diagnostic approach combining lung scans and venous studies may have considerable validity. Unfortunately, the clinical trials to date have been small and have not been applicable to large numbers of ill hospitalized patients. In particular, the McMaster series did not include patients with cardiopulmonary disease. Furthermore, there is now confusion over the diagnostic accuracy of the various noninvasive techniques for venous imaging. Unanswered questions are whether the conventional IPG test is highly accurate and its relative role compared to color flow Doppler ultrasound.

These questions are crucial in deciding whether a combined noninvasive approach to diagnosing PE will be clinically useful. A great deal may be riding on this issue, since most hospitals cannot afford to offer the "gold standard" diagnostic technology of pulmonary angiography. On the other hand, noninvasive venous studies are straightforward and widely available, and can be easily applied in conjunction with conventional lung scanning. Therefore, the correct noninvasive diagnostic approach to PE must be resolved within the forthcoming decade.

Also unknown is the role of clinical assessment in conjunction with noninvasive imaging. Clinical estimates of probability may have an important role in sharpening diagnostic technology and more research in this area needs to be conducted to better understand such interactive effect.

Other technological approaches to diagnosing PE have yet to reach fruition. Innovative imaging techniques such as radioactive labeling of clot and magnetic resonance imaging may prove to be useful in the future. However, as with all new techniques, their expense relative to accuracy must be clearly documented. There has been a long-standing quest for an accurate serum screening test for thromboembolism. The most commonly quoted is an assay of the D-dimer, a byproduct of coagulation. To date, there is no convincing study or large series which shows that a widely accepted determination of any serum test is sufficiently sensitive or specific to be used in the diagnosis of PE. Nonetheless, finding such a serum marker for PE would be an important adjunct to other noninvasive tests.

The current decade may also feature more of an emphasis on clinical outcomes in PE. In the previous three decades, research in PE has focused on the accuracy of documenting clot. However, there is now accumulating evidence that many patients, particularly those in the postoperative period, experience asymptomatic clot which seems to have a clinically benign outcome. As suggested by Hirsh,[31] future diagnostic research may emphasize outcome rather than image acquisition per se. It may no longer be important enough to document that an abnormality exists, but to ask the question whether this abnormality will significantly influence the patient's overall clinical condition. For example, if IPG misses nonocclusive clot in the proximal venous system and yet such clot is not associated with clinically-significant PE, the sensitivity of IPG for detecting this abnormality is unimportant.

The final challenge in all this research will be assuring that research findings will be incorporated into clinical practice. This has not always been the case. For example, there is unquestioned evidence that the prophylaxis of thromboembolism is highly effective, relatively inexpensive, and associated with very few side-effects. However, there is ample documentation that clinicians still are not using such prophylaxis appropriately. The reasons for this are unclear, but more research must be done to learn how to implement scientific findings of therapeutic or diagnostic trials into clinical practice. Specifically, in diagnosing PE, the use of noninvasive studies, the interpretation of lung scans, and the role of clinical judgment, etc. must be packaged into simple, clear guidelines which are unambiguous. How these guidelines are developed and promoted will determine their acceptability by the clinical community.

REFERENCES

1. Goldhaber SZ, Morpurgo M. For the WHO/ISFC Task Force on Pulmonary Embolism. Diagnosis, treatment, and prevention of pulmonary embolism. JAMA 1992;268: 1727–1733.

2. Anderson FA, Wheeler B, Goldberg RJ, Hosmer DW, Forcier A. The prevalence of risk factors for venous thromboembolism among hospital patients. Arch Intern Med 1992;152:1660–1664.

3. Bedell SE, Fulton EJ. Unexpected findings and complications at autopsy after cardiopulmonary resuscitation (CPR). Arch Intern Med 1986;146:1725–1728.

4. Goldman L, Sayson R, Robbins S. Diagnostic yield of the autopsy in a university hospital and a community hospital. N Engl J Med 1983;308:1000–1005.

5. Carson JL, Kelley MA, Duff A, et al. The clinical course of pulmonary embolism. N Engl J Med 1992;326:1240–1245.

6. Anderson FA, Wheeler HB, Goldberg RJ, et al. Physician practices in the prevention of venous thromboembolism. Ann Intern Med 1991;115:591–595.

7. Dalen JE, Alpert JS. Natural history of pulmonary embolism. Prog Cardiovasc Dis 1975;17:259–270.

8. Virchow R. Die Verstopfung der Lungenarterie und ihre Folgen. Br Exp Pathol Physiol 1846;2:227.

9. Barritt DW, Jordan SC. Anticoagulation drugs in the treatment of pulmonary embolism. Lancet 1960;1:1309–1312.

10. Havig GO. Deep vein thrombosis and pulmonary embolism: An autopsy study with multiple regression analysis of possible risk factors. Acta Chir Scand 1977; 478(suppl):1–120.

11. Urokinase-streptokinase embolism trial and phase 2 results. A cooperative study. JAMA 1974;229:1606–1611.

12. Robin ED. Overdiagnosis and overtreatment of pulmonary embolism: the emperor may have no clothes. Ann Intern Med 1977;87:775–781.

13. Alderson PO, Rujanavech W, Secker-Walker RH, McKnight RC. The role of Xe-133 ventilation studies in the scintigraphic detection of pulmonary embolism. Radiology 1976;120:633–640.

14. Biello DR, Mattar AG, McKnight RC, Siegel BA. Ventilation-perfusion studies in suspected pulmonary embolism. Am J Roentgenol 1979;133:1033–1037.

15. Cheely R, McCartney WH, Perry JR, et al. The role of noninvasive tests versus pulmonary angiography in the diagnosis of pulmonary embolism. Am J Med 1981;70:17–22.

16. Hull RD, Hirsh J, Carter CJ, et al. Diagnostic value of ventilation-perfusion lung scanning in patients with suspected pulmonary embolism. Chest 1985;88:819–828.

17. The PIOPED Investigators. Value of the ventilation/perfusion scan in acute pulmonary embolism: Results of the prospective investigation of pulmonary embolism diagnosis (PIOPED). JAMA 1990;263:2753–2759.

18. Moser KM. Venous thromboembolism: State of the art. Am Rev Respir Dis 1990;141:235–249.

19. Huisman MV, Büller HR, ten Cate JW, et al. Unexpected high prevalence of silent pulmonary embolism in patients with deep venous thrombosis. Chest 1989;95:498–502.

20. Hull RD, Hirsh J, Carter CJ, et al. Pulmonary angiography, ventilation lung scanning, and venography for clinically suspected pulmonary embolism with abnormal perfusion lung scan. Ann Intern Med 1983;98:891–899.

21. Huisman MV, Büller HR, ten Cate JW, Vreeken J. Serial impedance plethysmography for suspected deep venous thrombosis in outpatients. The Amsterdam General Practitioner Study. N Engl J Med 1986;314:823–828.

22. Hull RD, Raskob GE, Coates G, Panju AA, Gill GJ. A new noninvasive management strategy for patients with suspected pulmonary embolism. Arch Intern Med 1989;149: 2549–2555.

23. Alavi A, Palevsky HI, Gupta N, et al. Radiolabeled antifibrin antibodies in the detection of venous thrombosis. Radiology 1990;175:79–85.

24. Becker DM, Philbrick JT, Schoonover FW, Teates CD. Suspected pulmonary embolism and lung scan interpretation: Trial of a Bayesian reporting method. J Gen Intern Med 1990;5:285–291.

25. Knaus WA, Wagner DP, Draper EA, et al. The APACHE III prognostic system: Risk prediction of hospital mortality for critically ill hospitalized adults. Chest 1991;100: 1619–1636.

26. Kelley MA, Carson JL, Palevsky HI, Schwartz JS. Diagnosing pulmonary embolism: New facts and strategies. Ann Int Med 1991;114:300–306.

27. Prandoni P, Lensing AWA, Büller HR, et al. Failure of computerized impedance plethysmography in the diagnostic management of patients with clinically suspected deep-vein thrombosis. Thromb Haemost 1991;65:233–236.

28. Davidson BL, Elliott CG, Lensing AWA. For the RD Heparin Arthroplasty Group. Low accuracy of color doppler ultrasound in the detection of proximal leg vein thrombosis in asymptomatic high-risk patients. Ann Int Med 1992;117:735–738.

29. Agnelli G, Cosmi B, Ranucci V, et al. Impedance plethysmography and asymptomatic deep-vein thrombosis. Arch Intern Med 1992;151:2167–2171.

30. Anderson DR, Lensing AWA, Wells PS, Levine MN, Weitz JI, et al. Limitations of impedance plethysmography in the diagnosis of clinically suspected deep-vein thrombosis. Ann Int Med 1993;118:25–30.

31. Hirsh J. Reliability of non-invasive tests for the diagnosis of venous thrombosis. Thromb Haemost 1991;65:221–222.

21

The Clinical Diagnosis of Acute Pulmonary Embolism

Paul D. Stein

INTRODUCTION

The bedside evaluation of patients with suspected acute pulmonary embolism (PE) is important in calling attention to the potential diagnosis and assessing the extent to which the diagnosis should be pursued,[1] and for making a probability assessment which may lead to treatment on the basis of a noninvasive diagnosis.[2,3(I),4,5] Some lack of confidence in the clinical diagnosis of PE has resulted from clinical studies which showed that patients with acute PE had manifestations that did not differ from those in whom PE was suspected, but excluded by angiography.[6(I)] In the study of the Prospective Investigation of Pulmonary Embolism Diagnosis (PIOPED), for example, entry into the study was triggered by physicians who were sufficiently suspicious of PE to request a ventilation/perfusion lung scan or a pulmonary angiogram.[7] This suspicion of PE was based on well-known clinical features. Characteristic manifestations of PE, therefore, were also present in patients in whom PE was excluded by laboratory tests. In this set of patients, therefore, in whom the diagnosis was suspected by primary care physicians, the diagnostic features appear nonspecific. Indeed, the clinical manifestations are not pathognomonic. In the vast population of patients seen by physicians, however, the clinical manifestations serve well in identifying patients who are likely to have PE. The absence of clinical manifestations makes the likelihood of PE remote.[8]

Another reason that clinical characteristics may seem frustratingly nonspecific, possibly relates to confusion with the characteristics of underlying disease. It has been relatively recent that the clinical electrocardiographic and radiographic manifestations were examined in patients with no prior or associated cardiopulmonary disease.[9,10(I),11] Only in such a population can the character-

istics of PE be identified and separated from the confounding manifestations of associated illness.

Finally, some unavoidable problems in the selection of patients for study have contributed to incomplete information regarding the clinical diagnosis of PE. Studies of the clinical characteristics of PE based on data from investigations of diagnostic modalities or therapeutic trials[7,12,13(I)] may miss patients who die of PE, or patients in whom PE was not suspected. Autopsy studies, on the other hand, are likely to be biased because of the selection of patients that come to autopsy, namely those who died of unexplained causes. Both clinical studies and nonspecialized autopsy studies would miss patients who had small, subclinical PE. Presumably such patients do not require treatment.

In this chapter, two categories of patients will be described. The first category is those without prior or accompanying cardiopulmonary disease. This group allows us to identify the manifestations of acute PE in a population in which the characteristics of PE are not confounded by the characteristics of associated disease. The second category is all patients irrespective of prior or accompanying cardiac or pulmonary disease. These are the patients who confront physicians in daily practice.

SYNDROMES OF ACUTE PULMONARY EMBOLISM

In regard to making the clinical diagnosis of PE, it is useful to consider the presenting manifestations of PE in terms of the syndrome or mode of presentation.[9] Pulmonary embolism may present as: (1) pulmonary hemorrhage or infarction associated with pleuritic pain or hemoptysis, (2) circulatory collapse associated with arrhythmia or shock, and (3) isolated dyspnea, not compli-

Table 1
Presenting Syndromes of Acute Pulmonary Embolism

Presenting Syndrome	No Prior Cardiopulmonary Disease* (n = 117)	All Patients** (n = 260)
Pulmonary hemorrhage/pulmonary infarction	65%	59%
Circulatory collapse	8%	9%
Dyspnea not accompanied by pulmonary hemorrhage/infarction or circulatory collapse	22%	27%

An unexplained low P_aO_2 was observed in 1%. An additional 1% had unexplained atelectasis or parenchymal abnormality on the chest radiograph and might be considered in the pulmonary hemorrhage/infarction syndrome. Approximately 3% of patients had tachypnea that was identified by an observer and triggered diagnostic study. These patients perhaps could have been included in the uncomplicated dyspnea syndrome.
* Data from Stein et al.[6]
** Unpublished data from PIOPED.[14]

cated by pleuritic pain, hemoptysis, or circulatory collapse. The syndrome of pulmonary hemorrhage or infarction is the most frequent (or perhaps most frequently diagnosed), occurring in about 65% of patients with no prior cardiopulmonary disease.[6,9] Among the entire population of patients, irrespective of associated cardiopulmonary disease, the pulmonary hemorrhage/infarction syndrome occurred in 59%[14] (Table 1). Circulatory collapse occurred in 9% of patients with PE, and the syndrome of isolated dyspnea (not accompanied by pulmonary infarction or circulatory collapse) occurred in 27% (Table 1). Circulatory collapse, in the PIOPED experience among patients with no prior cardiopulmonary disease (8%), was less frequent than reported, among such patients in the Urokinase Pulmonary Embolism Trial and the Urokinase-Streptokinase Embolism Trial (19%).[6(I),9] This may reflect the selection of more severe

patients in the Urokinase Pulmonary Embolism Trial and in the Urokinase-Streptokinase Embolism Trial. Patients in these trials were selected for study only if the PE was massive or submassive.[12,13]

PREDISPOSING FACTORS

More than half of patients with PE were immobilized within three months of the acute episode (Table 2). The usual cause of immobilization was recent surgery. Among patients with no prior cardiopulmonary disease who were immobilized, 65% were immobilized ≤2 weeks and 7% were immobilized only one or 2 days.[6(I)] Short duration immobilization, therefore, is an important predisposing factor for PE.

Coronary heart disease was present in 20% of patients with acute PE[14] (Table 2). Recent acute myocardial

Table 2
Predisposing Factors in Patients With Acute Pulmonary Embolism

	Patients with No Prior Cardiopulmonary Disease* (n = 117)	All Patients** (n = 260)
Immobilization (≤3 months)	56%	54%
Surgery (≤3 months)	54%	43%
Malignancy	23%	21%
Coronary Disease (ever)	NA	20%
Thrombophlebitis (ever)	14%	18%
Lung Disease (COPD, asthma, interstitial)	NA	16%
Myocardial Infarction (≤3 months)	NA	14%
CHF (Right or Left) (≤3 months)	NA	12%
Trauma (lower extremities) (≤3 months)	10%	10%
Estrogen (at onset of PE)	9%	5%
Stroke	7%	9%
History of PE	NA	8%
Postpartum (≤3 months)	4%	2%

NA = Not applicable; COPD = Chronic obstructive pulmonary disease; CHF = Congestive heart failure.
* Data from Stein et al.[6]
** Unpublished data from PIOPED.[14]

infarction (≤3 months) was present in 67% of patients with coronary heart disease, and heart failure within 3 months (unspecified if left or right ventricular failure), was present in 29% of patients with coronary heart disease. Among patients with coronary heart disease, therefore, recent myocardial infarction seemed to predispose to PE more than heart failure. Lung disease (asthma, chronic obstructive pulmonary disease, or interstitial lung disease) was associated with PE in 16% of the patients. (Table 2)

SYMPTOMS OF ACUTE PULMONARY EMBOLISM

Among patients with PE and no prior cardiac or pulmonary disease, dyspnea was the most common symptom, occurring in 73%[6(1)] (Table 3). Pleuritic pain (66%) occurred more often than hemoptysis (13%). Hemoptysis was characterized as blood streaked, blood tinged or pure blood. Cough was common (37%), and was sometimes nonproductive, and sometimes productive of clear, bloody or occasionally purulent sputum. Purulent sputum was present in 7% of the patients.

Angina-like chest pain occurred in only 4% with PE and no prior cardiopulmonary disease.[6(1)] It was usually located in the anterior chest and it did not radiate to either arm or to the jaw in any of the patients with PE. The frequency of the various symptoms associated with PE was comparable in patients who had prior cardiopulmonary disease. The frequency of symptoms of acute PE was comparable among patients with no prior cardiopulmonary disease and all patients.[14] (Table 3)

SIGNS OF ACUTE PULMONARY EMBOLISM

Tachypnea (respiratory rate ≥20/min) was the most common sign of acute PE among patients with no cardiac or pulmonary disease, occurring in 70%[6] (Table 4).

Table 3
Symptoms of Acute Pulmonary Embolism

	Patients with No Prior Cardiopulmonary Disease (n = 117)* (%)	All Patients (n = 260)** (%)
Dyspnea	73	79
Pleuritic pain	66	58
Cough	37	40
Leg swelling	28	30
Leg pain	26	27
Hemoptysis	13	16
Palpitations	10	12
Wheezing	9	13
Angina-like pain	4	6

* Data from Stein et al.[6]
** Unpublished data from PIOPED.[14]

Tachycardia (heart rate >100/min) occurred in 30% of patients with PE. The pulmonary component of the second sound was accentuated in 23% of patients with PE. Deep venous thrombosis was clinically apparent in 11% of the patients. A right ventricular lift, third heart sound, or pleural friction rub were uncommon, each occurring ≤4% of patients with PE and no prior cardiopulmonary disease. The frequency of signs of PE was comparable among all patients, irrespective of prior cardiopulmonary disease[14] (Table 4).

Rales (crackles) were heard in 51% with no prior cardiopulmonary disease. Most patients with PE who had rales (88% of patients with rales) had pulmonary parenchymal abnormalities, atelectasis or a pleural effusion on the chest radiograph.[6(1)] Rales, therefore, appeared to be caused by the effects of pulmonary infarction or atelectasis.

An impression of the severity of PE associated with some clinical manifestations can be obtained from patients in the Urokinase Pulmonary Embolism Trial, although this study included only patients with massive or submassive PE.[12] The spectrum of severity, therefore, was somewhat narrow. Among patients with no prior cardiopulmonary disease, the most severe PE, as assessed by pulmonary arteriography, occurred in patients with shock or syncope.[9] In patients with uncomplicated dyspnea, the severity of PE was almost as great. Patients with the pulmonary hemorrhage/infarction syndrome had the least severe PE.[9]

Table 4
Signs of Acute Pulmonary Embolism

	Patients with No Prior Cardiopulmonary Disease (n = 117)* (%)	All Patients (n = 260)** (%)
Tachypnea (≥20/min)	70	73
Rales (crackles)	51	59
Tachycardia (>100/min)	30	28
Fourth heart sound	24	27***
Increased P2	23	21
Deep venous thrombosis	11	15
Diaphoresis	11	11
Temperature >38.5°C	7	7
Wheezes	5	8
Homan's sign	4	3
Right ventricular lift	4	3***
Pleural friction rub	3	4
Third heart sound	3	6
Cyanosis	1	3

P2 = Pulmonary component of second sound.
* Data from Stein et al.[6]
** Unpublished data from PIOPED.[14]
*** Approximate value.

Syncope was more frequent in patients with massive PE than submassive PE (17% versus 4%).[9] Apprehension, diaphoresis and tachypnea were also more frequent with massive PE. However, patients with massive PE, in comparison to patients with submassive PE, less often had pleuritic pain (67% versus 85%) or a pleural friction rub (14% versus 26%). Strikingly, among patients in shock from PE, only 71% were dyspneic and only 38% had pleuritic pain. Among all patients, irrespective of the presence or absence of prior cardiopulmonary disease, syncope, accentuated pulmonary component of the second sound, third or fourth heart sound (S_3 or S_4), and cyanosis were more frequent among patients with massive PE than submassive.[15(I)] Pleuritic pain, however, was less frequent among patients with massive PE than submassive PE.

PATIENTS WITH CHRONIC OBSTRUCTIVE PULMONARY DISEASE

Among patients with chronic obstructive pulmonary disease (COPD), one intuitively would predict that the clinical diagnosis would be more difficult than in uncomplicated patients, because dyspnea and tachypnea result from underlying disease. Worsening, that is unresponsive to bronchodilator therapy, may suggest PE.[16] In spite of the potential difficulty in reaching a clinical diagnosis, the clinical assessment by physicians, when they were confident that PE was present or confident that it was absent, was as likely to be correct among patients with COPD as among patients with no prior cardiopulmonary disease.[6(I),17(I)] The percent of uncertain clinical diagnoses was also similar in the assessment of patients with COPD and patients with no prior cardiopulmonary disease.[6(I),17(I)]

ELDERLY PATIENTS

Elderly patients (≥70 yrs) with no prior or associated cardiopulmonary disease, contrary to prior thought,[18–20] showed no significant difference among signs, symptoms, chest radiographs, and most ECG manifestations in comparison to young patients (<40 yrs) or patients in their middle years (age 40–69).[21(I)] Eleven percent of elderly patients, however, contrary to younger age groups, were identified on the basis of unexplained radiographic findings of atelectasis, pleural effusion, or pleural based opacities.[21(I)]

PLAIN CHEST RADIOGRAPH

The plain chest radiograph was abnormal in 84% of patients with PE and no prior cardiac or pulmonary disease[6] (Table 5). Atelectasis or pulmonary parenchymal abnormalities were the most common radiographic abnormalities (68%). A pleural effusion occurred in 48%. Among patients with a pleural effusion, only blunting of the costophrenic angle was shown in 86%. No patients with PE and no associated cardiopulmonary disease had pleural effusions that occupied more than one third of a hemithorax. Parenchymal abnormalities were more frequently observed than vascular abnormalities.[6,11]

Interstitial edema occurred in 3% of patients with pulmonary embolism and no prior cardiopulmonary disease.[6] Alveolar pulmonary edema occurred in only 1% of patients with PE and no prior cardiopulmonary disease. None of the radiographic abnormalities were specific for PE. Even the Westermark sign (prominent central pulmonary artery with decreased pulmonary vascularity) was not specific.[6]

Among patients with no prior cardiopulmonary disease, the lowest pulmonary artery mean pressures were in patients with a normal chest radiograph.[22] Such patients had lower pulmonary artery mean pressures than those with an elevated diaphragm, pleural-based opacity, decreased pulmonary vascularity, prominent central pulmonary artery, Westermark's sign or cardiomegaly.

The highest pulmonary artery mean pressures,

Table 5
Chest Radiograph in Patients With Acute Pulmonary Embolism*

	Patients with No Prior Cardiopulmonary Disease All Patients	All Patients (n = 260) (%)
Atelectasis or pulmonary parenchymal abnormality	68	69
Pleural effusion	48	78
Pleural based opacity	35	38
Elevated diaphragm	24	26
Decreased pulmonary vascularity	21	21
Prominent central PA	15	21
Cardiomegaly	12	18
Westermark's sign**	7	7
Pulmonary edema	4	11

PA = Pulmonary artery.
* Data from Stein et al.[6] and unpublished data from PIOPED.
** Prominent central pulmonary artery and decreased pulmonary vascularity.

Table 6
Combinations of Clinical Findings in Patients With Acute Pulmonary Embolism

	Patients with No Prior Cardiopulmonary Disease (n = 117)**	All Patients (n = 260)***
Dyspnea or tachypnea*	90%	92%
Dyspnea, tachypnea or pleuritic pain	97%	97%
Dyspnea, tachypnea, pleuritic pain, or x-ray atelectasis/parenchymal	98%	99%

* Tachypnea = respiratory rate ≥20 beats/min.
** Data from Stein et al.[6]
*** Unpublished data from PIOPED.[14]

among patients with no prior cardiopulmonary disease, were in patients with a prominent central pulmonary artery or cardiomegaly.[22] Patients with a prominent central pulmonary artery had higher pulmonary artery mean pressures than those of patients with atelectasis/pulmonary parenchymal abnormality or pleural effusion.[22] Patients with cardiomegaly also had higher pulmonary artery mean pressures than patients with atelectasis/pulmonary parenchymal abnormality, pleural effusion, pleural-based opacity, elevated diaphragm, or decreased pulmonary vascularity. Patients with cardiomegaly and a dilated central pulmonary artery had higher pulmonary artery mean pressures than patients with a prominent central pulmonary artery not accompanied by cardiomegaly.

COMBINATIONS OF CLINICAL CHARACTERISTICS

Combinations of clinical characteristics are useful in the assessment of PE (Table 6). Patients were rarely diagnosed if these clinical characteristics were absent. Dyspnea or tachypnea (respiratory rate ≥20/min) was present in 90% to 92%.[6,8,14] Dyspnea or tachypnea or pleuritic pain was present in 97 percent. Dyspnea or tachypnea or pleuritic pain or radiographic evidence of atelectasis or a parenchymal abnormality was present in 98% to 99%. An additional 1% had an unexplained low P_aO_2.

ELECTROCARDIOGRAM

The majority of patients (90% with no prior cardiopulmonary disease), were in sinus rhythm.[6(I)] Atrial flutter occurred in 1% and atrial fibrillation occurred in 4%. Atrial premature contractions were present in 4% and ventricular premature contractions were also present in 4%.

The electrocardiogram in patients with PE and no prior cardiopulmonary disease showed definite abnormalities which, however, were nonspecific.[6(I),10(I)] The most frequent abnormality was nonspecific changes of the ST segment or T wave (49%) (Table 7).[6(I)] Left axis deviation (left anterior hemiblock) occurred as often, or more often than right axis deviation and, therefore, should not lead to an exclusion of the clinical diagnosis of pulmonary embolism.[6(I),10(I),23,24] Right atrial enlargement (P pulmonale), right ventricular hypertrophy, right

Table 7
Electrocardiogram in Patients With Acute Pulmonary Embolism

	Patients with No Prior Cardiopulmonary Disease* (n = 89) (%)	All Patients** (n = 205) (%)
ST segment or T wave changes	49	54
Left axis deviation (left anterior hemiblock)	13	12
Complete right bundle branch block	6	4
Left ventricular hypertrophy	6	9
Incomplete right bundle branch block	4	3
Acute myocardial infarction pattern	3	6
Low voltage QRS	3	5
P pulmonale	2	1
Right axis deviation	2	3
Right ventricular hypertrophy	2	3

* Data from Stein et al.[6]
** Unpublished data from PIOPED.[14]

axis deviation and right bundle branch block occurred in ≤6% of patients with PE.[6(I)]

PARTIAL PRESSURE OF OXYGEN IN ARTERIAL BLOOD

The partial pressure of oxygen in arterial blood (P_aO_2) in patients with acute PE, has been shown to be a helpful adjunct in the diagnostic assessment.[25] It was, however, normal (≥80 mm Hg) in 26% of patients with PE who had no prior cardiopulmonary disease and were able to have their blood gases measured on room air.[6(I)] This percentage may be deceivingly large, however, because patients who required oxygen during the blood gas analysis were eliminated from this calculation. Even if the patients who could not have their blood gases measured on room air were considered as part of the entire group, 20% of patients with PE had a P_aO_2 ≥80mm Hg. Even some patients with submassive or massive PE may have had a normal P_aO_2.[15(I)]

ALVEOLAR ARTERIAL OXYGEN GRADIENT

The alveolar arterial oxygen gradient, in patients with no prior cardiopulmonary disease, was 37 ± 17 mm Hg (mean ± standard deviation) among patients with PE and no associated cardiopulmonary disease. It was ≤10 mm Hg in 8% of patients and 11–20 mm Hg in 6% of patients.[6] A normal alveolar-arterial oxygen gradient, therefore, does not exclude the diagnosis of PE.[6(I),26]

D-DIMER

An ancillary laboratory test that appears to have promise for excluding the diagnosis of PE is the measurement of D-dimer.[27] D-dimer is a degradation product of fibrin that is present only after stabilization of the fibrin network and subsequent lysis by plasmin.[28] It increases in any circumstance which may result in thrombus formation and lysis. An elevated level of D-dimer (>500 μg/L) is highly sensitive for PE, but not specific and therefore, not very useful for making a diagnosis of PE. On the other hand, studies, not yet fully confirmed, suggest that PE is unlikely if plasma D-dimer is lower than 500 μg/L.[27] D-dimer, therefore, potentially may be useful in excluding PE.

COMPUTER-BASED PATTERN RECOGNITION

Neural network computer-based pattern recognition has been shown to be able to predict the clinical likelihood of PE with an accuracy comparable to physicians who are experienced with PE.[29] The neural network was based on 50 input variables, which can be readily obtained by physicians or physician's assistants. These included data from the history, physical examination, chest radiograph, electrocardiogram, and arterial blood gases. The potential was shown in this investigation, therefore, for computer-based pattern recognition to assist physicians who are inexperienced with PE to reach a clinical impression with the same validity as physicians experienced with PE.[29]

Finally, an allusion should be made to the concept of diagnosis of deep venous thrombosis, rather than the diagnosis of pulmonary embolism. If proximal deep venous thrombosis is diagnosed, it should be treated, and the recommended antithrombotic treatment is the same as for PE.[30] The risk of a first PE in treated patients with deep venous thrombosis is comparable to the risk of a recurrent PE in treated patients with PE.[31,32(I)] These studies are not quite comparable, however, because the duration of follow-up differed, and there may have been differences of antithrombotic treatment. It would seem useful for comprehensive management, including an evaluation of possible residual impairments of perfusion,[34(I)] to obtain ventilation/perfusion scans whenever possible in patients with suspected PE. The ventilation/perfusion scan reading combined with clinical judgment permits an assessment of the probability of PE, which is useful even if deep venous thrombosis has been diagnosed by objective tests.

REFERENCES

1. Stein PD, Willis PW, Dalen JE. Importance of clinical assessment in the selection of patients for pulmonary arteriography. Am J Cardiol 1979;43:669–671.
2. Stein PD, Hull RD, Saltzman HA, Pineo G. Strategy for diagnosis of patients with suspected acute pulmonary embolism. Chest 1993;103:1553–1559.
(I)3. Stein PD, Henry JW, Gottschalk A. The addition of prior clinical assessment to stratification according to prior cardiopulmonary disease further optimizes the interpretation of ventilation/perfusion lung scans in pulmonary embolism. Chest 1993;104:1472–1476.
4. Stein PD, Hull RD. Relative risks of anticoagulant treatment of acute pulmonary embolism based upon an angiographic diagnosis versus a ventilation/perfusion scan diagnosis. Chest 1994;106:727–730.
5. Stein PD, Hull RD, Raskob G. Risks for major bleeding from patients with acute pulmonary embolism: consideration of noninvasive management. Annals Intern Med 1994;12:313–317.
(I)6. Stein PD, Terrin ML, Hales CA, Palevsky HI, Saltzman HA, et al. Clinical, laboratory, roentgenographic and electrocardiographic findings in patients with acute pulmonary embolism and no pre-existing cardiac or pulmonary disease. Chest 1991;100:598–601.
(I)7. The PIOPED Investigators. Value of the ventilation/perfusion scan in acute pulmonary embolism: Results of the Prospective Investigation of Pulmonary Embolism Diagnosis (PIOPED). J Am Med Assoc 1990;263:2753–2759.
8. Stein PD, Saltzman HA, Weg JG. Clinical characteristics of patients with acute pulmonary embolism. Am J Cardiol 1991;68:1723–1724.
9. Stein PD, Willis PW III, DeMets DL. History and physical examination in acute pulmonary embolism in patients

without pre-existing cardiac or pulmonary disease. Am J Cardiol 1981;47:218–223.

(I)10. Stein PD, Dalen JE, McIntyre KM, Sasahara AA, Wenger NK, et al. The electrocardiogram in acute pulmonary embolism. Prog Cardiovasc Dis 1975;17:247–257.

(I)11. Stein PD, Willis PW III, DeMets DL, Greenspan RH. Plain chest roentgenogram in patients with acute pulmonary embolism and no pre-existing cardiac or pulmonary disease. Am J Noninvas Cardiol 1987;1:171–176.

12. National Cooperative Study. The Urokinase Pulmonary Embolism Trial. Design of the trial. Circulation 1973; 47/48(Suppl II):II-18-II-24.

(I)13. National Cooperative Study: Urokinase-Streptokinase Embolism Trial. Phase 2 results. JAMA 1974;229: 1606–1613.

14. Stein PD. Unpublished data from the Prospective Investigation of Pulmonary Embolism Diagnosis (PI-OPED).

(I)15. National Cooperative Study. The Urokinase Pulmonary Embolism Trial. Associated laboratory and clinical findings. Circulation 1973;47/48(Suppl II):II-81-II-85.

16. Lippmann M, Fein A. Pulmonary embolism in the patient with chronic obstructive pulmonary disease: a diagnostic dilemma. Chest 1981;79:39–42.

(I)17. Lesser BA, Leeper KV, Stein PD, Saltzman HA, Chen J, et al. The diagnosis of pulmonary embolism in patients with chronic obstructive pulmonary disease. Chest 1992;102: 17–22.

18. Taubman LB, Silverstone FA. Autopsy proven pulmonary embolism among the institutionalized elderly. J Am Geriatr Soc 1986;34:752–756.

19. Morrell MT. The incidence of pulmonary embolism in the elderly. Geriatrics 1970;25:138–153.

20. Busby W, Bayer A, Pathy J. Pulmonary embolism in the elderly. Age Aging 1988;17:205–209.

(I)21. Stein PD, Gottschalk A, Saltzman HA, Terrin ML. Diagnosis of acute pulmonary embolism in the elderly. J Am College Cardiol 1991;18:1452–1457.

22. Stein PD, Athanasoulis C, Greenspan RH, Henry JW. Relation of plain chest radiographic findings to pulmonary arterial pressure and arterial blood oxygen levels in patients with acute pulmonary embolism. Am J Cardiol 1992;69:394–396.

23. Lynch RE, Stein PD, Bruce TA. Leftward shift of frontal plane QRS axis as a frequent manifestation of acute pulmonary embolism. Chest 1972;61:443–446.

24. Stein PD, Bruce TA. Left axis deviation as an electrocardiographic manifestation of acute pulmonary embolism. J Electrocardiol 1971;4:67–69.

25. Szucs MM, Brooks HL, Grossman W, Banas JR, Jr., Meister SG, et al. Diagnostic sensitivity of laboratory findings in acute pulmonary embolism. Ann Intern Med 1971;74:161–166.

26. Overton DT, Bocka JJ. The alveolar-arterial oxygen gradient in patients with documented pulmonary embolism. Arch Int Med 1988;148:1617–1619.

27. Bounameaux H, Cirafici P, DeMoerloose P, Schneider PA, Slosman D, et al. Measurement of D-dimer in plasma as diagnostic aid in suspected pulmonary embolism. Lancet 1991; 337:196–200.

28. Gaffney PJ, Creighton LJ, Callus M, Thorpe R. Monoclonal antibodies to crosslinked fibrin degradation products (XL-FDP). Br J Haematol 1988;68:83–96.

29. Patil S, Henry JW, Rubenfire M, Stein PD. A neural network in the clinical diagnosis of acute pulmonary embolism. Chest 1993;37:13–24.

30. Hyers TM, Hull RD, Weg JG. Antithrombotic therapy for venous thromboembolic disease. Chest 1992;102(Suppl): 408S-425S.

(I)31. Hull RD, Raskob GE, Hirsh J, Jay RM, Leclerc JR, et al. Continuous intravenous heparin compared with intermittent subcutaneous heparin in the initial treatment of proximal-vein thrombosis. N Engl J Med 1986;315: 1109–1114.

(I)32. Hull R, Hirsh J, Jay R, Carter C, England C, et al. Different intensities of oral anticoagulant therapy in the treatment of proximal-vein thrombosis. N Engl J Med 1982;307: 1676–1681.

33. Carson JL, Kelley MA, Duff A, Weg JG, Fulkerson WJ, et al. The clinical course of pulmonary embolism. N Engl J Med 1992;326:1240–1245.

(I)34. A National Cooperative Study: Perfusion lung scanning. (Chapter VIII of The Urokinase Embolism Trial). Circulation 1973;47/48(Suppl.II):II-46-II-50.

22

Ventilation-Perfusion Lung Scans for the Diagnosis of Acute Pulmonary Embolism

Alexander Gottschalk, Mark A. Bisesi, Paul D. Stein

INTRODUCTION

In the early 1960's George Taplin developed a way of generating and radiolabeling macroaggregated particles of albumin which ranged from 5 to 20 microns in size.[1] This was the first step towards accurate imaging tests. These microemboli could be injected intravenously and would lodge in the first small vascular bed they encountered, the pulmonary microcirculation. By imaging the lungs and locating the radioactivity following intravenous injection, pulmonary artery perfusion (Q) could be determined. Early trials determined the feasibility of this technique in clinical situations.[2–4] Further specificity of the perfusion scan was obtained by defining regional ventilation (V) abnormalities. A radioactive gas, xenon-133, is the agent most commonly used. Several other agents that have been developed and remain in clinical use are also discussed: technetium-99-M-diethylenetriaminepentaacetic acid (DTPA); and technetium-99-M-methylene diphosphonate (MDP); or pyrophosphate (PYP) aerosols, Krypton 81m, and technetium-labelled aerosolized carbon particles (Technegas).

Most pulmonary diseases such as obstructive pulmonary disease, lung masses, and pneumonia result in decreased pulmonary arterial perfusion. The development of ventilation-perfusion (V/Q) criteria have allowed investigators to distinguish pulmonary embolism (PE) from other diseases. When pulmonary emboli are present, both the regional chest radiograph and ventilation scan should, in theory, be normal, but perfusion is decreased in a pulmonary segmental configuration. This is called a mismatched segmental defect. A matched defect, where both perfusion and ventilation abnormalities are congruent, occurs in such diseases as emphysema.[5–7]

This chapter discusses the following aspects of lung scanning: (a) a review of the technical considerations for obtaining ventilation-perfusion images, (b) V/Q scan interpretation, and (c) new developments, both diagnostic and technical, which may further improve the clinician's ability to identify patients with PE.

TECHNICAL CONSIDERATIONS

For most patients, lung scanning is readily performed and almost innocuous. The patient requires no specific preparation. Studies of the highest technical quality are obtained in patients who are alert enough to follow directions and who have some mobility or are, at least, able to sit in an erect position. However, if patients are too ill, chest radiographs and V/Q images can be performed in the supine position. This may limit the diagnostic value to some extent, but if the patient receives the necessary supportive care, the study will be of value.

CHEST RADIOGRAPHY

A recent chest radiograph is an integral part of any V/Q scan protocol. Evaluation of the chest radiograph is necessary for the interpretation of lung scans and helps rule out the possibility of coexisting disease processes. A posterior-anterior and lateral radiograph should be obtained with the patient erect, but a supine, portable radiograph can be used in seriously ill patients. The V/Q study and the chest radiograph should be obtained at the same time.

VENTILATION SCANS

Xenon-133

Obtaining good quality ventilation images is usually the most difficult part of V/Q imaging. When xenon-133 is used, 15 to 20 mCi of the radiogas are used and there are three phases.[8] First, a single breath image is performed after a bolus is injected into the spirometer. The patient must be able to inhale deeply on command and hold his breath for 20 seconds. This view is obtained with the patient's back to a wide field (usually at least 38 cm in diameter) gamma camera. A ventilation defect is shown as a "cold spot" (a void) on this image.

Next, the patient breathes normally while the xenon is circulated within a closed spirometer for four minutes (equilibrium phase). The face mask must be tightly sealed to be sure equilibrium is reached.[9] During this time, collateral air drift as well as normal ventilation occurs, and this portion of the study shows the total aerated lung volume. Although many centers obtain only posterior views during this interval, we prefer to obtain a posterior view and both posterior obliques to maximize the ability to assess whether any lung zones have not been ventilated by radioxenon.

Finally, the patient must continue to breathe normally while the xenon is vented from the system (wash-out phase). The wash-out phase usually lasts about five minutes, and is accomplished by turning the spirometer valves such that the patient inhales room air, while exhaling into a shielded charcoal trap that catches the xenon-133. This phase demonstrates areas of slow wash-out ("air trapping") which are now shown as "hot spots". "Hot spots" represent areas of abnormal ventilation in which lung that was ventilated initially by the slow process of collateral air drift cannot get rid of xenon-133 by expiration as fast as normal lung. The resulting "unevenness" is characteristic of abnormal ventilation seen in diseases like chronic obstructive pulmonary disease. Images should be taken at about 45-second intervals during the wash-out phase, and posterior oblique views should be obtained during this interval as well. Because the photon energy of xenon-133 (80 keV) is lower then that of technetium-99m (140 keV, used to label the macroaggregates for perfusion scans), the xenon ventilation study is usually done before the perfusion scan to avoid confusing down-scatter from technetium-99m. Consequently, it is not known where in the lung the perfusion defect, if any, will be. To maximize the lung volume seen, the posterior view is used primarily for the xenon-133 study. The posterior oblique views should also be obtained to improve detection of areas of retention and to locate them in the anterior posterior plane. The wash-out phase is the most likely phase of the xenon-133 study to show ventilation abnormalities.[8,10(I)]

Radioaerosol Ventilation Scanning

Some centers use alternative tracers to assess ventilation. It has recently become possible to use technetium aerosols since disposable, easily shielded, efficient nebulizers are now commercially available.[11,12,13(I)] These make possible the delivery of small radiolabeled particles which impact in the central airways, but sediment more distally and diffuse into the alveoli.[14] Currently available nebulizers produce submicronic droplets which provide better penetration into the lung periphery than previous nebulizers which produced droplets in the three to five micron range that were often deposited in the central airway.[15]

The aerosol of Tc-99m-DPTA which comes in contact with alveoli, adheres to alveolar walls, crosses the epithelium, is absorbed into the blood stream, and is excreted by the kidneys. The half-time of this process of lung clearance is normally about one hour. In smokers, however, lung clearance is often faster and can cause the count rate to decrease during the ventilation study. To avoid this, aerosols of Tc-99m-MDP or Tc-99m-PYP have been used. These have a significantly longer lung clearance time.[15]

Aerosol ventilation imaging can be performed either before or after the perfusion scan, and images can be made in views precisely comparable to the perfusion images, allowing direct comparisons to be made. These advantages are offset by some problems: (1) because of central deposition, the aerosol has limited peripheral penetration in some patients, especially those with chronic bronchitis; (2) there is no wash-out phase with aerosol imaging since the aerosol is not exhaled, but is excreted by the kidney; and (3) aerosols can be swallowed and cause confusion in the interpretation if the reader mistakes gastric for pulmonary activity (Figure 1).

Ventilation imaging uses about 30 mCi of Tc-99m-DTPA in 2 to 3 ml of saline and the submicron particle nebulizer is aerated at a flow rate of 8 to 10 L/minute.[13(I)] The patient is positioned with his back to the camera and inhales the aerosol until an appropriate count rate is achieved (e.g., 50,000 counts/minute). If the ventilation scan is obtained after the perfusion scan (post-perfusion imaging), the nebulizer dose is raised to about 45 mCi of Tc-99m-PYP (or DTPA), and the inhalation of the aerosol is continued until the count rate is double that of the residual counts from the perfusion scan.[15]

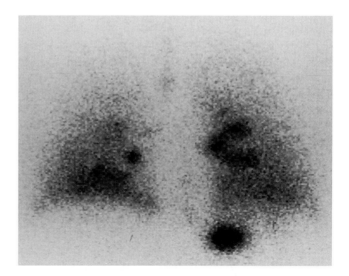

Figure 1. Ventilation scan made with Tc-99m-methylene diphosphonate aerosol. Note the central airway deposition, which is especially prominent on the left, and the swallowed radioactivity in the stomach. (Reproduced with permission from WB Saunders Co, Philadelphia, PA).

Other Ventilation Techniques

Krypton-81m, an inert radiogas tracer, has been used for ventilation imaging.[16] Because of its short half-life (13 seconds), images must be acquired rapidly, but they can also be repeated if necessary. Although krypton imaging is quite accurate, clinical use is limited in North America by the short half-life of the generator parent (Rb-81, half-life 4.7 hours), availability, and high cost.

Technegas, a new agent of technetium-labelled ultrasmall carbon particles (described as radioactive soot) has been used with increasing frequency in Australia and Europe.[17–20] There is good distribution due to the ultrasmall particle size, but there are still some reservations about its use. For example, transient symptomatic hypoxia has been observed.[20] It has not yet been approved by the FDA for use in the United States.

In spite of the many ventilation agents available, none has a clear diagnostic advantage. Cost, availability, and imaging logistics determine which is best suited for each institution.[9]

Perfusion Imaging

Perfusion imaging is performed after technetium-99m-labelled macroaggregated albumin has been injected into a peripheral vein. The average particle size of the aggregates is about 40 to 60 microns. Approximately 200,000 to 500,000 particles are injected. These temporarily lodge as microemboli in the small arterioles and occlude about one out of every 10,000.[21] After several hours, the particles are broken down mechanically to a size small enough to pass through the pulmonary vascular system, about one to two microns. They are then phagocytosed by the reticuloendothelial system and ultimately metabolized by the liver. Pulmonary complications are extremely rare. Because the microembolic aggregates are only temporarily impacted in the lung, the pulmonary microcirculation ultimately returns to normal.

To minimize any gravitational gradient to blood flow, the perfusion macroaggregates are injected when the patient is in the supine position.[10(I)] During this time the particles embolize the pulmonary arterioles and become "fixed." The images are then obtained with the patient sitting erect when possible. Just as an erect chest radiograph is easier to interpret then a supine one (especially to evaluate lung bases), an erect V/Q scan is preferable to a supine one.[10(I)]

Perfusion images are obtained in multiple views.[22–24] In the Prospective Investigation of Pulmonary Embolism Diagnosis (PIOPED) study, anterior, posterior, anterior oblique, and posterior oblique views were made with 750,000 counts/image using an all-purpose low-energy collimator on the gamma camera. The lateral images were timed views. The time to obtain 500,000 counts on the side with the best perfusion was used as the imaging time for the other side.[10(I)] The usual dose of Tc-99m-macroaggregates is 4 mCi. The perfusion images require about 15 minutes to complete. The overall examination time is approximately 30 minutes. The images are acquired with a gamma camera and printed on standard radiographic film. When the study is completed, the ventilation and perfusion images are interpreted together with a chest radiograph preferably obtained at the same time as the lung scan.

INTERPRETATION OF THE VENTILATION-PERFUSION SCAN

General Considerations

Interpretation of V/Q lung scans begins with a review of the chest radiograph. Often the radiograph has a normal appearance, but there are several radiographic findings that are suggestive of embolism. These include regional oligemia (especially with associated hilar vascular engorgement), peripheral infiltrates, and pleural effusions. However, none of these is specific. The main value of the chest radiograph is that other disease processes that might be causing the patient's symptoms can be evaluated.

To evaluate perfusion defects accurately, it must be ascertained if there is an abnormality on the chest radiograph in the region of the perfusion defect. For a V/Q abnormality to be considered characteristic of PE, the radiograph must be clear in the same area, emphasizing the importance of obtaining the chest radiograph at the same time as the lung scan. The maximal requirement is that it should have been performed within the 12 hours preceding the lung scan.[10] Chest radiography obtained prior to that time may result in an inaccurate correlation because of the rapid changes that can occur on the radiograph in the presence of evolving disease.

The appearance of the V/Q scan in a normal patient is illustrated in Figure 2. The perfusion scan shows homogenous uptake throughout the aerated lung. The wash-out views on the xenon-133 study may show mild but symmetric retention of tracer in the upper lung zones early during the wash-out phase.

Inflammation and other causes of pulmonary consolidation typically result in perfusion defects with matching radiographic and ventilation abnormalities. For example, pulmonary hemorrhage from thromboembolism (the radiographic pulmonary "infarct") cannot be differentiated on V/Q scans from other causes of consolidation.[9] Chronic obstructive pulmonary disease, chronic bronchitis, and most restrictive diseases cause matched ventilation and perfusion defects.

Segmental V/Q mismatched lesions with clear radiographic regions are NOT pathognomonic of PE. Diseases and conditions that mimic PE do occur. Nonembolic pulmonary vascular occlusion can occur from neoplastic compression of the pulmonary arteries

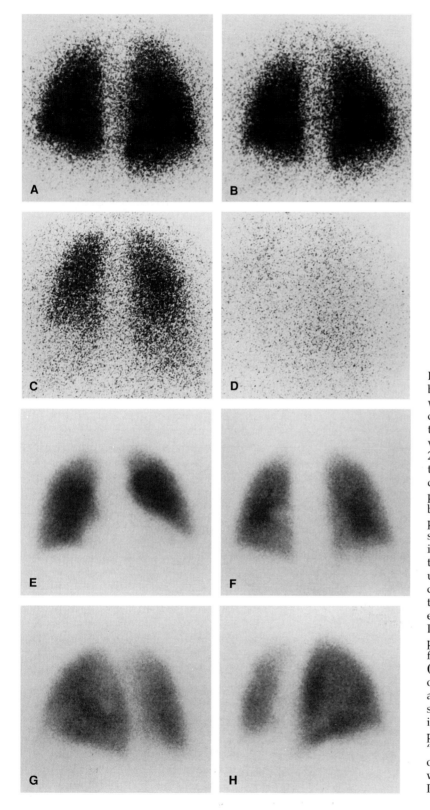

Figure 2. Normal Xe-133 ventilation and Tc-99m albumin macroaggregate perfusion scan in a patient who has mild cardiomegaly and an otherwise normal chest radiograph. The first four views (A-D) are from the xenon-133 study. **(A),** The posterior single breath view from the inhaled xenon bolus. Usually about 20,000 counts are obtained in about 20 seconds for this image. **(B),** A posterior equilibrium image taken during the 4-minute rebreathing xenon-equilibration period. About 15–20 mCi of xenon-133 are equilibrated by breathing in a closed spirometer in this phase of the study. **(C),** Early wash-out phase (45–90 seconds). This posterior view shows more retention in the upper lung zones than the bases. Note the uptake below the right diaphragm. Xenon-133 is fat-soluble and if the patient has a fatty liver, hepatic uptake can be seen. In this case, liver uptake is mild. In addition, the lung uptake is symmetrical showing no "unevenness" which would indicate air trapping. **(D),** Late wash-out phase (180–225 seconds). No air trapping is seen with virtually all the xenon-133 exhaled from the lungs. Slight hepatic uptake is still present. **(E), (F), (G), (H)** are anterior, posterior, left posterior oblique, and right posterior oblique perfusion images. The heart and prominent hilar structures can be seen on all the images causing focal or diffuse diminished activity which is particularly prominent on the posterior scan. Comparison of the way these areas "rotate" between views indicates their mediastinal origin. The lungs perfuse normally. (Reproduced with permission from WB Saunders Co, Philadelphia, PA).

(Figure 3). This is often seen with bronchogenic carcinoma which may even cause a lack of perfusion in an entire lung. This would be unusual for PE which usually causes bilateral segmental lesions.[25] Collagen disease with pulmonary vasculitis can mimic PE. Embolism of nonthrombotic material injected by intravenous drug abusers can mimic PE. The list of other causes of PE mimics is extensive, but most are rare, and many can be diagnosed from a good chest radiograph.[9,26]

Bronchial constriction may result from PE and cause a matched, rather than a mismatched, defect on the V/Q scan. This might result from substances released by the embolic material. Bronchial constriction is usually a transient response in PE, however, and is rare by the time the patient presents for V/Q scintigraphy.[27–29]

On occasion, patients present with a diffuse generalized abnormality on the chest radiograph. It is usually pulmonary edema, but might be diffuse reticulonodular disease. Because the process is so symmetrical, the perfusion scan may be normal. In one series, 73% of 55 patients with diffuse pulmonary disease had normal or nearly normal perfusion scans. These scans can be used to exclude PE and guide management decisions in such patients who are frequently critically ill.[30]

VENTILATION-PERFUSION SCAN DIAGNOSTIC CRITERIA

The characteristic finding of PE is a segmental rectangular, square, or triangular pleural-based perfusion defect in a REGION of the lung that has both a normal radiograph and normal ventilation scan (Figure 4). The diagnostic scan categories commonly used can be ranked: high probability has precedence over intermediate probability, which has precedence over low probability, which has precedence over normal. For example, if a scan has findings in some area that are those of intermediate probability, the study could never be called low probability.

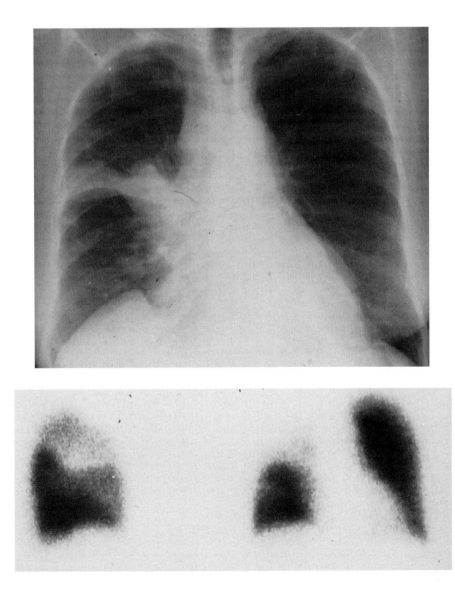

Figure 3. Top: Posterior-anterior chest radiograph showing a right hilar bronchogenic carcinoma with slight peripheral right upper lobe atelectasis, but most of the right upper lung is normally aerated on the radiograph. On the xenon-133 ventilation study, the right upper lobe ventilated normally. **Bottom**: Right lateral and anterior perfusion images show a solitary right upper lobar perfusion defect. Note some "shine through" activity from the left lung on the lateral view in the region of the upper-lobe defect. This is a lobar mismatched perfusion defect. The defect is also substantially larger than the radiographic findings (i.e., Q≫ than x-ray, see Table 1). This is a PE mimic. (Reproduced with permission from WB Saunders Co, Philadelphia, PA).

However, it might be called high probability if mismatched segmental lesions were found in other areas.

Many investigators have either developed criteria for V/Q scan interpretation, or their publications have led to the establishing of criteria. Some of these are listed in Tables 1 to 3. The probability for the various scan categories using these criteria is comparable and is shown in Table 4.[31] When the chest radiograph and the ventilation scan are called normal according to these criteria, it must be emphasized that this designation refers to the REGION of the chest radiograph or ventilation scan in which the perfusion defect is found. The chest radiograph or ventilation scan may show an abnormality elsewhere.

Xenon-133 was the ventilation agent used when many of these criteria were developed. Consequently, ventilation scans were performed primarily using posterior images with only posterior oblique views to provide anterior posterior localization. It was not always possible to define precisely in which lung segment the ventilation defect occurred. Thus, many ventilation studies were interpreted using lung zones obtained by dividing the lung craniocaudally (that is, upper, middle, and lower zones). Table 1 notes the slight variations in terminology used by different investigators.

Most of the studies evaluating V/Q scan efficacy were done using retrospective analysis of patients who had both V/Q scans and pulmonary angiography. Only in the PIOPED[10(I)] and McMaster[32(I)] studies were patients prospectively recruited for V/Q scan and angiography, and only in the PIOPED study were their *diagnostic criteria* evaluated prospectively.

Both the pulmonary angiogram and the V/Q scan were described in a computer-compatible format in the PIOPED study.[33] As a result, the criteria used in the study could be reevaluated and the PIOPED nuclear medicine working group has recommended changes from the original criteria.[25] These can be found in Tables 1 to 3.

In the PIOPED study, a high-probability diagnosis indicated PE in 87% of patients.[10(I)] Other series ranged from a positive predictive value of 86% to 92% (Figure 5 and Table 4).[32(I),34,35] Similarly, Table 4 shows that 20% to 40% of patients have PE when intermediate or indeterminate probability is diagnosed, a range that is not clinically useful.

A low-probability V/Q scan diagnosis correctly excluded PE in 86% in the PIOPED study, and 90% or more using the other criteria listed (Figure 6). There were 21 cases in the PIOPED study called normal. None of these

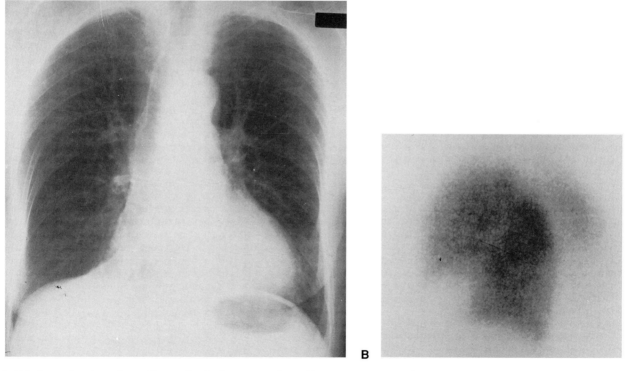

Figure 4. (A), Posterior-Anterior radiograph, the lungs are clear. The xenon-133 ventilation study was normal in this patient. **(B),** Left posterior oblique perfusion image. There is a solitary anterior basal segmental defect in the left lower lobe. No other abnormality was present on other views. This is a single mismatched segmental lesion. Table 2 shows that although this is a characteristic mismatched segmental perfusion defect, with only one such lesion, the V/Q scan will be called intermediate/indeterminate probability in most of the interpretive criteria listed. In this case, the pulmonary angiogram showed no PE. (Reproduced with permission from WB Saunders Co, Philadelphia, PA).

Table 1
Criteria for High Probability in the Interpretation of Ventilation/Perfusion Scans for Pulmonary Embolism

Biello 1987[35]	Biello et al, 1979[34]	Sullivan et al,[54] based on McNeil 1980[55]	PIOPED[10]	PIOPED Revised[25]	Hull et al,[32]
≥2 Large V/Q mismatches with N1 X-ray or ≥2 Mod V/Q mismatches with N1 X-ray or ≥1 Q >> X-ray*	≥1 Large V/Q mismatches with N1 X-ray or ≥2 Mod V/Q mismataches with N1 X-ray or ≥1 Q >> X-ray*	Multiple V/Q mismatches largest being ≥ segmental	≥2 Large V/Q mismatches or 1 large V/Q and ≥3 Mod V/Q mismatches or ≥4 Mod V/Q mismatches	>2 Large V/Q mismatches (2 Large V/Q are borderline high prob) or 1 Large V/Q and ≥2 Mod V/Q mismatches or ≥4 Mod V/Q mismatches	≥1 Segmental mismatch
Mod: 25–90% Seg Large: >90% Seg V/Q mismatch = N1 V in region of Q defect	Mod: 25–75% Seg Large: >75% Seg V/Q mismatch = N1 V in region of Q defect	V/Q mismatch = N1 or mildly reduced V with N1 X-ray in region of Q defect	Mod: 25–75% Seg Large: >75% Seg V/Q mismatch = N1 V and N1 X-ray or Q > V or X-ray in region of Q defect	Mod: 25–75% Seg Large: >75% Seg V/Q mismatch = N1 V and N1 X-ray or Q > V or X-ray in region of Q defect	
V/Q match = abnormal V in region of Q defect	V/Q match = abnormal V in region of Q defect				

* Our interpretation of Biello's articles.
N = normal; V/Q = ventilation/perfusion; X-ray = radiographic abnormality in region of perfusion abnormality; Mod = moderate; Seg = segment.
Reprinted from Stein PD and Gottschalk A. Critical Review of Ventilation/Perfusion Lung Scans in Acute Pulmonary Embolism. Progress in Cardiovascular Disease 1994;37:13–24.

Table 2
Criteria for Intermediate Probability in the Interpretation of Ventilation/Perfusion Scans for Pulmonary Embolism

Biello 1987[35]	Biello et al, 1979[34]	Sullivan et al,[54] based on McNeil 1980[55]	PIOPED[10]	PIOPED Revised[25]	Hull et al,[32]
≥1 Q = X-ray or 1 Large V/Q mismatch or 1 Mod V/Q mismatch or Severe COPD with Q defects	≥1 Q = X-ray or 1 Mod V/Q mismatch with N1 X-ray or Severe COPD with Q defects	1 Seg V/Q mismatch or ≥1 Q = X-ray or Mixed V/Q mismatched and matched defects or 1 V/Q mismatch ≥ lobar size or Multiple subsegmental V/Q mismatches	1 Large V/Q mismatch ± 1 Mod V/Q mismatch or 2 or 3 Mod V/Q mismatches	1 Large ± 1 Mod V/Q mismatch or 1 to 3 Mod V/Q mismatches or 1 matched V/Q defect with N1 X-ray (2 Large V/Q mismatches are borderline intermediate to high prob)	≥1 subsequental* V/Q mismatch or ≥1 segmental V/Q match or ≥1 subseqmental V/Q match

Abbreviations as in Table 1.
* Our interpretation of Hull's criteria.
Reprinted from Stein PD and Gottschalk A. Critical Review of Ventilation/Perfusion Lung Scans in Acute Pulmonary Embolism. Progress in Cardiovascular Disease 1994;37:13–24.

Table 3
Criteria for Low Probability in the Interpretation of Ventilation/Perfusion Scans for Pulmonary Embolism

Biello 1987[35]	Biello et al, 1979[34]	Sullivan et al,[54] based on McNeil 1980[55]	PIOPED[10]	PIOPED Revised[25]	Hull et al,[32]
Small V/Q mismatches or V/Q matches with N1 X-ray or Q << X-ray	Small V/Q mismatches or V/Q matches with N1 X-ray or Q << X-ray	1 Subseg V/Q mismatch or ≥1 V/Q match	1 Mod V/Q mismatch with N1 X-ray or Q << X-ray or V/Q matches with N1 X-ray or X-ray << Q involving ≤4 segments in 1 lung and ≤3 segments in 1 lung region or Perfusion defects due to pleural effusion, cardiomegaly, enlarged aorta, hilum, mediastinum, and elevated diaphragm or >3 Small Q with N1 X-ray or Very low probability ≤3 Small Q with N1 X-ray	Q << X-ray defect or ≥2 V/Q matches with N1 X-ray and some areas of normal perfusion in lung or Perfusion defects due to pleural effusion, cardiomegaly, enlarged aorta, hilum, mediastinum, and elevated diaphragm or Any small perfusion defects and N1 X-ray	Not reported
Small: <25% Seg	Small: <25% Seg	Small: <25% Seg			

Abbreviations as in Table 1.
Reprinted from Stein PD and Gottschalk A. Critical Review of Ventilation /Perfusion Lung Scans in Acute Pulmonary Embolism. Progress in Cardiovascular disease 1994;37:13–24.

Table 4
Probability of Pulmonary Embolism Obtained with Different Criteria for the Interpretation of Ventilation/Perfusion Scans for Pulmonary Embolism

	Biello 1987[35]	Biello et al, 1979[34]	PIOPED[10]	Hull et al,[32]
High	90%	87–92%	87%	86%
Intermediate	30%	20–33%	30%	21–40%
Low	10%	0–8%	14%	—
Normal	0%	0%	0%	0%

Reprinted from Stein PD and Gottschalk A. Critical Review of Ventilation/Perfusion Lung Scans in Acute Pulmonary Embolism. Progress in Cardiovascular Disease 1994;37:13–24.

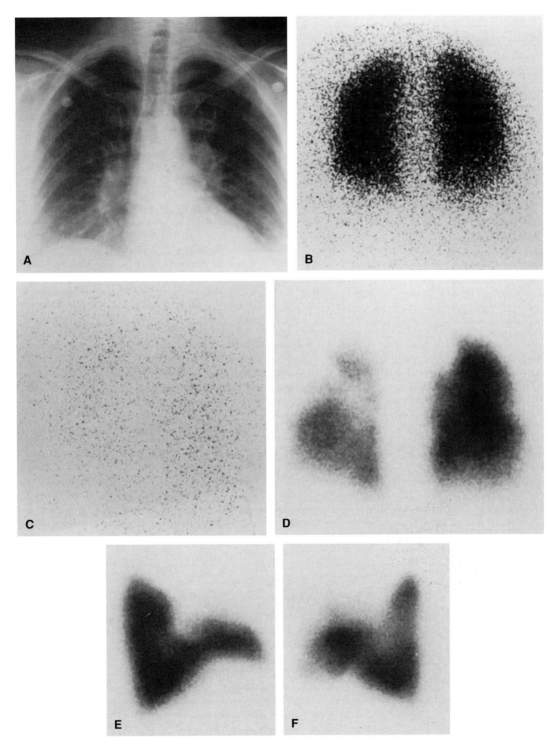

Figure 5. (A), Posterior-Anterior chest radiograph with hilar fullness and possible increased vascularity in the bases compared to the mid and upper lung zones. **(B), (C),** Posterior single breath and 90- to 135-second wash-out view from the xenon-133 ventilation study. These are normal. **(D), (E), (F),** Posterior, right lateral, and left lateral views from the perfusion study. The right lateral view has a peculiar shape because all of the right upper lobe and some of the middle lobe are NOT perfused. A similar appearance is seen on the left with most of the apical lower lobe segment also unperfused. On the posterior view, additional moderate-sized segmental defects are seen on the right side. If the height of the lungs on the perfusion scan is measured and compared to the height on the single breath xenon image **(B)** the upper lung zones will be missing from the perfusion scan. This is a high-probability V/Q scan with multiple bilateral mismatched segmental defects. Pulmonary angiogram was terminated when a large right upper-lobe embolus was identified. (Reproduced with permission from WB Saunders Co, Philadelphia, PA.)

had PE. There were 121 cases in the PIOPED study called "near normal" (best thought of as very low probability) and PE was correctly excluded in 95%.[10] This result is comparable in precision to that obtained from pulmonary angiograms. In the PIOPED study, 72 pulmonary angiograms had intraobserver interpretation, the reader agreeing with himself 95 ± 5% of the time.[36]

The distribution of the scan category readings for the V/Q scans in PIOPED was 13% high probability, 39% intermediate/indeterminate probability, 34% low probability, and 14% were nearly normal (very low probability) or normal. A high-probability interpretation was 97% specific but only 41% sensitive.[10]

The ventilation scan is considered a cornerstone of the diagnostic technique, permitting the separation of perfusion defects in diseases such as chronic obstructive pulmonary disease and PE, but it is not always obtainable, especially in very ill or uncooperative patients. The perfusion scan compared to the chest radiograph alone still has diagnostic value. In a series of 98 patients with perfusion scans and chest x-rays but no ventilation scans, the diagnostic reliability of both high- and low-probability interpretations were comparable to patients with a complete V/Q scan. There was an increase, however, in the number of intermediate/indeterminate cases.[37(I)]

Associated cardiopulmonary disease increases the number of intermediate/indeterminated readings of V/Q scans. Using PIOPED study criteria, the number of such readings was 13% in patients with normal chest radiographs,[38(I)] 33% in patients with no clinical assessment of prior cardiac or pulmonary disease,[39(I)] 43% in patients with any cardiac or pulmonary disease,[39] and 60% in patients with chronic obstructive pulmonary disease.[40(I)]

Among elderly patients (over 70 years old) the V/Q scan performed as well as it did in younger patients. Sensitivity and specificity were comparable in the two groups for high-probability readings.[41(I)]

CLINICAL ASSESSMENT AND LUNG SCAN INTERPRETATION IN COMBINATION

The PIOPED study has demonstrated that if there is congruence between the clinical probability assessment of PE and the V/Q scan interpretation, the results are reliable enough to guide therapy without further patient evaluation. However, this concordance occurred in only 28% of the patients in the PIOPED study.[10(I)] Furthermore, in that study, the clinical probability of PE was determined by experienced physicians interested in this problem. Objective clinical information obtained by any physician or physician's assistant can be processed

Figure 6. (A), Posterior-Anterior chest radiograph showing clear lungs. **(B), (C), (D),** Posterior single breath, early equilibrium, and 180- to 225-second wash-out views from the xenon-133 ventilation study. On the single-breath image **(B)** there is marked decrease in ventilation in both lower lung zones. This is beginning to fill in by collateral air drift on the early equilibrium image **(C)**. On the wash-out view **(D)** there is air trapping in both lower lung zones. **(E), (F),** Posterior and left posterior oblique views from the perfusion study. These illustrate perfusion defects in both lower lung zones which match the air trapping seen on ventilation.

Tables 2 and 3 show that according to the PIOPED study, this case would be called intermediate probability, but according to the revised PIOPED criteria, it would be cased low probability since there are two areas of V/Q match, a clear chest x-ray, and normally perfused lung elsewhere (the mid and upper lungs in this case). The pulmonary angiogram showed no emboli. (Reproduced with permission from WB Saunders Co, Philadelphia, PA.)

with neural network computer intelligence to yield a clinical assessment as accurate as that of an experienced physician.[42(I)]

The use of scan categories lumps together scans that may have different diagnostic power. For example, high probability is usually considered to represent an 80% to 100% likelihood of PE.[32(I)] However, it is now possible to give a discrete probability based on the number of mismatched defects.[43(I), 44(I), 45(I)]

An important new diagnostic refinement is possible if clinical stratification for the presence or absence of cardiopulmonary disease is used in conjunction with V/Q scan analysis. Fewer mismatched defects are necessary to diagnose PE with confidence in patients with no prior cardiopulmonary disease then are needed if cardiopulmonary disease is present (Figure 7).[43] No added benefit is obtained, however, if further stratification is made into either cardiac or pulmonary disease.[43(I)]

Criteria from the PIOPED study and others use the concept of segmental equivalents, the idea that a large segmental perfusion defect is equivalent to two moderate segmental perfusion defects.[6] A large perfusion defect is defined as one that is larger than 75% of a segment; a moderate perfusion defect is one that involves 25% to 75% of a segment. Deciding whether a perfusion defect is large or moderate is subjective, and even for experienced observers precision is not ideal, the defect size often being underestimated.[46] Recent data show that a moderate-size perfusion defect has the same diagnostic power as a large perfusion defect.[44(I)] Therefore, if either a moderate or a large segmental perfusion defect is considered to be a vascular perfusion defect, a positive predictive value for PE comparable to that for segmental equivalents is obtained.[44(I)] The use of vascular defects should make V/Q scans easier to read, and could decrease the number of intermediate/indeterminate interpretations.

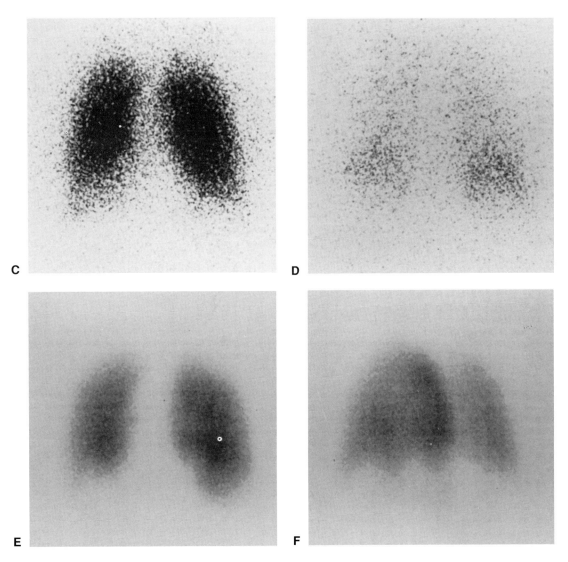

Figure 6. *(continued)*

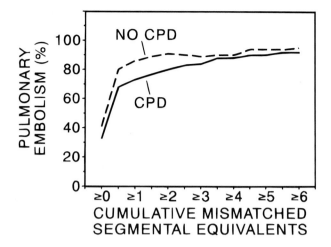

Figure 7. Predictive value of PE relative to the cumulative number of mismatched segmental equivalents among patients without prior cardiopulmonary disease (NO CPD) and among patients with any prior cardiopulmonary disease (CPD). Significant differences occurred with ≥0.5 and ≥1.0 segmental equivalents (P<.01) and with ≥1.5 segmental equivalents (P<.05). (Reproduced from Stein PD, et al,[43] with permission.)

DEVELOPING NEW CONCEPTS AND MODALITIES

An interesting new development in diagnostic imaging is the use of neural networks to aid in the interpretation of V/Q scans. It appears that trained neural networks can successfully arrive at the diagnosis of high, low or intermediate probability when the scintigraphic findings are entered.[47] It remains to be seen if this technology will evolve to the point where digitized images of the V/Q scan and chest radiographs can be accurately assessed in this way.

Noninvasive diagnosis of PE by new imaging modalities is currently being studied. Conventional, spiral, and electron beam computed tomography (CT) have recently been suggested as possible tools for the diagnosis of PE.[48–50] Conventional CT can detect proximal emboli in the pulmonary artery, but this is usually an incidental finding and not the purpose for which the CT scan was ordered. Spiral CT takes advantage of the speed of spiral imaging, and good images of the proximal branches of the pulmonary artery can be obtained during transit of a bolus of contrast material. Theoretically, this will permit the diagnosis of embolic intraluminal filling defects using essentially the same criteria as pulmonary angiography. Electron beam CT also makes it possible to scan faster, which also provides improved visualization of the pulmonary arteries.

Another area of technical advance is magnetic resonance angiography. Progress has been extremely rapid over the past several years. Flow-imaging techniques to evaluate the pulmonary arteries for PE or leg veins for deep venous thrombosis have been developed.[51,52]

Increasingly fast imaging techniques and improvements in image post-processing of magnetic resonance angiography may permit the reliable evaluation of intraluminal filling defects, oligemia, or vascular cut-offs with magnetic resonance angiography. The inherent advantages are that it is noninvasive, does not require contrast media, and does not involve ionizing radiation.

In conclusion, diagnostic approaches to the problem of PE continue to improve. Currently V/Q imaging is an important screening test to evaluate patients with suspected PE. If the scan is normal or very low probability, or high probability for PE, then no further evaluation is needed. Therapy can be started, or efforts can be directed toward other possible diagnoses. In the presence of an intermediate-probability scan or a low-probability scan with a high clinical suspicion, a diagnosis of deep venous thrombosis or angiographically proven PE is needed before starting definitive therapy. Many centers are now looking at the lower extremities in an effort to diagnose deep venous thrombosis and avoid pulmonary angiography.[53]

The PIOPED study has provided a large, prospective computerized data base that will allow continued refinement of the diagnostic criteria of the V/Q scan for PE. As technological advances continue in spiral CT, magnetic resonance imaging, and computer processing, they may find a role in the diagnosis of PE. At this time, however, V/Q lung scans continue to have an important role in the assessment of PE.

REFERENCES

1. Taplin GV, Johnson DE, Dore EK, Kaplan HS. Suspensions of radioalbumin aggregates for photoscanning the liver, spleen, lung and other organs. J Nucl Med 1964;5:259–275.
2. Wagner HN Jr, Sabiston DC Jr, Iio M, McAfee JG, Meyer JK, et al. Regional pulmonary blood flow in man by radioisotope scanning. JAMA 1964;187:601–603.
3. Wagner HN Jr, Sabiston DC Jr, McAfee JG, Tow D, Stern HS. Diagnosis of massive pulmonary embolism in man by radioisotope scanning. N Engl J Med 1964;271:377–384.
4. Quinn JL 3rd, Whitley JE, Hudspeth AS, Watts FC. An approach to the scanning of pulmonary infarcts. J Nucl Med 1964;5:1–8.
5. McNeil BJ, Holman L, Adelstein J. The scintigraphic definition of pulmonary embolism. JAMA 1974;227:753–756.
6. Neumann RD, Sostman HD, Gottschalk A. Current status of ventilation-perfusion imaging. Semin Nucl Med 1980;10:198–217.
7. Alderson PO, Line BR. Scintigraphic evaluation of regional pulmonary ventilation. Semin Nucl Med 1980;10:218–242.
8. Alderson PO, Biello DR, Khan AR, Barth KH, McKnight RC, et al. Comparison of 133-Xe single-breath and washout imaging in the scintigraphic diagnosis of pulmonary embolism. Radiology 1980;137:481–486.
9. Gottschalk A, Alderson PO, Sostman HD. Nuclear medicine techniques and applications. In: JF Murray, JA Nadel (eds.): Textbook of Respiratory Medicine, 2nd Edition,

Chapter 25, Philadelphia, WB Saunders Co. 1994: pp.682–710.

(I)10. A Collaborative Study by the PIOPED Investigators. Value of the ventilation/perfusion scan in acute pulmonary embolism—results of the prospective investigation of pulmonary embolism diagnosis (PIOPED). JAMA 1990;263:2753–2759.

11. Smith R, Maher JM, Miller RI, Alderson PO. Clinical outcomes of patients with suspected pulmonary embolism and low-probability aerosol-perfusion scintigrams. Radiology 1987;164:731–733.

12. Alderson PO, Line BR. Scintigraphic evaluation of regional pulmonary ventilation. Semin Nucl Med 1980;10:218–242.

(I)13. Alderson PO, Biello DR, Gottschalk A, et al. Tc-99m-DTPA aerosols and radioactive gases compared as adjuncts to perfusion scintigraphy in patients with suspected pulmonary embolism. Radiology 1984;153:515–521.

14. Stuart BO. Deposition of inhaled aerosol. Arch Intern Med 1973;131:60–73.

15. Krasnow AZ, Isitman AT, Collier BD, Effros RM, Hellman RS, et al. Diagnostic applications of radioaerosols in nuclear medicine. In: LM Freeman (ed.): Nuclear Medicine Annual 1993. Raven Press Ltd, NY, 1993, pp.123–193.

16. Miller TR, Biello DR, Lee JI, Davis HH, Mattar AG, et al. Ventilation imaging with Kr-81m: A comparison with Xe-133. Eur J Nucl Med 1981;6:11–16.

17. James JM, Herman KJ, Lloyd JJ, Shields RA, Testa RA, et al. Evaluation of Tc-99m Technegas ventilation scintigraphy in the diagnosis of pulmonary embolism. Br J Radiol 1991;64:711–719.

18. Cook G, Clarke SEM. An evaluation of Technegas as a ventilation agent compared with krypton-81m in the scintigraphic diagnosis of pulmonary embolism. Eur J Nucl Med 1992;19:770–774.

19. James JM, Lloyd JJ, Leahy BC, Church S, Hardy CC, et al. Tc-99m Technegas and krypton-81m ventilation scintigraphy: a comparison in known respiratory disease. British Journal of Radiology 1992;65:1075–1082.

20. James JM, Lloyd JJ, Leahy BC, Shields RA, Prescott MC, et al. The incidence and severity of hypoxia associated with Tc-99m Technegas ventilation scintigraphy and Tc-99m MAA perfusion scintigraphy. British Journal of Radiology 1992;65:403–408.

21. Miller WS. The structure of the lungs. J Morphol 1893;8:165. Quoted by: Dalen JE, Haynes FW, Hoppin FG Jr, Evans GL, Bhardwaj P, Dexter L. Cardiovascular responses to experimental pulmonary embolism. Am J Cardiol 1967;20:3–9.

22. Wellman HN, Mack JF, Saenger EL, Friedman BI. Clinical experience with oblique views in pulmonary perfusion scintiphotography in normal and pathological anatomy. J Nucl Med 1968;9:374–379.

23. Mack JF, Wellman HN, Saenger EL. Oblique pulmonary scintiphotography in the analysis of perfusion abnormalities due to embolism. J Nucl Med 1969;10:420.

24. Caride VJ, Puri S, Slavin JD, Lange RC, Gottschalk A. The usefulness of posterior oblique views in perfusion lung imaging. Radiology 1976;121:669–672.

25. Gottschalk A, Sostman HD, Coleman RE, Juni JE, Thrall J, et al. Ventilation-perfusion scintigraphy in the PIOPED study. Part II. Evaluation of the scintigraphic criteria and interpretations. J Nucl Med 1993;34:1119–1126.

26. Velchik MG, Tobin M, McCarthy K. Non-thromboembolic causes of high-probability lung scans. Am J Physiol Imaging 1989;4:32–36.

27. Thomas D, Stein M, Tanabe G, Rege V, Wessler S. Mechanism of bronchoconstriction produced by thromboemboli in dogs. Am J Physiol 1964;206:1207–1212.

28. Kessler RM, McNeil BJ. Impaired ventilation in a patient with angiographically demonstrated pulmonary embolism. Radiology 1975;114:111–112.

29. Epstein J, Taylor A, Alazraki NP, Coel M. Acute pulmonary embolus associated with transient ventilatory defect. J Nucl Med 1976;16:1017–1020.

30. Newman GE, Sullivan DC, Gottschalk A, Putman CE. Scintigraphic perfusion patterns in patients with diffuse lung disease. Radiology 1982;143:227–231.

31. Stein PD, Gottschalk A. Critical Review of Ventilation/Perfusion Lung Scans in Acute Pulmonary embolism. Progress in cardiovascular disease 1994;37:13–24.

(I)32. Hull RD, Hirsh J. Carter CJ, et al. Diagnostic value of ventilation-perfusion lung scanning in patients with suspected pulmonary embolism. Chest 1985;88:819–828.

33. Gottschalk A, Juni JE, Sostman HD, Coleman RE, Thrall J, et al. Ventilation-Perfusion scintigraphy in the PIOPED study. Part I. Data collection and tabulation. J Nucl Med 1993;34:1109–1118.

34. Biello DR, Mattar AG, McKnight RC, Siegel BA. Ventilation perfusion studies in suspected pulmonary embolism. Am J Radiol 1979;133:1033–1037.

35. Biello DR. Radiological (scintigraphic) evaluation of patients with suspected pulmonary thromboembolism. JAMA 1987;257:3257–3259.

36. Gottschalk A. Unpublished data from PIOPED. Presented to the Radiological Society of North America, December, 1992.

(I)37. Stein PD, Terrin ML, Gottschalk A, Alavi A, Henry JW. Value of ventilation/perfusion scans compared to perfusion scans alone in acute pulmonary embolism. Am J Cardiol 1992;69:1239–1241.

(I)38. Stein PD, Alavi A, Gottschalk A, Hales CA, Saltzman HA, et al. Usefulness of noninvasive diagnostic tools for diagnosis of acute pulmonary embolism in patients with a normal chest radiograph. Am J Cardiol 1991;67:1117–1120.

(I)39. Stein PD, Coleman RE, Gottschalk A, Saltzman HA, Terrin ML, et al. Diagnostic utility of ventilation/perfusion lung scans in acute pulmonary embolism is not diminished by preexisting cardiac or pulmonary disease. Chest 1991;100:604–606.

(I)40. Lesser BA, Leeper KV, Stein PD, Saltzman HA, Chen J, et al. The diagnosis of acute pulmonary embolism in patients with chronic obstructive pulmonary disease. Chest 1992;102:17–22.

(I)41. Stein PD, Gottschalk A, Saltzman HA, Terrin ML. Diagnosis of acute pulmonary embolism in the elderly. J Am Coll Cardiol 1991;18:1452–1457.

(I)42. Patil S, Henry JW, Rubenfire M, Stein PD. Neural network in the diagnosis of acute pulmonary embolism. Chest 1994;37:13–24.

(I)43. Stein PD, Gottschalk A, Henry JW, Shivkumar K. Stratification of patients according to prior cardiopulmonary disease and probability assessment based upon the number of mismatched segmental equivalent perfusion defects: Approaches to strengthen the diagnostic value of ventilation/perfusion lung scans in acute pulmonary embolism. Chest 1993;104:1461–1467.

(I)44. Stein PD, Henry JW, Gottschalk A. Mismatched vascular defects: A new approach to the interpretation of ventilation/perfusion lung scans in pulmonary embolism. Chest 1993;104:1468–1471.

(I)45. Stein PD, Henry JW, Gottschalk A. The addition of prior clinical assessment to stratification according to prior cardiopulmonary disease further optimizes the interpretation of ventilation/perfusion lung scans in pulmonary embolism. Chest 1993;104:1472–1476.

46. Morrell NW, Nijran KS, Jones BE, Biggs T, Seed WA. The underestimation of segmental defect size in radionuclide lung scanning. J Nucl Med 1993;34:370–374.

47. Scott JA, Palmer EL. Neural network analysis of ventilation-perfusion lung scans. Radiology 1993;186:661–664.

48. Verschakelen JA, Vanwijck E, Bogaert J, Baert AL. Detection of unsuspected central pulmonary embolism with conventional contrast-enhanced CT. Radiology 1993;188:847–850.

49. Tiegen CL, Maus TP, Sheedy PF, Johnson CM, Stanson AW, et al. Pulmonary embolism: diagnosis with electron-beam CT. Radiology 1993;188:839–845.

50. Remy-jardin M, Remy J, Wattinne L, Giraud F. Central pulmonary thromboembolism: diagnosis with spiral volumetric CT with single breath-hold technique: comparison with pulmonary angiography. Radiology 1992;185:381–387.

51. Sostman HD. Deep venous thrombosis: experience with new techniques. In EJ Potchen, RG Grainger, R Green (eds.): Pulmonary Radiology. Philadelphia: WB Saunders, 1993;107–112.

52. Sostman HD, MacFall JR, Foo TKF. Pulmonary arteries and veins. In EK Potchen, EM Haacke, JE Siebert, A Gottschalk (eds.): Magnetic Resonance Angiography: Concepts and Applications. St. Louis, MO: Mosby, 1993, pp. 546–572.

53. Stein PD, Hull RD, Saltzman HA, Pineo G. Strategy for diagnosis of patients with suspected acute pulmonary emoblism. Chest 1993;103:1553–1559.

54. Sullivan DC, Coleman RE, Mills SR, Ravin CE, Hedlund LW. Lung scan interpretation: effect of different observers and different criteria. Radiology 1983;149:803–807.

55. McNeil BJ. Ventilation-perfusion studies and the diagnoses of pulmonary embolism: concise communication. J Nucl Med 1980;21:319–323.

23

Pulmonary Angiography

G.V.R.K. Sharma, Arthur A. Sasahara

INTRODUCTION

Since its introduction in 1964,[1] selective pulmonary angiography has continued to be the definitive method of establishing the diagnosis of pulmonary embolism (PE) during life. All other tests for PE are indirect and at best suggest a level of probability of the diagnosis high enough to warrant initiation of therapy. However, the seriousness of the disease and the significant risks of anticoagulant or thrombolytic treatment justify the use of angiography whenever the diagnosis is in reasonable doubt. When performed within 72 hours of the suspected embolic episode, pulmonary angiography has been shown to have high sensitivity, specificity, and predictive accuracy. Although autopsy correlations in close proximity to angiography are limited, available data indicate nearly 100% accuracy.[2,3] Pulmonary angiography is also employed in the evaluation of other abnormalities of the pulmonary vasculature, congenital or acquired. This report, however, focuses on its most frequent clinical indication—the diagnosis of PE.

TECHNIQUE

Although pulmonary angiography was initially performed from the arm (usually by venotomy), in modern practice the procedure is performed most often by the transfemoral route. The introduction of the pigtail catheter in 1970,[4] has facilitated transfemoral catheterization of the pulmonary artery, and helped to prevent the occasional complication of right ventricular perforation, associated with the use of the stiff NIH and Gensini catheters. Percutaneous cannulation of the femoral vein also eliminates the possibility of veno-spasm sometimes encountered in the brachial approach. Although some angiographers have raised the issue of the potential dislodgement of proximal venous thrombi, the concern has remained minimal and experience has established the

safety of the transfemoral route. Introduction of the angled pigtail catheter such as Grollman's,[5] has further enhanced the feasibility and safety of selective pulmonary angiography with the result that the procedure, once the domain of the cardiologist, is now performed by radiologists in most institutions.

The preferred approach is through the right femoral vein which may be easier than the left, as the latter may join the inferior vena cava at a right angle. It is important to enter the femoral vein on the first attempt because failure to do so can result in the development of a groin hematoma.[6] Once the vein is entered, a side-arm sheath is inserted to facilitate easy maneuverability and exchange of catheters.

Hemodynamic measurements are essential prior to angiography: pressures from the right atrium, right ventricle, and the pulmonary artery. Measurement of the pulmonary capillary wedge pressure is not essential; if desired, it may be obtained with a routine Swan-Ganz catheter prior to the introduction of the angiography catheter.

Once the right ventricle is entered, the straight pigtail catheter is directed into the outflow tract, where it can be advanced easily into the main pulmonary artery. If an angled pigtail catheter is used, slight rotation will direct the catheter away from the apex and towards the outflow tract. A few deep breaths by the patient may facilitate this maneuver and advance the pigtail into the pulmonary artery. If difficulty is encountered in crossing the tricuspid valve with the straight pigtail, the catheter can be reshaped temporarily with a guidewire.

The catheter can be selectively positioned in the right or left pulmonary artery; a straight pigtail catheter usually tends to advance into the left. Knowledge that the left pulmonary artery arises more cephalad than the right helps in maneuvering the catheter to the desired side. If difficulty is encountered, a guidewire may be inserted to bend the catheter and direct it towards the appropriate location.

Alternatively, a double-lumen Swan-Ganz catheter may be positioned in the pulmonary artery and then a pigtail catheter threaded over an exchange guidewire. The catheter is parked in the desired vessel based on the location of the defects on the perfusion lung scan.

A test dose of 5 ml to 10 ml of contrast material is administered prior to angiography. Also a plain scout film should be obtained to ascertain proper field of view and exposure. The patient should be informed that the injection of contrast material is associated with a transient, generalized, hot sensation and that it may cause chest discomfort and an urge to cough. However, the patient should be instructed to hold the breath in deep inspiration during filming and resist the urge to cough.

Pulmonary angiograms are conventionally filmed by large film seriography. Positioning of the patient, degree of obliquity, and the radiographic setting are based on the results of the scout film. Attention to these details can significantly improve the quality of the angiogram and its readability and reduce the need for multiple injections. The posterior oblique views are generally preferred as they open up the lower lobe vessels, which are the most common targets for emboli (Figure 1). Short exposure times of 50 msec or less will enhance angiographic quality, even in the presence of tachycardia and resultant motion artifact.[5] The filming rate that we employ is 3 per second for 3 seconds and one per second for 3 seconds so that the maximum number of pictures in the arterial and capillary phases are obtained (Figure 2).

The amount of contrast material employed for the angiogram varies with its "selectivity." For the opacification of the entire right or the left lung, 40 to 50 mls of contrast material are injected at a rate of 20 to 25 mls per second, with the flow rate dependent on the heart rate. For the more selective sequences (e.g., right lower or left lower pulmonary artery), smaller amounts (20 to 40 mls) and lower rates of injection (10 to 15 mls per second) are used. Main pulmonary artery injections are rarely employed now since they have been associated with most of the early reports of mortality and morbidity of pulmonary angiography.[7] After completion of filming, pressures in the pulmonary artery and right-sided pull-back pressures are recorded.

In patients with severe pulmonary hypertension, or in other situations where large amounts of contrast may not be tolerated well, balloon-occlusion pulmonary an-

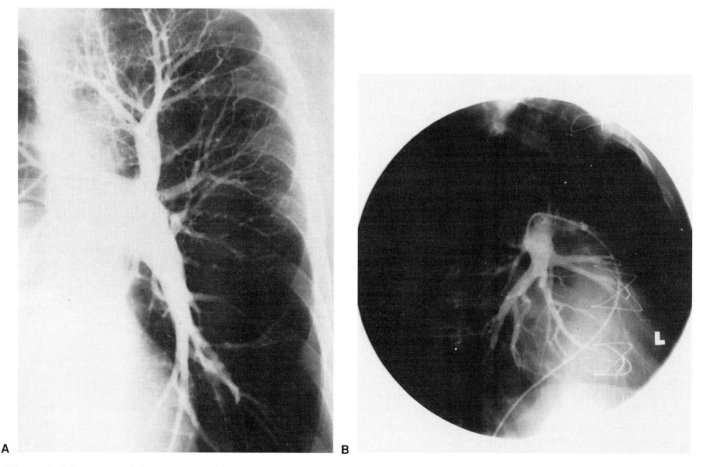

A **B**

Figure 1. Advantage of the posterior oblique view over the anterior oblique view. In the latter **(1A)** the lower lobe vessels are crowded, but separated and displayed better in the posterior oblique view **(1B)**.

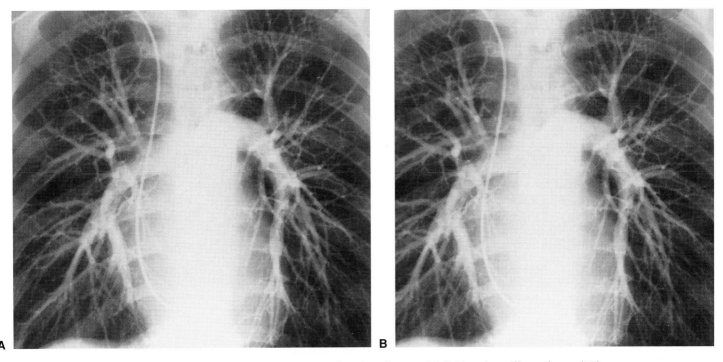

Figure 2. Normal pulmonary angiogram showing the arterial **(2A)** and capillary phases **(2B)**.

giography can be performed.[8,9] A **#7** French pulmonary wedge balloon catheter is passed into the lobar or segmental vessel in question. The balloon is inflated and 5 to 10 mls of contrast material are injected slowly. Once the vessel and its branches are opacified, angiograms are obtained by spot filming (Figure 3) or by the cineangiographic technique.[10] The balloon is deflated immediately after the filming.

COMPLICATIONS

The risks of pulmonary angiography have been overestimated. The most important complications reported in four large series[11–13] are shown in Table 1. The overall mortality rate is 0.22% (11 of 4927) which is similar to the 0.25% mortality rate reported by the Registry of the Society for Cardiac Angiography for patients over 60 years of age.[14] Most of the deaths occurred in patients with severe pulmonary hypertension or in those with perforations of the right ventricular outflow tract. Mills reported that in patients who had a high right ventricular end-diastolic pressure (20 mmHg or more), pulmonary angiography is likely to result in irreversible hypotension and death.[13] More recent reports, however, have indicated that even in the presence of severe pulmonary hypertension, angiography can be successfully performed if proper precautions are taken.[15] Perforation of the right ventricular outflow tract has not been a problem since the advent of the pigtail catheter and the discontinuation of the use of stiff catheters.

The other complications of pulmonary angiography can be classified as those incidental to right heart catheter-

Table 1
Mortality and Morbidity of Pulmonary Angiography

Series	Number of Angiograms	Fatal	Non-fatal Perforations	Arrhythmias
Pre-UPET analysis[11]	2347	5	15	8
UPET experience[12]	310	0	1	5
Mills et al[13]	1350	3	14	11
West Roxbury Series[7]	920	3	4	6
Total	4927	11(0.22%)	34(0.69%)	30(0.61%)

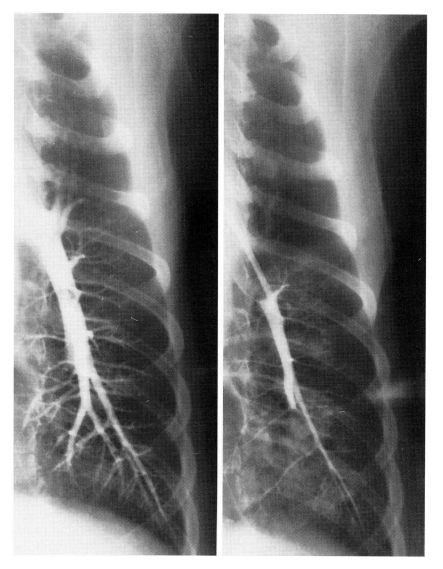

Figure 3. Balloon-occlusion pulmonary angiography. Left panel shows a balloon-occlusion angiogram of the left lower lobe with embolic occlusion of a segmental vessel which is not apparent in a conventional left selective angiogram (left panel).

ization and those secondary to injection of contrast material. Tachyarrhythmias, complete heart block (especially in patients with left bundle branch block), and endocardial or myocardial injury come under the former category. These are not unique to pulmonary angiography and can be avoided or managed by appropriate precautionary measures (e.g., insertion of a temporary pacemaker or a pacing catheter in patients with a left bundle branch block). Complications related to contrast media are allergic reactions and myocardial staining. Allergic reactions such as urticaria, bronchospasm and hypotension can be easily treated with standard antianaphylactic measures. Myocardial staining is usually innocuous and needs no special treatment. Use of nonionic contrast agents can further lower the risk for morbid events during angiography.

INTERPRETATION

Adequate training is required to perform pulmonary arteriography safely and to interpret the angiograms accurately. Since conventional pulmonary angiography attempts to portray the vasculature of a three-dimensional organ in a single plane, changes in the caliber and direction of vessels are not easy to interpret. Knowledge of the pulmonary vascular anatomy and an understanding of the radiographic techniques and pitfalls are important prerequisites for a valid interpretation. If the angiograms are suboptimal, appreciation of the inadequacy of the angiographic technique at the time of the procedure can help in the procurement of better images, thereby reducing the frequency of equivocal studies. If angiograms are properly done, the incidence of equivocal angiograms can be as low as 15%.[7]

Although a number of angiographic abnormalities have been reported, only two have been accepted as diagnostic for PE: persistent, intravascular filling defects and arterial vessel cut-offs (Figure 4). Other signs such as vessel pruning, oligemia, asymmetrical filling and prolonged arterial opacification with delayed emptying are less specific for PE as they are seen in various other cardiopulmonary diseases such as chronic cor pulmonale, obstructive airways disease, and congestive heart failure.

Angiographic scoring systems have been developed for quantification of the severity of PE and assessment of therapeutic efficacy. The Miller index,[16] which has been used mostly in Europe, can overestimate the extent of pulmonary vascular obstruction in patients with massive PE. On the other hand, the Walsh Scoring System,[17] which has been used in the Urokinase-Streptokinase PE trials, does not account for the loss of peripheral perfusion. Both indices are semiquantitative and fail to separate the elements of clot size and degree of occlusion. A method that accounts for both these elements and provides a more accurate means of quantitating the severity of occlusion has been described.[18]

ROLE OF PULMONARY ANGIOGRAPHY IN THE DIAGNOSIS OF PULMONARY EMBOLISM

Not only are the risks of pulmonary angiography generally overestimated[19] but the risks of mistreatment of suspected PE are also significantly underestimated.[20] Because the therapy for venous thromboembolism (VTE) has both considerable benefits and hazards, proper understanding of the relative risks of the diagnostic and therapeutic interventions is essential for optimal patient management. On the one hand, failure to treat PE exposes the patient to a threefold greater mortality and recurrence rate than when proper therapy is instituted, while on the other, the risks of the definitive forms of therapy for PE are sufficiently high to require an accurate diagnosis before embarking on a specific therapeutic strategy, such as thrombolytic therapy or inferior vena caval interruption.[21]

The recent report of the prospective investigation of pulmonary embolism diagnosis (PIOPED) study,[22] has provided important information as to the value of pulmonary angiography in patients with different degrees of probability of PE by the ventilation-perfusion (V/Q) scan. The relevant observations can be summarized as follows:

1. A negative pulmonary angiogram rules out clinically important PE (substantiates the earlier observation of Novelline, et al.)[23]
2. Interobserver variability even among expert nuclear radiologists, is as high as 30% for classifying intermediate and low-probability scan results.[22] A pulmonary angiogram is essential to provide an accurate diagnosis in this context, especially in the presence of a reasonable clinical suspicion.

3. Even a high-probability lung scan has false-positive results in 15% of the patients. More important, in patients with a low clinical suspicion of PE, the predictive value of a high-probability lung scan fell to 56%, indicating the need for angiographic verification.[24]

While the observations of the PIOPED study reestablish the important role of pulmonary angiography in the documentation of PE, there are other well-recognized advantages that merit reemphasis. These pertain to the usefulness and necessity of the angiogram in patients with prior cardiopulmonary disease,[25] the postoperative patient suspected of having PE, patients with significant risks for anticoagulation and those who are candidates for inferior vena caval interruption procedures. The problem of suspected recurrent PE also deserves special mention. Comparison of the baseline angiogram and the one obtained after the suspected recurrence (Figure 5) is the only reliable method of distinguishing between true and spurious embolization, (secondary to fragmentation of the original proximal clot and distal migration).[21]

Last but definitely not the least, hemodynamic observations made at the time of angiography are invaluable guides to evaluate the pathophysiological consequences of PE and its response to therapy (Figure 6).

CONTRAINDICATIONS (TABLE 2)

There are no absolute contraindications to pulmonary angiography. If there is a prior history of allergic reaction to contrast material and angiography is considered essential to patient management, pretreatment with steroids and antihistamines can acceptably reduce the risk. In patients with severe pulmonary hypertension and elevated right ventricular end-diastolic pressure (20 mm Hg or more), there is an increased mortality from the procedure. The risk of lethal right ventricular failure, systemic hypotension and cardiac arrhythmias can be minimized by administration of oxygen throughout the procedure, small injections of contrast with cinefluoroscopy to ensure patency of the main pulmonary trunks, and limiting the field of opacification to a lobar or even a segmental level.[15] The use of a temporary pacemaker can obviate the danger of precipitating complete heart block in patients with left bundle branch block. The hazards of fetal radiation decrease in the later stages of pregnancy and can be further reduced by proper shielding; they probably constitute a lower fetal and maternal risk than unnecessary anticoagulation.

In regard to the other contraindications such as right-sided bacterial endocarditis, decisions must be made on an individual basis weighing the risks of angiography against those of inappropriate therapy. A practical problem, however, remains unsolved. Although selective pulmonary angiography is definitive for the diagnosis of PE and can be safely carried out, it requires special equip-

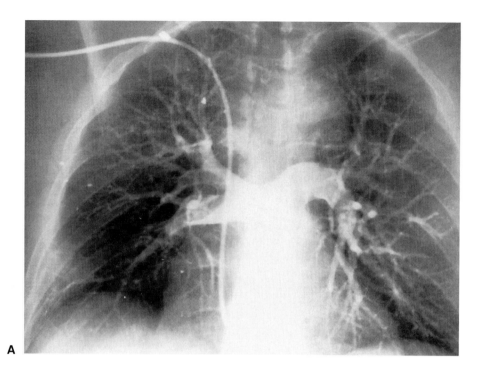

A

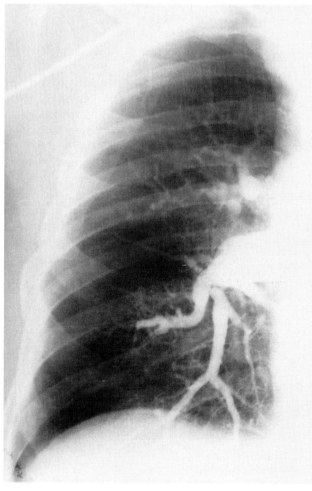

B

Figure 4. (A): Acute massive pulmonary embolism involving the right main pulmonary artery (saddle) and left upper and lower segmental vessels. **(B)**: Chronic pulmonary embolism of the right lung.

ment and expertise which are not available in many institutions. If the logistical issues surrounding pulmonary angiography—the costs, the time and the limited availability—are not resolved, one may have to rely on a noninvasive strategy, utilizing one of the newer, more promising techniques.

OTHER IMAGING TECHNIQUES[26]

Digital subtraction angiography (DSA) is useful for diagnosing massive PE involving the proximal vessels, but motion artifacts and lack of adequate resolution render evaluation of peripheral (segmental and subsegmental) emboli difficult. The only clinical situation in which DSA may help is when patients are suspected to have life-threatening PE and are too ill to undergo conventional angiography. The diagnosis of massive PE that is hemodynamically significant can also be established by means of two-dimensional echocardiography. Magnetic resonance imaging (MRI) is a promising noninvasive technique that

Table 2
Relative Contraindications to
Pulmonary Arteriography

Allergy to contrast material
Severe pulmonary hyptertension
Uncontrolled ventricular ectopy
Left bundle branch block
Pregnancy
Right-sided bacterial endocarditis
Severe congestive failure
Anticoagulated state (PT > 18 sec)
Severe renal insufficiency

is awaiting wider clinical use. Computed tomography (CT) has been effectively used to document chronic pulmonary emboli in patients with pulmonary hypertension. The advantage of MRI and CT is their applicability for serial noninvasive evaluation.

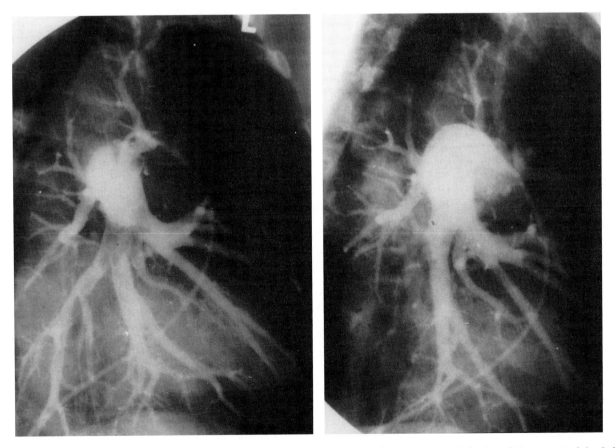

Figure 5. Fragmentation of proximal clot and distal migration. The left panel shows proximal clot involving most of the left lower segmental vessels. The right panel shows a follow-up pulmonary angiogram after a "clinical recurrence." The proximal clot has been lysed but part of the clot has migrated distally and completely occluded the posterior-basal segmental artery.

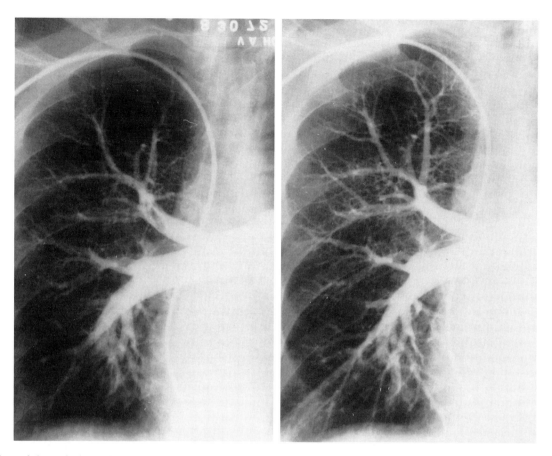

Figure 6. Effect of thrombolytic therapy. **(8A)** shows multiple sites of embolic occlusion involving both the right pulmonary vasculature. **(8B)** shows almost complete clearance after 12 hours of streptokinase therapy.

REFERENCES

1. Sasahara AA, Stein M, Simon M, Littmann D. Pulmonary angiography in the diagnosis of thromboembolic disease. N Engl J Med 1964;270:1075–1081.
2. Dalen JE, Brooks HL, Johnson LW, Meister SG, Szucs MM, et al. Pulmonary angiography in acute pulmonary embolism: indications, techniques and results in 367 patients. Am Heart J 1971;81:175–185.
3. Bell WR, Simon TL. A comparative analysis of pulmonary perfusion scans with pulmonary angiograms. Am Heart J 1976;92:700–706.
4. Grollman JH Jr, Gyepes MT, Helmer E. Transfemoral selective bilateral pulmonary artery-seeking catheter. Radiol 1970;96:202–204.
5. Grollman JH Jr. Pulmonary arteriography. Cardiovasc & Intervent Radiol 1992;15:166–170.
6. Meyerowitz MF. How to maximize the safety of coronary and pulmonary angiography in patients receiving thrombolytic therapy. Chest 1990;97(4):1325–1355.
7. Sharma GVRK, Sasahara AA. (Unpublished data)
8. Sharma GVRK, McIntyre KM. Subselective balloon occlusion pulmonary angiography. Am J Cardiol 1974;33:154(Abstract).
9. Bynum LJ, Wilson JE III, Christensen EE, Sorensen C. Radiographic techniques for balloon occlusion pulmonary angiography. Radiol 1979;133:518–520.
10. Benotti JR, Ockene IS, Alpert JS, Dalen JE. Balloon occlusion pulmonary cineangiography to diagnose pulmonary embolism. Cathet Cardiovasc Diagn 1984;10:519.
11. Manual of operations: Urokinase pulmonary embolism trial, National Heart Institute, October 1968.
12. The urokinase pulmonary embolism trial: A national cooperative study. Circ 1973;47(Suppl II):11–108.
13. Mills SR, Jackson DC, Older RA, Heaston DA, Moore AV. The incidence, etiologies, and avoidance of complications of pulmonary angiography in a large series. Radiol 1980;136:295–299.
14. Kennedy JW. Complications associated with cardiac catheterization and angiography. Cathet Cardiovasc Diagn 1982;8:5–12.
15. Nicod P, Peterson K, Levine M, et al. Pulmonary angiography in severe chronic pulmonary hypertension. Ann Int Med 1987;107:565–568.
16. Miller GAH, Sutton GC, Kerr IH, Gibson RV, Honey M. Comparison of streptokinase and heparin in treatment of isolated acute massive pulmonary embolism. Br Med J 1971;2:681–683.
17. Walsh PN, Greenspan RH, Simon M, Simon AL, Hyers TM, et al. An angiographic severity index for pulmonary embolism. Circ 1973;47(Suppl II):11–101.
18. Simon M, Sharma GVRK, Sasahara AA. An angiographic method for quantitating the severity of pulmonary embolism. Internat Angiol 1984;3:389–392.
19. Dalen JE. Pulmonary angiography is not indicated in all patients with suspected pulmonary embolism. In: E Rapaport (ed.): Current Controversies in Cardiovascular Disease. Philadelphia, PA. WB Saunders Co, 1980; pp. 472–478.

20. Robin ED. Overdiagnosis and overtreatment of pulmonary embolism: The emperor may have no clothes. Ann Int Med 1977;87:775–781.
21. Messer JV. Pulmonary arteriography should be routinely performed in patients with suspected acute pulmonary emboli. In: E Rapaport (ed.): Current Controversies in Cardiovascular Disease. Philadelphia, PA, WB Saunders Co, 1980; pp. 445–471.
22. The PIOPED investigators. Value of the ventilation/perfusion scan in acute pulmonary embolism. Results of the prospective investigation of pulmonary embolism diagnosis (PIOPED). JAMA 1990;263:2753–2759.
23. Novelline RA, Baltarowich OH, Athanasoulis CA, Waltman AC, Greenfield AJ, et al. The clinical course of patients with suspected pulmonary embolism and a negative pulmonary arteriogram. Radiol 1978;126:561–567.
24. Kelley MA, Carson JL, Palevsky HI, Schwartz S. Diagnosing pulmonary embolism: New facts and strategies. Ann Int Med 1991;114:300–306.
25. Sharma GVRK, Sasahara AA. Diagnosis of pulmonary embolism in patients with chronic obstructive pulmonary disease. J Chronic Dis 1975;28:253–256.
26. Goldhaber SZ, Braunwald E. Pulmonary embolism. In: E Braunwald (ed.): Heart Disease, Philadelphia, PA, WB Saunders Co., 1992, pp. 1585–1587.

24

Role of Objective Tests for Deep-Vein Thrombosis in the Diagnosis of Pulmonary Embolism

Gary E. Raskob, Graham F. Pineo, Russell D. Hull

INTRODUCTION

The traditional approach to the patient with clinically suspected pulmonary embolism (PE) is based on the premise that all patients with PE require therapy to prevent death and morbidity from recurrent embolism or from thrombotic extension of the embolus. Therefore, the ability to accurately determine the presence or absence of PE has been considered crucial for good management.

Several factors have led to a rethinking of our approach to the patient with clinically suspected PE. These are:

1. The recognition, based on the findings of recent prospective studies,[1(I),2(I),3(I),4(I)] that ventilation-perfusion lung scanning has major diagnostic limitations.
2. The finding that combining the clinical assessment with the ventilation-perfusion scan is useful only for a minority of patients.[1(I),2(I),3(I)]
3. An improved understanding of the natural history of venous thromboembolism (VTE), and in particular, the strong association between PE and deep-vein thrombosis (DVT).[3(I),4(I),5,6] This has led to the conceptual advance that "Pulmonary embolism is not a disease; rather, Pulmonary embolism is merely a complication of deep venous thrombosis".[7]
4. The observation that PE usually originates from proximal-vein thrombosis (popliteal, femoral or iliac vein thrombosis),[5–10] and that thrombosis confined to the calf-veins does not produce clinically important PE.[5,6,11(I),12(I),13(I)]
5. The availability of accurate noninvasive objective tests for DVT.[14–16,17(I),18]

Recent editorials[19,20] suggest that more attention should be paid to the source of embolism, proximal DVT, in the work-up of patients with clinically suspected PE. Secker-Walker writes, "Clearly, we should be looking below the diaphragm—to venous thrombosis in the popliteal fossa or more proximally. When the perfusion scan is abnormal, consideration should be given to examining the deep veins, either by impedance plethysmography (IPG) or venography".[19] More recently, in an editorial[20] accompanying the PIOPED study, Bone states "In my opinion, the greatest recent advance has occurred in the noninvasive diagnosis of deep venous thrombi (which are the usual antecedents to pulmonary emboli), using either impedance studies or duplex ultrasound study of the legs" (Figure 1).

This chapter outlines the role of objective tests for DVT in the management of patients with clinically suspected PE. The chapter is organized into two sections. First, the background, rationale and clinical evidence for the use of objective tests for DVT is described. Second, a practical bedside approach is presented. This approach can be applied in a wide range of clinical settings, from the community hospital to the tertiary care center. The specific approach that is used depends on the availability of the objective tests for DVT. The technical details for the most widely available objective tests for DVT are described in chapters 12, 13 and 15.

BACKGROUND AND RATIONALE

Pulmonary embolism is strongly associated with proximal-vein thrombosis (thrombosis of the popliteal, femoral or iliac veins).[3(I),4(I),6] This association was first observed in autopsy studies[8,9] and in studies of patients with PE who were treated with deep venous thrombectomy.[10] More recently, prospective studies using pul-

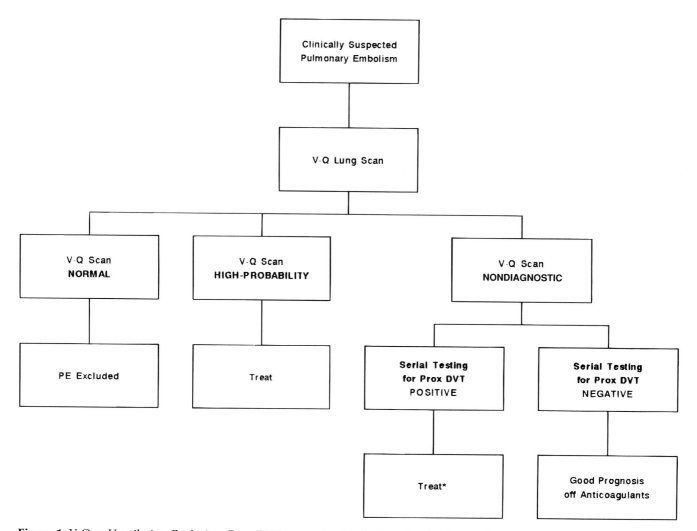

Figure 1. V-Q = Ventilation-Perfusion; Prox DVT = proximal-vein thrombosis. *In the absence of clinical conditions which may produce false-positive results. If such conditions are present, venography should be performed.

Serial testing for proximal-vein thrombosis can be used in patients with adequate cardiorespiratory reserve (see text for definition). Impedance plethysmography was the noninvasive test formally evaluated in our prospective study.[21] Data from studies in patients with venous thrombosis[17,18,26] suggest that B-mode ultrasonography can be substituted for impedance plethysmography, but this has not yet been formally evaluated in patients with suspected pulmonary embolism.

monary angiography and objective testing for venous thrombosis have established that residual proximal-vein thrombosis is present in 50% of patients with PE.[3(I),4(I)]

The prospective studies have documented a gradient for the frequency of proximal-vein thrombosis associated with the different ventilation-perfusion lung scan patterns.[3(I),4(I),21(I)] Proximal-vein thrombosis was found in 50% of patients with high probability lung scans,[3,4] in 8% to 25% of patients with low or intermediate probability lung scan findings,[3(I),4(I),21(I),22(I)] and in only 1% of patients with normal perfusion scans.[23(I)] Most patients with proximal-vein thrombosis do not have symptoms or signs of venous thrombosis at the time of presentation with symptoms of PE. The finding of proximal-vein thrombosis in 8% to 25% of patients with low probability lung scan patterns has important implications because these pa-

tients are at risk for clinically important recurrent venous thromboembolic events[24(I),25(I),26(I)] (see below).

Why is proximal-vein thrombosis absent at presentation in 50% of patients with PE? There are two possible explanations. Firstly, PE may have originated from a source other than the deep veins of legs, such as the right heart, axillary veins, renal veins, deep pelvic veins, or inferior vena cava. Alternately, the emboli originated from thrombosis in the deep veins of the legs, but all or most of the thrombus embolized, leaving no residual thrombosis. Recent data[21(I),22(I)] support the latter explanation. Regardless of the explanation however, the important clinical implication is that negative findings by objective testing for venous thrombosis do not exclude the presence of PE.[3(I),4(I)] Thus, patients with nondiagnostic lung scan findings who are negative by objective testing for

DVT on referral present a "diagnostic dilemma". Until recently, this "dilemma" could only be resolved by performing pulmonary angiography.

In 1984, we began a prospective study evaluating an alternative management strategy for patients with non-high probability lung scans. This alternative strategy is based on two key concepts:

(a) PE occurs in up to 50% of patients with confirmed proximal-vein thrombosis.[5,6]

This concept is supported by the findings of randomized trials which indicate that inadequate therapy for proximal-vein thrombosis is associated with a high risk (20% to 50%) of recurrent venous thrombosis and PE.[24(I),25(I),26(I)] Therefore, objective confirmation of proximal-vein thrombosis is an indication for treatment.

(b) Clinically important recurrent PE is unlikely in the absence of proximal-vein thrombosis.[5]

This concept is supported by the findings of prospective studies evaluating noninvasive testing in patients with clinically suspected DVT.[11(I),12(I),13(I),27(I)] These studies indicate that if proximal-vein thrombosis has been excluded by serial objective testing, the prognosis without treatment is excellent because of a low risk (<1%) of clinically evident PE.

The data in patients with DVT indicate that proximal-vein thrombosis is the important prognostic marker for recurrent VTE.[5,6,11–13,24–26] Our study sought to determine if this finding would hold in patients with clinically suspected PE. We tested the approach of using serial objective testing for proximal-vein thrombosis instead of pulmonary angiography in patients with nondiagnostic lung scan findings, providing the patient has adequate cardiorespiratory reserve (a specific definition is provided later in the chapter under the section "Practical Management Approach"). The hypothesis is that clinically important recurrent VTE is unlikely in the absence of proximal-vein thrombosis, and in such patients, treatment is not required, even though PE may be present. Thus, in patients with nondiagnostic lung scans, management hinges on the presence or absence of proximal DVT, a prognostic marker for recurrent VTE, rather than on the presence or absence of PE itself. This approach enables the clinician to make very good estimates of patient prognosis, and of the risks and benefits of therapy, even though in the individual patient, the presence or absence of PE often remains uncertain.

The use of serial testing for proximal-vein thrombosis is based on the following concepts, now confirmed by clinical observation[21(I),22(I)]:

1. In most patients, recurrent PE comes from proximal-vein thrombosis, which can be detected by currently available noninvasive tests.
2. Repeated testing is required for patients who have negative results initially. These patients may have had proximal-vein thrombosis that embolized in total; in the absence of repeated testing, proximal-

vein thrombosis that re-develops will go undetected, and could result in recurrent PE. Proximal-vein thrombosis could result from extension of calf-vein thrombosis[6,28(I)] (calf-vein thrombosis is not detected by the currently available noninvasive tests).
3. Calf-vein thrombosis or pelvic-vein thrombosis, which do not extend into the proximal venous segment, are not associated with clinically important PE.
4. Thrombotic extension of submissive PE is not an important cause of morbidity in patients with adequate cardiorespiratory reserve.

The approach of repeated testing for proximal-vein thrombosis is not recommended in patients with persistent inadequate cardiorespiratory reserve. These patients are at risk of serious morbidity or death from pulmonary emboli that may already be present (and responsible in part for the inadequate cardiorespiratory reserve), whereas in patients with adequate cardiorespiratory reserve, the primary clinical objective is to prevent recurrent thromboembolism.

CLINICAL EVIDENCE SUPPORTING THE APPROACH OF SERIAL TESTING FOR PROXIMAL-VEIN THROMBOSIS

The above concepts which were supported by the initial findings of our prospective study,[21(I)] have now been confirmed in an independent validation cohort.[22(I)] The study design and combined findings[21(I),22(I)] are summarized below.

Fifteen hundred and sixty-four consecutive patients with clinically suspected PE were entered into a prospective cohort study with long-term follow-up in all patients groups. Patients with nondiagnostic lung scan findings and adequate cardiorespiratory reserve were managed using serial objective testing for proximal-vein thrombosis. Anticoagulant therapy was withheld or withdrawn in all patients whose serial tests remained negative. The findings in patients negative by serial testing were compared with two concurrent control groups:

a. A negative control group made up of patients with normal perfusion lung scans (in whom PE is absent),[23(I)] and
b. a positive control group composed of patients with high probability lung scans, who have a high frequency (86% to 88%) of PE.[1(I),3(I)] These patients were given anticoagulant therapy.

Of 711 patients in the serial testing cohort, proximal-vein thrombosis was detected in 84 patients (12%). Only 12 of 627 patients (1.9%) negative by serial testing returned on follow-up with objectively documented symptomatic VTE, compared with four of 586 patients

(0.7%) with normal perfusion scans, and eight of 145 patients (5.5%) with high-probability lung scans.[22(I)] Thus, the outcome on follow-up in patients negative by serial testing for proximal-vein thrombosis was similar to the outcome in patients with normal lung scans, and better than (or at least equivalent to) the outcome in patients with high-probability lung scans who received anticoagulant therapy.

These findings indicate that serial objective testing for proximal-vein thrombosis can discriminate between two patient groups:

a. Patients who require treatment because proximal-vein thrombosis is detected, and
b. those whose serial tests are negative, who have a good prognosis without anticoagulant therapy.

The prognosis in patients whose serial tests were negative is similar to the 2% rate of PE on follow-up reported in two studies of patients with negative pulmonary angiograms.[29,30] Serial objective testing for proximal-vein thrombosis provides a practical noninvasive alternative to pulmonary angiography in many patients.

The study also assessed the relation between proximal-vein thrombosis and the number of predisposing factors for VTE that were identified from the clinical history.[21(I)] These predisposing factors were: age 40 years and more, a history of DVT or PE, surgery or trauma in the past 6 months, malignancy, congestive cardiac failure, leg paralysis, pregnancy, and oral contraceptive use. The findings are summarized in Table 1. The frequency of proximal-vein thrombosis detected at presentation, increased from 0% to 18% as the number of predisposing factors present increased from none to three or more (p = 0.013). The frequency of proximal-vein thrombosis detected on serial testing increased from 0% to 15% as the number of predisposing factors present increased from none to three or more (p<0.001). More than 90% of patients in the serial testing group had a predisposing factor for VTE. The overall rate of proximal-vein thrombosis in these patients ranged from 7% to 30% (Table 1). These rates indicate the patients were clearly at risk for clinically important recurrent venous thromboembolic events.

The finding of proximal-vein thrombosis on serial testing in 15% of patients with three or more predisposing factors suggests that serial testing is an important part of management for these patients. Repeated noninvasive testing is likely to be more effective than a single evaluation by venography at the time of presentation. A negative venogram is found in 30% of patients with PE by angiography.[4(I)] These patients may have had proximal-vein thrombosis that embolized in total. If a negative venogram is used to exclude VTE (without performing angiography), patients who re-develop proximal-vein thrombosis will not be detected, and will be exposed to the risk of recurrent PE.

The findings of this prospective study[21(I),22(I)] provide new insight into the natural history of VTE. Proximal-vein thrombosis was detected during initial testing in 12% of patients with nondiagnostic lung scans who had one or more predisposing factors for VTE (Table 1). Since the patients with proximal-vein thrombosis represent only half of the patients with PE, the data suggest that PE was present in 25% of these patients. One-half of these patients with PE were left untreated because proximal-vein thrombosis was absent. The frequency of VTE on follow-up was low (1.9%) in patients negative by serial testing for proximal-vein thrombosis (95% confidence interval 0.8% to 3.0%). These findings support the concept that if proximal-vein thrombosis is absent, treatment is not required, even though PE may be present. This is conditional on the patient having adequate cardiorespiratory reserve (see definition under "Practical Management Approach").

CURRENTLY AVAILABLE OBJECTIVE TESTS FOR DEEP-VEIN THROMBOSIS

The currently available objective tests for proximal-vein thrombosis include venography and several noninvasive tests which have become available over the past 15 years. Venography is the accepted diagnostic reference standard but it is not suitable for serial testing. Venography is useful for defining the presence and extent of venous thrombosis at a single point in time, but a negative venogram is less useful because it does not exclude PE. The technical details and methods for performing and interpreting venography are described in Chapter 13.

The noninvasive tests for DVT can be performed at the bedside or in the clinic and are readily repeated.

Table 1
Frequencies of Proximal-vein Thrombosis According to the Number of Predisposing Factors Present[21]

Proximal-vein Thrombosis	No. of Predisposing Factors			
	0	1	2	3 or more
At presentation	0/26(0%)	10/193(5%)	18/162(11%)	6/33(18%)
On serial testing	0/26(0%)	4/183(2%)	1/44(1%)	4/27(15%)
Total	0/26(0%)	14/193(7%)	19/162(12%)	10/33(30%)

Three approaches have been extensively evaluated: IPG,[11(I),12(I),13(I)16] Doppler ultrasonography,[31–36(I)] and venous imaging with real-time B-mode ultrasonography.[17(I),18,37] Because ultrasound technology has been widely disseminated to many hospitals, venous imaging using real-time ultrasonography is the real contender amongst the noninvasive tests in the 1990s. Impedance plethysmography is an effective low cost technology which continues to play an important role in centers in which this test is available. Doppler ultrasonography has had the disadvantage of subjective interpretation. Recently, an objective Doppler technique has become available[36(I)] that has high sensitivity and specificity for proximal-vein thrombosis (91% and 99% respectively); this objective Doppler technique may provide more reproducible results (see Chapter 16 for technical details and methods).

Of the available noninvasive tests for proximal-vein thrombosis, only IPG has undergone formal evaluation in patients with clinically suspected PE.[3(I),4(I),21(I),22(I)] The sensitivities and specificities of Doppler ultrasound and B-mode venous ultrasound imaging have to be inferred from the findings in patients with clinically suspected venous thrombosis.

Impedance plethysmography is sensitive and specific for proximal-vein thrombosis in patients with clinically suspected PE (sensitivity 86%; specificity 97%).[4(I)] Impedance plethysmography fails to detect most calf-vein thrombi, and may also fail to detect small, nonocclusive proximal-vein thrombi.[14–16] This potential limitation is overcome by performing serial testing. The technical details and methods for performing and interpreting occlusive cuff IPG are outlined in Chapter 14.

Impedance plethysmography does not distinguish between thrombotic and nonthrombotic obstruction to venous outflow. Therefore, falsely positive results may occur if the patient is positioned incorrectly or is inadequately relaxed with constriction of veins by contracting leg muscles, if the vein is compressed by an extravascular mass, or if venous outflow is impaired by raised central venous pressure. Reduced arterial inflow to the limb due to severe obstructive arterial disease may also produce a falsely positive result. Real-time B-mode ultrasound is highly sensitive and specific for proximal-vein thrombosis in symptomatic patients, but is insensitive for calf-vein thrombosis.[17(I),18,37] Therefore, serial testing is required to detect patients who develop proximal extension. B-mode venous ultrasound may fail to detect isolated iliac vein thrombi[17(I),18]; this is a practical limitation in patient groups in whom isolated iliac vein thrombosis is not uncommon (e.g., pregnant patients). B-mode ultrasound may also fail to detect thrombi in the segment of the superficial femoral vein which passes deep in the adductor canal. The technical details and methods for performing real-time B-mode ultrasound are outlined in Chapter 15.

B-mode venous imaging has a potential advantage in specificity over IPG in patients with raised central venous pressure, such as those with congestive cardiac failure (which may result in false-positive IPG findings). In addition, venous imaging may identify patients with extrinsic venous compression (e.g., due to Baker's cyst), which can lead to false-positive IPG results.

PRACTICAL MANAGEMENT APPROACH

A practical algorithm for the management of clinically suspected PE is shown in Figure 1. All patients undergo ventilation-perfusion lung scanning and objective testing for proximal-vein thrombosis on referral.

Normal Perfusion Scan

The finding of a normal perfusion scan excludes clinically important PE. Recent data indicate that proximal-vein thrombosis is found in only 1% of patients with normal perfusion scans,[23(I)] but if proximal-vein thrombosis is confirmed, treatment should be given.

High Probability Scan

Therapy can usually be commenced without further investigation in patients with one or more large perfusion defects (>75% of a lung segment) with ventilation mismatch (high probability scan). Proximal-vein thrombosis is present on referral in 50% of patients with high probability lung findings. The finding of a high probability lung scan together with objective evidence of proximal-vein thrombosis has very high predictive value for the presence of VTE. If objective testing for proximal-vein thrombosis is negative, the high probability scan is still associated with the high frequency of PE, except in patients in whom the initial clinical suspicion was low. In this latter group, and in patients at high risk of bleeding, pulmonary angiography should be considered.

In patients with nondiagnostic lung scan patterns, the management depends on the findings by objective testing for proximal-vein thrombosis and the patient's underlying cardiorespiratory reserve.

Nondiagnostic Scan: Management If Proximal-Vein Thrombosis Is Detected

The finding of proximal-vein thrombosis by objective testing is an indication for anticoagulant therapy,[24(I),25(I),26(I)] regardless of the cause of the patient's respiratory symptoms. In most patients, the treatment of DVT and PE is the same, so the objective confirmation of proximal-vein thrombosis avoids the need for pulmonary angiography. The presence of proximal-vein thrombosis does not necessarily establish a diagnosis of PE because venous thrombosis may have occurred in association with another underlying respiratory illness, which placed the patient at high risk for VTE. If therapy is started on the basis of documented proximal-vein thrombosis, the patient's respiratory status should be closely monitored to detect other disorders, such as pneumonia, that may be present but not evident at the time of presentation. If respiratory symptoms persist and the cause remains uncertain, pulmonary angiography can distinguish between PE and other respiratory problems.

Nondiagnostic Scan: Management If Proximal-Vein Thrombosis Is Absent

If objective testing for proximal-vein thrombosis is negative on referral, anticoagulant therapy can be withheld or withdrawn, and the patient followed with serial testing. This applies if the patient has adequate cardiorespiratory reserve.

The cardiorespiratory reserve is defined as adequate if *none* of the following are present[21(I),22(I)] : pulmonary edema, right ventricular failure, hypotension (systolic <90 mmHg), syncope, acute tachyarrhythmias, or respiratory failure shown by severely abnormal spirometry (FEV_1 <1.0 or VC <1.5) or blood gas measurements (PO_2 <50 mmHg or PCO_2 >45 mmHg on room air). Objective testing should be repeated four to five times over the 14 days following presentation (eg. the day after presentation and then on the 3rd, 5th to 7th, 10th and 14th days). Anticoagulant therapy can be safely withheld if the results by serial testing remain negative.[21(I),22(I)]

Serial testing for proximal-vein thrombosis can also be used in patients with temporary inadequate reserve, if the reserve improves to adequate within 10 days. In these patients, intravenous heparin is given during the period of inadequate cardiorespiratory reserve. When adequate cardiorespiratory reserve is achieved (as defined above), heparin therapy is withdrawn, and the patient followed with serial testing for the next 14 days (as outlined above).

The strategy of repeated testing for proximal-vein thrombosis is *not* recommended in patients with persistent inadequate cardiorespiratory reserve. This is to avoid the risk of serious morbidity or death from pulmonary emboli already present, and responsible in part for the inadequate cardiorespiratory reserve. These patients are usually readily identified at the time of presentation because of clinically overt underlying cardiorespiratory disorders, such as severe chronic obstructive pulmonary disease or severe congestive cardiac failure. If pulmonary angiography is contraindicated or impractical, then it may be prudent to err on the side of treatment in patients with persistent inadequate cardiorespiratory reserve, rather than risk death from PE.

REFERENCES

(I)1. PIOPED Investigators. Value of the ventilation-perfusion scan in acute pulmonary embolism: results of the Prospective Investigation of Pulmonary Embolism Diagnosis (PIOPED). JAMA 1990;263:2753–2759.

(I)2. Hull RD, Raskob GE, Pineo GF, Brant RF. The low-probability lung scan. A need for change in nomenclature. Arch Intern Med 1995;155:1845–1851.

(I)3. Hull RD, Hirsh J, Carter CJ, et al. Diagnostic value of ventilation-perfusion lung scanning in patients with suspected pulmonary embolism. CHEST 1985;88:819–828.

(I)4. Hull RD, Hirsh J, Carter CJ, et al. Pulmonary angiography, ventilation lung scanning, and venography for clinically suspected pulmonary embolism with abnormal perfusion lung scan. Ann Intern Med 1983;98:891–899.

5. Moser KM, LeMoine JR. Is embolic risk conditioned by location of deep venous thrombosis. Ann Intern Med 1981;94:439–444.

6. Kakkar VV, Flanc C, Howe CT, et al. Natural history of post-operative deep-vein thrombosis. Lancet 1969;2:230–233.

7. Moser KM. Venous thromboembolism. Am Rev Respir Dis 1990;141:235–249.

8. Sevitt S, Gallagher N. Venous thrombosis and pulmonary embolism: a clinico-pathological study in injured and burned patients. Br J Surg 1961;48:475–489.

9. Havig GO. Source of pulmonary emboli. Acta Chir Scan 1977;478(Suppl):42–47.

10. Mavor GE, Galloway JMD. The iliofemoral venous segment as a source of pulmonary emboli. Lancet 1967;1:871–874.

(I)11. Hull RD, Hirsh J, Carter CJ, et al. Diagnostic efficacy of impedance plethysmography for clinically suspected deep-vein thrombosis: a randomized trial. Ann Intern Med 1985;102:21–28.

(I)12. Huisman MV, Buller HR, ten Cate JW, Vreeken J. Serial impedance plethysmography for suspected deep venous thrombosis in outpatients: the Amsterdam General Practitioner Study. N Engl J Med 1986;314:823–828.

(I)13. Huisman MV, Buller HR, ten Cate JW, Heijermans HSF, van der Loan J, et al. Management of clinically suspected acute venous thrombosis in outpatients with serial impedance plethysmography in a community hospital setting. Arch Intern Med 1989;149:511–513.

14. Wheeler HB. Impedance phlebography. Technique, interpretation and results. Arch Surg 1972;104:164–169.

15. Hull RD, Van Aken WG, Hirsh J, et al. Impedance plethysmography using the occlusive cuff technique in the diagnosis of venous thrombosis. Circulation 1976;53:696–700.

16. Hull RD, Taylor DW, Hirsh J, et al. Impedance plethysmography: the relationship between venous filling and sensitivity and specificity for proximal-vein thrombosis. Circulation 1978;58:898–902.

(I)17. Lensing AW, Prandoni P, Brandjes D, et al. Detection of deep-vein thrombosis by real-time B-mode ultrasonography. N Engl J Med 1989;320:342–345.

18. White RH, McGahan JP, Daschbach MM, Hartling RP. Diagnosis of deep-vein thrombosis using Duplex ultrasound. Ann Intern Med 1989;111:297–304.

19. Secker-Walker RH. On purple emperors, pulmonary embolism, and venous thrombosis. Ann Intern Med 1983;98:1006–1008.

20. Bone RC. Ventilation/perfusion scan in pulmonary embolism. The emperor is incompletely attired. JAMA 1990;263:2794–2795.

(I)21. Hull RD, Raskob GE, Coates G, Panju AA, Gill GJ. A new non-invasive management strategy for patients with suspected pulmonary embolism. Arch Intern Med 1989;149:2549–2555.

(I)22. Hull RD, Raskob GE, Ginsberg JS, et al. A noninvasive strategy for the management of patients with suspected pulmonary embolism. Arch Intern Med 1994;154: 289–297.

(I)23. Hull RD, Raskob GE, Coates G, Panju AA. Clinical validity of a normal perfusion lung scan in patients with suspected pulmonary embolism. CHEST 1990;897:23–26.

(I)24. Hull RD, Delmore T, Genton E, et al. Warfarin sodium versus low-dose heparin in the long-term treatment of venous thrombosis. N Engl J Med 1979;301:855–858.

(I)25. Hull RD, Raskob GE, Hirsh J, et al. Continuous intravenous heparin compared with intermittent subcutaneous heparin in the initial treatment of proximal-vein thrombosis. N Engl J Med 1986; 315:1109–1114.

(I)26. Brandjes DPM, Buller HR, Heijboer H, Jagt J, de Rijk M, et al. Comparative trial of heparin and oral anticoagulants in the initial treatment of proximal deep-vein thrombosis. N Engl J Med 1992;327:1485–1489.

(I)27. Heijboer H, Buller HR, Lensing AWA, et al. A comparison of real-time B-mode ultrasonography with impedance plethysmography for the diagnosis of deep-vein thrombosis in symptomatic outpatients. N Engl J Med 1993;329:1365–1369.

(I)28. Lagerstedt CI, Olsson CG, Fagher B, Oqvist BW. Albrechlsson U. Need for long-term anticoagulant treatment in symptomatic calf-vein thrombosis. Lancet 1985;2:515–518.

29. Novelline RA, Oksana HB, Athanasoulis CA, et al. The clinical course of patients with suspected pulmonary embolism and a negative pulmonary arteriogram. Radiology 1978;126:561–567.

30. Cheely R, McCartney WH, Perry JR, et al. The role of noninvasive tests versus pulmonary angiography in the diagnosis of pulmonary embolism. Am J Med 1981;70: 17–22.

31. Strandness DE, Sumner DS. Ultrasonic velocity detector in the diagnosis of thrombophlebitis. Arch Surg 1972;104: 180–183.

32. Sumner DS, Lambeth A. Reliability of Doppler ultrasound in the diagnosis of acute venous thrombosis both above and below the knee. Am J Surg 1979;138:205–210.

33. Meadway J, Nicolaides AN, Walker CJ, O'Connell JD. Value of Doppler ultrasound in diagnosis of clinically suspected deep-vein thrombosis. Br Med J 1975;4: 552–554.

34. Barnes RW, Russell HE, Wilson MR. Doppler ultrasonic evaluation of venous disease. 2nd ed. Iowa City, Iowa: University of Iowa Press; 1975;1–251.

35. Flanigan DP, Goodreau JJ, Burnham SJ, Bergen JJ, Yao JS. Vascular-laboratory diagnosis of clinically suspected acute deep-vein thrombosis. Lancet 1978;2:331–334.

(I)36. Lensing AWA, Levi MM, Buller HR, et al. Diagnosis of deep-vein thrombosis using an objective Doppler method. Ann Intern Med 1990;113:9–13.

37. Becker DM, Philbrick JT, Abbitt PL. Real-time ultrasonography for the diagnosis of lower extremity deep venous thrombosis. The wave of the future? Arch Intern Med 1989;149:1731–1734.

25

A Strategy for the Treatment of Patients with Suspected Pulmonary Embolism using Noninvasive Tests

Russell D. Hull, Gary E. Raskob, Graham F. Pineo

INTRODUCTION

Pulmonary embolism (PE) is a common disorder in the United States, as demonstrated in a population-based study reported in 1991.[1] In that study, the incidence of PE was 21 patients per 100,000. The diagnosis of PE is a formidable problem because of the nonspecificity of the clinical findings associated with this disorder,[2-7] as well as the diagnostic uncertainties and challenges presented by both ventilation-perfusion lung scanning[2,3,5-14] and pulmonary angiography.[2,3,8,15,16]

The use of objective tests to detect venous thrombosis and substantial improvements in recent years have enhanced the clinician's ability to deal more effectively with the diagnostic challenges presented by PE. Many patients with PE have residual deep-vein thrombosis (DVT) in the lower extremities.[7,8] Indeed, as Bone has stated,[17] the greatest recent advance has occurred in the noninvasive diagnosis of deep-venous thrombi (which are the usual antecedents to pulmonary emboli), using either impedance studies or duplex ultrasound study of the legs. Today, the clinical history, used in conjunction with evaluation of arterial blood gas levels, ventilation-perfusion scans, and noninvasive studies of the deep veins of the legs, can markedly improve the clinician's ability to diagnose pulmonary embolic disease. In contrast, it was shown recently, in consecutive patients with suspected PE, that ventilation-perfusion lung scanning alone is diagnostically helpful in only a minority of patients.[5-8]

Studies of the natural history of DVT have established that new PE occurs in up to 50% of patients in whom proximal-vein thrombosis is confirmed, but is unlikely in its absence.[18,19] Further support for these observations are that: (1) inadequate therapy for proximal-vein thrombosis is associated with a high risk (20% to 50%) of recurrent venous thrombosis and PE,[20-22] and (2) if proximal-vein thrombosis has been excluded by serial objective testing in patients with symptomatic DVT, the prognosis without treatment is excellent because of a low risk (<1%) of clinically evident PE.[23-28]

Secker-Walker[10] has suggested studying the lower extremities with objective testing for proximal-vein thrombosis in patients with suspected PE and abnormal perfusion scans. Confirmation of proximal-vein thrombosis is an indication for treatment.[20-22] Noninvasive objective tests for proximal-vein thrombosis, that is, impedance plethysmography (IPG)[23-27] and duplex ultrasound imaging,[27-30] have become readily available. These tests can be performed at the bedside or in the clinic and are readily repeated.[23-30]

As we have reported previously, serial objective testing provides a practical noninvasive alternative to pulmonary angiography in patients with non-high-probability (nondiagnostic) lung scans and adequate cardiorespiratory reserve.[31] Because this inference was based on a single study,[31] a prospective study was carried out. The rational was twofold: (1) confirming or refuting our original observation[31] would be done in an independent prospective cohort, and (2) increasing the number of patients would provide narrow confidence limits for the observed outcomes of subsequent fatal and nonfatal venous thromboembolism in patients referred with suspected PE.

We performed a prospective comparative study in 1564 consecutive patients with suspected PE who underwent ventilation-perfusion lung scanning and objective testing for proximal-vein thrombosis. The primary goal was to assess the prognosis in patients: (1) who had abnormal lung scans that were not high probability for pulmonary embolism (nondiagnostic lung scans), (2) who

---

From *Venous Thromboembolism: An Evidence-Based Atlas* edited by Russell Hull, Gary Raskob, Graham Pineo © 1996, Futura Publishing Co., Armonk, NY.

201

were not taking anticoagulant therapy, and (3) whose serial noninvasive test results were negative for proximal-vein thrombosis.

PATIENTS AND METHODS

Study Population

A prospective study was performed on 1564 consecutive patients with suspected PE who were referred from both the community and hospital settings to the Thromboembolism Service at Chedoke and McMaster Hospitals, Hamilton, Ontario. Patients were referred between September 1984 and December 1991. The thromboembolism unit was structured to allow immediate access to diagnostic strategies. The study was performed in two independent consecutive phases and the first phase was reported previously.[31]

Each patient was examined on the day of referral by the consultant physician and study nurse who confirmed and recorded (on special forms) the clinical history and physical findings. These are listed in Table 1.

Each patient had an electrocardiogram and a chest roentgenogram, and underwent IPG (to detect proximal-vein thrombosis) and ventilation-perfusion lung scanning. Impedance plethysmography is a sensitive test for the presence of proximal-vein thrombosis in patients with clinically suspected PE.[8] Venography was performed in patients with abnormal IPG results to confirm the presence and extent of proximal-vein thrombosis.

The ventilation-perfusion scans were interpreted by a nuclear medicine physician (G.C.) and a thromboembolism consultant physician (R.D.H.) at the time lung scanning was performed. The two physicians conferred on the lung-scan findings and, based on their consensus, the patients were entered into one of the three cohorts listed below.

STUDY PROTOCOL

The study was designed and performed as a prospective cohort analytic clinical trial with long-term follow-up in all patient groups. One cohort was managed using serial noninvasive leg testing (impedance plethysmograph) and the findings were compared with those from two

Table 1
Clinical Characteristics, Demographic Findings, and Proximal-Vein Thrombosis on Initial Testing in the Study Cohorts

Demographic Findings	Study Cohort		
	Nondiagnostic Lung Scan (Serial Noninvasive Leg Testing) (n = 711)	Normal Lung Scan (n = 586)	High-Probability Lung Scan (n = 150)
Age, y (mean ± SD)	63 ± 24	43 ± 23	62 ± 15
Males/females	303/408	150/436	74/76
Inpatients/outpatients	284/427	163/423	49/101
Symptoms on presentation, No. (%)			
Pleuritic chest pain	292 (41)	279 (48)	62 (41)
Central chest pain	120 (17)	140 (24)	23 (15)
Dyspnea at rest	375 (53)	227 (39)	80 (53)
Dyspnea on mild or moderate exertion	425 (60)	293 (50)	104 (69)
Hemoptysis	52 (7)	25 (4)	10 (7)
Syncope	37 (5)	22 (4)	19 (13)
Signs on presentation, No. (%)			
Pleural friction rub	35 (5)	22 (4)	5 (3)
Elevated jugular venous pulse	128 (18)	41 (7)	30 (20)
Central cyanosis	25 (4)	2 (0.3)	1 (0.7)
Respiratory rate, >20/min	463 (65)	274 (47)	98 (65)
Chest wall tenderness	47 (7)	55 (9)	10 (7)
Left parasternal heave	2 (0.3)	0	3 (2)
Abnormal physical examination of chest	385 (54)	106 (18)	72 (48)
Other findings, No. (%)			
History of pulmonary embolism	28 (4)	14 (2)	15 (10)
History of deep-vein thrombosis	70 (10)	36 (6)	26 (17)
Surgery in past 6 mo.	165 (23)	91 (16)	42 (28)
Ischemic heart disease	140 (20)	66 (11)	31 (21)
Congestive heart failure	113 (16)	40 (7)	6 (4)
Chronic obstructive lung disease	144 (20)	25 (4)	16 (11)
Pneumonia	67 (9)	17 (3)	5 (3)
Carcinoma	73 (10)	34 (6)	26 (17)
Proximal-vein thrombosis on initial testing, No. (%)	84 (12)	10 (2)	38 (25)

(Reproduced with permission from Hull, et al. Arch Int Med 1994;154:252).

concurrent control groups: (1) a negative control group made up of patients with normal perfusion lung scans (in whom PE is absent),[5,32,33] in whom anticoagulant therapy was withheld, and (2) a positive control group composed of patients with high-probability lung scans (defined below), who had a high frequency of PE (90%)[5,7] and who were treated with anticoagulant therapy.

IDENTIFICATION OF STUDY COHORTS

Nondiagnostic Lung Scan Cohort (Serial Noninvasive Leg-Testing Cohort)

Patients were entered into the serial noninvasive leg-testing cohort if they had a nondiagnostic lung scan and their cardiorespiratory reserve was defined as adequate (see below), either at the time of presentation or during the first 10 days after presentation.

A lung scan was defined as nondiagnostic if one or more perfusion defects were associated with a corresponding ventilation defect (ventilation-perfusion match), were subsegmental (excluding large defects with ventilation mismatch), or corresponded to the chest roentgenographic defect.

Cardiorespiratory reserve was defined as adequate if none of the following were present: pulmonary edema, right ventricular failure, hypotension (systolic <90 mm Hg), syncope, acute tachyarrhythmias, or respiratory failure shown by severely abnormal spirometry (forced expiratory volume in 1 second <1.0, or vital capacity <1.5) or blood gas measurements (PO_2 <50 mm Hg, or PCO_2 >45 mm Hg breathing room air).

Impedance plethysmography was performed at presentation and, if negative, was performed serially with the patient's consent for 14 days as follows: it was repeated the day after presentation and on the 3rd, 5th or 7th, 10th, and 14th days. Anticoagulant therapy was withheld or withdrawn in all patients whose serial IPG remained negative. Anticoagulant therapy using previously described protocols[34,35] was indicated in patients with confirmed proximal-vein thrombosis.

The patients with nondiagnostic lung scans and persistent inadequate cardiorespiratory reserve for 10 days or more were managed by the responsible attending physician, and serial noninvasive leg testing was not performed in this group. Repeated testing for proximal-vein thrombosis was not recommended in these patients. It was important to avoid the risk of serious morbidity or death from pulmonary emboli which might already be present and be responsible in part for the poor cardiorespiratory reserve, particularly in patients with pulmonary hypertension. These patients could usually be readily identified at the time of presentation because of clinically overt underlying cardiorespiratory disorders, such as severe chronic obstructive pulmonary disease or congestive cardiac failure. The study team recommended that pa-

tients with persistent inadequate cardiorespiratory reserve either undergo pulmonary angiography or be given anticoagulant therapy. The management was left to the discretion of the responsible attending physician. This strategy allowed us to test the impact of intuitive clinical decision-making on the patient's long-term outcome. Intuitive clinical decision making was based on the clinical findings, ancillary tests, and lung scanning. The findings in this group are reported separately.

Normal Lung-Scan Cohort (Negative Control Group)

Patients were entered into the normal lung-scan cohort if perfusion defects were absent in all the views. These patients were considered to be free of PE.[5,32,33] Anticoagulant therapy was withheld or withdrawn immediately in all patients with normal lung scans, regardless of the clinical findings (except in the occasional patient with associated proximal-vein thrombosis).

High-Probability Lung-Scan Cohort (Positive Control Group)

Patients were entered into the high-probability lung-scan cohort if the ventilation-perfusion scan demonstrated either segmental or greater mismatched defects[5–8,12], or large subsegmental defects with ventilation mismatch. These patients were considered to have PE[5,7,8] and were managed by anticoagulant therapy[34,35] or, if anticoagulant therapy was contraindicated, by a Greenfield filter.[36]

Long-term Follow-up

The outcome in each of the study cohorts was assessed by long-term follow-up for 3 months. In all patients in each study cohort follow-up was successful.

All patients were asked to return at once if they developed symptoms or signs suggesting PE or DVT. Those with clinically suspected PE underwent ventilation-perfusion lung scanning. Pulmonary angiography was performed in patients with new perfusion defects that were not high-probability for PE.[5,7] The technique for performing pulmonary angiography and the diagnostic criteria for PE have been described previously.[8,15,37] Patients with clinically suspected DVT underwent noninvasive leg testing (IPG) and venography, according to previously described protocols.[24,38]

All patients were available for follow-up and re-evaluated routinely at 3 months. An interim history was taken. It addressed general health and specific symptoms (including chest pain, dyspnea, hemoptysis, or syncope, as well as leg pain, tenderness, or swelling), hospital admission, and the use of anticoagulants. The majority of patients were seen in the clinic, and testing with IPG was repeated. If patients were geographically inaccessible, follow-up was carried out by telephone. If patients died, the cause of death was documented from autopsy, coroner's report, or independent clinical review.

Techniques and Interpretation of Lung Scanning, Impedance Plethysmography, and Venography

The techniques for performing and interpreting ventilation-perfusion lung scanning, IPG, and venography have been previously described in detail.[7,8,39–42] Ventilation lung scanning using technetium Tc 99m sulfur colloid aerosol was described by Coates et al.[42] Perfusion lung scanning was performed after ventilation imaging as previously described.[7,8] The perfusion lung scan was considered either normal or abnormal if a perfusion defect was present in one or more views. In patients with abnormal perfusion scans the findings were classified as either high-probability according to previously described criteria or nondiagnostic.

METHODOLOGIC CONSIDERATIONS

The correctness of withholding anticoagulant therapy in patients whose serial noninvasive leg-test results were negative was tested by long-term follow-up. The validity of this approach is based on the observation that inadequate management of proximal-vein thrombosis is associated with a high frequency (20% to 50%) of recurrent venous thromboembolic events that can be readily measured.[20–22] These venous thromboembolic events on follow-up can be used as end points for comparing study cohorts. Long-term follow-up has been used previously in several studies to validate negative findings by objective testing for DVT[24–27,43] or PE.[5–8,16,32,33,44]

BIOLOGICAL CONSIDERATIONS

Proximal-vein thrombosis is strongly associated with PE[7,8] and provides a useful marker for the presence of PE. Previous prospective studies have shown that residual proximal-vein thrombosis is detected by pulmonary angiography in 50% of patients with PE.[7,8] Therefore, the expected rate of PE in any group of symptomatic patients is estimated by doubling the observed frequency of proximal-vein thrombosis.

The risk of developing venous thromboembolism is increased by predisposing factors.[45] Furthermore, there is an increased risk of recurrent venous thromboembolism in patients with established proximal-vein thrombosis who have predisposing factors.[20,38] For these reasons, we evaluated the relationship between proximal-vein thrombosis detected at presentation and on serial testing, and the number of predisposing factors present in patients entered into the serial noninvasive leg-testing cohort. The results of the risk-factor analysis

for the total cohort are beyond the scope of this article and are reported separately.

STATISTICAL CONSIDERATIONS

In each of the study cohorts, the frequencies of proximal-vein thrombosis and the frequencies of venous thromboembolism (VTE) on follow-up were compared using the X^2 test or Fisher's Exact Test. The confidence limits for the true incidence of VTE on follow-up were calculated from the binomial distribution; confidence limits for the difference in this incidence between the serial noninvasive leg-testing cohort and the control groups were calculated using the normal approximation to the binomial distribution.

RESULTS

Study Population

There were 1564 consecutive patients with suspected PE. Age ranged from 12 to 96 years (mean, 56 years); 585 were men (37%) and 979 were women (65%). At the time of presentation, 1027 were outpatients (66%) and 537 were inpatients (34%). An additional 99 patients were ineligible for the study: in 93, IPG could not be performed owing to leg casts, leg amputation, or other reasons, and in six ventilation lung scanning could not be performed.

Of the 1564 patients, 711 (46%) with nondiagnostic lung scans were entered into the serial noninvasive leg-testing cohort, 586 (38%) into the normal lung-scan cohort (negative cohort group), and 150 (10%) into the high-probability lung-scan cohort (positive control group). The remaining 117 patients (8%) had nondiagnostic lung scans and persistent inadequate cardiorespiratory reserve.

Table 1 shows clinical characteristics, demographic findings, and the frequency of proximal-vein thrombosis at entry in the study cohorts. Because the findings on entry for phases I and II are similar, the findings for the total population are presented.

Clinical Characteristics and Demographic Findings

The serial noninvasive leg-testing cohort differed from the normal lung-scan cohort in that the average age was greater and there were more males. Also, there was more underlying cardiorespiratory disease, and the proportions of patients with congestive cardiac failure, chronic obstructive pulmonary disease, pneumonia, and abnormal findings on chest examination were two to three times higher (Table 1).

The serial noninvasive leg-testing and high-probability lung-scan cohorts were comparable on presentation, except for the following clinical characteristics which occurred more frequently in the high-probability lung-scan cohort: dyspnea on exertion, a history of carcinoma, prior venous thromboembolism, and prior surgery (Table 1).

Proximal-Vein Thrombosis on Initial Testing

There was a gradient in the frequency of proximal-vein thrombosis detected at presentation in the study cohorts. The frequency was highest in the high-probability lung-scan cohort (38 [25.3%] of 150 patients), intermediary in the nondiagnostic lung-scan cohort (84[11.8%] of 711 patients), and lowest in the normal lung-scan cohort (10 [1.7%] of 586 patients) (P<0.0001).

Findings from Serial Noninvasive Testing for Proximal-Vein Thrombosis

Serial noninvasive leg testing detected proximal-vein thrombosis in 16 (2.3%) of the 711 patients with nondiagnostic lung scans. Eighty-four (11.8%) of the 711 patients had associated proximal DVT, of which 16 (19.1%) were detected on serial follow-up. Of the 16 patients detected by serial testing, 3 were detected on day 2 (the day after presentation) and the remainder were detected on day 3 (1 patient), day 4 (3 patients), day 5 (1 patient), day 6 (1 patient), day 8 (3 patients), day 10 (3 patients), and day 13 (1 patient), respectively. None of the 16 patients detected by serial testing died from PE before anticoagulant therapy had been started.

Long-Term Outcomes in the Study Cohorts

Of the 627 patients whose serial noninvasive test results remained negative, 12 patients (1.9%) returned with objectively documented symptomatic venous thromboembolism on follow-up (95% confidence limits, 0.8% to 3.0%). One of these patients died of PE (confirmed by autopsy). This patient underwent a hemicolectomy for carcinoma of the colon during the fourth week and died of PE one week later, despite having received prophylaxis with low-dose heparin.

In those patients whose serial noninvasive leg-test results were negative, the frequency of venous thromboembolism on follow-up was compared with each of the other cohorts. The long-term outcomes in the normal lung-scan cohort (negative control group) and high-probability lung-scan cohort (positive control group) are presented in turn below and in comparison with the serial noninvasive leg-testing cohort. Table 2 summarizes the outcomes on follow-up.

Of the 586 patients in the normal lung-scan cohort, four (0.7%) (95% confidence limits, 0.02% to 1.3%) had objectively documented symptomatic venous thromboembolism on follow-up (P = 0.10) (compared with 12 [1.9%] of the 627 patients [95% confidence limits, 0.8% to 3.0%] whose serial noninvasive leg-test results were negative). Since the observed difference in the frequency of venous thromboembolism on follow-up in the two cohorts was 1.2% in favour of the normal lung-scan cohort, it is unlikely (P<0.05) that a true difference in favor of this group would be higher than 2.5%, and the difference could be as much as 0.03% in favor of the serial noninvasive leg-testing cohort. No patients in the normal lung-scan cohort died of PE.

One hundred and forty-five of the 150 patients in the high-probability lung-scan cohort received anticoagulant therapy. Eight patients in this cohort had objectively documented symptomatic venous thromboembolism on follow-up and all eight had received anticoagulant therapy. Thus, eight (5.5%) of the 145 treated patients (95% confidence limits, 1.8% to 9.2%) had objectively documented symptomatic venous thromboembolism on follow-up (P = 0.036, Fisher's Exact Test) compared with 12 (1.9%) of the 627 patients (95% confidence limits, 0.8% to 3.0%) whose serial noninvasive leg-test results remained negative. Since the observed difference in the frequency of venous thromboembolism in the two cohorts was 3.6% in fa-

Table 2
Long-term Outcome in the Study Cohorts*

	Serial Noninvasive Leg Testing Negative n = 627			Normal Lung Scan n = 586			High-Probability Lung Scan n = 145		
	Phase I n = 371	Phase II n = 256	Total Cohort, n = 627	Phase I n = 315	Phase II n = 271	Total Cohort, n = 586	Phase I n = 66	Phase II n = 79	Total Cohort, n = 145
Frequency of VTE on follow-up, No (%)	10 (2.7)	2 (1)	12 (1.9)	3 (1.0)	1 (0.4)	4 (0.7)	5 (7.6)	3 (3.8)	8 (5.5)
Type of event Time of event since entry, wk	4 PE; 6 DVT ...	2 DVT 2, 4, 5, 5 2, 4, 4, 5, 6, 6 12, 12	4 PE; 8 DVT ...	1 PE; 2 DVT ...	1 PE 7, 9	2 PE; 2 DVT ... 2, 3	3 PE; 2 DVT ...	1 PE; 2 DVT 1, 4d, 5d, 2; 3, 5, 6, 10	4 PE; 4 DVT ...

Table 3
Number and Causes of Deaths in the Study Cohorts*

Cause of Death	Nondiagnostic Scan (Serial Noninvasive Leg Testing) (n = 711)		Normal Scan (n = 586)		High Probability Scan (n = 150)	
	Patients	Time	Patients	Time	Patients	Time
Confirmed pulmonary embolism	1	5	0	. . .	1	1 d
Suspected but not confirmed pulmonary embolism	2+	5, 8	0	. . .	1†	3 d
Myocardial infarction	6‡	1 d, 3, 3, 4, 5, 8	6	1, 1, 4, 8, 10, 10	1	8
Disseminated carcinoma	20	2 d, 1, 1, 2, 2, 2, 2, 3, 3, 3, 5, 5, 5, 6, 7, 7, 8, 9, 11, 14	6	1, 2, 3, 6, 7, 10	5	2, 11, 12, 12, 14
Bronchopneumonia	5	1, 4, 4, 6, 10	2	3, 5	0	. . .
Cerebrovascular accident	3	3, 4, 7	0	. . .	1	9
Acute renal failure	4	2, 2, 6, 9	0	. . .	0	. . .
Cardiomyopathy	2	1, 14	2	4, 8	1	2
Acute or chronic obstructive lung disease	3	2, 3, 7	0	. . .	0	. . .
Septicemia	3	5, 9, 10	0	. . .	0	. . .
Aortic aneurysm	1	2	0	. . .	0	. . .
Lymphoma	0	. . .	0	. . .	1	5
Adrenal insufficiency	1	4	0	. . .	0	. . .

* The time is given in weeks, unless otherwise stated.
† These three patients had proximal deep-vein thrombosis at entry.
‡ One patient had an unconfirmed cause of death due to myocardial infarction (possibly pulmonary embolism).
(Reproduced with permission from Hull, et al. Arch Int Med 1994:254).

vor of the serial noninvasive leg-testing cohort, a true difference in favor of this group could have been as much as 7.5% and it is unlikely (P<0.05) that the difference would be more than 0.3% in favor of the high-probability lung-scan cohort. One of the patients in the high-probability lung-scan cohort died of PE (confirmed by autopsy) within 24 hours of entry.

DEATHS

Table 3 shows the number and causes of deaths in the study cohorts.

COMMENT

Our findings support the use of serial noninvasive leg testing in patients with suspected PE who have nondiagnostic lung-scan findings. The management approach evaluated in this prospective study separated patients with suspected PE into four prognostic cohorts: the normal lung-scan cohort, the high-probability lung-scan cohort, the nondiagnostic lung-scan cohort with adequate reserve, and the nondiagnostic lung-scan cohort with chronically inadequate reserve. Because of the broad scope of the study, the findings in patients with chronically inadequate cardiorespiratory reserve and nondiagnostic lung-scan findings will be reported separately.

The findings we present reflect cohort comparisons for patients with suspected PE who had adequate cardiorespiratory reserve and nondiagnostic lung-scan findings. Both the normal lung-scan and serial noninvasive leg-testing cohorts had a low frequency of VTE on follow-up (0.7% and 1.9%, respectively). When the serial leg-testing and normal lung-scan cohorts were compared, the 95% confidence limits showed that a true difference on follow-up in the frequency of VTE in favor of the normal lung-scan cohort was unlikely (P<0.05) to be more than 2.5%. The difference could have been as much as 0.03% in favor of the serial noninvasive leg-testing cohort. Compared to the normal lung-scan cohort (Table 1), the serial noninvasive leg-testing cohort was older, there was more underlying cardiorespiratory disease, and there was a much higher frequency of proximal-vein thrombosis on initial testing. Although the findings favor a poorer prognosis in the serial leg-testing cohort, the clinical outcome was good, with a low frequency of VTE on follow-up. The one patient in the serial noninvasive leg-testing cohort who died of confirmed PE did so on the fifth week of follow-up, after exposure to a new high risk of PE by surgery for colon cancer one week earlier.

When the serial noninvasive leg testing and high-probability lung-scan cohorts were compared, the respective frequencies of VTE were 1.9% and 5.5% (P = 0.036) including one death from PE in the high-probability lung-scan cohort. The 95% confidence limits showed that the true frequency of VTE on follow-up in favor of the serial noninvasive leg-testing cohort could have been as much as 7.5%, and was unlikely (P<0.05) to be more than 0.3% in favor of the high-probability lung-scan group. The above findings indicate that, in patients in whom serial noninvasive leg testing is negative and who do not receive anticoagulant therapy, the long-term outcome is better than, or at least equivalent to, the outcome in patients with high-probability lung scans who receive anticoagulants. In the high-probability lung-scan cohort, there was a higher proportion of patients with carcinoma or a history of VTE than in the serial leg-testing cohort (Table 1). These clinical characteristics predispose patients to recurrent VTE[38,45] and may account for the higher frequency of VTE on follow-up observed in the high-probability lung-scan cohort.

Proximal-vein thrombosis was detected and confirmed in 11.8% of patients in the serial leg-testing cohort. This rate indicates that these patients were at high risk for clinically important PE. The rate of 11.8% is not low. It is similar to the rate observed in a broad spectrum of patients who presented with symptoms and signs of venous thrombosis.[24] Further, the 11.8% rate of proximal-vein thrombosis places these patients in the accepted high-risk category for fatal PE.[46] In the nondiagnostic lung-scan cohort, proximal-vein thrombosis was detected at presentation in 9.5% of patients and in 2.5% of patients on serial testing. In the high-probability lung-scan cohort, proximal-vein thrombosis was detected on initial testing in 25% of patients. This rate is not low because a considerable proportion of patients in this cohort had a history of DVT or PE that results in a persistent high-probability pattern (Table 1). Previous prospective studies[5] have shown that the predictive value of the high-probability lung scan for the presence of PE declines markedly in patients with a history of VTE.[5]

Our findings indicate that a practical noninvasive strategy in patients with adequate cardiorespiratory reserve and nondiagnostic lung scans is available to the clinician that: (1) avoids pulmonary angiography, (2) identifies patients with proximal-vein thrombosis who require treatment, and (3) avoids the need for treatment and further investigation in the majority of patients. In this study, repeated leg testing was performed five times over the 14 days following presentation. In previous studies in patients with suspected DVT, fewer repeated evaluations were carried out over a shorter period of time (7 to 10 days).[25–27] Excellent long-term outcomes were obtained in these patients in whom serial testing was negative. It may be sufficient to carry out fewer repeated evaluations than we did. On the other hand, of the 16 patients in whom proximal-vein thrombosis was detected on serial testing, seven were detected between days 8 and 14, and 4 between days 10 and 14. Assessment of the clinical factors predisposing to VTE will likely play a practical role, because serial noninvasive leg testing in patients with

multiple risk factors frequently identifies evolving proximal-vein thrombosis which was absent on initial testing.[31] We have shown previously that, in patients with multiple risk factors in the serial noninvasive leg-testing cohort in whom initial leg testing was negative, there was a high frequency (15%) of proximal DVT detected on serial testing.[31] (The results of the risk factor analysis for the total cohort are beyond the scope of this article and are reported separately).

This study entered a sufficient number of patients to provide narrow confidence intervals for the long-term outcomes observed in the serial noninvasive leg-testing cohort. This study used a cohort analytic design, a design appropriate for a study that evaluates prognosis.[47] Care was taken to ensure that bias did not influence the outcomes in the study. Selection bias was avoided by entering consecutive patients with suspected PE. The entering of patients into the study cohorts was based on their lung-scan findings and cardiorespiratory reserve, using criteria defined before the study began. Biased allocation due to other selection processes was thereby avoided. The lung-scan and cardiorespiratory-reserve criteria used are readily reproducible. Bias due to a low prevalence of VTE at entry in the serial noninvasive leg-testing cohort did not occur.[31]

Long-term follow-up was used to assess the prognosis of each of the study cohorts. This approach is valid because inadequate management of VTE is associated with a high frequency (20% to 50%) of recurrent venous thromboembolic events that can be readily measured.[20–22] To avoid diagnostic suspicion bias,[47,48] objective testing was performed in all patients who, on follow-up, presented with symptoms or signs suggesting PE or DVT.

The aggregate data for patients with DVT indicate that proximal-vein thrombosis is the important prognostic marker for recurrent VTE.[18–27] Our findings are consistent with two bodies of existing literature: (i) studies of the natural history of DVT indicate that PE is unlikely in the absence of proximal-vein thrombosis,[18,19] and (ii) recent studies evaluating objective testing in patients with suspected DVT indicate that clinically evident PE is rare (<1% to 2%) in patients whose serial objective test results were negative for proximal DVT.[24–27] Our study extends this concept to the treatment of patients with suspected PE. In patients with adequate cardiorespiratory reserve and nondiagnostic lung scans, noninvasive leg testing separated patients into 2 cohorts: those with proximal-vein thrombosis and those without. In the latter cohort, the prognosis without anticoagulant therapy was excellent. Only 12 (1.9%) of the 627 patients with nondiagnostic lung scan results and serial negative noninvasive leg testing suffered subsequent VTE on long-term follow-up.

Our findings support the concept suggested by Moser and LeMoine[19] that the presence or absence of proximal-vein thrombosis "provides a framework for selecting patients who require therapy." Clinical trials indicate that proximal-vein thrombosis is a marker for the presence of PE. In initial testing, half of the patients with confirmed PE had proximal-vein thrombosis.[7,8] Thus, the expected rate of PE on presentation in our nondiagnostic lung-scan cohort of patients with adequate cardiorespiratory reserve is twice the observed proximal-vein thrombosis rate: 11.8% x 2 = 23.6% with PE.

Of the 1564 patients presenting with suspected PE, 711 (45.5%) had nondiagnostic lung scans and adequate cardiorespiratory reserve. Our findings are consistent with recent studies indicating that ventilation-perfusion lung scanning alone is not helpful in many patients.[5-8] In addition, recent studies indicate that the use of clinical intuition combined with knowledge of the lung-scan findings is useful in only a minority of patients.[5,7] Noninvasive serial leg testing, now based on rigorous evidence, provides an alternative to pulmonary angiography in these patients. It provides a practical alternative strategy for patients with suspected PE in institutions where pulmonary angiography is unavailable or of limited access.

Our study entered a broad spectrum of patients with a wide variety of clinical characteristics, comorbid conditions, and predisposing factors. Patients were referred from both the community and hospital settings, and many patients were assessed. For these reasons, our patients should be representative of those presenting to other community and hospital-based practices.

Our findings reinforce two biological concepts. First, thrombotic extension of submassive PE is not an important cause of morbidity in patients with adequate cardiorespiratory reserve. Because residual proximal-vein thrombosis was present in only half of patients with PE, it is evident that there was a similar number of patients in the serial leg-testing cohort who had submassive PE but who did not receive anticoagulant therapy. The outcomes on follow-up indicate that patients whose serial leg-testing results remain negative do well without anticoagulant therapy. Second, in most patients, recurrent PE comes from proximal-vein thrombosis. Isolated pelvic-vein thrombosis or calf-vein thrombosis are not associated with clinically important PE, as long as they do not extend into the proximal venous segment. It should be possible to generalize the use of noninvasive serial leg testing to other methods of interpreting ventilation-perfusion lung scanning[5,9,13,49] and to other methods of noninvasive leg testing. Duplex ultrasound with B-mode imaging is widely available and, based on the principles outlined by our study, should be readily interchangeable with IPG. Because it is also sensitive and specific for proximal-vein thrombosis, B-mode imaging offers an attractive alternative to IPG.[28-30] Whichever noninvasive leg test is used, it is important that the validity of the noninvasive test is confirmed in the center of use.

A recent retrospective study[50] suggested that B-mode imaging may be superior to IPG. However, it is not clear whether the findings reported reflect problems with ascending contrast venography, which was used for comparison with the noninvasive tests, or to quality assurance problems with IPG. In some patients venography was classified as inadequate because of nonfilling venous segments.[41] However, in the presence of a positive B-mode ultrasound test, such segments were found to be indicative of venous thrombosis. The findings of the retrospective study by Anderson et al,[50] are contradicted by a prospective comparison of ultrasound and IPG. The latter study reported that compression ultrasound and IPG have similar high sensitivities for proximal-vein thrombosis (97% and 96%, respectively).[51] A recent large study of outpatients from the Netherlands[27] confirmed that IPG and B-mode imaging have similar negative predictive values for proximal-vein thrombosis. B-mode imaging, however, is not affected by congestive cardiac failure, which produces false-positive IPG results.[39,40] The clinician's choice of which noninvasive test to use will depend on local availability. A cost-effectiveness analysis is being carried out to further elucidate these issues.

REFERENCES

1. Anderson FA, Wheeler HB, Goldberg RJ, et al. A population-based perspective of the hospital incidence and case-fatality rates of deep vein thrombosis and PE: the Worcester deep-vein thrombosis Study. Arch Intern Med 1991;151:933–938.
2. Moser KM. Venous thromboembolism. Am Rev Respir Dis 1990;141:235–249.
3. Kelly MA, Carson JL, Palevsky HI, Schwartz JS. Diagnosing pulmonary embolism: new facts and strategies. Ann Intern Med 1991;114:300–306.
4. Stein PD, Saltzman HA, Weg JG. Clinical characteristics of patients with acute pulmonary embolism. Am J Cardiol 1991;68:1723–1724.
5. Prospective Investigation of Pulmonary Embolism Diagnosis Investigators. Value of the ventilation-perfusion scan in acute pulmonary embolism: results of the Prospective Investigation of Pulmonary Embolism Diagnosis (PIOPED). JAMA 1990;263:2753–2759.
6. Hull R, Raskob G. Low probability lung scan findings: a need for change. Ann Intern Med 1991;114:142–143.
7. Hull RD, Hirsh J, Carter CJ, et al. Diagnostic value of ventilation-perfusion lung scanning in patients with suspected pulmonary embolism. Chest 1985;88:819–828.
8. Hull RD, Hirsh J, Carter CJ, et al. Pulmonary angiography ventilation lung scanning and venography for clinically suspected pulmonary embolism with abnormal perfusion lung scan. Ann Intern Med 1983;98:891–899.
9. Gottschalk A. Lung scan interpretation: a physiologic, user friendly approach. J Nucl Med 1992;33:1422–1424.
10. Secker-Walker RH. On purple emperors, pulmonary embolism and venous thrombosis. Ann Intern Med 1983;98:1006–1008.
11. Cheely R, McCartney WH, Perry JR, et al. The role of noninvasive tests vs pulmonary in the diagnosis of pulmonary embolism. Am J Med 1981;70:17–22.
12. McNeil BJ. Ventilation-perfusion studies and the diagnosis of pulmonary embolism: concise communication. J Nucl Med 1980;21:319–323.
13. Biello DR, Mattar AG, McKnight RC, Siegel BA. Ventilation-perfusion studies in suspected pulmonary embolism. Am J Roentgenol 1979;133:1033–1037.
14. Alderson PO, Rujanavech N, Secker-Walker RH, McKnight RC. The role of ^{133}Xe ventilation studies in the

scintigraphic detection of pulmonary embolism. Radiology 1976;120:633–640.

15. Dalen JE, Brooks HL, Johnson LW, Meister SG, Szucs MM, et al. Pulmonary angiography in acute pulmonary embolism: indications, techniques, and results in 367 patients. Am Heart J 1971;81:175–185.

16. Stein PD, Athanasoulis C, Alavi A, et al. Complications and validity of pulmonary angiography in acute pulmonary embolism. Circulation 1992;85:462–468.

17. Bone RC. Ventilation-perfusion scan in pulmonary embolism: the emperor is incompletely attired. JAMA 1990;263:2794–2795.

18. Kakkar VV, Flanc C, Howe CT, Clarke MB. Natural history of post-operative deep vein thrombosis. Lancet 1969;2: 230–232.

19. Moser KM, LeMoine JR. Is embolic risk conditioned by location of deep venous thrombosis? Ann Intern Med 1981;94:439–444.

20. Hull RD, Delmore T, Genton E, et al. Warfarin sodium vs low dose heparin in the long-term treatment of venous thrombosis. N Engl J Med 1979;301:855–858.

21. Hull RD, Raskob GE, Hirsh J, et al. Continuous intravenous heparin compared with intermittent subcutaneous heparin in the initial treatment of proximal-vein thrombosis. N Engl J Med 1986;315:1109–1114.

22. Brandjes DPM, Heijboer H, Buller HR, De Rijk M, Jagt H, et al. Acenocoumarol and heparin compared with acenocoumarol alone in the initial treatment of proximal-vein thrombosis. N Engl J Med 1992;327:1485–1489.

23. Wheeler HB, Anderson FA Jr. Can noninvasive tests be used as the basis for treatment of deep-vein thrombosis? In: Berstein EF (ed.): Noninvasive Diagnostic Techniques in Vascular Disease. 3rd ed. St. Louis, Mo, Mosby-Year Book, 1985, pp. 805–818.

24. Hull RD, Hirsh J, Carter CJ, et al. Diagnostic efficacy of impedance plethysmography for clinically suspected deep-vein thrombosis: a randomized trial. Ann Intern Med 1985;102:21–28.

25. Huisman MV, Buller HR, ten Cate JW, Vreeken J. Serial impedance plethysmogrpahy for suspected deep venous thrombosis in outpatients: the Amsterdam General Practitioner Study. N Engl J Med 1986;814:823–828.

26. Huisman MV, Buller HR, ten Cate JW, Heijermans HS, Van der Laan J, et al. Management of clinically suspected acute venous thrombosis in outpatients with serial impedance plethysmography in a community hospital setting. Arch Intern Med 1989;149:511–513.

27. Heijboer H, Brandjes D, Lensing AW, Buller HR, ten Cate JW. Efficacy of real-time B-mode ultrasonography vs impedance plethysmography in the diagnosis of deep-vein thrombosis in symptomatic outpatients. Thromb Haemost 1991;65:436.

28. White RH, McGahan JP, Daschbach MM, Harlting RP. Diagnosis of deep-vein thrombosis using Duplex ultrasound. Ann Intern Med 1989;111:297–304.

29. Lensing AW, Prandoni P, Brandjes DPM, et al. Detection of deep-vein thrombosis by real-time B-mode ultrasonography. N Engl J Med 1989;320:342–345.

30. Cronan JJ. Ultrasound evaluation of deep venous thrombosis. Semin Roentgenol 1992;27:39–52.

31. Hull R, Raskob G, Coates G, Panju A, Gill GJ. A new noninvasive management strategy for patients with suspected pulmonary embolism. Arch Intern Med 1989;149: 2549–2555.

32. Hull R, Raskob G, Coates G, Panju A. Clinical validity of a

33. normal perfusion lung scan in patients with suspected pulmonary embolism. Chest 1990;97:23–26.

33. Kipper MS, Moser KM, Kortman KE, Ashburn WL. Long-term follow-up of patients with suspected pulmonary embolism and a normal lung scan. Chest 1982;82:411–415.

34. Hull R, Raskob G, Rosenbloom D, et al. Heparin for 5 days compared with 10 days in the initial treatment of proximal venous thrombosis. N Engl J Med 1990;322:1260–1264.

35. Hull R, Hirsh J, Jay R, et al. Different intensities of oral anticoagulant therapy in the treatment of proximal-vein thrombosis. N Engl J Med 1982;307:1676–1681.

36. Greenfield LJ. Current indications for and results of Greenfield filter placement. J Vasc Surg 1984;1:502–504.

37. Bookstein JJ, Silver TM. The angiographic differential diagnosis of acute pulmonary embolism. Radiology 1974;110:25–33.

38. Hull RD, Carter CJ, Jay RM, et al. The diagnosis of acute recurrent deep-vein thrombosis: a diagnostic challenge. Circulation 1983;67:901–906.

39. Hull RD, Van Aken WG, Hirsh J, et al. Impedance plethysmography using the occlusive cuff technique in the diagnosis of venous thrombosis. Circulation 1976;53:696–700.

40. Hull RD, Taylor DW, Hirsh J, et al. Impedance plethysmography: the relationship between venous filling and sensitivity and specificity for proximal-vein thrombosis. Circulation 1978;58:898–902.

41. Rabinov K, Paulin S. Roentgen diagnosis of venous thrombosis in the leg. Arch Surg 1972;104:134–144.

42. Coates G, Dolovich M, Koehler D, Newhouse J. Ventilation scanning with technetium labelled aerosols: DTPA or sulfur colloid? Clin Nucl Med 1985;10:835–838.

43. Hull RD, Hirsh J, Sackett DL, et al. Clinical validity of a negative venogram in patients with clinically suspected venous thrombosis. Circulation 1981;64:622–625.

44. Noveline RA, Baltarowich OH, Athanasoulis CA, Waltman A, Greenfield AJ, et al. The clinical course of patients with suspected pulmonary embolism and a negative pulmonary arteriogram. Radiology 1978;126:561–567.

45. Carter C, Gent M, Leclerc JR. The epidemiology of venous thrombosis. In: Coleman RW, Hirsh J, Marder J, Salzman EW (eds.): Hemostatsis and Thrombosis: Basic Principles and Clinical Practice. Philadelphia, Pa, JB Lippincott, 1987, pp. 1185–1198.

46. Salzman EW, Hirsh J. Prevention of venous thromboembolism. In: Coleman RW, Hirsh J, Marder V, Salzman EW, eds. Hemostasis and Thrombosis: Basic Principles and Clinical Practice. 2nd ed. Philadelphia, Pa, JB Lippincott, 1987, pp. 1252–1265.

47. Sacket DL, Haynes RB, Tugwell P. Clinical Epidemiology: A Basic Science for Clinical Medicine. Boston, Mass, Little Brown & Co. Inc, 1985, pp. 159–169.

48. Sackett DL. Bias in analytic research. J Chronic Dis 1979;32: 51–63.

49. Palevsky HI, Alavi A. A noninvasive strategy for the managment of patients suspected of pulmonary embolism. Semin Nucl Med 1991;21:325–331.

50. Anderson DR, Lensing AW, Wells PS, Levine MN, Weitz JI, et al. Limitations of impedance plethysmography in the diagnosis of clinically suspected deep-vein thrombosis. Ann Intern Med 1993;118:25–30.

51. Heijboer H, Cogo A, Buller HR, Prandoni P, ten Cate JW. Detection of deep-vein thrombosis with impedance plethysmography and real-time compression ultrasonography in hospitalized patients. Arch Intern Med 1992;152: 1901–1903.

26

Cost Effectiveness of Pulmonary Embolism Diagnosis

Russell D. Hull, William Feldstein, Paul D. Stein, Graham F. Pineo

INTRODUCTION

A 1991 population study found the incidence of pulmonary embolism (PE) to be 21 patients per 100,000 (.021%).[1] The nonspecificity of clinical findings[2-7] and the diagnostic uncertainties and challenges presented by both ventilation-perfusion lung scanning[2,3,5-14] and pulmonary angiography,[2,3,8,15,16] have made this frequent disorder a significant diagnostic problem for clinicians.

A key element in the diagnosis of PE in symptomatic patients is ventilation-perfusion lung scanning.[2,3,5-14] The concept of high-, intermediary-, indeterminate-, and low-probability lung scan patterns have resulted from pioneering retrospective studies.[12,13] In recent prospective studies, it has been found that the low-probability lung scan pattern is associated with an unacceptably high frequency of PE (14% to 30%).[5-8] These rigorous studies suggest that it would be more appropriate to categorize patients with abnormal perfusion lung scans as either high-probability or nondiagnostic, as suggested by Moser.[2]

In recent years, objective tests to detect venous thrombosis and improvements in clinical-trial methodology have improved the clinician's abilty to diagnose PE. Many patients with PE have residual deep-vein thrombosis (DVT) in the lower extremities.[7,8] A major advance in the diagnosis of PE has been the noninvasive diagnosis of deep venous thrombi (the usual antecedents to pulmonary emboli), using either impedance studies or duplex ultrasound studies of the legs, as noted by Bone.[17] Incorporating lower limb diagnostics for venous thrombosis enhances the clinician's ability to achieve a cost-effective diagnosis of PE, as noted by Dalen.[18]

We have recently reported a practical noninvasive strategy,[19] in patients with adequate cardiorespiratory re-

serve and nondiagnostic lung scans. The advantages of this strategy are that it: (1) avoids pulmonary angiography, (2) identifies patients with proximal-vein thrombosis who require treatment, and (3) avoids the need for treatment and further investigation in the majority of patients. We have found that: (1) in patients with adequate cardiorespiratory reserve, local thrombotic extension in the lung of submassive pulmonary embolism is not an important cause of morbidity or mortality, and (2) in most patients, recurrent pulmonary embolism comes from proximal-vein thrombosis of the lower extremities. Our findings cannot be applied to patients with nondiagnostic lung scans and inadequate cardiorespiratory reserve who require either treatment or further investigation with selective pulmonary angiography.

To maximize the health of the population served, subject to the available resources, decision-makers employ the techniques of economic evaluation.[20-25] Cost-effectiveness analysis is an economic tool which ranks alternative approaches to the same health problem to determine "which is best". The best approach in economic terms is the approach that: (1) accomplishes the desired health effect at minimum cost (cost minimization), (2) produces maximum health benefit for a given cost, or (3) carries the maximum effectiveness/cost ratio.

In performing a cost-effectiveness analysis of the recommended strategies for PE diagnosis and management, two criteria of effectiveness were used: (1) the correct identification of pulmonary embolism, and (2) the correct identification of the number of patients in whom treatment was correctly withheld.

In an era of healthcare cost constraints guided by managed care, our findings provide a rational comparison of the commonly used strategies for PE diagnosis and management in symptomatic patients.

From *Venous Thromboembolism: An Evidence-Based Atlas* edited by Russell Hull, Gary Raskob, Graham Pineo © 1996, Futura Publishing Co., Armonk, NY.

METHODS

Objective Tests for Pulmonary Embolism

Methods for diagnosing PE in symptomatic patients include clinical findings, ventilation-perfusion lung scanning, pulmonary angiography, and noninvasive leg tests.[4–20] Therapy can be withheld or withdrawn if serial noninvasive leg testing is negative in patients with a nondiagnostic lung scan pattern and adequate cardiorespiratory reserve.[19] In such patients, serial testing detects recurrent venous thrombosis, thus preventing the morbidity and mortality associated with recurrent venous thromboembolism (VTE).[19]

Our cost-effectiveness analysis is based on data from a decision analysis which has been published separately, "Prospective Investigation Of Pulmonary Embolism Diagnosis (PIOPED)",[5,26] a collaborative study in which 662 patients participated. Patients were prospectively evaluated by ventilation-perfusion lung scanning and pulmonary angiography. Three diagnostic strategies were used.

Strategy 1: Ventilation-Perfusion Lung Scans and Pulmonary Angiography

If patients had a high-probability lung scan, they would be treated. If patients had a near-normal lung scan, treatment would be withheld or withdrawn. If patients had nondiagnostic lung scans (irrespective of cardiorespiratory reserve), they would receive pulmonary angiography and treatment would be based on the result of the angiogram.

Strategy 2: Ventilation-Perfusion Lung Scans, Single Noninvasive Leg Test, and Pulmonary Angiography

If patients had a high-probability lung scan, they would be treated. If patients had a near-normal lung scan, treatment would be withheld or withdrawn. If patients had nondiagnostic lung scans, they would receive a single noninvasive leg test. Those patients with a positive noninvasive leg test would receive treatment, and those with a negative test would receive pulmonary angiography.

Strategy 3: Ventilation-Perfusion Lung Scans, Serial Noninvasive Leg Tests, and Pulmonary Angiography

If patients had a high-probability lung scan, they would be treated. If patients had a near-normal lung scan, treatment would be withheld or withdrawn. If patients had nondiagnostic lung scans and had poor cardiorespiratory reserve, they would receive pulmonary angiography. If patients had nondiagnostic lung scans and had adequate cardiorespiratory reserve, they would receive serial noninvasive leg tests.

COST-EFFECTIVENESS

Cost

The cost of each diagnostic alternative was defined as the direct cost of administering the diagnostic test plus the treatment cost associated with a positive test. All diagnostic testing charges included physician/specialist charges for interpretation. Treatment costs consisted of: (1) the cost of anticoagulant therapy (drugs, laboratory tests for monitoring anticoagulant therapy, and physician fees), and (2) the "hotel" costs of hospitalization (rooming, laundry, food, etc.). The costs of complications and side effects associated with anticoagulant therapy, as measured empirically in a recent double-blind, multicenter clinical trial, are included and discussed within the Appendix. The costs of treating the complications and side effects of pulmonary angiography were relatively minor and are not included.[27]

The economic viewpoint of this analysis[22] was that of a third-party payer (in the United States, an insurance company in Canada, the Ministry of Health). The cost-effectiveness findings shown in the Results section are expressed both in 1992 American and Canadian dollars (to the nearest dollar), according to the charges at an urban-based hospital site in the United States and one in Canada, respectively.

Unit Charges At An Urban Teaching Hospital In the United States

The cost data are based on actual quantities. The costs were derived from the operating charges incurred in a midwestern urban hospital affiliated with a university medical school and details are shown in the Appendix. Because clinical examination was the starting point for all patients in each strategy, the charge for the initial physician's fee was not included. This facility's charges were US $575 per day for hotel charges, US $510 for ventilation-perfusion lung scans, US $2,553 for pulmonary angiography (which includes two additional days in hospital), US $150 for a single impedance plethysmograph, US $300 for a single Doppler ultrasonograph with B-mode imaging, and US $750 and US $1,500 for serial IPG or serial Doppler ultrasonography with B-mode imaging, respectively. The total charges for treating each patient with intravenous heparin therapy followed by long-term warfarin sodium were US $6,522, and are detailed in the Appendix.

Unit Costs At An Urban Teaching Hospital in Canada

This economic analysis was also performed using actual 1992 costs in Canadian dollars at an urban hospital in western Canada. Although the Canadian costs are lower, the ranking of the costs is similar to the ranking of charges in the United States (for example, this facility's hotel charge was CDN $543 per day, compared with US $575 per day, for the facility in the United States).

This facility's costs were CDN $258 for ventilation-perfusion lung scans, CDN $828 for pulmonary angiography (which includes two additional days in hospital), CDN $30 for a single IPG, CDN $80 for a single Doppler ultrasonograph with B-mode imaging, and CDN $150 and CDN $400 for serial IPG or serial Doppler ultrasonography with B-mode imaging, respectively. The total costs for treating each patient with intravenous heparin therapy followed by long-term warfarin sodium were CDN $4,160, and are detailed in the Appendix.

Effectiveness

Two criteria of effectiveness were used. They involved: (1) the correct identification of pulmonary embolism, and (2) the correct identification of the number of patients in whom treatment was correctly withheld.

SENSITIVITY ANALYSIS

Multiple sensitivity analyses[20,22] were performed. The variables examined were charges for the hospital bed, charges for treatment, and charges for diagnostic tests. For prevalence, a range of 10 to 80 cases of PE per 100 symptomatic patients with clinically suspected PE was used. This range exceeds the prevalence of PE reported in the literature. For the charges for the hospital bed and treatment, a range of 40% to 300% was used, and for objective testing, a range of 55% to 195% was used, reflecting regional variations in charges in the United States.

The impact of false-positive results by noninvasive testing was also examined by sensitivity analysis.

The costs incurred by ancillary investigations such as chest x-rays, electrocardiograms, and baseline biochemistry during the initial work-up were the same for all strategies. These minor costs were evaluated by sensitivity analysis.

RESULTS

Table 1 summarizes the results of applying the three strategies to this group of 662 patients. The Appendix presents a detailed analysis of the charges in the United States (or costs in Canada).

In all three strategies, each of the 662 patients would have undergone ventilation-perfusion lung scanning. Eighty-nine would have had high-probability, 105 near-normal, and 468 nondiagnostic (intermediate- and low-probability) lung scans.

Strategy 1: Ventilation-Perfusion Lung Scans and Pulmonary Angiography

Patients with a high-probability lung scan (89) would receive treatment. Patients with a near-normal lung scan (105) would receive no treatment. Patients with a nondiagnostic lung scan (468) would have undergone pulmonary angiography, resulting in positive angiograms in 105 patients who would then receive treatment. Patients with a negative pulmonary angiogram would not receive treatment. In total, Strategy 1 would result in 194 patients requiring treatment, and 468 patients in whom treatment would have been correctly withheld or withdrawn.

Table 1
U.S. Dollar Charges, Canadian Dollar Costs, and Effectiveness of the Alternative Strategies for Diagnosing Pulmonary Embolism in 662 Patients

Strategy	No. of Patients Requiring Treatment		Total US $ Charges or CDN $ Costs	US $ Charge or CDN $ Cost Per Patient Requiring Treatment	US $ Charge or CDN $ Cost Per Patient Correctly Withheld from Treatment
#1	194	US	$2,797,692	$14,421	$5,978
		CDN	$1,873,120	$ 9,655	$4,002
#2a	195	US	$2,739,105	$14,047	$5,865
		CDN	$1,789,931	$ 9,179	$3,833
#2b	195	US	$2,809,305	$14,407	$6,016
		CDN	$1,813,331	$ 9,299	$3,883
#3a	169	US	$2,135,967	$12,639	$4,333
		CDN	$1,283,725	$ 7,596	$2,604
#3b	169	US	$2,339,367	$13,842	$4,745
		CDN	$1,351,525	$ 7,997	$2,741

Strategy Descriptions:
#1 = Ventilation-perfusion lung scans and pulmonary angiography.
#2a = Ventilation-perfusion lung scans, single noninvasive leg test with Doppler ultrasonography with B-mode imaging, and pulmonary angiography.
#2b = Ventilation-perfusion lung scans, single noninvasive leg test with Doppler ultrasonography with B-mode imaging, and pulmonary angiography.
#3a = Ventilation-perfusion lung scans, serial noninvasive leg tests with impedance plethysmography, and pulmonary angiography.
#3b = Ventilation-perfusion lung scans, serial noninvasive leg tests with Doppler ultrasonography with B-mode imaging, and pulmonary angiography.
(Reproduced with permission from Hull, et al. Arch Int Med 1996;156:68–72.)

The total U.S. dollar charges (or Canadian dollar costs) for administering this strategy to yield a diagnosis of PE in 194 patients in 1992, would be US $2,797,692 (or CDN $1,873,120). Therefore, the charges in the U.S. (or costs in Canada) for each patient requiring treatment would be US $14,421 (or CDN $9,655). The charges (or costs) incurred per patient correctly withheld from treatment would be US $5,978 (or CDN $4,002).

Strategy 2: Ventilation-Perfusion Lung Scans, Single Noninvasive Leg Test, and Pulmonary Angiography

Patients with a high-probability lung scan (89) would receive treatment. Patients with a near-normal lung scan (105) would receive no treatment. Patients with a nondiagnostic lung scan (468) would have undergone a single noninvasive leg test (IPG or Doppler ultrasound with B-mode imaging), resulting in positive outcomes in 53 patients who would then receive treatment. Patients with a negative single noninvasive leg test (415) would have pulmonary angiography resulting in 53 patients with positive angiograms who would then receive treatment. Patients with a negative pulmonary angiogram would not receive treatment. In total, Strategy 2 would would result in 195 patients requiring treatment, and 468 patients in whom treatment would have been correctly withheld or withdrawn.

The total U.S. dollar charges (or Canadian dollar costs) for administering this strategy to yield a diagnosis of PE in 195 patients in 1992 would be US $2,739,105 (or CDN $1,789,931) if IPG were used, and would be US $2,809,305 (or CDN $1,813,331) if Doppler ultrasonography were used. Therefore, the charges in the U.S. (or costs in Canada) for each patient requiring treatment would be US $14,047 (or CDN $9,179) if IPG were used, and would be US $14,407 (or CDN $9,299) if Doppler ultrasonography were used. The charges (costs) incurred per patient in whom treatment were correctly withheld would be US $5,865 (CDN $3,833) if impedance plethysmography were used, and would be US $6,016 (CDN $3,883) if Doppler ultrasonography were used.

Strategy 3: Ventilation-Perfusion Lung Scans, Serial Noninvasive Leg Tests, and Pulmonary Angiography

Patients with a high-probability lung scan (89) would receive treatment. Patients with a near-normal lung scan (105) would receive no treatment. Patients with a nondiagnostic lung scan (468) would have undergone a single noninvasive leg test (IPG or Doppler ultrasound with B-mode imaging), resulting in positive outcomes for 53 patients who would then require treatment. Of the patients with a negative single noninvasive leg test (415), 222 would have adequate cardiorespiratory reserve and would then undergo serial noninvasive leg testing; this

would result in seven patients with positive outcomes who would then require treatment. The 193 patients who would have inadequate cardiorespiratory reserve would receive pulmonary angiography; this would result in 20 patients with positive angiogram,s who would then require treatment. Those patients with adequate cardiorespiratory reserve who had negative results subsequent to serial noninvasive leg testing, as well as those patients with inadequate cardiorespiratory reserve, who had a negative pulmonary angiogram would not receive treatment. In total, Strategy 3 would result in 169 patients requiring treatment, and 493 patients in whom treatment would be correctly withheld or withdrawn.

The total U.S. dollar charges (or Canadian dollar costs) for administering this strategy to the 662 patient group would be US $2,135,967 (or CDN $1,283,725) if IPG were used, and would be US $2,339,367 (or CDN $1,351,525) if Doppler ultrasonography were used. Therefore, the charges in the U.S. (or costs in Canada) for each patient requiring treatment would be US $12,639 (or CDN $7,596) if IPG were used, and would be US $13,842 (or CDN $7,997) if Doppler ultrasonography were used. The charges (or costs) incurred per patient in whom treatment were correctly withheld would be US $4,333 (or CDN $2,604) if IPG were used, and would be US $4,745 (CDN $2,741) if Doppler ultrasonography were used.

SENSITIVITY ANALYSIS

Sensitivity analysis showed that ventilation-perfusion lung scans, serial noninvasive leg tests using IPG, and pulmonary angiography is the most cost-effective approach. The ranking of the other strategies is less stable and may vary according to the variations in charges (or costs) for IPG, ultrasonography, pulmonary angiography, or treatment. It is probable, however, that any potential change in charges or costs will be proportionately similar at participating centers, so that leaving the actual ranking observed by cost-effectiveness analysis remains unchanged.

DISCUSSION

The strategy requiring pulmonary angiography in the least number of patients proved to be a combination of ventilation-perfusion lung scans and serial noninvasive leg testing.[2–5,10] It was effective in identifying those patients requiring anticoagulant therapy and those not requiring treatment and was the least costly.

A diagnostic strategy which minimizes the need for pulmonary angiography (which is invasive and requires expertise for safe and effective imaging[5]) has considerable clinical appeal. The combination of ventilation-perfusion lung scanning with noninvasive leg testing has gained widespread acceptance.[3,17,19,28]

If all patients with nondiagnostic lung scans receive pulmonary angiography, such invasive technology will be used in up to 70% of symptomatic patients. This is a costly approach. The need for pulmonary angiography in 70% or more of patients with suspected PE can be avoided by using ventilation-perfusion lung scans and serial noninvasive leg tests. This is the most cost-effective approach. The use of a single noninvasive leg test to detect DVT avoids the need for pulmonary angiography in approximately 20% of patients with nondiagnostic scans. The cost-effectiveness of this approach is intermediate.

It is evident that noninvasive leg testing with serial IPG is less expensive than Doppler ultrasonography with B-mode imaging. Serial IPG can be carried out in the outpatient clinic, ward, or emergency room.[19] In many centers, B-mode imaging is carried out in a centralized facility. Serial B-mode imaging is more costly than serial IPG. It has been shown that B-mode imaging and IPG are equally effective in ruling out DVT.[29] However, B-mode imaging has the advantage that a bedside examination is not required to rule out clinical disorders known to produce false-positive results as is the case with IPG.[30] In patients who do not have disorders that might produce false-positive IPG results, it would be clinically and economically advantageous to use serial IPG. In some patient subgroups, for example in the intensive care unit where patients frequently suffer from cardiac failure, the use of serial B-mode imaging would avoid the otherwise high false-positive rates associated with IPG testing.

B-mode imaging may be more sensitive to popliteal extension of calf-vein thrombosis than IPG as recent observations suggest.[31] Large outcome studies, however, have shown that serial IPG and ultrasonography are equally safe in symptomatic patients with negative outcomes.

Our cost-effectiveness analyses suggest that IPG and B-mode imaging, if selected appropriately for various populations, would maximize effectiveness without the excessive costs associated with the routine use of B-mode imaging in all patients. A strategy which would optimize cost and effectiveness would be the employment of B-mode ultrasonography as the initial noninvasive leg test, followed by IPG if serial leg tests are necessary. Our cost-effectiveness analysis suggest that Doppler ultrasonography with B-mode imaging and IPG are complementary rather than competitive.

Serial testing is only feasible in patients who can and will return for follow-up. Otherwise, pulmonary angiography remains the diagnostic method of choice. Furthermore, if it is necessary to determine whether PE has occurred, pulmonary angiography will be required if lung scanning is nondiagnostic.

Although the actual cost of each component in the diagnostic strategies will be dictated by regional differences and will change in the future, the proportion that each parameter contributes to the total cost will remain linked.

Thus, ranking the strategies from most to least expensive, as determined by cost-effectiveness analysis, should continue to be relevant.

APPENDIX

U.S. CHARGES:

Diagnostic Testing:

The charges were US $510 for ventilation-perfusion lung scans, US $150 for IPG, US $300 for Doppler ultrasonography with B-mode imaging, and US $2,553 for pulmonary angiography. All diagnostic charges included physician/specialist charges.

Hotel Charge:

US $575 per day.

Charges for Treatment with Intravenous Heparin and Warfarin Sodium:

The total charge per patient for 6 days of intravenous heparin therapy in the hospital and 3 months of out-patient long-term treatment with warfarin sodium was US $6,522. The charges per patient were US $966 for intravenous heparin therapy (physician fee, drug bolus, infusion bags, and PTT tests), US $3,450 for a 6–day hospital stay and $1,649 for long-term therapy with warfarin sodium (including PT/INR and physician fees). This total charge also includes the charges incurred (empirically derived from our treatment data) for the approximately 6% of patients who had a recurrent venous thromboembolic event as well as for the 5% of patients who had a major bleeding event. Minor bleeding occurred infrequently, as did other side effects of anticoagulant therapy (e.g., thrombocytopenia) and were unimportant compared with the other charges.

Strategy 1: Ventilation-Perfusion Lung Scans and Pulmonary Angiography

The total charge for administering Strategy 1 to 662 patients was US $2,797,692 and consisted of US $337,620 for ventilation-perfusion lung scans (662 × $510), US $1,194,804 for pulmonary angiography (468 × $2,553), and US $1,265,268 for treatment charges (194 × $6,522). The charge per patient requiring treatment was US $14,421 ($2,797,692 ÷ 194), and the charge per patient in whom treatment was correctly withheld or withdrawn because of negative angiography or near-normal lung scans was US $5,978 ($2,797,692 ÷ 468).

Strategy 2: Ventilation-Perfusion Lung Scans, Single Noninvasive Leg Test, and Pulmonary Angiography

The total charge for administering Strategy 2 using IPG to 662 patients was US $2,739,105 and consisted of US

$337,620 for ventilation-perfusion lung scans (662 × $510), US $70,200 for impedance plethysmography (468 × $150), US $1,059,495 for pulmonary angiography (415 × $2,553), and US $1,271,790 for treatment charges (195 × $6,522). The charge per patient requiring treatment was US $14,047 ($2,739,105 ÷ 195), and the charge per patient in whom treatment was correctly withheld or withdrawn was US $5,865 ($2,739,105 ÷ 467).

The total charge for administering Strategy 2 using Doppler ultrasonography with B-mode imaging to 662 patients was US $2,809,305 and consisted of US $337,620 for ventilation-perfusion lung scans (662 × $510), US $140,400 for IPG (468 × $300), US $1,059,495 for pulmonary angiography (415 × $2,553), and US $1,271,790 for treatment charges (195 × $6,522). The charge per patient requiring treatment was US $14,407 ($2,809,305 ÷ 195), and the charge per patient in whom treatment was correctly withheld or withdrawn was US $6,016 ($2,809,305 ÷ 467).

Strategy 3: Ventilation-Perfusion Lung Scans, Serial Noninvasive Leg Testing, and Pulmonary Angiography

The total charge for administering Strategy 3 using IPG to 662 patients was US $2,135,967 and consisted of the following charges: US $337,620 for ventilation-perfusion lung scans (662 × $510), US $70,200 for the initial IPG performed on all patients with a nondiagnostic lung scan (468 × $150), US $133,200 for the subsequent IPG performed serially on the 222 patients with adequate cardiorespiratory reserve (222 × 4 × $150), US $492,729 for pulmonary angiography performed on the 193 patients with inadequate cardiorespiratory reserve (193 × $2,553), and US $1,102,218 for treatment charges (169 × $6,522). The charge per patient requiring treatment was US $12,639 ($2,135,967 ÷ 169), and the charge per patient in whom treatment was correctly withheld or withdrawn was US $4,333 ($2,135,967 ÷ 493).

The total charge for administering Strategy 3 using Doppler ultrasonography with B-mode imaging to 662 patients was US $2,339,367 and consisted of the following charges: US $337,620 for ventilation-perfusion lung scans (662 × $510), US $140,400 for the initial Doppler ultrasound with B-mode imaging performed on all patients with a nondiagnostic lung scan (468 × $300), US $266,400 for the subsequent Doppler ultrasonography performed serially on the 222 patients with adequate cardiorespiratory reserve (222 × 4 × $300), US $492,729 for pulmonary angiography performed on the 193 patients with inadequate cardiorespiratory reserve (193 × $1,403), and US $1,102,218 for treatment charges (169 × $6,522). The charge per patient requiring treatment was US $13,842 ($2,339,367 ÷ 169), and the charge per patient in whom treatment was correctly withheld or withdrawn was US $4,745 ($2,339,367 ÷ 493).

CANADIAN COSTS:

Diagnostic Testing:

The costs were CDN $258 for ventilation-perfusion lung scans, CDN $30 for IPG, CDN $80 for Doppler ultrasonography with B-mode imaging, and CDN $1,913 for pulmonary angiography. All diagnostic costs included physician/specialist costs.

Hotel Cost:

CDN $543 per day.

Costs for Treatment with Intravenous Heparin and Warfarin Sodium

The total cost per patient for 6 days of intravenous heparin therapy in the hospital and 3 months of out-patient long-term treatment with warfarin sodium was CDN $4,160. The costs per patient were CDN $143 for intravenous heparin therapy (physician fee, drug bolus, infusion bags, and PTT tests), CDN $3,255 for a 6–day hospital stay, and CDN $472 for long-term therapy with warfarin sodium (including PT/INR and physician fees). The total cost also includes the costs incurred (empirically derived from our treatment data) for the approximately 6% of patients who had a recurrent venous thromboembolic event as well as for the 5% of patients who had a major bleeding event. Minor bleeding occurred infrequently, as did other side effects of anticoagulant therapy (e.g., thrombocytopenia) and were unimportant compared with the other costs.

Strategy 1: Ventilation-Perfusion Lung Scans and Pulmonary Angiography

The total cost for administering Strategy 1 to 662 patients was CDN $1,873,120 and consisted of CDN $170,796 for ventilation-perfusion lung scans (662 × $258), CDN $895,284 for pulmonary angiography (468 × $1,913), and CDN $807,040 for treatment costs (194 × $4,160). The cost per patient requiring treatment was CDN $9,655 ($1,873,120 ÷ 194), and the cost per patient in whom treatment was correctly withheld or withdrawn because of negative angiography or near-normal lung scans was CDN $4,002 ($1,873,120 ÷ 468).

Strategy 2: Ventilation-Perfusion Lung Scans, Single Noninvasive Leg Test and Pulmonary Angiography

The total cost for administering Strategy 2 using IPG to 662 patients was CDN $1,789,931 and consisted of CDN $170,796 for ventilation-perfusion lung scans (662 × $258), CDN $14,040 for IPG (468 × $30), CDN $793,895 for pulmonary angiography (415 × $1,913), and CDN $811,200 for treatment costs (195 × $4,160). The cost per patient requiring treatment was CDN $9,179 ($1,789,931

÷ 195), and the cost per patient in whom treatment was correctly withheld or withdrawn was CDN $3,833 ($1,789,931 ÷ 467).

The total cost for administering Strategy 2 using Doppler ultrasonography with B-mode imaging to 662 patients was CDN $1,813,331 and consisted of CDN $170,796 for ventilation-perfusion lung scans (662 × $258), CDN $37,440 for IPG (468 × $80), CDN $793,895 for pulmonary angiography (415 × $1,913), and CDN $811,200 for treatment costs (195 × $4,160). The cost per patient requiring treatment was CDN $9,299 ($1,813,331 ÷ 195), and the cost per patient in whom treatment was correctly withheld or withdrawn was CDN $3,883 ($1,813,331 ÷ 467).

Strategy 3: Ventilation-Perfusion Lung Scans, Serial Noninvasive Leg Tests, and Pulmonary Angiography

The total cost for administering Strategy 3 using IPG to 662 patients was CDN $1,283,725 and consisted of CDN $170,796 for ventilation-perfusion lung scans (662 × $258), CDN $14,040 for the initial IPG performed on all patients with a nondiagnostic lung scan (468 × $30), CDN $26,640 for the subsequent IPG performed serially on the 222 patients with adequate cardiorespiratory reserve (222 × 4 × $30), CDN $369,209 for pulmonary angiography performed on the 193 patients with inadequate cardiorespiratory reserve (193 × $1,913), and CDN $703,040 for treatment costs (169 × $4,160). The cost per patient requiring treatment was CDN $7,596 ($1,283,725 ÷ 169), and the cost per patient in whom treatment was correctly withheld or withdrawn was CDN $2,604 ($1,283,725 ÷ 493).

The total cost for administering Strategy 3 using Doppler ultrasonography with B-mode imaging to 662 patients was CDN $1,351,525 and consisted of CDN $170,796 for ventilation-perfusion lung scans (662 × $258), CDN $37,440 for the initial Doppler ultrasound with B-mode imaging performed on all patients with a nondiagnostic lung scan (468 × $80), CDN $71,040 for the subsequent Doppler ultrasonography performed serially on the 222 patients with adequate cardiorespiratory reserve (222 × 4 × $80), CDN $369,209 for pulmonary angiography performed on the 193 patients with inadequate cardiorespiratory reserve (193 × $1,913), and CDN $703,040 for treatment costs (169 × $4,160). The cost per patient requiring treatment was CDN $7,997 ($1,351,525 ÷ 169), and the cost per patient in whom treatment was correctly withheld or withdrawn was CDN $2,741 ($1,351,525 ÷ 493).

REFERENCES

1. Anderson FA, Wheeler HB, Goldberg RJ, et al. A population-based perspective of the hospital incidence and case-fatality rates of deep vein thrombosis and pulmonary embolism: The worcester DVT study. Arch Intern Med 1991;151:933–938.
2. Moser KM. Venous thromboembolism. Am Rev Respir Dis 1990;141:235–249.
3. Kelley MA, Carson JL, Palevsky HI, Schwartz JS. Diagnosing pulmonary embolism: new facts and strategies. Ann Intern Med 1991;114:300–306.
4. Stein PD, Saltzman HA, Weg JG. Clinical characteristics of patients with acute pulmonary embolism. Am J Cardiol 1991;68:1723–1724.
5. Prospective investigation of pulmonary embolism diagnosis investigators. Value of the ventilation-perfusion scan in acute pulmonary embolism: results of the prospective investigation of pulmonary embolism diagnosis (PIOPED). JAMA 1990;263:2753–2759.
6. Hull R, Raskob G. Low probability lung scan findings: a need for change. Ann Intern Med 1991;114:142–143.
7. Hull RD, Hirsh J, Carter CJ, et al. Diagnostic value of ventilation-perfusion lung scanning in patients with suspected pulmonary embolism. Chest 1985;88:819–828.
8. Hull RD, Hirsh J, Carter CJ, et al. Pulmonary angiography ventilation lung scanning and venography for clinically suspected pulmonary embolism with abnormal perfusion lung scan. Ann Intern Med 1983;98:891–899.
9. Gottschalk A. Lung scan interpretation: a physiologic, user-friendly approach. J Nucl Med 1992;33:1422–1424.
10. Secker-Walker RH. On purple emperors, pulmonary embolism and venous thrombosis. Ann Intern Med 1983;98:1006–1008.
11. Cheely R, McCartney WH, Perry JR, et al. The role of noninvasive tests versus pulmonary in the diagnosis of pulmonary embolism. Am J Med 1981;70:17–22.
12. McNeil BJ. Ventilation-perfusion studies and the diagnosis of pulmonary embolism: Concise Communication. J Nucl Med 1980;21:319–323.
13. Biello DR, Mattar AG, McKnight RC, Siegel BA. Ventilation-perfusion studies in suspected pulmonary embolism. Am J Roentgenol 1979;133:1033–1037.
14. Alderson PO, Rujanavech N, Secker-Walker RH, McKnight RC. The Role of ^{133}Xe ventilation studies in the scintigraphic detection of pulmonary embolism. Radiology 1976;120:633–640.
15. Dalen JE, Brooks HL, Johnson LW, Meister SG, Szucs MM, et al. Pulmonary angiography in acute pulmonary embolism: indications, techniques, and results in 367 patients. Am Heart J 1971;81:175–185.
16. Stein PD, Athanasoulis C, Alavi A, et al. Complications and validity of pulmonary angiography in acute pulmonary embolism. Circulation 1992;85:462–468.
17. Bone RC. Ventilation-perfusion scan in pulmonary embolism: the emperor is incompletely attired. JAMA 1990;263:2794–2795.
18. Dalen J. When can treatment be withheld in patients with suspected pulmonary embolism. Arch Int Med 1993;153:1415–1418.
19. Hull R, Raskob G, Ginsberg J, et al. A noninvasive strategy for the treatment of patients with suspected pulmonary embolism. Arch Int Med 1994;154:289–297.
20. Weinstein MC. Economic assessment of medical practices and technologies. Medical Decision Making 1981;1:309–330.
21. Weinstein MC, Stason WB. Foundations of cost-effectiveness analysis for health and medical practices. N Engl J Med 1977;296:716–721.
22. Drummond MF, Stoddart GL, Torrance GW. Methods for the Economic Evaluation of Health Care Programs. Oxford University Press 1987, Oxford, UK.

23. Eddy DM. Principles for making difficulty decisions in difficult times. JAMA 1994;271:1792–1798.

24. Eisenberg JM. Clinical economics: a guide to economic analysis of clinical practices. JAMA 1989;262:2879–2886.

25. Detsky AS, Naglie IG. A clinical guide to cost-effectiveness analysis. Ann Int Med 1990;113:147–54.

26. Stein PD, Hull RD, Pineo GF. Strategy that includes serial noninvasive leg tests for diagnosis of thromboembolic disease in patients with suspected acute pulmonary embolism based on data from PIOPED. Arch Int Med 1995;155:2101–2104.

27. Hull RD, Raskob GE, Pineo GF, Green D, Trowbridge AA, et al. Subcutaneous low-molecular-weight heparin compared with continuous intravenous heparin in the treatment of proximal-vein thrombosis. N Engl J Med 1992;326:975–982.

28. Oupkerk M, Van Breek EJR, Van Putten WLJ, Buller HR. Cost-effectiveness of various strategies in the diagnostic management of pulmonary embolism. Ann Int Med 1993;153:947–954.

29. Heijboer H, Buller HR, Lensing AWA, Turpie AG, Colly LP, et al. A randomized comparison of the clinical utility of real-time compression ultrasonography versus impedance plethysmography in the diagnosis of deep-vein thrombosis in symptomatic outpatients. N Engl J Med 1993;329:511–513.

30. Huisman MV, Buller HR, ten Cate JW, Vreeken J. Serial impedance plethysmography for suspected deep venous thrombosis in outpatients: The Amsterdam General Practitioner Study. N Engl J Med 1986;814:823–828.

31. Kearon C, Hirsh H. Factors influencing the reported sensitivity and specificity of impedance plethysmography for proximal deep vein thrombosis. Thromb Haemost 1994;72:652–658.

SECTION V

Treatment

27

Overview of Treatment of Venous Thromboembolism

Russell D. Hull, Gary E. Raskob, and Graham F. Pineo

Over the past two decades, objective tests have become available for the diagnosis of primary or recurrent venous thromboembolism (VTE).[1,2,3,4,5,6,7,8,9,10,11,12,13,14,15,16,17,18] The advent of these objective tests and the development of clinical trial methodology has permitted the performance of a number of Level I clinical trials assessing the use of various agents in the treatment of VTE.[19,20,21,22,23,24,25,26,27,28,29,30,31,32,33,34,35,36,37,38,39,40,41,42] There are few disorders that have been the subject of more Level I clinical trials than VTE and the impact of these trials on the pattern of practice has been dramatic. In the past, patients with a diagnosis of deep-vein thrombosis (DVT) or pulmonary embolism (PE) (often poorly documented), would be placed on intravenous or subcutaneous unfractionated heparin for 10 or more days without the use of any kind of quality assurance monitoring to ensure that the appropriate level of the monitoring test (usually APTT) was being achieved. When quality assurance was monitored, it usually applied only to the achievement of a therapeutic APTT without reference to the incidence of bleeding complications or recurrent VTE.

After a period of heparin treatment, oral anticoagulants were commenced, often with the use of a loading dose and the targeted therapeutic range was a prothrombin time of two to three times the control value. The optimal duration of oral anticoagulant treatment for primary or recurrent VTE was largely based on clinical intuition rather than on data from clinical trials, and there was little documentation to support any particular therapeutic range of oral anticoagulation for the prevention of recurrent disease.

Thrombolytic agents have been used for some time now in patients with proximal venous thrombosis or submassive PE in an effort to prevent the development of the postphlebitic syndrome or the serious consequences of PE, i.e., death or the development of thromboembolic pulmonary hypertension. Although the ability of thrombolytic drugs to lyse pulmonary emboli was established by Level I clinical trials in the early 1970s (Urokinase Pulmonary Embolism Trial),[34] subsequent studies have used a variety of thrombolytic agents in different dosage schedules and usually required the use of invasive diagnostic tests to establish the diagnosis (e.g., pulmonary angiography).[34-41] Treatment was usually given in an intensive care unit setting. The high incidence of bleeding complications and the questionable benefit of thrombolytic agents as compared with heparin alone have discouraged most physicians from using these agents in patients with venous thromboembolism except in unusual circumstances.

A number of devices have been designed for the interruption of the inferior vena cava in patients with recurrent VTE despite adequate anticoagulant treatment, or in patients in whom anticoagulation is hazardous. Information on the effectiveness and complications of these devices have been derived solely from retrospective case series. Therefore the incidence of serious complications such as thrombosis, displacement, or dislodgement have been poorly studied and the clinical outcomes with or without placement of an inferior vena cava filter remain to be conclusively demonstrated. The effectiveness and safety of inferior vena cava filters therefore will remain uncertain until prospective randomized clinical trials are performed.

Many of the uncertainties being faced by the clinician with respect to the treatment of VTE have been clarified by Level I clinical trials.

With respect to heparin treatment, it is now clear that adequate heparinization in the initial 24 to 48 hours of treatment of proximal venous thrombosis is required to prevent an unacceptably high incidence of recurrent disease during the subsequent 3 months.[21,26,29] The use of a continuous intravenous infusion of heparin following a bolus injection is the most efficient way to achieve adequate heparinization and it is clear from Level I clinical trials that the use of a heparin nomogram is mandatory if adequate heparinization is to be achieved, i.e., an APTT greater than one and a half times the mean of the control value.[24,29] There is a wide variability in the APTT measurements derived from different commercial thromboplastin reagents as well as with the instruments used for measuring the value so that each institution must establish that the therapeutic APTT range corresponds with therapeutic heparin levels (0.2 to 0.4 units/mL).

As opposed to the concern about the lower therapeutic range for heparin treatment, there is less agreement with the concern that a supratherapeutic APTT may predispose to bleeding. Information from prospective clinical trials indicates that bleeding is more closely associated with underlying clinical conditions which predispose to bleeding rather than the level of the APTT.[24] In any event, with the use of a heparin nomogram, the length of time that patients are exposed to a supratherapeutic level of heparin as measured by the APTT can be minimized.[24,29]

The use of low-molecular-weight heparin (LMWH) will eliminate many of the problems associated with the use of intravenous unfractionated heparin in the treatment of venous thromboembolism.[25,27–31] The LMWHs have a much higher bioavailability (>90%), the half life is prolonged permitting a once-a-day subcutaneous injection and the biological response is closely related to body weight permitting fixed dosage treatment. Level I clinical trials to date have shown that a number of LMWHs,[25,27–31] and one heparinoid[32] given by either subcutaneous or intravenous injection, are at least as effective as unfractionated heparin in the prevention of recurrent venous thromboembolism (VTE) [25,27–31] and some have shown a decreased incidence of major bleeding as well as a decrease in mortality rate over the subsequent 3-months follow-up.[25,27] The ease of once-a-day subcutaneous administration without laboratory monitoring has permitted the development of clinical trials using LMWHs in the outpatient setting, a practice that will further improve the cost-effectiveness of these agents. The incidence and severity of complications of the LMWHs such as heparin induced thrombocytopenia or osteoporosis, are the subject of ongoing clinical trials.

The mystery of the higher warfarin doses and higher bleeding complications in patients treated with warfarin in North American as opposed to Europe, was unravelled with the advent of the International Normalized Ratio (INR).[20] It was shown that the high bleeding rates that were found with the use of the higher INR (3.0 to 4.5) could be eliminated with the use of a lower INR (2.0 to 3.0) or the use of adjusted-dose subcutaneous heparin every 12 hours without loss of effectiveness with respect to recurrent VTE.[20] The INR of 2.0 to 3.0 has become the standard for warfarin therapy except in patients with mechanical prosthetic heart valves (INR 2.5 to 3.5) and war-

farin can safely be started at the time of initiating heparin therapy in the vast majority of patients.[22,23] The exceptions to this rule include patients who are unstable and may require further interventions including thrombolytic therapy or surgical procedures so that intravenous heparin alone is more appropriate than intravenous heparin plus warfarin, because heparin alone can be more rapidly reversed.[22,23]

The management of warfarin therapy is fraught with difficulty because of the unpredictability of warfarin dosage in individual patients. The use of a warfarin nomogram for the induction of warfarin therapy either with or without heparin, permits the rapid achievement of a therapeutic INR. Innovations such as the use of prothrombin home monitoring or the use of the native prothrombin antigen for the regulation of warfarin dosage have also simplified warfarin treatment. Warfarin is usually started without the use of heparin in patients for whom anticoagulation is initiated for atrial fibrillation, or when warfarin is used as a prophylactic agent as in high-risk orthopedic surgery.

The advent of objective tests which have high specificity and sensitivity when compared to "gold standards" such as ascending venography or pulmonary angiography, has permitted the use of these diagnostic tests in the treatment of patients with venous thromboembolism.[8,9,12,16,18] Therefore, patients who present with suspected PE and a nondiagnostic ventilation/perfusion lung scan, may be managed with the use of serial noninvasive leg tests without the need for anticoagulant therapy.[9,18] In centers where noninvasive leg tests (impedance plethysmography or Doppler ultrasound) are available, and where the use of LMWH is available for treatment of venous thromboembolism, a strategic plan of outpatient management can be designed. The use of noninvasive leg tests can significantly decrease the need for invasive tests, thereby eliminating their associated risks and permitting a more cost-effective approach to the management of many patients.[9,18]

In recent years, it has been shown that thrombolytic agents can be given as a pulse or a bolus infusion over 15 to 60 minutes, thereby decreasing the risk of bleeding while maintaining the therapeutic benefit as measured by 2-D echocardiography.[42] Furthermore, the use of 2-D echocardiography to identify patients with right ventricular impairment who may benefit from thrombolysis, decreases the need for pulmonary angiography and decreases the threat of bleeding as a result of invasive intervention. Thrombolytic agents can now be used on a regular medical ward. The use of this simplified approach to thrombolytic therapy as compared with intravenous heparin or subcutaneous LMWH will be the subject of further clinical trials. At this time there is little enthusiasm for the use of thrombolytic agents in the treatment of proximal venous thrombosis except in unusual circumstances.

CONCLUSION

Our knowledge regarding the appropriate management of VTE has been revolutionized by the results of a large number of Level I clinical trials. Although questions remain, the clinician is in a much better position to manage VTE in a safe and effective manner, and this will undoubtedly lead to improved patient care and a decreased threat of medical liability. The use of similar methodology for the evaluation of new antithrombotic agents including LMWH and the specific antithrombin agents as well as the newer thrombolytic agents, e.g. recombinant pro-urokinase or recombinant bat tissue plasminogen activator will be awaited with interest.

REFERENCES

(I)1. Hull RD, Van Aken WG, Hirsh J, et al. Impedance plethysmography using the occlusive cuff technique in the diagnosis of venous thrombosis. Circulation 1976;53: 696–700.

(I)2. Salzman EW, Deykin D, Shapiro RM, et al. Management of heparin therapy: controlled prospective trial. N Engl J Med 1976;292:1046–1050.

(I)3. Hull RD, Taylor DW, Hirsh J, et al. Impedance plethysmography: the relationship between venous filling and sensitivity and specificity for proximal-vein thrombosis. Circulation 1978;58:898–902.

(I)4. Hull RD, Hirsh J, Sackett DL, et al. Clinical validity of a negative venogram in patients with clinically suspected venous thrombosis. Circulation 1981;64:622–625.

(I)5. Hull RD, Hirsh J, Carter CJ, et al. Pulmonary angiography ventilation lung scanning and venography for clinically suspected pulmonary embolism with abnormal perfusion lung scan. Ann Intern Med 1983;98:891–899.

(I)6. Hull RD, Hirsh J, Carter CJ, et al. Diagnostic value of ventilation-perfusion lung scanning in patients with suspected pulmonary embolism. Chest 1985;88:819–828.

(I)7. Hull RD, Hirsh J, Carter CJ, et al. Diagnostic efficacy of impedance plethysmography for clinically suspected deep-vein thrombosis: a randomized trial. Ann Intern Med 1985;102:21–28.

(I)8. Huisman MV, Buller HE, ten Cate JW, et al. Serial impedance plethysmography for suspected deep venous thrombosis in outpatients. The Amsterdam General Practitioner Study. N Engl J Med 1986;314:823–828.

(I)9. Hull R, Raskob G, Coates G, Panju A, Gill GJ. A new noninvasive management strategy for patients with suspected pulmonary embolism. Arch Intern Med 1989;149: 2549–2555.

(I)10. Huisman MV, Buller HR, ten Cate JW, et al. Unexpected high prevalence of silent pulmonary embolism in patients with deep venous thrombosis. Chest 1989;95: 498–502.

(I)11. Lensing AW, Prandoni P, Brandjes DPM, et al. Detection of deep-vein thrombosis by real-time B-mode ultrasonography. N Engl J Med 1989;320:342–345.

(I)12. Huisman MV, Buller HR, ten Cate JW, et al. Management of clinically suspected acute venous thrombosis in outpatients with serial impedance plethysmography in a community hospital setting. Arch Int Med 1989;149:511–513.

(I)13. Hull R, Raskob G, Coates G, Panju A. Clinical validity of a normal perfusion lung scan in patients with suspected pulmonary embolism. Chest 1990;97:23–26.

(I)14. Prospective Investigation of Pulmonary Embolism Diagnosis Investigators. Value of the ventilation-perfusion scan in acute pulmonary embolism: results of the Prospective Investigation of Pulmonary Embolism Diagnosis. JAMA 1990;263:2753–2759.

(I)15. Hull R, Raskob G. Low probability lung scan findings: a need for change. Ann Intern Med 1991;114:142–143.

(I)16. Heijboer H, Cogo A, Buller HR, Prandoni P, ten Cate JW. Detection of deep-vein thrombosis with impedance plethysmography and real-time compression ultrasonography in hospitalized patients. Arch Intern Med 1992;152:1901–1903.

(I)17. Heijboer H, Buller HR, Lensing AWA, Turpie AG, et al. A comparison of real-time compression ultrasonography versus impedance plethysmography for the diagnosis of deep-vein thrombosis in symptomatic outpatients. N Engl J Med 1993:329:1365–1369.

(I)18. Hull R, Raskob G, Ginsberg J, et al. A noninvasive strategy for the treatment of patients with suspected pulmonary embolism. Arch Intern Med 1994;154:289–297.

(I)19. Hull RD, Delmore T, Genton E, et al. Warfarin sodium vs low dose heparin in the long-term treatment of venous thrombosis. N Engl J Med 1979;301:855–858.

(I)20. Hull R, Hirsh J, Jay R, et al. Different intensities of oral anticoagulant therapy in the treatment of proximal-vein thrombosis. N Engl J Med 1982; 307:1676–1681.

(I)21. Hull RD, Raskob GE, Hirsh J, et al. Continuous intravenous heparin compared with intermittent subcutaneous heparin in the initial treatment of proximal-vein thrombosis. N Engl J Med 1986;315:1109–1114.

(I)22. Gallus A, Jackaman J, Tillett J, et al. Safety and efficacy of warfarin started early after submassive venous thrombosis or pulmonary embolism. Lancet 1986;2:1293–1296.

(I)23. Hull R, Raskob G, Rosenbloom D, et al. Heparin for 5 days compared with 10 days in the initial treatment of proximal venous thrombosis. N Engl J Med 1990;322: 1260–1264.

(I)24. Hull RD, Raskob GE, Rosenbloom DR, et al. Optimal therapeutic level of heparin therapy in patients with venous thrombosis. Arch Int Med 1992;152:1589–1595.

(I)25. Hull RD, Raskob GE, Pineo GF, et al. Subcutaneous low-molecular-weight heparin compared with continuous intravenous heparin in the treatment of proximal-vein thrombosis. N Engl J Med 1992;326:975–982.

(I)26. Brandjes DPM, Heijboer H, Buller HR, et al. Acenocoumarol and heparin compared with acenocoumarol alone in the initial treatment of proximal-vein thrombosis. N Engl J Med 1992;327:1485–1489.

(I)27. Prandoni P, Lensing AW, Buller HR, et al. Comparison of subcutaneous low-molecular-weight heparin with intravenous standard heparin in proximal deep-vein thrombosis. Lancet 1992;339:441–445.

(I)28. Lopaciuk S, Meissner AJ, Filipecki S, et al. Subcutaneous low-molecular-weight heparin versus subcutaneous unfractionated heparin in the treatment of deep vein thrombosis: a Polish multicentre trial. Thromb Haemost 1992;68:14–18.

(I)29. Raschke RA, Reilly BM, Guidry JR, et al. The weight-based heparin dosing nomogram compared with a "standard care" nomogram. Ann Int Med 1993;119:874.

(I)30. Simonneau G, Charbonnier B, Decousus H, et al. Subcutaneous low-molecular-weight heparin compared with continuous intravenous unfractionated heparin in the treatment of proximal deep vein thrombosis. Arch Int Med 1993;153:1541–1546.

(I)31. Lindmarker P, Holmstrom M, Granqvist S, Johnsson H,

Locner D. Comparison of once-daily subcutaneous Fragmin with continuous intravenous unfractionated heparin in the treatment of deep venous thrombosis. Thromb Haemost 1994:72:186–190.

(I)32. de Valk HW, Banga JD, Wester JWJ, et al. Comparing subcutaneous danaparoid with intravenous unfractionated heparin for the treatment of venous thromboembolism. Ann Int Med 1995;123(1):1–9.

(I)33. Schulman S, Rhedin AS, Lindmarker P, et al. A comparison of six weeks with six months of oral anticoagulant therapy after a first episode of venous thromboembolism. N Engl J Med 1995;332:1661–1665.

(I)34. The Urokinase Pulmonary Embolism Trial. A national cooperative study. Circulation 1973;47-I:1–108.

(I)35. Sharma GVRK, Burleson VA, Sasahara AA. Effect of thrombolytic therapy on pulmonary-capillary blood volume in patients with pulmonary embolism. N Engl J Med 1980;303:842–845.

(I)36. The UKEP Study Research Group. The UKEP study: multicentre clinical trial on two local regimens of urokinase in massive pulmonary embolism. Eur Heart J 1987;8: 2–10.

(I)37. Verstraete M, Miller GAH, Bounameaux H, et al. Intravenous and intrapulmonary recombinant tissue-type plasminogen activator in the treatment of acute massive pulmonary embolism. Circulation 1988;7: 353–360.

(I)38. Goldhaber SZ, Kessler CM, Heit J, et al. A randomized controlled trial of recombinant tissue plasminogen activator versus urokinase in the treatment of acute pulmonary embolism. Lancet 1988;2:293–298.

(I)39. Levine MN, Hirsh J, Weitz J, et al. A randomized trial of a single bolus dosage regimen of recombinant tissue plasminogen activator in patients with acute pulmonary embolism. Chest 1990;98:1473–1479.

(I)40. Dalla-Volta S, Palla A, Santolicandro A, et al. PAIMS 2: Alteplase combined with heparin versus heparin in the treatment of acute pulmonary embolism. Plasminogen Activator Italian Multicentre Study 2. J Am Coll Cardiol 1992;20:520–526.

(I)41. Meyer G, Sors H, Charbonnier B, et al, on behalf of the European Cooperative Study Group for Pulmonary Embolism. Effects of intravenous urokinase versus alteplase on total pulmonary resistance in acute massive pulmonary embolism: a European multicentre double-blind trial. J Am Coll Cardiol 1992;19:239–245.

(I)42. Goldhaber SZ, Haire WD, Feldstein ML, et al. Alteplase versus heparin in acute pulmonary embolism: randomized trial assessing right ventricular function and pulmonary perfusion. Lancet 1993;341:507–511.

28

Heparin Treatment of Venous Thromboembolism

Russell D. Hull, Graham F. Pineo

INTRODUCTION

A combination of continuous intravenous heparin and oral warfarin sodium is the standard anticoagulant therapy for venous thromboembolism (VTE) (deep-vein thrombosis (DVT) and/or pulmonary embolism (PE)).[1–3(I)] Heparin and warfarin used simultaneously is standard clinical practice for all patients with VTE who are medically stable.[4(I),5(I)] Exceptions are patients who require immediate medical or surgical intervention (such as thrombolysis or insertion of a vena cava filter), patients in the intensive care unit who have multiple invasive lines, and patients with conditions that predispose them to major bleeding. A shortening of the hospital stay to 5 days for initial intravenous heparin therapy has led to significant cost savings.[4(I),5(I)] Although heparin and warfarin are given together, they are discussed separately in this review.

HEPARIN THERAPY FOR VENOUS THROMBOEMBOLISM

Because the onset of action of standard unfractionated heparin is immediate when it is administered intravenously, it is the anticoagulant of choice for the treatment of acute thrombotic disorders.[1–3(I)] The basic biochemistry, pharmacology, and pharmacokinetics of heparin have recently been reviewed,[6,7] and the uses of heparin in the prevention of venous thrombosis have been well established by consensus conferences.[8,9] Well-designed randomized clinical trials conducted over the past 10 years have led to important advances in heparin therapy.[4(I),5(I),10(I),11(I)] Most of the uncertainties commonly encountered in selecting an appropriate course of heparin therapy have now been resolved.

HEPARIN: MECHANISM OF ACTION AND PHARMACOLOGY

The anticoagulant activity of unfractionated heparin depends upon a unique pentasaccharide which binds to antithrombin III (ATIII) and potentiates the inhibition of thrombin and activated factor X (X_a) by ATIII.[12–15] Heparin also catalyzes the inactivation of thrombin by another plasma cofactor, heparin cofactor II, which acts independently of ATIII.[16] Other effects of heparin are that it binds to numerous plasma and platelet proteins, to endothelial cells and leukocytes, and it increases vascular permeability.[7] These latter effects may explain some of the nonanticoagulant effects as well as the hemorrhagic effects of heparin, and may also help to explain why relative heparin resistance develops in some individuals.[7] It has been shown that there is wide variability in the response of individuals to heparin and that frequent monitoring with laboratory tests (e.g., activated partial thromboplastin time [APTT]) is necessary.

HEPARIN THERAPY FOR VENOUS THROMBOEMBOLISM

Two developments have led to clinical trials for evaluating heparin therapy for VTE: the availability of accurate objective tests to detect VTE, and advances in clinical trial methodology.[4(I),5(I),10(I),11(I)] Such clinical trials have established the need for initial heparin treatment,[10(I),17(V)] the optimal duration of this treatment,[4(I),5(I)] and the need for adequate intensity of heparin treatment to prevent recurrent VTE.[5(I)] Because the anticoagulant response to a standard dose of heparin varies widely between patients, the anticoagulant response to heparin must be monitored and the dose must be titrated in the individual patient.[19,20] Most recently, clinical trials have provided im-

From *Venous Thromboembolism: An Evidence-Based Atlas* edited by Russell Hull, Gary Raskob, Graham Pineo © 1996, Futura Publishing Co., Armonk, NY.

portant new information on the appropriate therapeutic range for laboratory monitoring of heparin therapy.[11(I)]

LABORATORY MONITORING AND THERAPEUTIC RANGE

The laboratory test most commonly used to monitor heparin therapy is the APTT. In a traditional and widely used approach, the heparin infusion dose is adjusted to maintain the APTT within a defined "therapeutic range". Over the years, it has been customary to use an upper and lower limit (that is, an APTT ratio of 1.5 to 2.5 times control). Maintaining the APTT response within this range is based on two concepts: (1) maintaining the APTT ratio above the lower limit of 1.5 minimizes recurrent venous thromboembolic events, and (2) maintaining the APTT ratio below the upper limit of 2.5 minimizes the risk of bleeding complications. More recently, rigorously designed clinical trials have led to firm recommendations about the appropriate therapeutic range for the APTT. Failure to exceed the lower limit (an APTT ratio of 1.5) is associated with an unacceptably high risk of recurrent VTE[5(I)]; in contrast, no association exists between supratherapeutic APTT responses (an APTT ratio of 2.5 or more) and the risk of bleeding.[11(I)]

VARIABILITY OF APTT RESULTS AND HEPARIN BLOOD LEVELS WITH DIFFERENT APTT REAGENTS

The efficacy of heparin therapy depends upon achieving a critical therapeutic level of heparin within the first 24 hours of treatment, as shown by experimental studies and clinical trials. The critical therapeutic level of heparin as measured by the APTT is 1.5 times the mean of the control value, or a heparin blood level of 0.2 to 0.4 units/mL measured by the protamine sulphate titration assay.[19] Different reagents and even different batches of the same reagent can cause the APTT and heparin blood levels to vary widely. It is, therefore, vital that each laboratory establish the minimal therapeutic level of heparin (measured by the APTT) that will provide a heparin blood level of at least 0.2 units/mL (measured by the protamine titration assay) for each batch of thromboplastin reagent being used, and particularly if the reagent is provided by a different manufacturer.

Variability in the APTT response to different heparin blood levels supports the need for an aggressive approach to heparin therapy to ensure that all patients achieve adequate therapy early in the course of their treatment. This problem can be eliminated by using low-molecular-weight heparin which does not require laboratory monitoring. However, until these agents are approved for use, the problem of APTT standardization remains.

EVIDENCE FOR THE LOWER LIMIT OF THE THERAPEUTIC RANGE

Data from three randomized clinical trials[5(I),21(I),22(I)] have provided firm support for using an APTT ratio of 1.5 as the lower limit of the therapeutic range.

The first randomized trial evaluated clinical outcomes in patients with proximal-vein thrombosis who were treated either with continuous intravenous heparin or with intermittent subcutaneous heparin which was adjusted to prolong the APTT to > 1.5 times the control value.[5(I)] When the subcutaneous regimen was used, the initial anticoagulant response was below the lower limit in the majority (63%) of patients. There was also a high frequency of recurrent VTE (11 of 57 patients, 19.3%); this was virtually confined to patients with a subtherapeutic anticoagulant response.[5(I)] In contrast, when continuous intravenous heparin was used, there was an adequate anticoagulant response in the majority (71%) of patients, and a low frequency of recurrent thromboembolic events (three of 58 patients, 5.2%); the recurrences in this group were also limited to patients with an initial subtherapeutic anticoagulant response.[5(I)] Thirteen of 53 patients (24.5%) who had an APTT response below the lower limit for 24 hours or more had recurrent VTE; in contrast, only one of 62 patients (1.6%) in whom the APTT ratio was 1.5 or more had recurrent thromboembolism (p < 0.001). The relative risk for recurrent VTE was 15 : 1. Similar results were found when a weight-based heparin-dosing nomogram (starting dose 80 units/kg bolus and 18 units/kg/hour infusion) was compared with a standard-care nomogram (starting dose 5,000 units bolus and 1,000 units/hour infusion).[22(I)] When the weight-based nomogram was used, the therapeutic threshold was exceeded in 60 of 62 patients (97%) within 24 hours compared with 37 of 48 (77%) of patients in the standard care group (p<0.002). Recurrent thromboembolism in the 3-month treatment period was more frequent in the standard care group; relative risk was 5.0 (95% CI 1.1–21.9).[22(I)]

These findings are strongly supported by a recent randomized trial in which intravenous heparin was compared with oral anticoagulants alone for the initial treatment of patients with proximal-vein thrombosis.[21(I)] Because of the nature of treatment in the latter group, the APTT response was inadequate for at least the first 48 hours because the onset of the anticoagulant effect of oral anticoagulants was delayed. Recurrent VTE occurred in 12 of 60 patients (20%) treated with oral anticoagulants alone over the subsequent 3 months; only four of 60 patients (6.7%) who received initial intravenous heparin plus oral anticoagulants had recurrent VTE (p = 0.058).[21(I)]

Because recurrent thromboembolism typically occurred between 3 and 12 weeks in all these trials, it may not be recognized that these recurrent clinical events relate to the failure of initial therapy.

LACK OF ASSOCIATION BETWEEN THE UPPER LIMIT OF THE THERAPEUTIC RANGE AND THE RISK OF BLEEDING

In contrast to the strong association between a subtherapeutic APTT response and recurrent VTE, evidence supporting the use of an upper limit for the therapeutic range is weak. Randomized clinical trials were not able to provide clear guidelines for an upper limit to the therapeutic range until recently. The use of an upper limit, and the clinical practice of reducing the heparin dose when the APTT results exceed this limit, have been based on clinical custom and the intuitive belief that this practice minimizes the risk of bleeding.

Important new information on the upper limit of the therapeutic range for the APTT has been obtained from a recent randomized trial.[11(I)] Patients with proximal-vein thrombosis were randomized to receive initial treatment with either intravenous heparin alone, or intravenous heparin with simultaneous warfarin sodium, and clinical outcomes were evaluated. The group that was treated with combined heparin and warfarin received more intensive anticoagulation, and the majority of patients exceeded the predefined upper limit (an APTT ratio of 2.5) for sustained periods of time.[11(I)] This was demonstrated by the finding that 69 of 99 patients (69%) in the combined group had a supratherapeutic APTT value (a ratio of 2.5 or more) persisting for 24 hours or more, compared with 24 of 100 patients (24%) in the heparin-alone group ($p < 0.001$). Despite the more intense therapy in the combined group, bleeding complications occurred with similar frequency in the two groups: nine of 99 patients in the combined group (9.1%) had bleeding complications, compared with 12 of 100 patients (12%) in the heparin-alone group.[11(I)] Major bleeding occurred in 3 of 93 patients (3.2%) with supratherapeutic APTT findings, compared with 10 of 106 patients (9.4%) without supratherapeutic APTT findings (relative risk 0.3, $p = 0.09$).[11(I)]

These results indicate a lack of association between a supratherapeutic APTT result (ratio 2.5 or more) and the risk of clinically important bleeding complications. On the other hand, when the incidence of major bleeding was related to the clinical risk of bleeding, patients considered at low risk for bleeding who received the higher heparin dose had a low frequency of major bleeding (1%); those considered at high risk for bleeding who received a lower dose of heparin had a higher frequency of major bleeding (11%) ($p = 0.007$).[11(I)]

THE NEED FOR QUALITY ASSURANCE OF HEPARIN THERAPY

Surveys of heparin therapy suggest that administration of intravenous heparin is always difficult,[17(V),23(IV),24] and that using an ad hoc or intuitive approach to heparin dose-titration frequently results in inadequate therapy. For example, physician practices at three university-affiliated hospitals were examined.[24] Adequate APTT responses (a ratio of 1.5) were not obtained during the initial 24 hours of therapy. Furthermore, 30% to 40% of patients remained subtherapeutic over the next 3 to 4 days.

A frequent factor in inadequate therapy is the clinician's exaggerated fear of bleeding complications. Consequently, it has been common practice for many clinicians to start treatment with a low heparin dose and to cautiously increase this dose over several days to achieve the therapeutic range. Clinical trial data indicate that this practice is inappropriate, and indeed dangerous, because it places the patient at an unacceptably high risk for recurrent VTE.[11(I)]

APPROACHES TO QUALITY ASSURANCE OF INTRAVENOUS HEPARIN THERAPY

A prescriptive protocol for administering intravenous heparin therapy has been evaluated in three studies in patients with VTE.[11(I),22(I),23(IV)]

Cruickshank et al,[23(IV)] evaluated a dosing nomogram for intravenous heparin that was designed to achieve an early therapeutic APTT response, to prevent prolonged periods of inadequate anticoagulation, and to avoid periods of overanticoagulation. Compared with a historical control group, the use of the nomogram resulted in differences that are clinically important and statistically significant. There was an increase in the proportion of patients in whom the APTT result was within the therapeutic range at 24 hours (an increase from 37% to 66%) and at 48 hours (an increase from 58% to 81%). Even when the dosing nomogram was used, however, a relatively high proportion (19%) of patients had subtherapeutic APTT responses early in therapy which persisted for 24 hours or more. This study did not report on recurrent VTE and bleeding. In a recently reported clinical trial, patients were randomized to receive heparin therapy alone (100 patients) or heparin therapy with simultaneous warfarin sodium therapy (99 patients).[11(I)] The two objectives were: (1) to validate a prescriptive approach designed to minimize the proportion of patients receiving subtherapeutic doses of heparin within the first 24 hours in the presence or absence of oral anticoagulant therapy; and (2) to determine the effectiveness and safety of decreasing the amount of heparin infused (based on the prolongation of the APTT) to reflect both the heparin effect and alteration of the vitamin K clotting factors due to warfarin sodium. This prescriptive approach is summarized in Tables 1 and 2.

Table 1
Intravenous Heparin Protocol for Patients with Venous Thromboembolism*

1. Initial intravenous heparin bolus: 5000 units.
2. Continuous intravenous heparin infusion: commence at 42 mL/hour of 20,000 units (1680 units/hour) in 500 mL of diluent (a 24-hour heparin dose of 40,320 units), except in the following patients, in whom the heparin infusion is commenced at a rate of 31 mL/hour (1240 units/hour) (i.e., a 2-hour dose of 29,760 units).
   a. Patients who have undergone surgery within the previous 2 weeks.
   b. Patients with a previous history of peptic ulcer disease, gastrointestinal bleeding, or genitourinary bleeding.
   c. Patients with recent stroke (i.e., thrombotic stroke within the previous 2 weeks).
   d. Patients with a platelet count $< 150 \times 10^9$ per liter.
   e. Patients with miscellaneous reasons for a high risk of bleeding (e.g., invasive line, hepatic failure, etc.)
3. The APTT is performed in all patients as outlined below:
   a. 4 hours after commencing heparin; the heparin dose is then adjusted according to the nomogram shown in Table 3.
   b. 4 to 6 hours after implementing the first dosage adjustment.
   c. The APTT is then performed as indicated by the nomogram (Table 3) for the first 24 hours of therapy.
   d. Thereafter, the APTT is performed once daily, unless the patient is subtherapeutic, in which case the APTT should be repeated 4 hours after increasing the heparin dose.

---

* From Hull R, Raskob G, Rosenbloom D, et al. Optimal therapeutic level of heparin therapy in patients with venous thrombosis. Arch Intern Med 152:1589–1595, 1992.

Only 2% and 1% of the patients received subtherapeutic doses for more than 24 hours in the combined heparin and warfarin group, and the heparin-alone group, respectively.[11(I)] Recurrent VTE (objectively documented) occurred infrequently in both groups (7%),[11(I)] rates similar to those previously reported.[4(I),5(I),11(I)] Subtherapy was avoided in most patients, and the prescriptive heparin protocol resulted in effective delivery of heparin therapy in both groups. Further, because of the influence of warfarin on the APTT response, patients in the combined treatment group received less heparin per 24 hours than those in the heparin-alone group, with no adverse outcome.[11(I)]

The frequencies of bleeding were 9% in the group treated with heparin and warfarin simultaneously, and 12% in the heparin-alone group.[11(I)] These frequencies are similar to previously reported rates of bleeding.[3(I),4(I),5(I)] The heparin nomogram was also used in a randomized clinical trial in which fixed-dose subcutaneous LMWH was compared with continuous intravenous heparin in the initial treatment of proximal venous thrombosis.[25(I)] Warfarin was started on day 2 in all patients. In all 15 different treatment centers, use of the heparin nomogram insured that the vast majority of patients were within the therapeutic range within 24 hours. Findings from one of the treatment centers indicated that 91% of patients were within the therapeutic range (PTT > 1.5 × control) within 24 hours compared with only 60% of the patients who were treated without the use of a heparin protocol.[26(I)]

In another randomized clinical trial, a weight-based heparin-dosing nomogram was compared with a standard-care nomogram.[22(I)] Patients on the weight-based heparin nomogram received a starting bolus of 80 units/kg and infusion of 18 units/kg/hour. Patients on the standard-care nomogram received a bolus of 5,000 units and infusion of 1,000 units/hour The heparin dose was planned to maintain an APTT of 1.5 to 2.3 times control. The results to be measured were: (1) the time to exceed the therapeutic threshold of an APTT > 1.5 times control, and (2) the time to achieve the therapeutic range (an APTT of 1.5 to 2.3 times control). In the weight-based

Table 2
Intravenous Heparin Dose-Titration Nomogram Using the APTT for Patients with Venous Thromboembolism*

APTT (secs)	IV Infusion		Additional Action
	Rate Change (mL/hr)	Dose Change (units/24 hrs)	
≤ 45	+6	+5,760	Repeat APTT in 4–6 hrs
46–54	+3	+2,880	Repeat APTT in 4–6 hrs
55–85	0	0	None***
86–110	−3	−2,880	Stop heparin for 1 hour / Repeat APTT 4–6 hours after restarting heparin
>110	−6	−5,760	Stop heparin for 1 hour / Repeat APTT 4–6 hours after restarting heparin

* Using Actin-FS thromboplastin APTT reagent (Dade). From Hull R, Raskob G, Rosenbloom D, et al. Optimal therapeutic level of heparin therapy in patients with venous thrombosis. Arch Intern Med 1992; 152:1589–1595.

** Heparin concentration 20,000 units in 500 mL = 40 units/mL.

*** During the first 24 hours, repeat APTT in 4–6 hours. Thereafter, the APTT is done once daily, unless subtherapeutic.

heparin group, 97% of patients exceeded the therapeutic threshold within 24 hours compared with 77% in the standard-care group (p = 0.082).[22(I)] In the weight-based group, 89% of patients achieved the therapeutic range within 24 hours compared with 75% in the standard-care group.[22(I)] The risk of recurrent thromboembolism was more frequent in the standard-care group. This study also included patients with unstable angina and arterial thromboembolism (in addition to patients with VTE) indicating that the principles used in the heparin nomogram for treating VTE may be generalized to other clinical conditions.

SUMMARY

Clinical trials performed over the past decade have revolutionized the use of heparin and warfarin in the treatment of VTE. The use of a heparin nomogram, as opposed to the intuition-based ordering of heparin, guarantees that virtually all patients will achieve a therapeutic heparin level as measured by the APTT within the first 24 hours. The threat of recurrent VTE is minimized. In the past, fear of bleeding if the APTT level rose above the therapeutic range frequently led to inadequate treatment. However, bleeding on heparin depends more on underlying clinical risk factors rather than on the level of the APTT. It is more important, therefore, to avoid subtherapeutic doses of heparin than to be overly concerned about achieving supratherapeutic APTT levels. Furthermore, the APTT will vary widely with different reagents and even with different batches of the same reagent. It is vital, therefore, that each laboratory establish the minimal therapeutic level of heparin (as measured by the APTT) that will provide a heparin blood level of at least 0.2 units/mL as measured by the protamine titration assay. This exercise must be repeated with each batch of thromboplastin reagent being used, especially if the reagent is provided by a different manufacturer.

Unfractionated heparin remains the drug of choice for the initial management of VTE. Intravenous heparin is, however, labor-intensive and expensive because the dose must be titrated for each patient. The advent of the LMWHs, some of which have been shown to be effective and safe and to have the convenience of a once daily subcutaneous injection without laboratory monitoring, indicates that unfractionated heparin will soon be relegated to a secondary role in the treatment of VTE.[25(I)]

REFERENCES

1. Hyers TM, Hull RD, Weg J. Antithrombotic therapy for venous thromboembolic disease. Chest 1992;102:408S-425S.
2. Moser KM. Venous thromboembolism. Am Rev Respir Dis 1990;141:235–249.
(I)3. Salzman EW, Deykin D, Shapiro RM, et al.

Management of heparin therapy: controlled prospective trial. N Engl J Med 1976;292:1046–1050.
(I)4. Gallus A, Jackaman J, Tillett J, et al. Safety and efficacy of warfarin started early after submassive venous thrombosis or pulmonary embolism. Lancet 1986;2:1293–1296.
(I)5. Hull RD, Raskob GE, Rosenbloom D, et al. Heparin for 5 days as compared with 10 days in the initial treatment of proximal venous thrombosis. N Engl J Med 1990;322:1260–1264.
6. Colvin BT, Barrowcliffe TW on behalf of BCSH Haemostasis and Thrombosis Task Force. The British Society for Haematology Guidelines on the use and monitoring of heparin 1992; second revision. J Clin Path 1993;46:97–103.
7. Hirsh J, Dalen JE, Deykin D, et al. Heparin: mechanism of action, pharmacokinetics, dosing consideration, monitoring, efficacy, and safety. Chest 1992;102(4):337S-351S.
8. Clagett GP, Anderson FA Jr, Levine MN, et al. Prevention of venous thromboembolism. Chest 1992;102(4):391S-407S.
9. Nicolaides AN (Chairman), European Consensus Statement 1–5 Nov 1991: Prevention of venous thromboembolism. Int Angiol 1992;11(3):151–159.
(I)10. Hull RD, Raskob GE, Hirsh J, et al. Continuous intravenous heparin compared with intermittent subcutaneous heparin in the initial treatment of proximal-vein thrombosis. N Engl J Med 1986;315:1109–1114.
(I)11. Hull RD, Raskob GE, Pineo GF, et al. Subcutaneous low-molecular weight heparin compared with continuous intravenous heparin in the treatment of proximal-vein thrombosis. N Eng J Med 1992;326:975–982.
12. Bjork I, Lindahl U. Mechanism of the anticoagulant action of heparin. Mol Cell Biochem 1982;48:161–182.
13. Lindahl U, Backstrom G, Cook M, et al. Structure of the antithrombin-binding site of heparin. Proc Natl Acad Sci USA 1979;76:3198–3202.
14. Rosenberg RD, Damus PS. The purification and mechanism of action of human antithrombin-heparin cofactor. J Biol Chem 1973;248:6490–6506.
15. Rosenberg RD, Lam L. Correlation between structure and function of heparin. Proc Natl Acad Sci USA 1979;76:1218–1222.
16. Tollefsen DM, Majerus DW, Blank MK. Heparin cofactor II: purification and properties of thrombin in human plasma. J Bio Chem 1982;257:2162–2169.
(V)17. Fennerty A, Thomas P, Backhouse G, et al. Audit of control of heparin treatment. Br Med J 1985;290:27–28.
18. Cipolle RJ, Seifert RD, Neilan BA, et al. Heparin kinetics: variables related to disposition and dosage. Clin Pharmacol Ther 1981;29:387–393.
19. Brill-Edwards P, Ginsberg S, Johnston M, Hirsh J. Establishing a therapeutic range for heparin therapy. Ann Int Med 1993;119:104–109.
20. Hirsh J, van Aken WG, Gallus AS, et al. Heparin kinetics in venous thrombosis and pulmonary embolism. Circulation 1976;53:691–695.
(I)21. Brandjes DPM, Heijboer H, Buller HR, et al. Acenocoumarol and heparin compared with acenocoumarol alone in the initial treatment of proximal-vein thrombosis. N Engl J Med 1992;327:1485–1489.
(I)22. Raschke RA, Reilly BM, Guidry JR, et al. The weight-based heparin dosing nomogram compared with a "standard care" nomogram. Ann Intern Med 1993;119:874–881.
(IV)23. Cruickshank MK, Levine MN, Hirsh J, et al: A standard

nomogram for the management of heparin therapy. Arch Intern Med 1991;151:333–337.

24. Wheeler AP, Jaquiss RD, Newman JH. Physician practices in the treatment of pulmonary embolism and deep-venous thrombosis. Arch Intern Med 1988;148:1321–1325.

(I)25. Hull RD, Raskob GE, Rosenbloom DR, et al. Optimal therapeutic level of heparin therapy in patients with venous thrombosis. Arch Intern Med 1992;152:1589–1595.

(I)26. Elliott CG, Hiltunen SJ, Suchyta M, et al. Physician guided treatment compared with a heparin protocol for deep vein thrombosis. Arch Int Med 1994;154:999–1004.

29

The Treatment
of Venous Thromboembolism
with Low-Molecular-Weight Heparin

Graham F. Pineo, Russell D. Hull

INTRODUCTION

Certain low-molecular-weight heparins (LMWHs) can now be justified for the initial treatment of venous thromboembolism (VTE), in place of continuous intravenous unfractionated heparin. The LMWHs are given subcutaneously and have a predictably high absorption rate and a prolonged duration of action. This means that they can be administered by injection once or twice daily for the prevention or treatment of venous thrombosis. Another advantage is that treatment does not require laboratory monitoring. Eliminating the need for continuous IV infusion and for laboratory monitoring will allow patients to be discharged earlier, and eventually lead to the outpatient treatment of VTE. Studies indicate that LMWH is more cost-effective than unfractionated heparin. This cost-effectiveness will be further increased by out-of-hospital treatment. Because the findings associated with any individual LMWH preparation cannot be extrapolated to different LMWHs, each preparation must be evaluated in separate clinical trials. The information to date is that LMWH is safer and more effective than continuous intravenous unfractionated heparin in the treatment of proximal venous thrombosis. An unexpected decrease in mortality rate has been observed in two clinical trials, particularly in patients with metastatic cancer. Larger prospective randomized trials are necessary to confirm this finding.

BACKGROUND

Acute VTE is usually treated as follows: intravenous heparin is given continuously for 5 to 6 days[1(I),2(II),3(I)] and warfarin is started on day 1 or 2[(I)4,5(I)] and continued for 3 months. The therapeutic range for heparin is indicated by an APTT value of 1.5 to 2.5 times the mean of the control value to provide a heparin blood level of 0.2 to 0.4 units/mL (using the protamine sulphate titration assay). The targeted INR for warfarin is 2.0 to 3.0.

Evaluation of various methods for the treatment of VTE have resulted from improvements in clinical-trials methodology as well as the availability of accurate objective tests for detecting VTE. From this series of randomized clinical trials, therapeutic ranges for intravenous heparin and oral warfarin have been established. As a result, the recurrence rate of VTE has decreased and brought the incidence of major bleeding to acceptably low levels. If the APTT does not reach a therapeutic level (> 1.5 times the control value) within the initial 24 hours or more, patients have a much greater tendency to develop recurrent VTE during the following 3-month period.[3(I),8(I),9(I)] Most symptomatic recurrences occurred after the first month of treatment. A less intense form of warfarin (INR 2.0 to 3.0) was as effective as higher intensity warfarin (INR 3.0 to 4.5) and there was a markedly reduced incidence of major bleeding.[7(I)] Although bleeding in patients on warfarin can be directly related to elevation of the INR above its therapeutic range,[7(I)] there is little evidence that bleeding in patients on heparin is associated with an APTT above its therapeutic range (>2.5 times control).[6(I)] There is, however, a direct correlation between bleeding in patients on heparin and the existence of a clinical risk for bleeding (such as recent surgery, peptic ulcer disease, or recent stroke) in these patients.[6(I)] Unless a heparin protocol is used, many patients will remain subtherapeutic for extended periods of time. Consequently, they will be at significant risk for recurrent VTE and death.[10,11] A heparin protocol will ensure that the therapeutic range of APTT will be achieved in virtually all patients (98% to 99%) within the initial 24 hours of treatment. The chances of recurrent thromboembolism will be decreased with no added risk of bleeding.[6(I),9(I)]

A number of randomized clinical trials have compared the effectiveness and safety of subcutaneously injected heparin given twice daily with that of continuous intravenous heparin. Meta-analysis led to the conclusion that subcutaneous heparin is at least as effective and safe as intravenous heparin.[12] In view of the well-established need to achieve a lower limit for the therapeutic range of APTT or heparin level[6(I),9(I),13] and the demonstration that subcutaneous heparin frequently results in subtherapeutic therapy (as indicated by the APTT or heparin level), subcutaneous heparin cannot be recommended in the initial treatment of proximal venous thrombosis. Furthermore, there is growing evidence that if heparin is used inadequately in the initial stages, markedly increased heparin doses may be required over the subsequent 5 or 6 days. Such heparin resistance has been most evident in patients who have subsequently developed recurrent VTE.[14]

LOW-MOLECULAR-WEIGHT HEPARIN

The possible role of LMWH in the initial treatment of VTE has been eagerly awaited. Several LMWH derivatives of commercial heparin have been prepared in recent years. The mean molecular weight of these heparins ranges from 4,000 to 5,000 daltons (the molecular weight for unfractionated heparin is 12,000 to 16,000 daltons[15]). Pharmacokinetic studies[16–21] as well as recent small clinical trials in selected patients with venous thrombosis[22–24,25(II),26] have indicated that the availability of LMWH fractions after subcutaneous injection was very high. The bioavailability of LMWH after a single subcutaneous injection of 120 factor X_a units/kg was approximately 90% of an equivalent intravenous dose in studies on healthy volunteers.[18] Compared with unfractionated heparin,[16–19,21,27] this excellent bioavailability of LMWH, along with the longer half-life of its anticoagulant activity (as measured by antifactor X_a activity), suggested that an effective regimen for the initial treatment of VTE using a once-daily subcutaneous injection of LMWH might be possible. Furthermore, there was also a high correlation between body weight and the anticoagulant response (measured by factor X_a inhibitor units/mL) observed with a given dose of LMWH.[21] This suggested that LMWH could be given by a fixed dose (in terms of factor X_a units/kg) with no laboratory monitoring. Studies in experimental animal models of venous thrombosis have shown that some LMWH fractions have equal (or greater) antithrombotic efficacy and fewer hemorrhagic effects than unfractionated heparin.[15,28–31] Low-molecular-weight heparins have been shown to be effective prophylactic agents following a number of moderate to high-risk procedures.[32,33,34(I),35(I),36]

RANDOMIZED CLINICAL TRIALS—EVALUATING THE USE OF LOW-MOLECULAR-WEIGHT HEPARIN FOR THE TREATMENT OF PROXIMAL VENOUS THROMBOSIS

Low-molecular-weight heparin has been compared with unfractionated heparin in several randomized clinical trials for the initial treatment of patients with proximal venous thrombosis.[26(II),37(I),38(II),39(II),40(V),41(II),42(V),43(II),44(I),45(I),46(I),47(I),48(I),49(I)] Continuous intravenous LMWH was compared with continuous intravenous unfractionated heparin in many of these studies.[37–39,43] In two trials, subcutaneous LMWH was compared with subcutaneous unfractionated heparin,[26(II),49(I)] and in three studies subcutaneous LMWH was compared with continuous intravenous unfractionated heparin.[46(I),47(I),48(I),49(I)] The findings are summarized below.

An exploratory study evaluated the effectiveness of LMWH in the treatment of venous thrombosis. Patients with venographically proven deep-vein thrombosis (DVT) were randomized to receive continuous intravenous infusion of either LMWH or unfractionated heparin.[39(II)] The initial dose was 240 anti-X_a units/kg/12 hours. After 27 patients had been entered, this initial study was stopped because two postoperative patients in the LMWH group had major bleeding. The factor X_a levels assayed retrospectively were found to be much higher in the LMWH group than in the unfractionated heparin group (1.6 to 2.0 anti-X_a units/mL versus 0.5 to 0.8 anti-X_a/mL, respectively). A subsequent study in patients with venous thrombosis compared LMWH 120 anti-X_a units/kg/12 hours with unfractionated heparin 340 units/kg/12 hours, both given intravenously.[39(II)] In this study of 27 patients, the mean activity was higher in the LMWH group (0.9 to 1.2 anti-X_a units/mL) than in the unfractionated group (0.5 to 0.7 anti-X_a units/mL). Progression of thrombus size in three (11%) patients on unfractionated heparin in both these studies (n = 29) and improvement in 14 (48%) was demonstrated by repeat venography. There was no progression of thrombus size in any of the patients on LMWH; six (50%) had improved in the first study, and 10 (77%) had improved in the second study. However, the mean decrease of thrombus size score (according to the Marder classification)[50] during treatment did not differ between the three groups. Antithrombin III levels decreased significantly in the unfractionated heparin group but not in the LMWH groups. Amino transferase levels were transiently increased in all three groups. Mean capillary bleeding showed no differences in the three treatment groups.

Forty-four patients with venographically proven DVT were randomized to receive either intravenous unfractionated heparin (240 anti-X_a units/kg/12 hours) or LMWH (Fragmin) 120 or 240 anti-X_a units/12 hours.[43(II)] Improvement in 48% of patients treated with unfractionated heparin and in 50% and 77%, respectively, of the Fragmin-treated patients was demonstrated by repeat venography. Progression of thrombus size was seen in 11% of the unfractionated heparin-treated patients but not in patients on LMWH. Bleeding complications occurred in two patients receiving the high-dose of Fragmin (240 anti-X_a units/kg/12 hours). In the LMWH group there was no correlation between the anti-X_a activity in plasma and the APTT.

The efficacy and the safety of LMWH were studied by comparing intravenous Fragmin with unfractionated heparin in a prospective randomized double-blind trial in 194 unselected patients with acute VTE.[38(II)] Ninety-six patients received intravenous Fragmin and 98 patients received continuous intravenous heparin, both for five to 10 days. Doses were adjusted to maintain anti-X_a levels between 0.3 and 0.6 units/mL for patients with a high risk of bleeding, and between 0.4 and 0.9 units/mL for patients with a low risk of bleeding. When the therapeutic range was reached using warfarin (INR > 3.5), treatment was stopped. Thirteen patients on heparin and 10 patients on Fragmin had major bleeding . The difference in the combined incidence of major and minor bleeding complications was 10.4% (95% CI for the difference = −3.5 to +24.2%). This corresponds to a relative risk reduction of 21.2% for the patients on LMWH. New high-probability lung-scan defects were observed in six of the 46 patients in the heparin group and three of 34 patients in the Fragmin group (95% CI for the difference = −9.4 to +17.8%). It was concluded that, compared with unfractionated heparin, LMWH (Fragmin) given by adjusted continuous intravenous doses was safe and effective in the initial treatment of acute VTE. There was a trend in risk reduction for bleeding in favor of LMWH.

A collaborative European multicenter study[37(I)] compared subcutaneous LMWH (CY216 Fraxiparine) with intravenous heparin over a 10-day period. Unfractionated heparin was started at 20 IU/kg/hour and adjusted to maintain an APTT between 1.5 and 2.0 times control. Low-molecular weight heparin, 225 anti-X_a International Choay Units (ICU)/kg/12 hours was given and adjusted for high or low body weight. The trial was not double-blinded. Venograms on day 1 and day 10 were assessed to show quantitative and qualitative changes by measuring the Marder[50] and Arnesen[51] scores. Perfusion lung scans were also done on days 0 and 10. In the 166 patients, both an efficacy analysis and an intention-to-treat analysis showed that LMWH was more effective than continuous intravenous unfractionated heparin according to the Marder[50] and Arneson[51] venographic scores. There was no increase in the risk of pulmonary embolism (PE), hemorrhage, or extension of thrombosis.

Unmonitored LMWH given subcutaneously was found to be as effective and as safe as monitored continu-

ous intravenous heparin in three large randomized clinical trials. In the largest clinical trial carried out so far, patients with venographically proven DVT were randomized. One group received a fixed dose of LMWH (Logiparin: 175 X_a units/kg) once daily. The other group received intravenous unfractionated heparin by continuous infusion adjusted to maintain an APTT of 1.5 to 2.5 times the mean control value using a heparin nomogram.[46(I)] Warfarin sodium was started on day 2 and continued for three months. At presentation all patients had chest x-rays, ventilation-perfusion lung scans, and impedance plethysmography (IPG). The IPG was repeated every 3 weeks until it was normalized. The outcome events included objectively documented VTE (recurrence or extension of DVT or PE), major or minor bleeding, thrombocytopenia, and death.

Six of 213 patients receiving LMWH (2.8%) and 15 of 219 patients receiving intravenous unfractionated heparin (6.9%; p = 0.07; 95% CI for the difference = 0.02 to +8.1%) had new episodes of VTE.[46(I)] Major bleeding associated with initial therapy occurred in one patient receiving LMWH (0.5%) and in 11 patients receiving intravenous unfractionated heparin (5.0%), a reduction in risk of 95% (p = 0.006). During long-term warfarin therapy, major hemorrhage was seen in five patients who had received LMWH (2.3%) and in none of those receiving intravenous heparin (p = 0.028). There were 10 deaths in the group that received LMWH (4.7%) compared to 21 deaths in the group that received intravenous unfractionated heparin (9.6%), a risk reduction of 51% (p = 0.049).[46(I)] Analysis by the log rank test, taking into account the length of time to an event, demonstrated a significant difference (p = 0.024) in the frequency of thromboembolic events and deaths (Figure 1). The most striking difference was in abrupt deaths in patients with metastatic carcinoma, the majority of these deaths occurring within the first 3 weeks. It is possible that the long-term use of LMWH, rather than warfarin sodium, may have a greater impact on recurrent thromboembolic events, bleeding, and death, particularly in patients with metastatic carcinoma.

A cost-effectiveness analysis using real costs and a sensitivity analysis showed that LMWH was more cost-effective than unfractionated heparin in the treatment of proximal venous thrombosis.[52] Further substantial cost-saving was possible in that about 37% of these patients could have been treated on an outpatient basis, thus increasing the cost-effectiveness of LMWH.

Prandoni et al,[47(I)] reported a randomized trial in consecutive symptomatic patients with proximal-vein thrombosis. To assess the relative effectiveness and risk of bleeding, fixed-dose LMWH (CY216 Fraxiparine) was compared with adjusted-dose intravenous unfractionated heparin for 10 days followed by oral warfarin sodium for 3 months. Patients in the LMWH groups re-

Time-to-Event Analysis for Patients
Who Had Recurrent Venous Thromboembolism or Died

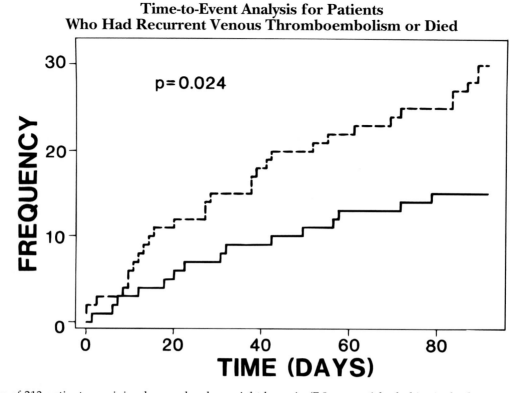

Figure 1. Fifteen of 213 patients receiving low-molecular-weight heparin (7.0 percent) had objectively documented recurrent venous thromboembolism or died, as compared with 30 of 219 patients receiving intravenous heparin (13.7 percent) (P = 0.024). In each group the majority of these events occurred within the first six weeks. (Reprinted with permission from Hull RD, et al. Subcutaneous Low-Molecular-Weight Heparin Compared With Continuous Intravenous Heparin in the Treatment of Proximal-Vein Thrombosis. NEJM 1992;326:975–982.)

ceived subcutaneous injections every 12 hours according to body weight (12,500 anti-X_a ICU for patients less than 55 kg; 15,000 anti-X_a ICU for patients between 55 and 80 kg; and 17,500 anti-X_a ICU for patients more than 80 kg). In patients on adjusted-dose intravenous heparin the APTT was maintained by continuous infusion at 1.5 to 2.0 times the mean normal control value. All patients had baseline perfusion lung scans and chest x-rays. Contrast venography was repeated on day 10 or earlier if new symptoms developed. The principle end-point to assess efficacy was symptomatic recurrent venous thrombosis or symptomatic PE. Secondary end-points to assess efficacy were changes between day 0 and day 10 in the venograms and perfusion lung scans.

There was no significant difference in the frequency of objectively diagnosed recurrent VTE between the unfractionated heparin and the LMWH groups (12 [14%] versus 6 [7%]; 95% CI = −3 to + 15%; p = 0.13).[47(l)] There was no significant difference in clinically evident bleeding between the two groups (3.5% for unfractionated heparin versus 1.1% for LMWH; p > 0.2).[47(l)] In the 6-month follow-up period, there were 12 deaths in the unfractionated heparin group and six in the CY216 group. This difference was largely due to cancer deaths (8 of 18 in the unfractionated heparin group and 1 of 15 in the LMWH).[47(l)]

The third multicenter randomized clinical trial compared subcutaneous Enoxaparin, 1 mg/kg subcutaneously every 12 hours, with continuous intravenous heparin starting at 500 U/kg/24 h. Both agents were continued for 10 days; at this time oral anticoagulation was started and continued for 3 months.[48(l)] The change in size of the thrombus shown by repeat venograms on day 10 was the primary assessment of efficacy. Major bleeding during the 10 days of treatment was the primary safety outcome measurement. Patients were assessed clinically at 3 months for recurrent thromboembolism, bleeding, or death. Patients on Enoxaparin showed greater venographic improvement after 10 days compared with those on heparin, and the incidence of recurrent thromboembolic disease during the 10-day treatment was higher in the heparin group (p < 0.002). There was no major bleeding and there were no deaths during the 10-day trial.

In the Polish multicenter trial, 149 consecutive patients with venographically proven venous thrombosis (proximal and/or distal), were randomized to receive fixed-dose LMWH (Fraxiparine) 225 anti-X_a IU/kg/12 hours or subcutaneous unfractionated heparin adjusted to maintain the APTT between 1.5 and 2.5 times the control value. Oral anticoagulants were started on day 7 and continued for 3 months. A repeat venogram on day 10 was the primary outcome assessment and major or minor bleeding was the main safety assessment. Patients were followed for 3 months to monitor their anticoagulant treatment and to assess thrombotic recurrence. In this study, the mean venographic score after 10 days was significantly decreased in both groups (p < 0.001), but there was no difference between the two groups. During follow-up, there were no recurrences in the LMWH group and two in the unfractionated heparin group. This study concluded that subcutaneous LMWH and unfractionated heparin are equally effective and safe.[49(I)]

FUTURE USES OF LOW-MOLECULAR-WEIGHT HEPARIN IN THE TREATMENT OF VENOUS THROMBOEMBOLISM

It has been shown that long-term use of LMWH is safe in patients who are unable to tolerate oral anticoagulants.[53(V)]

The use of LMWH has been reported in small case series of pregnant patients. Low-molecular-weight heparins are considered to be safe in pregnancy because anticoagulant activity does not cross the placenta.[54–58] Clinical trials in pregnant patients with active DVT or a history of previous DVT are awaited with interest. Low-molecular-weight heparins are also being studied at present in patients who have unstable angina or who have had coronary angioplasty.

SAFETY ISSUES

Thrombocytopenia was seen in 1.7% and 2.8% of patients receiving LMWH for either prophylaxis[34(I)] or treatment[46(I)] of venous thrombosis, respectively. Neither of these two trials resulted in thrombotic disease related to thrombocytopenia. However, the administration of LMWH has been associated with this complication.[59] Further prospective clinical trials are necessary to establish the exact incidence of heparin-induced thrombocytopenia related to LMWHs. Elevation of liver enzymes has been observed in patients receiving both LMWH and unfractionated heparin; however, the exact incidence and nature of this complication (compared with the use of unfractionated heparin) has not been established.[60(V)] The LMWHs have been shown to affect bone mineral metabolism in experimental models, but the relevance of these findings to patients on long-term LMWH is unclear.[61]

REFERENCES

(I)1. Salzman EW, Deykin D, Shapiro RM, et al. Management of heparin therapy: controlled prospective trial. N Engl J Med 1986;315:1109–1114.

(II)2. Wilson JR, Lampman J. Heparin therapy: a randomized prospective study. Am Heart J 1979;97:155–158.

(I)3. Hull RD, Raskob GE, Hirsh J, et al. Continuous intravenous heparin compared with intermittent subcutaneous heparin in the initial treatment of proximal vein thrombosis. N Engl J Med 1986;315:1109–1114.

(I)4. Gallus AS, Jackaman J, Tillett J, et al. Safety and efficacy of warfarin started early after submassive venous thrombosis or pulmonary embolism. Lancet 1986;2: 1293–1296.

(I)5. Hull RD, Raskob GE, Rosenbloom D, et al. Heparin for 5 days as compared with 10 days in the initial treatment of proximal venous thrombosis. N Engl J Med 1990;322: 1260–1264.

(I)6. Hull RD, Raskob GE, Rosenbloom D, et al. Optimal therapeutic levels of heparin therapy in patients with venous thrombosis. Arch Intern Med 1992;152: 1589–1595.

(I)7. Hull R, Hirsh J, Jay R, et al. Different intensities of oral anticoagulant therapy in the treatment of proximal-vein thrombosis. N Engl J Med 1982;307:1676–1681.

(I)8. Basu D, Gallus A, Hirsh J, et al. A prospective study of value of monitoring heparin treatment with the activated partial thromboplastin time. N Engl J Med 1972;287:324–327.

(I)9. Raschke P, Reilly BM, Guidry JR, et al. The weight-based heparin dosing nomogram compared with a "standard care" nomogram. Ann Intern Med 1992;327: 1128–1133.

10. Fennerty A, Thomas P, Backhouse G, et al. Audit of control of heparin treatment. Br Med J 1985;290:27.

11. Wheeler AP, Jaquiss RD, Newman JH. Physician practices in the treatment of pulmonary embolism and deep-venous thrombosis. Arch Intern Med 1988;148: 1321–1325.

12. Hommes DW, Bura A, Mazzolai L, et al. Subcutaneous heparin compared with continuous intravenous heparin administration in the initial treatment of deep vein thrombosis. Ann Intern Med 1992;116:279–284.

13. Brill-Edwards P, Ginsberg S, Johnston M, et al. Establishing a therapeutic range for heparin therapy. Ann Intern Med 1993;119:104–109.

14. Hull R, Brant R, Pineo G, et al. Heparin (H) resistance as a predictor of recurrent venous thromboembolism (RVTE). Blood 1993;82(10):406.(Abstract 1611)

15. Verstraete M. Pharmacotherapeutic aspects of unfractionated and low-molecular-weight heparin. Drugs 1990;40:498–530.

16. Bara L, Billaud E, Gramond G, et al. Comparative pharmacokinetics of a low-molecular-weight heparin and unfractionated heparin after intravenous and subcutaneous administration. Thrombosis Res 1985;39:631–636.

17. Bergqvist D, Hedner U, Sjorin E, et al. Anticoagulant effects of two types of low-molecular-weight heparin administered subcutaneously. Thrombosis Res 1983;32: 381–391.

18. Bratt G, Tornebohm E, Widlund L, et al. Low-molecular-weight heparin (Kabi 2165; Fragmin): pharmacokinetics after intravenous and subcutaneous administration in human volunteers. Thrombosis Res 1986;42: 613–620.

19. Frydman AM, Bara L, LeRoux Y, et al. The antithrombotic activity and pharmacokinetics of enoxaparine, a low-molecular-weight, in humans given single subcutaneous doses of 20 to 80 mg. J Clin Pharmacol 1988;28: 609–618.

20. Harenberg J, Wurzner B, Zimmermann R, et al. Bioavailability and antagonization of the low-molecular-weight heparin CY216 in man. Thrombosis Res 1986;44:549–554.

21. Matzsch T, Bergqvist D, Hedner U. Effects of an enzymatically depolymerized heparin as compared with conventional heparin in healthy volunteers. Thromb Haemost 1987;57:97–101.

22. Albada J, Neuwenhuis HK, Sixma JJ. Comparison of intravenous standard heparin and Fragmin in the treatment of venous thromboembolism: a randomized double-blind study. Thrombosis Res 1987;Suppl VI.(Abstract)

23. Arneson KE, Handeland GF, Abildgaard U, et al. What is the optimal dosage of LMW heparin in the subcutaneous treatment of deep vein thrombosis? Thromb Haemost 1987;58:214.(Abstract 794)

24. Bratt G, Aberg W, Tornebohm E, et al. Subcutaneous KABI 2165 in the treatment of deep venous thrombosis of the leg. Thrombosis Res Suppl 1987;VII:24 .(Abstract)

(II)25. Bratt G, Tornebohm E, Granqvist S, et al. A comparison between low-molecular-weight heparin (KABI 2165) and standard heparin in the intravenous treatment of deep venous thrombosis. Thromb Haemost 1985;54: 813–817.

(II)26. Holm HA, Ly B, Handeland GF, et al. Subcutaneous heparin treatment of deep venous thrombosis: a comparison of unfractionated and low-molecular-weight heparin. Haemost 1986;16:30–37.

27. Aiach M, Michaud A, Balian JL, et al. A new low-molecular-weight heparin derivative, in vitro and in vivo studies. Thrombosis Res 1983;31:611–621.

28. Cade JF, Buchanan MR, Boneau B, et al. A comparison of the antithrombotic and haemorrhagic effects of low molecular heparin fractions: the influence of the method of preparation. Thrombosis Res 1984;35: 613–625.

29. Carter CJ, Kelton JR, Hirsh J, et al. Relationship between the antithrombotic and anticoagulant effects of low-molecular-weight heparin. Thrombosis Res 1981;21: 169–174.

30. Carter CJ, Kelton JG, Hirsh J, et al. The relationship between the hemorrhagic and antithrombotic properties of low-molecular-weight heparin in rabbits. Blood 1982;59:1239–1245.

31. Holmer E, Mattsson C, Nilsson S. Anticoagulant and antithrombotic effects of heparin and low-molecular-weight heparin fragments in rabbits. Thrombosis Res 1982;25:475–485.

32. Nurmohamed MT, Rosendal FR, Buller HR, et al. Low-molecular-weight heparin in the prophylaxis of venous thrombosis: a meta-analysis. Lancet 1992;340:152–156.

33. Leizorovicz A, Haugh MC, Chapuis F-R, et al. Low-molecular-weight heparin in prevention of perioperative thrombosis. Br Med J 1992;305:913–920.

(I)34. Hull RD, Raskob GE, Pineo GF, et al. A comparison of subcutaneous low-molecular-weight heparin with warfarin sodium for prophylaxis against deep-vein thrombosis after hip or knee implantation. N Engl J Med 1993;329:1370–1376.

(I)35. Kakkar VV, Cohen AT, Edmonson RA, et al. Low molecular weight versus standard heparin for prevention of venous thromboembolism after major abdominal surgery. Lancet 1993;341;259–265.

36. Thomas DP. Prevention of post-operative thrombosis by low-molecular-weight heparin in patients undergoing hip replacement. Thromb Haemost 1992;67: 491–493.

(I)37. A Collaborative European Multicentre Study. A randomized trial of subcutaneous low-molecular-weight heparin (CY216) compared with intravenous unfractionated heparin in the treatment of deep-vein thrombosis. Thromb Haemost 1991;65:251–256.

(II)38. Albada J, Nieuwenhuis HK, Sixma JJ. Treatment of acute venous thromboembolism with low-molecular-weight heparin (Fragmin). Results of a double-blind randomized study. Circulation 1989;80:935–940.

(II)39. Bratt G, Aberg W, Johansson M, et al. Two daily subcutaneous injections of Fragmin as compared with intravenous standard heparin in the treatment of deep venous thrombosis (DVT). Thromb Haemost 1990;64:506–510.

(V)40. Handeland GF, Abildgaard U, Holm HA, et al. Dose-adjusted heparin treatment of deep venous thrombosis: a comparison of unfractionated and low-molecular-weight heparin. Eur J Clin Pharmacol 1990;39:107–112.

(II)41. Harenberg J, Huck K, Bratsch H, et al. Therapeutic application of subcutaneous low-molecular-weight heparin in acute venous thrombosis. Haemost 1990; 20(Suppl 1):205–219.

(V)42. Huet Y, Janvier G, Bendriss PH, et al. Treatment of established venous thromboembolism with Enoxaparin: preliminary report. Acta Chir Scand 1990;Suppl 556: 116–120.

(II)43. Lockner D, Bratt G, Tornebohm E, et al. Intravenous and subcutaneous administration of Fragmin in deep venous thrombosis. Haemost 1986;16:25–29.

(I)44. Prandoni P, Vigo M, Cattelan AM, et al. Treatment of deep venous thrombosis by fixed doses of a low-molecular-weight heparin (CY216). Haemost 1990;20(Suppl 1):220–223.

(I)45. Siegbahn A, Y-Hassan S, Boberg J, et al. Subcutaneous treatment of deep venous thrombosis with low-molecular-weight heparin. A dose finding study with LMWH-Novo. Thrombosis Res 1989;55:767–778.

(I)46. Hull RD, Raskob GE, Pineo GF, et al. Subcutaneous low-molecular-weight heparin compared with continuous intravenous heparin in the treatment of proximal-vein thrombosis. N Engl J Med 1992;326:975–983.

(I)47. Prandoni P, Lensing AW, Buller HR, et al. Comparison of subcutaneous low-molecular-weight heparin with intravenous standard heparin in proximal deep-vein thrombosis. Lancet 1992;339:411–415.

(I)48. Simonneau G, Charbonnier B, Decousus H, et al. Subcutaneous low-molecular-weight heparin compared with continuous intravenous unfractionated heparin in the treatment of proximal deep vein thrombosis. Arch Intern Med 1993;153:1541–1546.

(I)49. Lopaciuk S, Meissner AJ, Filipecki S, et al. Subcutaneous low-molecular-weight heparin versus subcutaneous unfractionated heparin in the treatment of deep vein thrombosis: a Polish multicentre trial. Thromb Haemost 1992;68(1):14–18.

50. Marder VJ, Soulen RL, Atchartakarn V, et al. Quantitative venographic assessment of deep vein thrombosis in the evaluation of streptokinase and heparin therapy. J Lab Clin Med 1977;89(5):1018–1029.

51. Arnesen H, Heilo A, Jakobsen E, et al. A prospective study of streptokinase and heparin in the treatment of deep vein thrombosis. Acta Med Scand 1978;203: 457–463.

52. Hull RD, Rosenbloom D, Pineo GF, et al. A cost-effectiveness analysis of low-molecular-weight heparin compared with continuous intravenous heparin in the treatment of proximal-vein thrombosis. Circulation 1993;88(4;part 2):I-516.(Abstract 2777)

(V)53. Harenberg J, Leber G, Dempfle CE, et al. Long-term anticoagulation with low-molecular-weight heparin in outpatients with side effects on oral anticoagulants. Nouv Rev Fr Hematol 1989;31:363–369.

54. Omri A, Delaloye JF, Andersen H, et al. Low-molecular-

weight heparin Novo (LHN-1) does not cross the placenta during the second trimester of pregnancy. Thrombosis Haemost 1989;61:55–56.

55. Bergqvist D, Hedner U, Sjorin E, et al. Anticoagulant effects of two types of low-molecular-weight heparin administered subcutaneously. Thrombosis Res 1983;32:381–391.

56. Forestier F, Daffos F, Capella-Pavlovsky M. Low-molecular-weight heparin (PK 10169) does not cross the placenta during the second trimester of pregnancy. Study by direct fetal blood sampling under ultrasound. Thrombosis Res 1984;34:557–560.

57. Forestier F, Daffos F, Rainaut M, et al. Low-molecular-weight heparin (CY 216) does not cross the placenta during the third trimester of pregnancy. Thromb Haemost 1987;57:234.

58. Andrew M, Cade J, Buchanan MR, et al. Low-molecular-weight heparin does not cross the placenta. Thromb Haemost 1983;50:225.(Abstract)

59. Mohr VD, Lenz J. Heparin-assoziierte thrombocytopenie, thrombose und embolie. Unerwünschte wirkung der thromboembolieprophylaxe mit dem niedermolekularen heparin Enoxaparin? Chirug 1991;62:686–690.

(V)60. Monreal M, Lafoz E, Salvador R, et al. Adverse effects of three different forms of heparin therapy: thrombocytopenia, increased transaminases, and hyperkalaemia. Eur J Clin Pharmacol 1989;37:415–418.

61. Matzsch T, Bergqvist D, Hedner U, et al. Effects of an enzymatically depolymerized heparin as compared with conventional heparin in healthy volunteers. Thromb Haemost 1987;57:97–101.

30

Oral Anticoagulant Therapy

Jack E. Ansell

INTRODUCTION

The coumarin-type oral anticoagulants have become well established weapons in the armamentarium against thrombotic disease, ever since their first clinical use in 1941.[1] They have proven beneficial for the prevention and treatment of venous thromboembolism (VTE) and for the prevention of cardiogenic embolism, as well as for the possible prevention of recurrent myocardial infarction.[2] Most physicians consider themselves well versed in the practical management of oral anticoagulant therapy, yet the literature[3] and personal experience suggests that the relatively high risk of therapy results from improper management, rather than from patient noncompliance or other aberrations. Thus, the following discussion emphasizes the practical aspects of anticoagulation management to help clinicians optimize their skills and improve the overall quality of anticoagulant care.

DISCOVERY OF DICUMAROL

The discovery and initial development of oral anticoagulants is an intriguing story and is worth reviewing as a prologue to a further discussion of drug pharmacology and use. In the early 1900s, a hemorrhagic disease of cattle developed in the plains area of the upper midwestern United States and adjacent Canada. Schofield, a veterinary pathologist, identified the cause of this disease in 1924 as the consumption of spoiled sweet clover.[4] Sweet clover, planted years earlier as one of the few crops able to grow on the exhausted, overfarmed land, would occasionally spoil during the ensilage process, and its consumption by cattle would lead to this disease. Roderick, another veterinary pathologist, confirmed Schofield's earlier work,[5] and found that affected cattle were deficient in prothrombin, one of the few coagulation factors known at that time.

At approximately the same time, Henrik Dam described a hemorrhagic disease in chickens, fed a specially formulated diet, free of sterols by ether and alcohol extraction.[6] In 1935, he postulated the existence of a vitamin K,[7] the lack of which predisposed to the bleeding tendency. Prothrombin deficiency was also noted to be present in these animals. During this time, Armand Quick also described the prothrombin time assay[8] which quickly became the basis for measuring the clotability of blood in animals with this disease,[9] and subsequently, the basis for monitoring oral anticoagulant therapy.

In 1933, Karl Paul Link, who was investigating the coumarin compounds responsible for the bitter taste, but sweet smell, of freshly cut hay, set off on a fascinating journey of discovery leading to the isolation of dicumarol (3–3'-methyl-bis-4–hydroxycoumarin) from spoiled sweet clover in 1939,[10,11] its synthesis in 1940,[10,12] and its first use in man in 1941.[1] The formation of this hemorrhagic agent resulted from the oxidation of coumarin to 4-hydroxycoumarin, which, upon coupling with formaldehyde and another 4-hydroxycoumarin led to the formation of dicumarol.

In the early 1940s, a number of related compounds were synthesized in Dr. Link's laboratory.[13] One of these, Compound #42 (sodium warfarin), emerged as an ideal rodenticide in the late 1940s, because of its greater effectiveness compared to dicumarol.[10] It was not long thereafter that the first case of warfarin use in man was encountered when a sailor unsuccessfully tried to commit suicide by ingestion of the rodenticide.[14] Warfarin's utility in man, however, did not become commonplace until after its use to treat President Eisenhower following a heart attack in the mid-1950s.[10]

PHARMACOLOGY

Even before the isolation of dicumarol, Link understood the importance of vitamin K in counter-balancing its anticoagulant effect. Subsequently, the mechanism of the coumarin anticoagulants was found to be intimately linked to the physiology of vitamin K as reviewed below.

From *Venous Thromboembolism: An Evidence-Based Atlas* edited by Russell Hull, Gary Raskob, Graham Pineo © 1996, Futura Publishing Co., Armonk, NY.

The discovery of vitamin K was an outgrowth of work first reported by Dam[6] in 1929, and its isolation was achieved by Dam[7] and Almquist[15] several years later. Doisy,[16,17] however, was the first to identify the structure of the vitamin, and Doisy and Dam shared in the Nobel Prize for their work in 1943. Although it was known that vitamin K was critical for the synthesis of specific coagulation factors (II, VII, IX and X), real progress in understanding vitamin K physiology took years to achieve.

In 1974, Stenflo et al,[18] and Nelsestuen et al,[19] described the essential posttranslational modification mediated by vitamin K, converting 10 specific N-terminal glutamic acid residues in precursor prothrombin to gamma carboxyglutamic acid (gla) to create functioning prothrombin (Figure 1). Similar modifications occur in the other vitamin K-dependent factors as well as in the coagulation inhibitors, proteins C and S, and the noncoagulation vitamin K-dependent proteins in bone, cartilage, and other tissue.[20,21] Gamma carboxylation confers the calcium mediated ability to bind to negatively charged phospholipid surfaces,[19,22,23] an essential requirement for normal coagulation. Evidence suggests that vitamin K serves as a cofactor for a membrane-bound vitamin K-depen-

dent gamma carboxylase, labilizing the gamma glutamyl hydrogen and leaving the carbon atom open to CO_2 attack.[21] Oxygen and CO_2 are needed in the reaction. In the process, vitamin K undergoes 2,3–epoxidation (Figure 1), and then undergoes reduction to the quinol form for recycling. It is this latter step that is interrupted by the coumarin anticoagulants.[24–27] The primary inhibitory effect appears to be on the vitamin K epoxide reductase enzyme which may also be the microsomal binding site for warfarin.[27,28] There appears to be less inhibitory potency directed toward the second enzymatic step, mediated by a vitamin K reductase enzyme. Oral anticoagulants lead to a decrease in functioning prothrombin and related factors due to synthesis of decarboxylated or partially carboxylated precursors.[29–32] The biological activity of the final protein will depend on the degree of carboxylation of its gla residues.[29–31] Thus, the prothrombin peptide with a decreasing number of gla residues from fully carboxylated 10-gla prothrombin to partially carboxylated 6-gla prothrombin loses over 90% of its activity.[31] Furthermore, particular gla residues may be more important than others as can be seen by the loss of almost 60% activity when simply going from the 9-gla to 8-gla containing peptide.[32]

There are a number of available oral anticoagulants but crystalline sodium warfarin is the major coumarin anticoagulant used in North America.[33] It replaced dicoumarol because of its favorable pharmacokinetic and pharmacodynamic properties initially recognized by Link when he developed it as a rodenticide in the 1940s. The indanediones are rarely used because of their much higher incidence of side effects and they will not be discussed. For a more detailed overview of other coumarin preparations, the reader is referred elsewhere.[33,34]

Warfarin is highly water soluble and rapidly absorbed from the gastrointestinal tract after an oral dose.[35] Peak absorption occurs in 60 to 90 minutes and peak effect occurs at 36 to 72 hours. The presence of food in the stomach is said to decrease the rate, but not the extent of absorption.[36] Personal experience, however, suggests that food may alter absorption, and thus, warfarin should be taken on an empty stomach.

Warfarin is a racemic mixture of stereo isomers.[37] The R isomer has a longer half-life, a reduced potency, and a different metabolic pathway compared to the S isomer.[37,38] Both are highly protein bound (97% to 99%) principally to albumin. They are initially metabolized in the liver (microsomal fraction) where the S isomer is converted to 7-hydroxywarfarin and excreted in the bile and the R isomer is coverted to warfarin alcohols and is excreted in the urine. Although the warfarin alcohols may have minimal anticoagulant activity, the metabolites are generally inactive, and renal failure does not necessitate a change in dose.

The S isomer has an average shorter plasma half-life of approximately 33 hours (range 18 to 34 hours) while the R isomer has a half-life of 45 hours (range 20 to 70

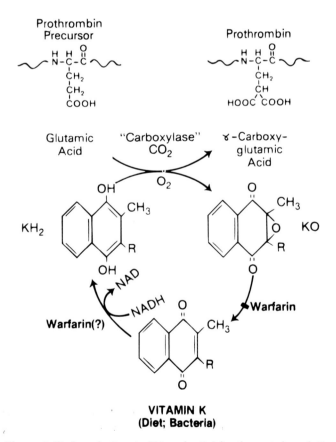

VITAMIN K
(Diet; Bacteria)

Figure 1. Reduced vitamin K is essential for the γ-carboxylation reaction of glutamiic acid residues in precursor prothrombin or other vitamin K-dependent factors. Reduced vitamin K is oxidized in the carboxylation reaction. Warfarin sodium interferes with the recycling (reduction) of oxidized vitamin K.

hours).[37] The average half-life of a racemic mixture can be anywhere from as brief as 15 hours to as long as 58 hours, with a mean of 42 hours.[39] There are many factors that influence an individual's response to warfarin as discussed below, but a principal factor is variability in warfarin half-life, due either to natural differences in warfarin metabolism or to disease and drug-induced alterations in metabolic half-life. Such differences account for marked variations in an individual's initial response to, or maintenance requirement for warfarin.

MANAGEMENT OF ORAL ANTICOAGULATION

Initial Dosing

The use of a loading dose of warfarin to initiate therapy is of historical interest only. A loading dose induces a rapid, but excessive reduction in factor VII activity, the factor with the shortest half-life (Figure 2), predisposing patients to hemorrhage in the first few days of therapy.[40] It fails to achieve a significantly more rapid decline of the other vitamin K-dependent coagulation factors (II, IX and X) above that achieved without a loading dose. Therefore, therapy is properly initiated using an average maintenance dose, or slightly higher, for those who might have a higher requirement, for the first 2 or 3 days, assessing the prothrombin time response and estimating a mainte-

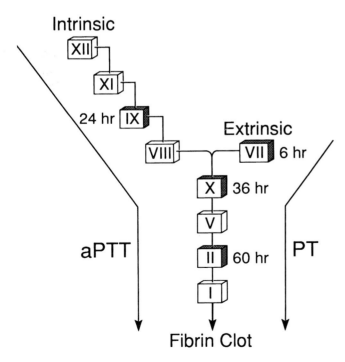

Figure 2. A simplified illustration of the coagulation cascade indicating those factors that are vitamin K dependent (shaded), their average metabolic half-life, and the limbs assessed by the prothrombin time (PT) and activated partial thromboplastin time (aPTT).

nance dose.[40] Most patients beginning warfarin therapy are already receiving heparin. Both medications must overlap for a period of 3 to 5 days since it requires that amount of time to reduce the vitamin K-dependent coagulation factors in the intrinsic (factor IX) and common pathways (factors II and X) of coagulation (Figure 2). In the setting of deep venous thrombosis (DVT) or pulmonary embolism (PE), a number of studies have shown that heparin and warfarin can be started together to limit the duration of hospitalization and associated costs without effecting the outcome.[41(I),42(I),43(I),44(II)]

Estimation of the maintenance dose is relatively easy for the experienced user of warfarin, but may be difficult for the novice. A number of pharmacokinetic formulas and computer assisted dosing programs have been developed,[37,45–47] but they are often not reliable enough to stand on their own,[48] nor are they particularly user friendly. Most physicians attempt to predict dose requirements based on observations of prothrombin time response following a fixed dose of warfarin over a few days interval.[49–51(II)] A simple guideline for estimating maintenance dose requirements is as follows. An individual who rapidly (after 2 doses of 10 mg) achieves a high therapeutic prothrombin time (INR > 2.5), is likely to be a slow metabolizer of warfarin and require a low maintenance dose. The opposite holds for those who show little elevation of the prothrombin time (INR < 1.5) after 2 doses. For a more detailed discussion of warfarin dosing from a pharmacokinetic perspective, the reader is referred to the chapter by Porter.[37]

Maintenance Dosing

Unlike many pharmaceuticals, the biological effect of warfarin has a slow onset and slow decline of action allowing a wide flexibility in dosing schedule. This is fortunate, because the fluctuations in biological response (i.e., prothrombin time) require frequent changes in warfarin dose. The goal of therapy should be simplicity and clarity without sacrificing effectiveness, especially in patients who are likely to be elderly, who may confuse tablet colors and tablet strengths, and who may be receiving numerous other medications. Personal experience suggests that these goals can best be achieved by predominantly using one tablet strength of warfarin, and fractions or multiples thereof to achieve varying doses, and by providing altering doses according to days of the week rather than calendar or odd/even days as illustrated in Figure 3. Dose adjustments can best be made by considering the weekly cumulative dose, increasing or decreasing it by 10% or 20%, and spreading that change over the course of a week.

Warfarin therapy is historically given in the early evening, at least in hospitalized patients. How this tradition evolved is unclear. It may be because the peak effect of a dose of dicoumarol (and warfarin) is approximately

Mon	Tue	Wed	Thu	Fri	Sat	Sun	Total Weekly Dose	
5	5	5	5	5	5	5	35	mg
5	5	5	5	5	5	2.5	32.5	mg
2.5	5	5	2.5	5	5	5	30	mg
2.5	5	2.5°	5	2.5	5	5	27.5	mg

Figure 3. Warfarin dosing schedule. A single-strength tablet is recommended for all patients. Fractions or multiples of the tablet can be used for different doses and/or alternative doses can be given based on days of the week. As illustrated, three alternative doses per week can be given on Monday, Wednesday and Friday; two on Monday and Thursday; and one on Sunday. Dose adjustments should be done based on total weekly dose with changes of 10% to 20% up or down that is spread out over the week.

36 hours but not all formulations have the same onset of peak effect. It may also be that 5:00 p.m. gives the physician adequate time to obtain the morning prothrombin time result and write the anticoagulant order. Given hospital routine, the medication is not available until late in the day. In either case, there is little justification to continue evening dosing once a patient is stabilized. Patients should be advised to take their warfarin at the same time each day, and morning dosing on an empty stomach may provide more reliable absorption and compliance.

Therapeutic Range and Monitoring

The concept of a therapeutic range for oral anticoagulation, above or below which the risk of hemorrhage or thrombosis is unacceptable, developed as a consequence of trial and error and clinical empiricism. Beginning with the use of anticoagulants in the 1940s, investigators selected what they thought best represented this therapeutic range.[52–54(III)] Based on an extensive clinical study by Wright[55] in the late 1940s, the American Heart Association recommended a therapeutic PT ratio of 2 to 2.5 times the control value.[55] A later study by Moschos and associates[56] considered this range too high, but Sevitt and Gallagher[54] found a range of two to three times control, optimal in their classic study of oral anticoagulation prophylaxis in patients with hip fractures. Comparison of PT ranges in these early studies, however, is difficult because the thromboplastin reagents used for the prothrombin time test were of unspecified sensitivity, even though their biological source was often identified. Such qualitative differences in thromboplastin were not unknown to these early investigators and Allen presages the future when he states in a 1947 study, "Attention must be given to the thromboplastic substances used, for they vary in potency. Identical prothrombin times for two lots of thromboplastin may indicate entirely different values for prothrombin."[57(V)]

Tissue thromboplastins are derived from lung, brain, or placental tissue, and depending on their source and method of preparation, exhibit marked differences in their response to a reduction in the vitamin K-dependent coagulation factors.[58,59] Beginning in the 1950s and 1960s, the major manufacturers of thromboplastin in North America supplied a rabbit brain-derived preparation of reduced sensitivity compared with the thromboplastins produced in many individual laboratories,[60] or compared with the human brain thromboplastin used in Great Britain. In spite of these differences, clinicians did not adjust their treatment by altering the therapeutic range. An international survey illustrated the consequences of this situation by finding considerable variation in thromboplastins, instrumentation, methods of reporting results, and even therapeutic ranges.[61] A subsequent survey also found that the mean dose of anticoagulant needed to achieve a therapeutic degree of anticoagulation differed considerably from country to country even if similar therapeutic ranges were used.[62]

The British were the first to act on this situation in the 1960s, by developing a national standard for anticoagulant therapy (the Manchester Comparative Reagent).[63] Over the years, others have made recommendations for standardization,[64,65] and in 1977, the World Health Organization adopted a scheme for calibrating thromboplastins based on an International Reference (human brain) Preparation.[66,67] This scheme was subsequently modified to the present system of thromboplastin calibration.[68]

Unfortunately, these initial efforts had little effect on the practice of anticoagulant care in North America until the important study by Hull and coworkers,[69(I)] which was instrumental in identifying the consequences of this practice. By managing two groups of patients in traditional therapeutic ranges with a more responsive and a less responsive thromboplastin, they found a greater incidence of hemorrhage in the more intensely treated group (less responsive thromboplastin) and no difference in the frequency of recurrent thromboembolism.

As a consequence of Hull's study, a lower but equivalent therapeutic range for the insensitive thromboplastins used in North America was recommended (PT ratio of 1.3 to 1.6) to equate to the therapeutic range with sensitive thromboplastins (PT ratio 2.0 to 3.0). The dilemma, however, is that tissue thromboplastins differ from laboratory to laboratory[70,71] and even within laboratories over time as manufacturers or supply lots change. In recognition of these differences, the British Society of Hematology[72] and a task force of the American College of Chest Physicians/National Heart Lung Blood Institute,[73] have recommended that all therapy be managed based on an international standard as described below.

The sensitivity of individual tissue thromboplastins is established by comparison to an international reference thromboplastin.[66,67] The comparative factor, known as the International Sensitivity Index (ISI), represents the slope of a regression line from a log plot of reference thromboplastin prothrombin times (in seconds), compared to an unknown thromboplastin prothrombin time on blood samples from patients who are stably anticoagulated.[68] The ISI is established by the manufacturer for each new lot of thromboplastin. The international reference has by definition an ISI of one. Thus, a prothrombin time twice control value with one reagent may be quite different with another reagent. Using the ISI, one prothrombin time can be compared to another by taking the ratio of the result divided by the mean of the normal range and raising it to the power of the ISI of the thromboplastin used (Table 1). The result, the so-called International Normalized Ratio (INR), provides the reference to which all therapy should be compared. Based on a number of studies and the recommendations of a national concensus group,[73] the therapeutic range for different categories of disease based on the INR is summarized in Table 2.

Consequently, use of the INR obviates the differences in prothrombin time response seen in multisite testing. Such differences might even account for a higher rate

Table 2
Indications and Recommended Therapeutic Range for Oral Anticoagulation

Indication	INR
Prophylaxis of venous thrombosis (high-grade surgery)	
Treatment of venous thrombosis	
Treatment of pulmonary embolism	
Prevention of systemic embolism	
Tissue heart valves	2.0–3.0
Acute myocardial infarction (to prevent systemic embolism)	
Valvular heart disease	
Atrial fibrillation	
Recurrent systemic embolism on warfarin	
Mechanical prosthetic valves	2.5–3.5
Post myocardial infarction	

of anticoagulation failure noted in one study, comparing the outcome of patients tested in different laboratories.[74] Although uniform use of an INR may lead to improved control, an INR is heavily dependent on the manufacturer's proficiency in establishing an ISI for a new batch of thromboplastin, and deficiencies in this regard can lead to problems.[75,76] Lastly, instrumentation is another consideration,[77–79] yet the ability to account for instrumentation differences is even less standardized than it is for reagents. Nevertheless, monitoring oral anticoagulation based on an INR should provide a significant enhancement in care, especially in those countries commonly using less responsive thromboplastins.

Alternatives to Prothrombin Time

Is the prothrombin time the most accurate guide to effective anticoagulant therapy? Over the years, various assays have been developed to provide a theoretical improvement to the prothrombin time,[80–83] but the advantages of these tests have not been proven. Recently, investigators have presented evidence that the ability to interfere with thrombin generation (prothrombinase activity) may be the most sensitive indicator of effective anticoagulation as well as an indicator of risk of hemorrhage.[84,85] Furie et al,[82(II)] recently showed in a prospective study that measuring and maintaining the concentration of native prothrombin antigen (i.e., the residual normal prothrombin present in warfarin treated subjects), in a previously determined therapeutic range, provided safer and more effective therapy compared to a control group managed by the prothrombin time. Additional studies need to be conducted to confirm these reports. Of concern is the cost of these more sophisticated assays and the ability to provide timely results. For the time being, the prothrombin time remains the assay of choice in managing oral anticoagulant therapy.

Table 1
Use of ISI to Calculate an INR

ISI = International Sensitivity Index
    A comparative rating of different thromboplastins
INR = Internal Normalized Ratio
    A comparative rating of prothrombin time ratios for individuals with stable therapeutic anticoagulation
To convert a prothrombin time (PT) ratio to an INR equivalent:
    $INR = PT\ Ratio^x\ (X = ISI)$
Example:
    17.9 s = PT
    12.2 s = Mean of Normal Range
    2.3 = ISI of Thromboplastin
Then:
$$\frac{17.9}{12.3} = 1.47\ PT\ Ratio$$
    $1.47^{23} = 2.4\ INR$

Nontherapeutic Prothrombin Times

Because of the fluctuation in anticoagulant response, warfarin therapy requires frequent monitoring. One of the challenges of such management is the problem of determining the cause of nontherapeutic prothrombin times, especially in patients who are stable for long periods of time.[86,87] Table 3 identifies two principal considerations when a nontherapeutic prothrombin time is encountered. Although warfarin and vitamin K are not biochemical antagonists, they clinically behave as such. Thus, the prothrombin time will vary inversely with the amount of vitamin K absorbed from the diet[88,89] and directly with the amount of warfarin absorbed. A simple history assessing these two variables will often clarify the cause of over- or under-responsiveness. Table 4 summarizes the approximate content of vitamin K in various food groups.

Anticoagulation can fail to be achieved because of resistance to warfarin not only on an acquired basis attributable to excessive or surreptitious vitamin K intake,[88] but also on a hereditary basis.[90–92] Fortunately, the latter is quite rare with only a few kindreds reported worldwide. Such individuals may respond to extremely high doses of warfarin (> 50 mg daily). The mechanism of hereditary resistance is unknown, but is presumed to result from a faulty interaction between warfarin and its receptor, the vitamin K epoxide reductase enzyme.

Of course, other factors can effect the prothrombin time response to warfarin therapy as identified in Table 3.

Table 3
Causes of Nontherapeutic Prothrombin Time (PTs)

Considerations	PT
Major	
Too much or too little vitamin K	
Decrease in dietary vitamin K	Increase
Malabsorption of vitamin K	Increase
Suppression of gut bacteria	Increase
Increase in dietary vitamin K	Decrease
Too much or too little warfarin sodium	
Decrease in absorption	Decrease
Changes in metabolism	Increase/decrease
Drug effects	Increase/decrease
Minor	
Changes in factor production/ metabolism	
Liver disease	Increase
Hypermetabolic states (fever)	Increase
Other illnesses	Increase
Technical/Laboratory factors: problems with:	
Phlebotomy	Increase/decrease
Evacuated collection tube	Increase/decrease
Handling	Increase/decrease
Instrumentation	Increase/decrease
Different thromboplastin reagents	Increase/decrease

Table 4
Vitamin K Content of Different Foods

Food	Vitamin K ug/100 gm
Vegetables	
Asparagus	57
Beans, green	14
Broccoli	200
Cabbage	125
Lettuce	129
Peas, green	19
Spinach	89
Turnip greens	650
Potato	3
Pumpkin	2
Tomato	5
Watercress	57
Fruits	
Applesauce	2
Banana	2
Orange	1
Peach	8
Raisins	6
Strawberries	–
Meat & Meat Products	
Ground beef	7
Beef	92
Pork liver	25
Ham	15
Pork tenderloin	11
Chicken liver	7
Bacon	46
Eggs	
Whole eggs (hens)	11
Milk & Milk Products	
Milk (cows)	3
Cheese	35
Butter	30
Cereal & Grain Products	
Rice	–
Maize	5
Whole wheat	17
Wheat flour	4
Bread	4
Oats	20
Fats	
Corn oil	10
Safflower oil	–
Beverages	
Coffee	38
Cola	2
Tea, green	712
Tea, black	–

One area of major concern for those managing oral anticoagulation is the problem of drug interactions with warfarin. Such interactions can lead to difficulty in achieving therapeutic anticoagulation[93] or predispose to instability of control.[94,95] Most drugs mediate their deleterious effects by altering warfarin pharmacokinetics and thus, the pharmacodynamic response.[96] Drugs can also effect other aspects of hemostasis resulting in an altered anticoagu-

Table 5
Warfarin-Drug Interactions and Mechanisms

Drug	Mechanism of Interaction
Prolongs Prothrombin Time	
Amiodarone[100,101]	Decreases clearance (nonstereoselective)
Anabolic steroids[102]	Unknown
Cephalosporins (2nd/3rd generation)[103,104]	Interferes with vitamin K recycling
Cimetidine[105,106]	Decreases clearance (inhibits R isomer)
Clofibrate[107]	Unknown
Disulfiram[108]	Decreases clearance (inhibits S isomer)
Erythromycin[109]	Unknown
Fluoroquinolones[110,111]	Displace binding to albumin
Fluconazole[112]	Unknown
Glucagon[113]	Unknown
Metronidazole[114]	Decreases clearance (inhibits S isomer)
Miconazole[115]	Decreases clearance (nonstereoselective)
Omeprazole[116]	Decreases clearance (inhibits R isomer)
Pheyntoin[99]	Unknown
Piroxican[99]	Unknown
Quinidine[117]	Unknown
Phenylbutazone[118]	Decreases clearance (inhibits S isomer)
Salicylates[119,120]	Enhances hypoprothrombinemia (large doses)
Sulfinpyrazone[121]	Decreases clearance (inhibits S isomer)
Tamoxifen[122]	Unknown; ? inhibits metabolism
Thyroxine[123]	Increases metabolism of coagulation factors
Trimethroprim-Sulfamethoxazole[124]	Decreases clearance (inhibits S isomer)
Vitamin E[125]	Unknown
Reduces Prothrombin Time	
Alcohol[99,126]	Increases clearance (stimulates metabolism)
Barbiturates[127]	Increases clearance (stimulates metabolism)
Carbamazepine[128]	Increases clearance (stimulates metabolism)
Cholestyramine[99]	Decreases absorption
Griseofulvin[129]	Increases clearance (stimulates metabolism)
Nafcillin[130]	Increases clearance (stimulates metabolism)
Rifampin[131]	Increases clearance (stimulates metabolism)
Sucralfate[132]	Decreases absorption
Enhances Risk of Bleeding	
Aspirin[133]	Inhibits platelet function
Heparin	Inhibits other coagulation factors
Penicillins[134]	Inhibits platelet function

lant response.[96] Numerous cases of drug interactions with warfarin are reported, but many are not well characterized as to the mechanism of interference. Table 5 lists most interactions and identifies those for which a mechanism seems well established.

Drug interactions commonly occur by affecting the pharmacokinetic behavior of warfarin.[96,97] Drug interactions may interfere with gastrointestinal absorption of warfarin resulting in a reduction in plasma levels, or interfere with the metabolism of warfarin leading to a reduction or increase in clearance, and consequently, higher or lower plasma warfarin levels. The latter effects may be stereospecific in that only one of the stereoisomers may be affected, or it may be nonspecific in that both isomers may be affected. Interference in the metabolism of the S isomer, usually by affecting the P450 cytochrome system,[98] is more common and has a greater potential for enhancing the intensity of anticoagulation since the S isomer is several times more potent than its counterpart. Drugs may also decrease plasma warfarin levels, by enhancing the metabolic clearance of racemic warfarin through induction of hepatic microsomal enzymes. Displacement of warfarin binding to albumin is another mechanism of drug interaction leading to an enhanced effect since unbound warfarin is the metabolically active form.

The pharmacodynamics of warfarin may also be altered when drugs interfere with other aspects of hemostasis or vitamin K homeostasis. A prime example are many of the third generation cephalosporins, those containing an N-methyl-thiotetrazole side chain, which causes an interference with the regeneration of reduced vitamin K from the 2,3 epoxide form. Some drugs or disease states (liver disease, hyperthyroidism) can alter the metabolism of coagulation factors, inhibit coagulation factor interactions by other mechanisms (heparin), or inhibit other aspects of hemostasis (aspirin's effect on platelet function) and lead to a greater risk of bleeding. In addition to these mechanisms, there are a number of reported drug interactions for which a well-defined mechanism has not been described, but for which the practitioner should be well aware when managing patients on oral anticoagulants.[99] In general, most interactions are not problematic unless medications are added or deleted from a patient's regimen.

Complications of Therapy and Their Management

Hemorrhage is obviously the major problem associated with therapy. The frequency of bleeding correlates with the elevation of the prothrombin time,[135,136(V),137(V), 138,139(V)] as well as other factors, such as history of stroke, gastrointestinal bleeding or a serious comorbid condition or instability of control.[139,140] Older age, however, is a controversial determinant of an increased risk of hemorrhage.[139,141(V),142(V)] In this regard, hemorrhage may also be related to the sensitivity of the thromboplastin reagent

Table 6
Pooled Data Showing Incidence of Hemorrhage During Long-Term Anticoagulant Therapy*

Indication	No. of Patients	Incidence of Bleeding, No. (%)			
		Total	Minor	Major	Fatal
Ischemic cerebrovascular	588	169 (28.7)	128 (21.8)	41 (7.0)	28 (4.8)
Prosthetic heart valves	405	23 (5.7)	13 (3.2)	10 (2.4)	7 (1.7)
Atrial fibrillation	302	46 (15.2)	43 (14.2)	3 (0.01)	1 (0.3)
Ischemic heart disease	1890	287 (19.1)	199 (10.5)	88 (4.7)	19 (1.0)
Venous thromboembolism	159	36 (22.6)	23 (14.4)	13 (8.1)	0

* Data from Levine and Hirsh.[138]

used. Thus, patients in the Unites States may have experienced more bleeding over the last two or three decades because of the pervasive use of a less sensitive rabbit brain thromboplastin compared to other populations.[60] Unfortunately, reports are difficult to interpret in this regard. Furthermore, the measurement of hemorrhagic frequency is quite variable, ranging from episodes per patient, per treatment course, per patient year, month, or day, per cumulative frequency, etc. Table 6 summarizes data from a number of studies and suggests that major hemorrhage occurs in approximately 5% of treatment courses.

Management of serious bleeding requires immediate correction of the prothrombin time by replacement of the vitamin K-dependent coagulation factors. This can be achieved by the administration of fresh frozen plasma, but sufficient plasma must be given to be effective. Approximately 15 ml/Kg is an appropriate estimated dose. Factor IX concentrates (concentrates of the vitamin K-dependent factors), should be avoided because of the risk of thrombotic or infectious complications, although rarely, in the face of life threatening bleeding due to severe over-anticoagulation, they may be indicated. Vitamin K can be given for less serious degrees of excessive anticoagulation, but small doses are recommended[143] (1 mg parenterally), since larger doses may predispose to relative degrees of warfarin resistance for patients who need to remain anticoagulated once excessive anticoagulation is corrected. Vitamin K will take 12 to 24 hours to improve the prothrombin time in individuals with normal hepatic function. Lastly, excessive prolongations of the prothrombin time without bleeding, can be corrected simply by withholding warfarin for a few days. Knowing the usual maintenance dose in a specific case will help determine how long the prothrombin time will remain excessively elevated—a high maintenance dose (≥7.5 mg daily) indicates a rapid metabolizer of warfarin, and thus, a rapid drug clearance and lowering of the prothrombin time. A slow metabolizer (≤2.5 mg daily) suggests the opposite.

Gastrointestinal (GI) and genitourinary bleeding in the presence of a therapeutic degree of anticoagulation may result from an unsuspected lesion of clinical significance. Coon and Willis,[144] identified occult lesions responsible for bleeding in 11% of 292 patients with hemorrhage. Jaffin et al,[145] uncovered occult GI lesions in 70% (15/21) of individuals with anticoagulant-related GI hemorrhage. Ten percent of these were malignant. Wilcox et al,[146] however, only found a source of GI bleeding in 50% of 50 patients studied retrospectively. Three cancers were found, and those with no identifiable lesion did well on follow-up. Finally, Landefeld et al,[137] identified occult lesions in 17% (22/130) of bleeding episodes of which 7% (3/130) were cancerous. Hematuria may also herald important underlying pathology as demonstrated by Schuster et al,[147] (17/29 important abnormalities) and Caralis et al.[148] Although the literature is far from uniform on this matter, it is generally recommended to investigate the cause of gastrointestinal or genitourinary bleeding, especially in the presence of a therapeutic level of anticoagulation. Other aspects of the patient's clinical condition and concomitant risk factors for bleeding will dictate how extensive an evaluation to pursue.

Warfarin-induced skin necrosis is another rare, but serious complication of therapy.[149] This tends to occur during the initiation phase of therapy and typically in areas of abundant subcutaneous fatty tissue.[150,151] In some cases it is related to an excessive reduction of protein C, a vitamin K-dependent inhibitor of activated coagulation factors V and VIII, that has a short metabolic half-life similar to factor VII (6 hours).[152,153] Individuals with heterozygous protein C deficiency (approximately 50% activity at baseline), seem to be at greatest risk. In such cases, protein C falls to very low levels before a commensurate reduction in the vitamin K-dependent coagulation factors leading to an initial hypercoagulable state before a hypocoagulable state is achieved.[154] Paradoxically, patients who develop this problem typically have a marked elevation of their prothrombin time.[155] Anticoagulation with heparin during a slowly progressive initiation of warfarin therapy may be adequate to prevent this sequela in patients known to be at risk,[156,157] but the cost effectiveness of screening patients for protein C deficiency or committing every patient to heparin therapy (and hospitalization) prior to oral anticoagulation is doubtful. The treatment of warfarin-induced skin necrosis has been successful with the prompt administration of vitamin K[158] as well as the use of prostacyclin.[159] A deficiency of protein S, a vitamin K-dependent cofactor for protein C, can also cause a similar syndrome.[160]

Invasive Procedures During Warfarin Therapy

With increasing frequency, physicians are confronted with the problem of handling anticoagulation in individuals requiring noncardiac surgery or other invasive procedures, especially in individuals with prosthetic heart valves. There is a paucity of critical studies examining the alternative choices for managing anticoagulation in this setting. Rustad and Myhre,[161] showed no major difference in blood loss during cholecystectomy or gastric resection in anticoagulated or nonanticoagulated individuals, none of whom had prosthetic heart valves. McIntyre,[162] showed that dental extractions can safely be performed in individuals with a therapeutic level of anticoagulation. Tinker et al,[163] in a small retrospective study, showed no difference in thromboembolism between patients who discontinued anticoagulation versus those who did not with either aortic or mitral prostheses. However, it is well known that individuals with a prosthetic valve in the mitral position are more prone to thromboembolism.[164,165] Katholi et al,[164] retrospectively showed a higher rate of postoperative thromboembolism in subjects with a prosthesis in the mitral position versus the aortic position when anticoagulants were discontinued perioperatively. In a subsequent prospective study,[166(V)] they found no difference in postoperative thromboembolism when anticoagulants were discontinued for those with aortic prostheses compared to the use of pre and postoperative heparin in those with mitral prosthesis. Eckman et al,[165] also question the cost effectiveness of prolonged hospitalization for heparin therapy in all such patients, and only recommend it for those with the most thrombogenic prostheses.

Lastly, Gazelle et al,[167] assessed the influence of anticoagulation on blood loss in an animal model of liver or kidney biopsies with different gauge needles. Kidney, but not liver biopsy, was adversely affected by anticoagulation resulting in a small increase in blood loss. Although these results may not be directly extrapolated to humans, they do suggest that one must take into consideration the needle size and target organ when planning a biopsy in the presence of anticoagulation.

There are essentially two basic questions to consider in subjects requiring invasive procedures. First, what is the type of procedure, the relative risk of bleeding, and the ability to control bleeding (i.e., percutaneous biopsies may be more dangerous than open procedures). Second, what is the risk of thromboembolism if an individual's anticoagulant therapy is reduced or temporarily halted.

This will vary depending on the indication for anticoagulation, the type of heart valve, its location, and other factors. After a risk assessment is considered the physician has one of three choices: (1) Discontinuing warfarin several days before the procedure to allow the prothrombin time to return to normal and reinstituting therapy shortly after surgery; (2) Lowering the warfarin dose so as to maintain the patient in a lower or subtherapeutic range during the procedure; (3) Discontinuing warfarin, admitting the patient to the hospital a few days before surgery, and instituting heparin therapy that will be discontinued 2 to 4 hours before surgery and reinstituted when considered safe after surgery, followed by oral anticoagulation. The last of these options provides the shortest interval free of anticoagulation if surgery cannot be done on an anticoagulated patient. The cost effectiveness of this latter approach in all cases is questionable,[165] and as others have shown,[163] many individuals can be entirely off anticoagulation for short periods of time without undue risk.

Anticoagulation During Pregnancy

The need for anticoagulant therapy during pregnancy to treat or prevent DVT or PE or to prevent systemic embolism in women with prosthetic heart valves may be even greater today, especially in light of the frequent use of prosthetic heart valves in young women over the last 20 years. The occurrence of a warfarin embryopathy is well documented when warfarin is used in the first trimester.[168–170] Consequently, warfarin has traditionally been recommended only during the second and early third trimesters, with heparin being used during the other times. In recent years, however, heparin has become the preferred choice of anticoagulation during the entire course of pregnancy.[169] Even though some studies suggest a similar rate of obstetrical complications with either heparin or warfarin,[170] heparin seems to be associated with less serious consequences.[171] Although the appropriate large scale prospective studies have not been done, retrospective data and knowledge of heparin safety suggests that for the prophylaxis of VTE, a fixed dose of subcutaneous heparin should be given twice daily (5000 units bid), perhaps with a larger dose near term to maintain the midinterval APTT 1.5 times the control value.[172] For treatment of acute venous thromboembolism, heparin should be given twice daily (subcutaneous) to achieve a mid interval APTT 1.5 times control value throughout pregnancy, following the usual brief course of inpatient full dose intravenous therapy as would be done in any patient with an acute deep venous thrombosis. In women with prosthetic heart valves, twice daily subcutaneous heparin (mid-interval APTT 1.5 times control) can be used, even though its protective effectiveness is still unclear, and the long duration of use may predispose to osteoporosis. The use of warfarin during the second and early third trimester is not recommended as an alternative to heparin, even though the risk of teratogenicity is reduced compared to the first trimester.

Patient Education and Anticoagulation Clinics

Given the many factors that influence the response to warfarin and the frequency of hemorrhagic complications, it is reasonable to assume that patient education will enhance the efficacy of therapy, even though this assumption has not been tested by rigorously designed studies. Effective education empowers patients to share in the responsibility for their own care. Major points of instruction include those items outlined in **Table 7**. Education and management may be initiated on an inpatient basis[173(IV),174] and continued in specialized "anticoagulation" clinics, which may provide better care[175(V),176,177] and be more cost effective[176] than traditional models of care. These clinics are often nurse[178(V)] or pharmacist[175,177(V)] directed, freeing the physician for other activities. Patient education is an important component of care in these settings,[178(V)] whether delivered by traditional one-on-one personal contact or by specially produced videotaped programs.[179(II)] Although anticoagulation clinics may result in better therapeutic control[175] and even reduce complications, the overall effect on long-term outcome remains unclear.[180]

Table 7
Major Points for Patient Education

Indication for Anticoagulation: Patients are more compliant when they understand the importance of warfarin.
Anticoagulant's Effect on Blood: Warfarin does not dissolve a clot nor thin the blood; it interferes with the ability to form additional clots.
Drug Administration: It is best to take the full dose of warfarin the same time once daily, preferably on an empty stomach. Know the strength (mg) and color of the tablet.
The Importance of PT Monitoring: Explain the importance of maintaining a specific therapeutic range and the need for frequent blood tests.
Signs of Bleeding: Discuss risks of therapy, what to look for, how to avoid, and what to do.
Medication Interactions: Drugs can alter the PT response. The patient is responsible for informing you of all changes in medications. Use of over-the-counter medications (aspirin) should be discussed. Avoiding aspirin products should be emphasized.
Diet: A stable diet, especially with foods rich in vitamin K is essential. Changes in diet can alter the PT response.
Alcohol: Because of its widespread use and ability to increase or decrease the PT response, alcohol always requires special comment. Abstinence is ideal, but minimal use can be tolerated.
Safety: Common sense is the rule. Avoid situations that increase the risk of hemorrhage. Patients are responsible for informing other physicians of their use of anticoagulants. Wear a Medic Alert bracelet or carry an identification card.
Thromboembolism: Discuss what to look for and how to avoid (e.g., thrombophlebitis).

THE FUTURE OF ANTICOAGULATION MANAGEMENT

Self Management of Oral Anticoagulation

Managing long-term oral anticoagulation is a labor intensive and often frustrating experience, both for the physician and the patient. Patients are often elderly, may be in poor health, nonambulatory, and are required to make frequent visits to their physician's office or to a nearby laboratory to have repetitive vena punctures. Physicians must coordinate multiple schedules with various laboratories, retrieve results of questionable accuracy, and contact patients for frequent dose adjustments. The possibility of error, just on the basis of faulty communication alone, is astounding. A potential mechanism to eliminate many of these roadblocks to effective therapy currently exists with the recent development of a hand-held portable instrument designed to measure a prothrombin time[181] or partial thromboplastin time[182] (for heparin monitoring) from a fingerstick sample of capillary whole blood. The accuracy and equivalency to standard prothrombin times have been verified[181,183(I),184,185] and its utility for patient self testing has been reported.[183(I),186(V)]

This instrument not only provides the possibility of immediate prothrombin time results in the physician's office, it can also be taken home by the patient after hospital discharge for self testing and reporting of results to the physician for instructions regarding dose adjustments.[183(I)] Lastly, this instrument provides the opportunity for individuals to monitor their own prothrombin time and adjust their own warfarin dose based on specific nomograms developed for this purpose, just as diabetics do in managing their own insulin therapy. A trial recently reported the feasibility of patient self management of anticoagulant therapy,[186(V)] and the author now has over five years of experience with a small group of patients managing their own therapy at home without untoward effects. The widespread use of this means of management might further enhance the quality of life during long-term warfarin therapy.[187]

REFERENCES

1. Butt HR, Allen EV, Bollman JL. A preparation from spoiled sweet clover which prolongs coagulation and prothrombin time of the blood: preliminary report of experimental and clinical studies. Mayo Clin Proc 1941;16:388–395.
2. Hirsh J, Dalen JE, Deykin D, Poller L. Oral anticoagulants: mechanism of action, clinical effectiveness, and optimal therapeutic range. Chest 1992;102(Suppl):312S–326S.
3. Harland CC, Walt RP. Warfarin therapy: Need for a protocol? Brit J Clin Prac 1988;42:196–197.
4. Schofield FW. Damaged sweet clover: the cause of a new disease in cattle simulating hemorrhagic septicemia and blackleg. J Amer Vet Asso 1924;64:553–575.

5. Roderick LM. Problems in the coagulation of the blood. Amer J Physiol 1931;96:413–425.

6. Dam H. Cholesterinstoffwechsel in huhnereiern und huhnchen. Biochem Z 1929;215:475–492.

7. Dam H. Antihemorrhagic vitamin of the chick: occurrence and chemical nature. Nature 1935;135:652–653.

8. Quick AJ, Stanley-Brown M, Bancroft FW. A study of the coagulation defect in hemophilia and in jaundice. Am J Med Sci 1935;190:501–511.

9. Quick AJ. The coagulation defect in sweet clover disease and in the hemorrhagic chick disease of dietary origin. Am J Physiol 1937;118:260–271.

10. Link KP. The discovery of dicumarol and its sequels. Circulation 1959;19:97–107.

11. Campbell HA, Link KP. Studies on the hemorrhagic sweet clover disease. IV. The isolation and crystallization of the hemorrhagic agent. J Biol Chem 1941;138:21–33.

12. Stahmann MA, Heubner CF, Link KP. Studies on the hemorrhagic sweet clover disease. V. Identification and synthesis of the hemorrhagic agent. J Biol Chem 1941;138:513–527.

13. Link KP. The anticoagulant from spoiled sweet clover hay. Harvey Lecture Series 1944;34:162–216.

14. Holmes RW, Love J. Suicide attempt with warfarin, a bishydroxycoumarin-like rodenticide. JAMA 1952;148:935–937.

15. Almquist JH, Stohstad ELR. Dietary hemorrhagic disease in chicks. Nature 1935;136:31.

16. Thayer SA, MacCorquadale DW, Brinkley SB, Doisy EA. Isolation of crystalline compound with vitamin K activity. Science 1938;88:243.

17. Brinkley SB, McKee RW, Thayer SA, Doisy EA. Constitution of vitamin K_2. J Biol Chem 1940;133:721–729.

18. Stenflo J, Fernlund P, Egan W, Roepstorft P. Vitamin K dependent modifications of glutamic acid residues in prothrombin. Proc Natl Acad Sci 1974;71:2730–2733.

19. Nelsestuen GL, Zytkovicz TH, Howard JB. The mode of action of vitamin K. Identification of gamma carboxyglutamic acid as a component of prothrombin. J Biol Chem 1974;249:6347–6350.

20. Lian JB, Hauschka PV, Gallop PM. Properties and biosynthesis of a vitamin K-dependent calcium binding protein in bone. Federation Proc 1978; 37:2615–2620.

21. Friedman PA, Przysiecki CT. Vitamin K-dependent carboxylation. Int J Biochem 1987;19:1–7.

22. Nelsestuen GL. Role of gamma-carboxyglutamic acid: an unusual protein transition required for calcium-dependent binding of prothrombin to phospholipid. J Biol Chem 1976;251:5648–5656.

23. Borowski M, Furie BC, Bauminger S, Furie B. Prothrombin requires two sequential metal-dependent conformational transitions to bind phospholipid. J Biol Chem 1986;261:14969–14975.

24. Whitlon DS, Sadowski JA, Suttie JW. Mechanism of coumarin action: significance of vitamin K epoxide reductase inhibition. Biochemistry 1978;17:1371–1377.

25. Bell RG. Metabolism of vitamin K and prothrombin synthesis: anticoagulants and the vitamin K-epoxide cycle. Federation Proc 1978;37:2599–2604.

26. Wallin R, Martin LF. Vitamin K dependent carboxylation and vitamin K metabolism in liver: effects of warfarin. J Clin Invest 1985;76:1879–1884.

27. Thijssen HHW, Baars LGM. Microsomal warfarin binding and vitamin K 2,3-epoxide reductase. Biochemical Pharmacol 1989;38:1115–1120.

28. Thijssen HHW, Baars LGM. Tissue distribution of selective warfarin binding sites in the rat. Biochem Pharmacol 1991;42:2181–2186.

29. Friedman PA, Rosenberg RD, Hauschta PV, Fitz-James A. A spectrum of partially carboxylated prothrombins in the plasmas of coumarin-treated patients. Biochem Biophys Acta 1977;494:271–276.

30. Malhotra OP, Nesheim ME, Mann KG. The kinetics of activation of normal and gamma-carboxyglutamic acid deficient prothrombins. J Biol Chem 1985;260:279–287.

31. Malhotra OP. Dicoumarol-induced prothrombins containing 6, 7 and 8 gamma carboxyglutamic acid residues: isolation and characterization. Biochem Cell Biol 1989;67:411–421.

32. Malhotra OP. Dicoumarol-induced 9 gamma carboxyglutamic acid prothrombin: isolation and comparison with 6, 7, 8 and 10 gamma carboxyglutamic acid isomers. Biochem Cell Biol 1990;68:705–715.

33. Sutcliffe FA, MacNicoll AD, Gibson GG. Aspects of anticoagulant action: a review of the pharmacology, metabolism, toxicology of warfarin and congeners. Drug Metab Interact 1987;5:225–271.

34. Poller L. Oral anticoagulant therapy. In: AL Bloom and DP Thomas (eds.):Hemostasis and Thrombosis. London, Churchill Livingstone, Ch 42 pp. 725–736.

35. Breckenridge A. Oral anticoagulant drugs: pharmacokinetic aspects. Semin Hematol 1978;15:19–26.

36. Anticoagulants: coumarin and indanedione derivatives. In: McEroy GK, McQuarrie GM (eds.): American Hospital Formulary Service, Drug Information 85, Bethesda, MD. Amer Soc Hosp Pharmacists 1985;559–565.

37. Porter RS, Sawyer WT, Lowenthal DT. Warfarin. In: WE Evans, JJ Schentag, WJ Jusko (eds.): Applied Pharmaco-Kinetics. 2nd Ed, Applied Therapeutics, Spokane, WA 1986, pp. 1057–1104.

38. Bell RG, Ren P. Inhibition by warfarin enantiomers of prothrombin synthesis, protein carboxylation, and the regeneration of vitamin K from vitamin K epoxide. Biochem Pharmacol 1981;30:1953–1958.

39. O'Reilly RA, Aggeler PM, Leong LS. Studies on the coumarin anticoagulant drugs: the pharmacodynamics of warfarin in man. J Clin Invest 1963;42:1542–1551.

40. O'Reilly RA, Aggeler PM. Studies on coumarin anticoagulant drugs: initiation of warfarin therapy without a loading dose. Circulation 1968;38:169–177.

(I)41. Gallus A, Jackaman J, Tillett J, Mills W, Wycherley A. Safety and efficacy of warfarin started early after submassive venous thrombosis or pulmonary embolism. Lancet 1986;2:1293–1296.

(I)42. Rosiello RA, Chan CK, Tencza F, Matthay RA. Timing of oral anticoagulation therapy in the treatment of angiographically proven acute pulmonary embolism. Arch Intern Med 1987; 147:1469–1473.

(I)43. Hull RD, Raskob GE, Rosenbloom D, et al. Heparin for 5 days as compared with 10 days in the initial treatment of proximal venous thrombosis. N Engl J Med 1990;322:1260–1264.

(II)44. Mohiuddin SM, Hillemen DE, Destache CJ, Stoysich AM, Gannon JM, et al. Efficacy and safety of early versus late initiation of warfarin during heparin therapy in acute thromboembolism. Am Heart J 1992;123:729–732.

45. Routledge PA, Bell SM, Davies DM, Cavanagh JS, Rawlins MD. Predicting patients' warfarin requirements. Lancet 1977;ii:854–855.

46. Williams DB, Karl RC. A simple technique for predicting daily maintenance dose of warfarin. Am J Surg 1979;137:572–576.

47. Sawyer WT. Digital computer-assisted warfarin therapy: comparison of two models. Comp Biomed Res 1979;12:221–231.

48. Carter BL, Reinders TP, Hamilton RA. Prediction of maintenance warfarin dosage from initial patient response. Drug Int Clin Pharm 1983;17:23–26.

49. Sawyer WT. Predictability of warfarin dose requirements: theoretical considerations. J Pharmaceut Sci 1979;68:432–434.

50. Miller DR, Brown MA. Predicting warfarin maintenance dosage based on initial response. Am J Hosp Pharm 1979;36:1351–1355.

(II)51. Doecke CJ, Cosh DG, Gallus AS. Standardized initial warfarin treatment: evaluation of initial treatment response and maintenance dose prediction by randomized trial, and risk factors for an excessive warfarin response. Aust NZ J Med 1991;21:319–324.

52. Allen EV. The clinical use of anticoagulants. JAMA 1947;134:323–329.

53. Wright IS, Marple CD, Beck DF. Anticoagulant therapy of coronary thrombosis with myocardial infarction. JAMA 1948;138:1074–1079.

(III)54. Sevitt S, Gallagher NG. Prevention of venous thrombosis and pulmonary embolism in injured patients. Lancet 1959;ii:981–989.

55. Wright IS. Myocardial infarction and its treatment with anti-coagulants. Lancet 1954;i:92–95.

56. Moschos CB, Wong PCY, Sise HS. Controlled study of the effective level of long-term anticoagulation. JAMA 1964;190:799–805.

(V)57. Allen EV. The clinical use of anticoagulants. Report of treatment with Dicumarol in 1,686 postoperative cases. JAMA 1947;134:323–329.

58. Poller L. The effect of the use of different tissue extracts on one-stage prothrombin times. Acta Haemat 1964;32:292–298.

59. Bailey EL, Harper TA, Pinkerton PH. The "therapeutic range" of the one-stage prothrombin time in the control of anticoagulant therapy: the effect of different thromboplastin preparations. CMA Journal 1971;105:1041–1043.

60. Hirsh J. Is the dose of warfarin prescribed by American physicians unnecessarily high? Arch Intern Med 1987;147:769–771.

61. Lam-Po-Tang PRLC, Poller L. Oral anticoagulant therapy and its control: an international survey. Thromb Haemostas 1975;34:419–425.

62. Poller L, Taberner DA. Dosage and control of oral anticoagulants: an international collaborative survey. Br J Haematol 1982;51:479–485.

63. Poller L. A national standard for anticoagulant therapy. The Manchester Comparative Reagent. Lancet 1967;i:491–493.

64. Biggs R, Denson KWE. Standardization of the one-stage prothrombin time for the control of anticoagulant therapy. Br Med J 1967;1:84–88.

65. Zucker S, Cathey MH, Sox PJ, Hall EC. Standardization of laboratory tests for controlling anticoagulant therapy. Am J Clin Pathol 1970;53:348–354.

66. WHO Expert Committee on Biological Standardization. 28th Report. WHO Tech Ser 1977;610:14–16, 45–51.

67. WHO Expert Committee on Biological Standardization. 31st Report. WHO Tech Ser 1981;658:185–205.

68. Kirkwood TBL. Calibration of reference thromboplastins and standardization of the prothrombin time ratio. Thromb Haemostas 1983;49:238–244.

(I)69. Hull R, Hirsh J, Jay R, et al. Different intensities of anticoagulation in the long term treatment of proximal venous thrombosis. N Engl J Med 1982;307:1676–1681.

70. Ansell JE. Imprecision of prothrombin time monitoring of oral anticoagulation: a survey of hospital laboratories. Am J Clin Pathol 1992;98:237–239.

71. Bussey HI, Force RW, Bianco TM, Leonard AD. Reliance on prothrombin time ratios causes significant errors in anticoagulation therapy. Arch Int Med 1992;152:278–282.

72. Poller L. Progress in standardization in anticoagulant control. Hematol Rev 1987;1:225–241.

73. Hirsh J, Dalen JE, Deykin D, Poller L. Oral anticoagulants: Mechanism of action, clinical effectiveness and optimal therapeutic range. Chest 1992; 102(Suppl):312S-326S.

74. Mennemeyer ST, Winkelman JW. Searching for inaccuracy in clinical laboratory testing using Medicare data: evidence for prothrombin time. JAMA 1993;269:1030–1033.

75. Gottfried EL, Ng VL, Lavin J, Corash L. Problems with the international normalized ratio. Blood 1992;80:2690–2691.

76. Poller L. Regulating the dosage of warfarin for anticoagulation. N Engl J Med 1987;316:1277–1278.

77. van den Besselaar AMHP, Evatt BL, Brogan DR, Triplett DA. Proficiency testing and standardization of prothrombin time: effect of thromboplastin instrumentation, and plasma. Am J Clin Pathol 1984;82:688–699.

78. Ray MJ, Smith IR. The dependence of the international sensitivity index on the coagulometer used to perform the prothrombin time. Thromb Haemostas 1990;63:424–429.

79. Poller L, Thompson JM, Taberner DA. Effect of automation on prothrombin time test in NEQAS surveys. J Clin Pathol 1989;42:97–100.

80. Owren PA. Thrombotest. A new method for controlling anticoagulant therapy. Lancet 1959;II:754.

81. Paulssen MMP, Kolhorn A, Rothuizen J, Planje MC. An automated amidolytic assay for thrombin generation: an alternative for the prothrombin time test. Clinica Chimica Acta 1979;92:465–468.

(II)82. Furie B, Duiguid CF, Jacobs M, Diuguid DL, Furie BC. Randomized prospective trial comparing the native prothrombin antigen with the prothrombin time for monitoring oral anticoagulant therapy. Blood 1990;75:344–349.

83. Lammle B, Bainamlaux H, Market GA, Eichlisberge R, Duckert F. Monitoring of oral anticoagulation by an amidolytic factor X assay. Thromb Hemostas 1980;44:150–153.

84. Xi M, Beguin S, Hemker HC. The relative importance of the factors II, VII, IX and X for the prothrombinase activity in plasma of orally anticoagulated patients. Thromb Haemostas 1989;62:788–791.

85. Furie B, Liebman HA, Blanchard RA, Coleman MS, Kruger SF, et al. Comparison of the native prothrombin antigen and the prothrombin time for monitoring oral anticoagulant therapy. Blood 1984;64:445–451.

86. Loeliger EA, van Dijk-Wierda CA, van den Besselaar AMHP, Broekmans AW, Roos J. Anticoagulant control and the risk of bleeding. In Meade TW, (ed.): Anticoagulants and Myocardial Infarction. John Wiley & Sons, Ltd. 1984, pp. 135–177.

87. Breckenridge AM. Interindividual differences in the response to oral anticoagulants. Drugs 1977;14: 367–375.

88. Qureshi GD, Reinders TP, Swint JJ, Slate MB. Acquired warfarin resistance and weight-reducing diet. Arch Intern Med 1981;141:507–509.

89. Udall JA. Human sources and absorption of vitamin K in relation to anticoagulation stability. JAMA 1965;194: 107–109.

90. O'Reilly RA, Aggeler PM, Hoag MS, et al. Hereditary transmission of exceptional resistance to coumarin anticoagulant drugs. N Engl J Med 1964;271:809–815.

91. O'Reilly RA. The second kindred with hereditary resistance to oral anticoagulant drugs. N Engl J Med 1970;282:1448–1451.

92. Alving BM, Strickler MP, Knight RD, Barr CF, Berenberg JL, et al. Hereditary warfarin resistance. Arch Intern Med 1985;145:499–501.

93. O'Malley K, Stevenson IHN, Ward CA, Wood AJJ, Crooks J. Determinants of anticoagulant control in patients receiving warfarin. Br J Clin Pharmac 1977;4: 309–314.

94. Williams JRB, Griffin JP, Parkins A. Effect of concomitantly administered drugs on the control of long term anticoagulant therapy. Quart J Med 1976;45:66–73.

95. O'Reilly RA, Aggeler PA. Determinants of the response to oral anticoagulant drugs in man. Pharmacol Rev 1970;22:35.

96. O'Reilly RA. Warfarin metabolism and drug-drug interactions. In: Wessler S, Becker CG, Nemerson Y (eds.) The new dimensions of warfarin prophylaxis. Vol 214 of Advances in Experimental Medicine and Biology. New York, Plenum, 1986, pp. 205–212.

97. Hirsh J. Oral anticoagulant drugs. N Engl J Med 1991;324:1865–1875.

98. Rettie AE, Korzekwa KR, Kunze KL, et al. Hydroxylation of warfarin by human cDNA-expressed cytochrome P-450: a role for P-4502C9 in the etiology of (S)-warfarin-drug interactions. Chem Res Toxicol 1992;5:54–59.

99. Hansten PD, Horn JR. Oral anticoagulant drug interactions. In: Hansten PD, Horn JR, (eds). Drug Interactions and Updates. Malvern PA, Lea & Febiger, 1990, pp. 115–162.

100. Kerin NZ, Blevins RD, Goldman L, Faitel K, Rubenfire M. The incidence, magnitude, and time course of the Amiodarone-Warfarin interaction. Arch Intern Med 1988;148:1779–1781.

101. Heimark LD, Wienkers L, Kunze K, et al. The mechanism of the interaction between amiodarone and warfarin in humans. Clin Pharmacol Ther 1992;51:398–407.

102. Lorentz SM, Weibert RT. Potentiation of warfarin anticoagulation by topical testosterone ointment. Clin Pharm 1985;4:332–333.

103. Sattler FR, Weitekamp MR, Ballard JO. Potential for bleeding with the new beta-lactam antibiotics. Ann Intern Med 1986;105:924–931.

104. Shearer MJ, Bechtold H, Andrassy K, et al. Mechanism of cephalosporin-induced hypoprothrombinemia: relation to cephalosporin side chain, vitamin K metabolism, and vitamin K status. J Clin Pharmacol 1988;28: 88–95.

105. Choonara IA, Cholerton S, Haynes BP, Breckenridge AM, Park BK. Stereoselective interaction between the R enantiomer of warfarin and cimetidine. Br J Clin Pharmac 1986;21:271–277.

106. O'Reilly RA. Comparative interaction of cimetidine and ranitidine with racemic warfarin in man. Arch Intern Med 1984;144:989–991.

107. O'Reilly RA, Sahud MA, Robinson AJ. Studies on the interaction of warfarin and clofibrate in man. Thrombo Diath Haemorrh 1972;27:309–318.

108. O'Reilly RA. Interaction of sodium warfarin and disulfiram in man. Ann Intern Med 1973;78:73–76.

109. Wiebert RT, Lorentz SM, Townsend RJ, Cook CE, Klauber MR, et al. Effect of erythromycin in patients receiving long-term warfarin therapy. Clin Pharm 1989;8:210–214.

110. Linville D, Emory C, Graves L. Ciprofloxacin and warfarin interaction. Am J Med 1991;90:765.

111. Roush MK, Bussey HL, Bianco TM. Do fluoroquinolones alter the effects of warfarin therapy? Arch Intern Med 1992;152:1533–1544.

112. Crussel-Porter LL, Rindone JP, Ford MA, Jaskar DW. Low-dose fluconazole therapy potentiates the hypoprothrombinemic response of warfarin sodium. Arch Intern Med 1993;153:102–104.

113. Koch-Weser J. Potentiation by glucagon of the hypoprothrombinemic action of warfarin. Ann Intern Med 1970;72:331–335.

114. O'Reilly RA. The stereoselective interaction of warfarin and metronidazole in man. N Engl J Med 1976;295:354–357.

115. O'Reilly RA, Goulart DA, Kunze KL, et al. Mechanisms of the stereoselective interaction between miconazole and racemic warfarin in human subjects. Clin Pharmacol Thera 1992;51:656–667.

116. Sutfin T, Balmer K, Bostrom H, et al. Stereoselective interaction of omeprazole with warfarin in healthy men. Ther Drug Monit 1989;11:176–184.

117. Koch-Weser J. Quinidine-induced hypoprothrombinemic hemorrhage in patients on chronic warfarin therapy. Ann Int Med 1968;68:511–517.

118. Lewis RJ, Trager WF, Chan KK, et al. Warfarin: stereochemical aspects of its metabolism and the interaction with phenylbutazone. J Clin Invest 1974;53: 1607–1617.

119. Roncaglioni MC, Ulrich MMW, Muller AD, Soute BAM, de Boer-van den Berg MAG, et al. The vitamin K-antagonism of salicylate and warfarin. Thromb Res 1986;42:727–736.

120. Littleton F. Warfarin and topical salicylates. JAMA 1990;263:2888.

121. Toon S, Low LK, Gibaldi M, et al. The warfarin-sulfinpyrazone interaction: stereochemical considerations. Clin Pharmacol Ther 1986;39:15–24.

122. Lodwick R, McConkey B, Brown AM. Life threatening interaction between tamoxifen and warfarin. Br Med J 1987;295:1141.

123. Owens JC, Neely WB, Owen WR. Effect of sodium dextrothyroxine in patients receiving anticoagulants. N Engl J Med 1962;266:76–79.

124. O'Reilly RA. Stereoselective interaction of trimethoprim-sulfamethoxazole with the separated enantiomorphs of racemic warfarin in man. N Engl J Med 1980;302:33–35.

125. Corrigan JJ. The effect of vitamin E on warfarin-induced vitamin K deficiency. Ann NY Acad Sci 1982;393:361–368.

126. O'Reilly RA. Lack of effect of fortified wine ingested during fasting and anticoagulant therapy. Arch Intern Med 1981;141:458–459.

127. O'Reilly RA, Trager WF, Motley CH, Howald W.

Interaction of secobarbital with warfarin pseudoracemates. Clin Pharmacol Ther 1980;28:187–195.

128. Hansen IM, Siersbock-Nielson K, Skovsted L. Carbamazepine-induced acceleration of diphenylhydantoin and warfarin metabolism in man. Clin Pharmacol Ther 1971;12:539–543.

129. Cullen SI, Catalano PM. Griseofulvin-warfarin antagonism. JAMA 1967;199:582–583.

130. Qureshi GD, Reinders TP, Somori GJ, Evans HJ. Warfarin resistance with nafcillin therapy. Ann Intern Med 1984;100;527–529.

131. O'Reilly RA. Interaction of chronic daily warfarin therapy and rifampin. Ann Intern Med 1975;83:506–508.

132. Parrish RH, Waller B, Gondalia BG. Sucralfate-warfarin interaction. Ann Pharmaco 1992;26:1015–1016.

133. Roth GJ, Majerus PW. The mechanism of the effect of aspirin on human platelets. I. Acetylation of a particulate fraction protein. J Clin Invest 1975;56:624–632.

134. Brown CH, Bradshaw MW, Natelson EA, Alfrey CP, Williams TW. Defective platelet function following the administration of penicillin compounds. Blood 1976;47:949–956.

135. Sise HS, Lavelle SM, Adamis D, Becker R. Relation of hemorrhage and thrombosis to prothrombin during treatment with coumarin-type anticoagulants. N Engl J Med 1958;259:266–271.

(V)136. Forfar JC. Prediction of hemorrhage during long-term oral coumarin anticoagulation by excessive prothrombin ratio. Am Heart J 1982;103:445–446.

(V)137. Landefeld CS, Rosenblatt MW, Goldman L. Bleeding in outpatients treated with warfarin: relation to the prothrombin time and important remedial lesions. Am J Med 1989;87:153–159.

138. Levine MN, Hirsh J. Hemorrhagic complications of anticoagulant therapy. Semin Thromb Hemostas 1986;12:39–57.

(V)139. Landefeld CS, Goldman L. Major bleeding in outpatients treated with warfarin: incidence and prediction by factors known at the start of outpatient therapy. Am J Med 1989;87:144–152.

140. Fihn SD, McDonell M, Martin D, et al. Risk factors for complications of chronic anticoagulation. Ann Int Med 1993;118:511–520.

(V)141. Gurwitz J, Goldberg R, Holden A, Knapic N, Ansell J. Age-related risks of long-term oral anticoagulant therapy. Arch Int Med 1988;148:1733–1736.

(V)142. Gurwitz JH, Avorn J, Ross-Degnan D, Choodnonskiy I, Ansell J. Aging and the anticoagulant response to warfarin therapy. Ann Int Med 1992;116:901–904.

143. Shetty HG, Backhouse G, Bentley OP, et al. Effective reversal of warfarin-induced excessive anticoagulation with low dose vitamin K1. Thromb Hemostas 1992;67:13–15.

144. Coon WW, Willis PW. Hemorrhagic complications of anticoagulant therapy. Arch Intern Med 1974;133:386–392.

145. Jaffin BW, Bliss CM, Lamart JT. Significance of occult gastrointestinal bleeding during anticoagulation therapy. Am J Med 1987;269–272.

146. Wilcox CM, Truss CD. Gastrointestinal bleeding in patients receiving long-term anticoagulant therapy. Am J Med 1988;84:683–690.

147. Schuster GA, Lewis GA. Clinical significance of hematuria in patients on anticoagulant therapy. J Urol 1987;137:923–925.

148. Caralis P, Gelbard M, Washer J, Rhamy R, Marcial E. Incidence and etiology of hematuria in patients on anticoagulant therapy. Clin Res 1989;37:791A.

149. Cole MS, Minifee PK, Wolma FJ. Coumarin necrosis: A review of the literature. Surgery 1988;103:271–276.

150. Davis CE, Wiley WB, Faulconer RJ. Necrosis of the female breast complicating oral anticoagulant treatment. Ann Surg 1972;175:647–656.

151. Lacy JP, Goodin RR. Warfarin-induced necrosis of skin. Ann Int Med 1975;82:381–382.

152. Broekmans AW, Bertina RM, Loeliger EA, Hofmann V, Klingemann HG. Protein C and the development of skin necrosis during anticoagulant therapy. Thromb Haemostas 1983;49:251.

153. McGehee WG, Klatz TA, Epstein DJ, Rapaport SI. Coumarin necrosis associated with hereditary protein C deficiency. Ann Int Med 1984;100:59–60.

154. D'Angelo SV, Comp PC, Esmon CT, D'Angelo A. Relationship between protein C antigen and anticoagulant activity during oral anticoagulation and in selected disease states. J Clin Invest 1986;77:416–425.

155. Green D. Warfarin. Ann Int Med 1984;311:1578–1579.

156. Zauber NP, Stark MW. Successful warfarin anticoagulation despite protein C deficiency and a history of warfarin necrosis. Ann Int Med 1986;104:659–660.

157. Enzenauer RJ, Campbell J. Progressive warfarin anticoagulation in protein C deficiency: a therapeutic strategy. Am J Med 1990;88:697–698.

158. van Amstel WJ, Boekhout-Mussert MJ, Loeliger EA. Successful prevention of coumarin-induced hemorrhagic skin necrosis by timely administration of vitamin K1. Blut 1978;36:89–93.

159. Norris PG. Warfarin skin necrosis treated with prostacyclin. Clin Exper Dermatol 1987;12:370–372.

160. Friedman KD, Marlar RA, Houston JG, Montgomery RR. Warfarin-induced skin necrosis in a patient with protein S deficiency. Blood 1986;68(Suppl 1):333a.

161. Rustad H, Myhre E. Surgery during anticoagulant treatment. Acta Med Scand 1963;173:115–119.

162. McIntyre H. Management during dental surgery of patients on anticoagulants. Lancet 1966;2:99–100.

163. Tinker JH, Tarhan S. Discontinuing anticoagulant therapy in surgical patients with cardiac valve prosthesis. JAMA 1978;239:738–739.

164. Katholi RE, Nolan SP, McGuire LB. Living with `prosthetic' heart valves: subsequent noncardiac operations and the risk of thromboembolism or hemorrhage. Am Heart J 1976;92:162–167.

165. Eckman MH, Beshansky JR, Durand-Zaleski I, Levine HJ, Pauker SG. Anticoagulation for noncardiac procedures in patients with prosthetic heart valves. JAMA 1990;263:1513–1521.

(V)166. Katholi RE, Nolan SP, McGuire LB. The management of anticoagulation during noncardiac operations in patients with prospective heart valves. Am Heart J 1978;96:163–165.

167. Gazelle GS, Haaga JR, Rowland DY. Effect of needle gauge, level of anticoagulation, and target organ on bleeding associated with aspiration biopsy. Radiol 1992;183:509–513.

168. Pettifor JM, Benson R. Congenital malformations associated with the administration of oral anticoagulants during pregnancy. J Pediatr 1975;86:459–462.

169. Stevenson RE, Burton OM, Ferlanto GJ, Taylor HA. Hazards of oral anticoagulants during pregnancy. JAMA 1980;243:1549–1551.

170. Hall JG, Pauli RM, Wilson KM. Maternal and fetal sequelae of anticoagulation during pregnancy. Am J Med 1980;68:122–140.

171. Ginsberg JS, Hirsh J. Anticoagulants during pregnancy. Ann Rev Med 1989;40:79–86.

172. Ginsberg JS, Hirsh J. Use of anticoagulants during pregnancy. Chest 1989;95(Suppl):156S-160S.

(IV)173. Ellis RF, Stephens MA, Sharp GB. Evaluation of a pharmacy-managed warfarin monitoring service to coordinate inpatient and outpatient therapy. Am J Hosp Pharm 1992;49:387–394.

174. Landefeld CS, Anderson PA. Guide-line based consultation to prevent anticoagulant-related bleeding. Ann Int Med 1992;116:829–837.

(V)175. Garabedian-Ruffalo SM, Gray DR, Sax MJ, Ruffalo RL. Retrospective evaluation of a pharmacist-managed warfarin anticoagulation clinic. Am J Hosp Pharm 1985;42:304–308.

176. Gray DR, Garabedian-Ruffalo SM, Chretien SD. Cost justification of a clinical pharmacist-managed anti-coagulation clinic. Drug Intel Clin Pharm 1985;19: 575–580.

(V)177. Bussey HI, Rospond RM, Quandt CM, Clark GM. The safety and effectiveness of long-term warfarin therapy in an anticoagulation clinic. Pharmacother 1989;9: 214–219.

(V)178. Kornblit P, Senderoff J, Davis-Ericksen M, Zenk J. Anticoagulation therapy: patient management and evaluation of an outpatient clinic. Nur Pract 1990;15: 21–32.

(II)179. Stone S, Holden A, Knapic N, Ansell J. Comparison between videotape and personalized patient education for anticoagulant therapy. J Fam Pract 1989;29:55–57.

180. Hamilton GM, Childers RW, Silvestein MD. Does clinic management of anticoagulation improve the outcome of prosthetic valve patients? Clin Res 1985;33:832A.

181. Lucas FV, Duncan A, Jay R, et al. A novel whole blood capillary technique for measuring the prothrombin time. Am J Clin Pathol 1987;88:442–446.

182. Ansell J, Tiarks C, Hirsh J, McGehee W, Adler D, et al. Measurement of the activated partial thromboplastin time from a capillary (fingerstick) sample of whole blood. Am J Clin Pathol 1991;95:222–227.

(I)183. White RH, McCurdy SA, von Marensdorff H, Woodruff DE, Leftgoff L. Home prothrombin time monitoring after the initiation of warfarin therapy. Ann Int Med 1989;111:730–737.

184. Jennings I, Luddington RJ, Baglin T. Coagulation monitor for the control of oral anticoagulation. J Clin Pathol 1991;44:950–953.

185. Yano Y, Kambayashi JI, Murata K, et al. Bedside monitoring of warfarin therapy by a whole blood capillary coagulation monitor. Thromb Res 1992;66:583–590.

(V)186. Ansell J, Holden A, Knapic N. Patient self-management of oral anticoagulation guided by capillary (fingerstick) whole blood prothrombin times. Arch Intern Med 1989;149:2509–2511.

187. Lancaster TR, Singer DE, Sheehan MA, et al. The impact of long-term warfarin therapy on quality of life. Arch Intern Med 1991;151:1944–1949.

31

Thrombolytic Therapy

C. Gregory Elliott

INTRODUCTION

After much investigation, the exact role of thrombolytic therapy in the treatment of venous thromboembolism (VTE) remains controversial. Uncertainty regarding the relative risks and benefits of thrombolysis fuels the controversy. Available data suggest that thrombolytic agents accelerate the dissolution of venous thromboemboli, but they also increase the risk of serious hemorrhage. Well designed clinical trials which demonstrate benefits in overall mortality or morbidity are not available. Thus medical opinion remains divided, and most practitioners rely upon thrombolytic agents only for the extremes of venous thromboembolic disease.

ENDOGENOUS FIBRINOLYSIS

The human body possesses a fibrinolytic system which dissolves intravascular clots. Plasmin is the active enzyme which digests fibrin. Plasminogen, its inactive precursor, is converted to active plasmin ("activated") by cleavage of a single peptide bond; a reaction which splits plasminogen into disulfide linked heavy and light chains, and allows the light chain to assume a conformation capable of fibrinolytic activity.[1]

Endogenous plasminogen activation originates with tissue injury which stimulates vascular endothelial cells to produce tissue plasminogen activator (tPA). Fibrin-bound plasmin then converts circulating pro-urokinase to urokinase which amplifies the activation of fibrin-bound plasminogen. In addition, endothelial injury activates factor XII which activates kallikrein which in turn converts fibrin-bound plasminogen to plasmin.[2]

Endogenous regulatory mechanisms balance plasminogen activation. The most important inhibitor of plasmin activity in the circulation is α_2-antiplasmin which the liver produces. Plasma concentrations of α_2-antiplasmin are sufficient to inhibit approximately one-half of available plasmin. Thus when massive plasminogen activation depletes α_2-antiplasmin, circulating plasmin causes a "systemic lytic state" in which hemostasis is impaired. Plasminogen activator inhibitors also inhibit endogenous fibrinolysis. The liver, endothelial cells, and platelets produce plasminogen activator inhibitors.

Pathological venous thromboemboli are subject to endogenous fibrinolysis. Thus partial or even complete dissolution of venous thromboemboli occurs with time. The rate and degree of thrombus dissolution remain extremely variable from patient to patient. Patients with chronic thrombotic obstruction of major pulmonary arteries, a rare sequel of pulmonary thromboembolism, illustrate failure of endogenous fibrinolysis. To date functional abnormalities of plasma fibrinolytic components (plasminogen and α_2-antiplasmin) have not been associated with chronic thrombotic obstruction of major pulmonary arteries.[3]

PHARMACOLOGY OF THROMBOLYTIC DRUGS

General Pharmacology

All thrombolytic agents convert plasminogen to plasmin (Figure 1). Plasmin, in turn, degrades cross-linked fibrin in thrombi as well as circulating fibrinogen. Degradation products of fibrin and fibrinogen can accelerate the fibrinolytic process. For example, fragment D enhances plasminogen activation. Plasminogen exists both bound to fibrin and fibrinogen as well as circulating in the plasma.[4] Thus it is possible for thrombolytic drugs to exhibit selectivity for the plasminogen which they activate. Thrombolytic agents may exhibit more activity upon fibrin-bound plasminogen than upon circulating plasminogen, hence earning the pharmacological distinction of fibrin selectivity. However the clinical benefits of fibrin selectivity remain unproven.

Thrombolytic drugs promote bleeding through actions on hemostatic plugs, impairment of coagulation, and impairment of platelet function. Activated plasmin cleaves adhesion proteins such as thrombospondin and

From *Venous Thromboembolism: An Evidence-Based Atlas* edited by Russell Hull, Gary Raskob, Graham Pineo © 1996, Futura Publishing Co., Armonk, NY.

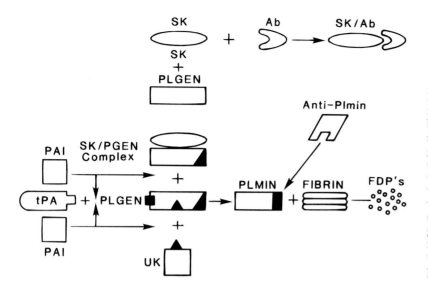

Figure 1. The activation of plasminogen to plasmin results from cleavage of the arginine560-valine561 bond, a reaction which allows a light chain to assume an active proteolytic conformation, and degrade fibrin to soluble fibrin degradation products (FDP's). Urokinase (UK) and tissue plasminogen activator (tPA) are direct activators of plasminogen, whereas streptokinase (SK) is an indirect activator which forms a complex with plasminogen (SK/PGEN). This complex activates other plasminogen molecules. Natural antibodies (Ab) can neutralize streptokinase (SK/Ab), and plasminogen activator inhibitors (PAI) can block the activation of plasminogen.

fibronectin. In addition, hypofibrinogenemia and fibrin degradation products inhibit fibrin polymerization. These actions cause the dissolution of fibrin plugs at sites of previous vascular injury. Thrombolytic agents decrease circulating coagulation factors V and VIII. Thrombolytic drugs also impair platelet adhesion and aggregation. Thus the pro-hemorrhagic effects of thrombolytic drugs rely not only upon hypofibrinogenemia. They also result from effects on platelets, the endothelial surface, and ability of these agents to dissolve platelet and fibrin plugs at sites of prior vascular injury.

Comparative Pharmacology (Table 1)

Streptokinase. In 1933, Tillet and Garner observed that a filtrate of Group C β-hemolytic streptococci lysed a human thrombus.[5] The filtrate was subsequently purified and refined to be a 47,000 Dalton protein which forms a stable complex with plasminogen, producing a conformational change to release free plasmin. This streptokinase-plasminogen complex is not inhibited by antiplasmin. However, failure to achieve a lytic state may result if most plasminogen is bound to streptokinase activator complex, leaving low concentrations of plasminogen for conversion to plasmin.[6]

Streptokinase is a foreign protein. Antibodies to streptococcal proteins, consequent to prior streptococcal infections, may neutralize the effect of a first dose of streptokinase by forming antigen-antibody complexes. For this reason clinicians give a large initial dose of streptokinase. A loading dose of 250,000 units of streptokinase overcomes antibody mediated resistance for more than 90% of patients. Furthermore, as early as 5 to 6 days after the initial administration of streptokinase, antistreptokinase antibody titers rise. These antibodies preclude retreatment for more than a year.

Table 1
Thrombolytic Agents-Basic Pharmacology

	Source	Molecular Weight Daltons	Antibody Formation	Half-Life Minutes	Fibrin Specificity
Streptokinase (SK)	Group C, beta-hemolytic Streptococci	47,000	Yes	30	No
Anisoylated Plasminogen Activator Complex (APSAC)	in vitro p-anisoylation of plasminogen and streptokinase	131,000	Yes	90	Partial
Urokinase (UK)	Purification from human urine or cultured fetal kidney cells	32,600	No	10	No
Prourokinase (single chain urokinase-type plasminogen activator) (Scu-PA)	Derived from urine using recombinant technology and e. coli	54,000	NK	5	Yes
Recombinant tissue plasminogen activator (rTPA)	recombinant DNA technology	72,000	NK	6	Yes

NK = not known

The streptokinase activator complex has a half-life of approximately 30 minutes. During this time the streptokinase activator complex rapidly converts circulating plasminogen and fibrinogen to circulating plasmin and fibrinogen breakdown products. Degradation of factors V and VIII accompanies the systemic lytic state.

Anisoylated Plasminogen-Streptokinase Activator Complex (APSAC). Anisoylated plasminogen-streptokinase activator complex (anistreplase) is formed by complexing streptokinase with plasminogen and inactivating the catalytic site with a P-anisoyl group. The complex is deacylated (activated) when given intravenously. The deacylation step occurs in the thrombus and is responsible for the partial fibrin specificity of APSAC. Intravenous APSAC can be administered rapidly without causing hypotension. APSAC has a somewhat longer half-life, approximately 90 minutes, than streptokinase. However like streptokinase, APSAC is antigenic.

Urokinase. Urokinase is a thrombolytic agent initially isolated from urine.[7] Currently urokinase is purified from cultured fetal kidney cells. It is a serine protease which directly activates plasminogen. Unlike streptokinase, urokinase is nonantigenic, and resistance due to antibody formation does not occur. Urokinase is not fibrin specific. Therefore, it decreases circulating fibrin and plasminogen, and produces a systemic lytic effect. Urokinase has a half-life of approximately 15 minutes.

Tissue Plasminogen Activator or TPA. Tissue plasminogen activator is a single chain glycoprotein. Tissue plasminogen activator has a stronger affinity for plasminogen in the presence of fibrin. Plasminogen and tissue plasminogen activator form a complex within fibrin clots which converts plasminogen into plasmin. This fibrin selectivity decreases the severity of fibrinogenolysis in the plasma. In addition, tissue plasminogen activator has a shorter half-life, of approximately six minutes, than other thrombolytic agents.

Available Preparations

Streptokinase, urokinase, and recombinant tissue plasminogen activator (rtPA) are the three thrombolytic drugs currently approved for the treatment of pulmonary embolism (PE) (Table 2). Urokinase and tissue plasminogen activator are more expensive than streptokinase.

Monitoring Thrombolytic Therapy

Thrombolytic treatment of VTE should begin after heparin has been discontinued, and the activated partial thromboplastin time is < 1.5 times control. Since the fibrinolytic state prolongs the activated partial thromboplastin time and thrombin time, it is customary to reinstitute heparin once the thrombin time or activated partial thromboplastin time are less than twice normal. This usually necessitates monitoring of the APTT or thrombin time at 4-hour intervals after discontinuing thrombolytic therapy. Additional *in vitro* monitoring does not appear warranted because neither bleeding nor the degree of clot lysis are predicted by *in vitro* tests; and present dosing regimens are fixed i.e., adjusting the dose in response to an *in vitro* test has not been shown to alter the outcome.[8,9]

CLINICAL OBSERVATIONS IN PATIENTS WITH PULMONARY THROMBOEMBOLISM

Comparison With Heparin

Several randomized clinical trials have compared thrombolytic drugs with heparin for the treatment of PE.[10(I),11(I),12,13(I),14(I)] The largest of these studies was the urokinase PE trial[10] which compared a 12-hour infusion of urokinase with intravenous heparin (Table 3). This trial demonstrated that urokinase accelerated thrombus dissolution when compared with heparin. Evidence for accel-

Table 2
Thrombolytic Treatment of Acute Venous Thromboembolism

Agent	Dose		Duration (hrs.)	Monitoring	Cost†	Comment
	Loading	Maintenance				
SK	250,000	—	0.5	TT, APTT, PT or Fibrinogen 4 Hrs. after start	$	May not be effective between 5 days and 12 months after acute streptococcal infections *or* prior SK treatment
	—	100,000 IU/Hr	24 (PE) 48–72 (DVT)			
UK	2000 IU/lb over 10 min.	2000 IU/lb/Hr	12 or 24 (PE or DVT)		$$$$	
	1×10^6 over 10 min.	2×10^6 over 110 min.	2 (PE)			As effective and safer than 24 Hr infusion
rt-PA	—	100 mg	2 (PE)		$$$	

Abbreviations: SK = streptokinase; UK = urokinase; rt-PA = recombinant tissue plasminogen activator; PE = pulmonary embolism; DVT = deep-vein thrombosis.

Table 3
Comparison of Urokinase with Heparin for Patients With Acute Pulmonary Embolism*

	Urokinase n = 82	Heparin n = 78
Mortality (%)	7	9
Bleeding (%)		
Overt	45	27
Severe †	27	14
Recurrent PE (%)	15	19
Angiographic improvement (%)	44	6
(24 hours)		
Lung perfusion scan improvement (%)		
24 Hours	6	2
Day 7	12	11

* Source reference #10.

† Severe Bleeding = ↓ in Hct of more than 10%; and/or transfusion of more than 2 units of packed red blood cells.

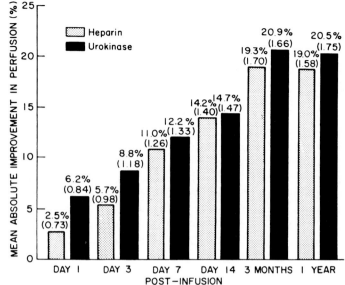

Figure 3. Comparison of the mean absolute improvement in perfusion lung scan defects for patients treated with heparin *or* urokinase. Note that by day 7 the degree of improvement was comparable, suggesting that urokinase accelerates the endogenous fibrinolytic process. (Reproduced with permission from reference 10.)

erated thrombolysis included quantitative measures of angiographic scores (Figure 2); quantitative scores of pulmonary perfusion scans (Figure 3), and measures of pulmonary vascular resistance (Figure 4). By the seventh day after treatment the improvement in lung perfusion scans was almost identical for the two treatment groups. Bleeding occurred frequently at sites of invasive procedures during the period of urokinase infusion.

The individual response to thrombolytic therapy varied. Almost one-third of urokinase treated patients had a "large" improvement in angiogram (Figure 5), lung perfusion scan, and pulmonary artery pressure within 24 hours of thrombolysis. In these trials no patient

who received heparin had comparable improvement. The investigators also noted that more massive thromboemboli treated within 48 hours of symptoms were more likely to respond to thrombolysis. Chronic severe pulmonary hypertension and cor pulmonale occur most commonly after unrecognized and untreated pulmonary emboli.[15] More modest abnormalities of pulmonary artery pressure and pulmonary vascular resistance may occur years after PE treated with anticoagulants.[16] Thrombolytic therapy may prevent late hemodynamic sequelae of acute PE,[17] and improve physiological tests of pulmonary function.[18(I)] However, the relative values of

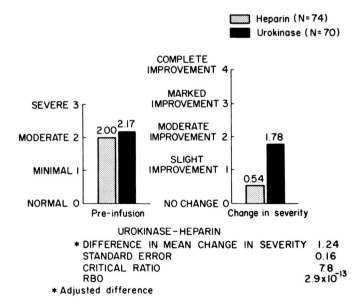

Figure 2. Comparison of the mean pretreatment angiographic severity score with the mean angiographic severity scores 24 hours after heparin or urokinase treatment. (Reproduced with permission from reference 10).

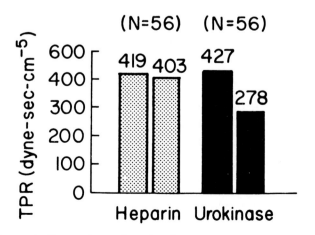

Figure 4. Comparison of total pulmonary resistance measurements before and 24 hours after either heparin *or* urokinase treatment. (Reproduced with permission from reference 10).

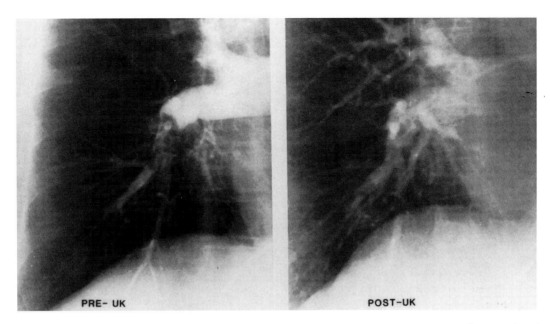

Figure 5. Marked lysis of proximal thromboembolus can occur after a 2-hour infusion 3×10^6 units of urokinase.

thrombolysis and anticoagulation upon late sequelae of PE remain largely undefined.[9]

Comparison of Thrombolytic Drugs and Dosing Regimens

To improve the efficacy and safety profile of thrombolytic therapy for PE investigators have evaluated a variety of dosing strategies as well as newer thrombolytic drugs. Increasing the duration of urokinase infusion from 12 to 24 hours did not produce significantly more thrombolysis.[19(I)] Furthermore, 24 hours of streptokinase proved comparable to urokinase. Recombinant tissue plasminogen activator (rtPA), delivered intravenously in 2 hours, produced more rapid angiographic resolution and hemodynamic improvement, than 12 or 24-hour infusions of urokinase.[20(I),21(I)] However, comparison of 2-hour infusions of urokinase (3 million units) with rtPA (100 mg) suggests that the shorter infusion is more important than the thrombolytic agent.[22(I)] Unfortunately, major bleeding complications; including intracerebral hemorrhage continue to occur, even with these shorter infusions, and newer thrombolytic agents.[22(I),23(I),14(I)]

Bolus infusion of rtPA may reduce the risk of severe hemorrhage. A bolus dose takes advantage of the fibrin specific properties of rtPA by promoting dissolution of thrombi while avoiding systemic plasma proteolysis.[24] To date, one well-designed clinical trial evaluated a bolus regimen of rtPA (0.6 mg/kg over 2 minutes).[13(I)] Tissue plasminogen activator produced accelerated reperfusion without major bleeding complications, although systemic proteolysis occurred. Because a small number of patients received bolus rtPA in this trial, the relative safety and efficacy of this dosing method remain uncertain.

Direct versus Peripheral Lytic Therapy

Direct administration of thrombolytic drugs to the thrombus would appear to concentrate the lytic effect and limit systemic bleeding complications. However, even one-tenth of a usual systemic dose administered into the pulmonary artery produces systemic fibrinolysis,[25] and low-dose regional infusions do not avoid bleeding complications at remote sites.[26(V)] At present infusion of thrombolytic drugs into the pulmonary artery does not appear safer or more efficacious than peripheral venous administration.[27(I)]

CLINICAL OBSERVATIONS IN PATIENTS WITH DEEP-VEIN THROMBOSIS

Comparison with Anticoagulants

A number of randomized clinical trials have compared thrombolytic therapy with anticoagulant treatment for acute deep-vein thrombosis (DVT).[28(I),29(III),30(III),31(I),32(I),33(I),34(II),35(I),36(I)] Collectively these studies demonstrate accelerated lysis of thrombi achieved at the cost of an increase in the incidence and severity of bleeding.[37] Overall, clot dissolution occurs for 60% to 75% of patients who receive 3 or more days of intravenous streptokinase within one week of the onset of symptoms. Neither tests of fibrinolysis nor the duration of symptoms reliably predict the degree of thrombolysis. Furthermore, thrombolysis does not improve the rate or degree of immediate symptomatic relief which occurs with adequate heparin therapy and bed rest; and, in spite of limited evidence to suggest preservation of venous valve function[28(I),30(III)]; thrombolytic therapy does not unequivocally improve postphlebitic symptoms. Bleeding complications, including fatal intracranial hemorrhage, occur more frequently with thrombolysis.[33](I) In addition febrile and allergic reactions commonly accompany streptokinase administration, even when patients are premedicated with corticosteroids.

Comparison of Thrombolytic Drugs and Dosing Regimens

The superiority of any specific thrombolytic medication for the treatment of DVT remains unproven.

The administration of shorter bolus infusions of tissue plasminogen-activator may improve the efficacy and safety of thrombolytic therapy for deep-vein thrombi. Limited data suggest that a 4-hour infusion of tPA (0.5 mg/kg) lyses deep-vein thrombi to the same degree as the same dose administered over 8 hours and repeated 24 hours later.[38](I) Seven of twelve patients who received a 4-hour infusion had more than 50% of the thrombus lysed. Clinically overt bleeding occurred in two of twelve patients, and fibrinogen concentrations decreased.

COMPLICATIONS

Bleeding

Bleeding is the principal complication of thrombolytic therapy. Invasive procedures, particularly arterial and venous catheterization, predispose patients to bleed following administration of thrombolytic drugs. These bleeding events can be minimized by assiduously avoiding invasive vascular procedures, and by using meticulous technique when such procedures are necessary.[39]

Similarly, careful patient selection for thrombolytic treatment reduces the risk of bleeding complications. Survey data suggest that approximately one-half of all patients with acute PE have conditions which preclude thrombolysis.[40] Surgery, major trauma or internal organ biopsy within 10 days represent common contraindications to thrombolysis (Table 4). Even when given more than 1 week after surgery, thrombolysis may trigger major bleeding complications in operative wounds which are difficult to manage (e.g., mediastinal wounds after coronary artery bypass grafting).[41](V) Therefore, the nature of the wound as well as the time since surgery deserve consideration in seeking to avoid the bleeding complications which accompany thrombolysis. For example, clinical investigators are reluctant to administer thrombolytic drugs after intracranial or intraspinal surgery or within 2 weeks of open heart surgery.[40] Intracranial hemorrhage is a particularly important complication of thrombolytic therapy for venous thromboembolism. Intracranial hemorrhage typically occurs within the first 24 hours of thrombolysis. Early symptoms often include headache, drowsiness and vomiting accompanied by neurological deficits. Diagnosis can be confirmed by com-

Table 4
Increased Risk for Thrombolysis

Cerebrovascular disease
Recent* major surgery or internal organ biopsy or obstetrical delivery
History of serious gastrointestinal bleeding
Positive stool guiac examination
Recent* trauma
Recent* cardiopulmonary resuscitation
Left heart (e.g. left atrial enlargement with atrial fibrillation) thrombus
Subacute bacterial endocarditis
Hemostatic defect including those due to severe hepatic or renal disease, platelets < 100,000/ml
Age ≥ 70 years
Pregnancy
Diabetic hemorrhagic retinopathy
Hypertension

* Recent = within 10 days. Longer durations are proposed for selected operations which involve anatomical spaces in which hemorrhage is difficult to control e.g., open heart surgery within 2 weeks.

puted tomography which typically shows hemorrhage into subcortical white matter (Figure 6). Treatment includes immediate cessation of thrombolytic and anticoagulant therapy.

Avoiding intracerebral hemorrhage is important, but difficult because such hemorrhages occur at sites of clinically silent cerebrovascular pathology. Thus risk factors for occult cerebrovascular disease (e.g., increasing age, hypertension, diabetes, lipid disorders or arteriosclerotic disease elsewhere) should be considered relative contraindications to thrombolytic therapy. Any history of stroke or transient ischemic attack increases the risk for intracerebral hemorrhage,[42] and is usually viewed as a strong relative contraindication, and any history of intracranial bleeding as an absolute contraindication.

Management of Bleeding. Most patients who bleed can be managed by discontinuing thrombolytic and anticoagulant therapy. Manual pressure with gauze soaked with epsilon aminocaproic acid can control troublesome superficial bleeding.[43] However, difficult internal bleeding requires aggressive replacement therapy. Because thrombolytic therapy can impair hemostasis pathways at several steps, different components are needed. Cryoprecipitate contains fibrinogen and factor VIII, both of which are depleted by thrombolysis. Transfusion of ten units of cryoprecipitate achieves a fibrinogen level of 1.0 gram/L and a factor VIII level of 30% for most adults. Fresh frozen plasma provides α2-antiplasmin, and factors V and VIII, as well as volume expansion. Continued active bleeding following cryoprecipitate and fresh frozen plasma infusion may require platelet transfusions or administration of antifibrinolytic drugs.[44]

Antifibrinolytic therapy with aminocaproic acid inhibits plasminogen activators and to a lesser extent plas-

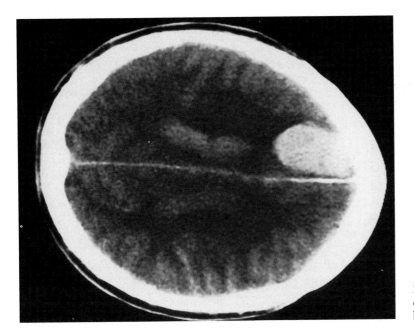

Figure 6. Intracranial hemorrhage at sites of clinically occult cerebrovascular disease may complicate thrombolytic therapy.

min. The drug may be given orally or intravenously. Rapid intravenous administration may cause hypotension. Such therapy is indicated only if active bleeding occurs during administration of fibrinolytic agents or within four half-lives of discontinuing thrombolytic therapy. Furthermore aminocapraic acid should not be given for upper urinary tract bleeding because intrarenal thrombotic obstruction may occur. With these precautions, the administration of a 5 gram loading dose followed by 1 gram hourly reverses fibrinolysis.

Reperfusion Pulmonary Edema

Reperfusion of lung tissue may result in pulmonary edema following surgical thromboendarterectomy and transplantation. Thus it is not surprising that successful thrombolysis of pulmonary emboli can lead to acute focal pulmonary edema.[45,46] Arterial hypoxemia and pulmonary arterial hypertension accompany this complication, but typically improve within 72 hours.

Allergic Reactions

Streptokinase and, less commonly, anistreplase can produce anaphylactic or anaphylactoid reactions. These range in severity from minor to severe dyspnea, periorbital swelling, angioneurotic edema or urticaria. Delayed hypersensitivity reactions such as vasculitis and interstitial nephritis may complicate streptokinase therapy. Fever also rarely complicates treatment with streptokinase or urokinase.

Management of allergic type reactions depends upon the nature and severity of the reaction. Acetaminophen rather than aspirin should be used for fever. Anti-histamines with or without corticosteroids are appropriate for mild to moderate reactions; whereas more severe clinical manifestations may require intravenous adrenergics and corticosteroids in addition to supportive management.

INDICATIONS AND CONTRAINDICATIONS

Definitions of the indications for thrombolytic treatment of PE vary.[9,47,48] Some physicians believe thrombolytic drugs are never indicated for PE. Others believe that thrombolysis can be recommended for patients with obstruction of blood flow to a lobe or multiple pulmonary segments.[47,48] A more widely-held view is that thrombolytic therapy is appropriate for patients with acute massive PE who are hemodynamically unstable, and who are not prone to bleed. This reflects the fact that patients with massive PE and shock are more likely to die shortly after presentation.[49(I)] Thus the increased risk for fatal or otherwise serious bleeding complications may be justified by accelerated thrombolysis for patients whose observed 2-week case fatality rate approximates 20 percent.[49(I)]

Definitions of the indications for use of thrombolysis for the treatment of DVT are less certain. Without proof that thrombolysis avoids late morbidity or mortality, use of thrombolytic therapy should be restricted. Potential candidates may include young patients who appear likely to sustain ischemic ulceration of the leg or internal organ (e.g., mesenteric vein thrombosis or the thrombosed renal vein of a transplanted kidney). As with acute pulmonary emboli, these patients should not be prone to bleed, so that the anticipated risk for morbidity from the venous thrombus exceeds the likelihood of major bleeding complications.

Contraindications to thrombolytic treatment of venous thromboemboli include situations for which bleeding poses a special risk. Active bleeding, particularly associated with a source which is difficult to manage (e.g., esophageal varices or in an anatomically dangerous area [e.g., mediastinal wounds]), represents an absolute contraindication to thrombolysis as does any history of intracranial bleeding. Surgery, trauma, and internal organ biopsies within 10 days; as well as history of stroke or other intracranial disease constitute strong contraindications for thrombolytic therapy. Similarly conditions which are associated with an increased risk for bleeding (e.g., prior gastrointestinal bleeding, bacterial endocarditis, diabetic retinopathy, poorly controlled hypertension, hemostatic defects, etc.) represent contraindications to thrombolysis.

REFERENCES

1. Marder VJ, Sherry S. Thrombolytic therapy: current status. N Engl J Med 1988;318:1512–1520.
2. Benedict CR, Mueller S, Anderson HV, Willerson JT. Thrombolytic therapy: a state of the art review. Hospital Practice 1992;61–72.
3. Rich S, Levitsky S, Brundage BH. Pulmonary hypertension from chronic pulmonary thromboembolism. Ann Intern Med 1988;108:425–434.
4. Haire WD. Pharmacology of thrombolysis. Chest 1992;101:92S-97S.
5. Tillet WS, Garner RL. The fibrinolytic activity of hemolytic streptococci. J Exp Med 1933;58:485–502.
6. Volgesang GB, Bell WR. Treatment of pulmonary embolism and deep vein thrombosis with thrombolytic therapy. Clinics in Chest Medicine 1984;5:487–494.
7. MacFarlane RG, Pilling J. Observations on fibrinolysis: plasminogen, plasmin, and antiplasmin content of human blood. Lancet 1946;2:562–565.
8. Hirsh DR, Goldhaber SZ. Laboratory parameters to monitor safety and efficacy during thrombolytic therapy. Chest 1991;99:113S-120S.
9. Hyers TM, Hull RD, Weg JG. Antithrombotic therapy for venous thromboembolic disease. Chest 1992;102:408S-425S.
(I)10. Urokinase Pulmonary Embolism Trial. A national cooperative study. Heart Association Monograph No. 39. Circulation 1973;47:108.
(I)11. Tibbutt DA, Davies JA, Anderson JA, et al. Comparison by controlled clinical trial of streptokinase and heparin in treatment of life-threatening pulmonary embolism. Br Med J 1974;1:343–347.
12. Ly B, Arnesen H, Eie H, Hol R. Controlled clinical trial of streptokinase and heparin in the treatment of major pulmonary embolism. Acta Med Scand 1978;203:465–470.
(I)13. Levine MN, Hirsh J, Weitz J, et al. A randomized trial of a single bolus dosage regimen of recombinant tissue plasminogen activator in patients with acute pulmonary embolism. Chest 1990;98:1473–1479.
(I)14. Dalla-Volta S, Palla A, Santo Licandro A, et al. PAIMS 2: alterplase combined with heparin versus heparin in the treatment of acute pulmonary embolism. J Am Coll Cardiol 1992;20:520–526.
15. Moser KM, Spragg RG, Utley J, Daily PO. Chronic thrombotic obstruction of major pulmonary arteries. Ann Intern Med 1983;99:299–304.
16. Riedel M, Stanek V, Widimsky J, Prerovisky I. Long term follow-up of patients with pulmonary thromboembolism: late prognosis and evaluation of hemodynamic and respiratory Data. Chest 1982;81:151–158.
17. Sharma GVRK, Folland ED, McIntyre KM, et al. Longterm hemodynamic benefit of thrombolytic therapy in pulmonary embolic disease. J Am Coll Cardiol 1990;15:65A.(Abstract)
(I)18. Sharma GVRK, Burleson VA, Sasahara AA. Effect of thrombolytic therapy on pulmonary-capillary blood volume in patients with pulmonary embolism. N Engl J Med 1980;303:842–845.
(I)19. Urokinase-Streptokinase Embolism Trial. Phase II Results. A cooperative study. JAMA 1974;229:1606–1613.
(I)20. Goldhaber SZ, Kessler CM, Heit J, et al. A randomized controlled trial of recombinant tissue plasminogen activator versus urokinase in the treatment of acute pulmonary embolism. Lancet 1988;2:293–298.
(I)21. Meyer G, Sors H, Charbonnier B, et al. Effects of intravenous urokinase versus alteplase on total pulmonary resistance in acute massive pulmonary embolism: a European multicenter double-blind trial. JACC 1992;19:239–245.
(I)22. Goldhaber SZ, Kessler CM, Heit JA, et al. Recombinant tissue-type plasminogen activator versus a novel dosing regimen of urokinase in acute pulmonary embolism: a randomized controlled multicentered trial. J Am Coll Cardiol 1992;20:24–30.
(I)23. A Collaborative Study by the PIOPED Investigators: Tissue plasminogen activator for the treatment of acute pulmonary embolism. Chest 1990;97:528–533.
24. Agnelli G. Rationale for bolus t-PA therapy to improve efficacy and safety. Chest 1990;97:161S-167S.
25. Leeper KV, Popovick J, Adams D, Stein PD. Treatment of massive acute pulmonary embolism with intrapulmonary artery low dose streptokinase combined with full heparinization. Chest 1986;89:453S.
(V)26. Dotter CT, Rosch J, Seaman AJ. Selective clot lysis with low-dose streptokinase. Radiology 1974;111:31–37.
(I)27. Verstraete M, Miller GAH, Bounameaux H, et al. Intravenous and intrapulmonary recombinant tissue-type plasminogen activator in the treatment of acute massive pulmonary embolism. Circulation 1988;77:353–360.
(I)28. Kakkar VV, Flanc C, Howe CT, O'Shea M, Flute PT. Treatment of deep vein thrombosis: a trial of heparin, streptokinase and arvin. Br Med J 1969;1:806–810.
(III)29. Robertson BR, Nilsson IM, Mylander G. Value of streptokinase and heparin in treatment of acute deep venous thrombosis: a coded investigation. Acta Chir Scand 1968;134:203–208.
(III)30. Robertson BR, Nilsson IM, Mylander G. Thrombolytic effect of streptokinase as evaluated by phlebography of deep venous thrombi of the leg. Acta Chir Scand 1970;136:173–180.
(I)31. Arnesen H, Heilo A, Jakobsen E, Ly B, Skaga E. A prospective study of streptokinase and heparin in the treatment of deep vein thrombosis. Acta Med Scand 1978;203:457–463.
(I)32. Elliot MS, Immelman EJ, Jeffrey R, et al. A comparative randomized trial of heparin versus streptokinase in the treatment of acute proximal venous thrombosis: an interim report of a prospective trial. Br J Surg 1979;66:838–843.

(I)33. Marder VJ, Soulen RL, Atichartakarn V, et al. Quantitative venographic assessment of deep vein thrombosis in the evaluation of streptokinase and heparin therapy. J Lab Clin Med 1977;89:1018–1029.

(II)34. Porter JM, Seaman AJ, Common HH, Rosch J, Eidemiller LR, et al. Comparison of heparin and streptokinase in the treatment of venous thrombosis. Am Surg 1975;41:511–519.

(I)35. Tsapagos MJ, Peabody RA, Wu KT, Karmondy Am, Dereraj KT, et al. Controlled study of thrombolytic therapy in deep vein thrombosis. Surgery 1973;74:973–984.

(I)36. Tibbutt OA, Williams EW, Walker MW, Cherteman CN, Holt JM, et al. Controlled trial of ancrod and streptokinase in the treatment of deep vein thrombosis of lower limbs. Br J Haematol 1974;27:407–414.

37. Goldhaber SZ, Buring JE, Lipnick RJ, Hennekens CH. Pooled analysis of randomized trials of streptokinase and heparin in phlebographically demonstrated acute deep venous thrombosis. Am J Med 1984;76:393–397.

(I)38. Turpie AG, Levine MN, Hirsh J, et al. Tissue plasminogen activator (rt-PA) vs heparin in deep vein thrombosis. Chest 1990;97:172S-175S.

39. Meyerovitz M. How to maximize the safety of coronary and pulmonary angiography in patients receiving thrombolytic therapy. Chest 1990;97:132S-135S.

40. Terrin M, Goldhaber SZ, Thompson B, and the TIPE Investigators. Selection of patients with acute pulmonary embolism for thrombolytic therapy. The thrombolysis in pulmonary embolism (TIPE) patient survey. Chest 1989;95:279S-281S.

(V)41. Goldhaber SZ, Vaughan DE, Markis JE, et al. Acute pulmonary embolism treated with tissue plasminogen activator. Lancet 1986;2:886–889.

42. Gore JM. Prevention of severe neurologic events in the thrombolytic era. Chest 1992;101:124S-130S.

43. Sharma GV, Cella G, Parisi AF, Sasahara AA. Thrombolytic therapy. N Engl J Med 1982;306:1268–1276.

44. Sane DC, Califf RM, Topal EJ, Mark DB, Greenberg CS. Bleeding during thrombolytic therapy for acute myocardial infarction: mechanisms and management. Ann Intern Med 1989;111:1010–1022.

45. Ward BJ, Pearse DB. Reperfusion pulmonary edema after thrombolytic therapy of massive pulmonary embolism. Am Rev Respir Dis 1988;138:1308–1311.

46. Martin TR, Sandblom RL, Johnson RJ. Adult respiratory distress syndrome following thrombolytic therapy for pulmonary embolism. Chest 1983;83:151–153.

47. Symposium: Thrombolytic therapy in thrombosis: A National Institute of Health Consensus Development Conference. Ann Inter Med 1980;93:141–143.

48. Goldhaber SZ. Thrombolysis for pulmonary embolism. Prog Cardiovasc Dis 1991;34:113–134.

(I)49. Urokinase Pulmonary Embolism Trial; Phase I Results. JAMA 1970;214:2163–2172.

32

A Noninvasive Strategy to Decrease Risk of Major Bleeding During Thrombolytic Therapy for Acute Pulmonary Embolism:
Consideration of Noninvasive Management

Paul D. Stein, Russell D. Hull, Gary E. Raskob

INTRODUCTION

Because patients with pulmonary embolism (PE) who receive thrombolytic therapy have a high frequency of major bleeding complications, physicians hesitate about administering thrombolytic agents in cases of acute PE. Because thrombolytic therapy is considered to be dangerous, pulmonary angiography is traditionally performed to confirm the diagnosis of PE. It would be a tragic error to administer thrombolytic therapy if PE were not present. However, major bleeding frequently occurs at the puncture site used for pulmonary angiography. The high rate of bleeding in such patients prompted us to assess the relative risks of bleeding with thrombolytic therapy in patients who were managed using pulmonary angiograms and in those managed using noninvasive tests, primarily the ventilation-perfusion lung scan.[1]

METHODS

Data from the literature were used to assess the risks associated with pulmonary angiography, and the risk of major bleeding from thrombolytic therapy in patients diagnosed invasively.[1] The risk of major bleeding from thrombolytic therapy in patients diagnosed noninvasively was assessed from studies on thrombolytic therapy in patients with acute myocardial infarction.

DEFINITION OF MAJOR BLEEDING

Major bleeding was defined as follows: a decrease in hemoglobin level of 20 g/L (2 g/dL) or more; a blood transfusion requirement of 2 units or more; intracerebral bleeding; retroperitoneal bleeding; pericardial bleeding; bleeding that required surgical intervention; bleeding into a major joint; or bleeding into the eye.

RISKS OF THROMBOLYTIC THERAPY IN PATIENTS DIAGNOSED BY PULMONARY ANGIOGRAPHY

Tissue plasminogen activator (tPA) was used in most investigations of thrombolytic therapy for acute PE. For consistency, only patients treated with tPA were studied. Data from several studies were averaged to obtain the frequency of major bleeding after tPA therapy in patients with acute PE who had pulmonary angiography.[2(I),3(I),4(I),5(I),6(I)] Data from patients who did and did not receive heparin were included, and the frequency of major bleeding in both groups did not differ significantly. Modest differences in dose, site of injection, and rate of injection were ignored in obtaining average values for the frequency of bleeding using tPA.

In the 1980s and more recently, trials of thrombolytic therapy in patients with PE showed lower rates of bleeding than did earlier studies, regardless of the thrombolytic agent used.[7(I)] Therefore, we have included only more recent studies in our analysis. Studies related to bleeding after the administration of urokinase over a 12-hour period or longer were not considered in this evaluation because the improvement of hemodynamic variables at 2 hours using tPA is potentially important in patients with life-threatening massive PE.[4,5(I),6(I),8(II)] It is possible that an accelerated regimen of urokinase given over 2 hours may be as effective as tPA in terms of lysis and hemodynamic improvement.[6(I)] However, data related to

From *Venous Thromboembolism: An Evidence-Based Atlas* edited by Russell Hull, Gary Raskob, Graham Pineo © 1996, Futura Publishing Co., Armonk, NY.

the bleeding rate with such a regimen are sparse and, therefore, all data using urokinase were excluded from our evaluation. Studies in which the description of bleeding complications did not specify the amount of blood transfused were also eliminated from our analysis.

The reported investigations excluded all patients at a high risk of bleeding, such as those with recent surgery, recent biopsy, peptic ulcer disease, blood dyscrasia, or severe hepatic or renal disease. Thus, all reported patients were at low risk for bleeding.

RISKS OF THROMBOLYTIC THERAPY IN PATIENTS DIAGNOSED USING NONINVASIVE PROCEDURES

There are few data on the use of thrombolytic agents for PE in patients who received treatment without an angiographically proven diagnosis.[9(I),10(I)] Goldhaber and associates[9(I)] treated 40 of 46 patients (87%) according to diagnoses based on ventilation-perfusion lung scans. Three of the 46 patients (6.5%) had major bleeding after receiving 100 mg of tPA administered over 2 hours. Levine and associates[10(I)] diagnosed 11 of 33 patients (33%) on the basis of a ventilation-perfusion lung scans. All 33 patients were treated with a bolus regimen of tPA (a different mode of administration of tPA) and there was no major bleeding.

Because data on the use of tPA in patients with PE who were diagnosed noninvasively were insufficient, the risk of bleeding after a noninvasive diagnosis was assessed from the Thrombolysis in Myocardial Infarction (TIMI) IIA study.[11(I)] The relative risk of bleeding was assessed after comparing invasive and noninvasive evaluations of acute myocardial infarction. We assumed that this risk ratio applied to the relative risks for invasive compared with noninvasive management of acute PE.[1] In the TIMI-IIA study, patients were randomly assigned to receive coronary arteriography within 2 hours of the administration of tPA or to receive tPA in the absence of coronary arteriography (which was subsequently done after 18 to 48 hours). Major bleeding (intracranial hemorrhage or transfusion of 2 or more units of blood) occurred in 23 of 195 (11.8%) patients who had immediate coronary arteriography and in 7 of 194 (3.6%) who did not have this invasive procedure at the time of tPA administration. The risk ratio was 3 : 3 (11.8 ÷ 3.6 [CI, 1.5 to 9.8]) for major bleeding (invasive management of myocardial infarction compared with noninvasive management of myocardial infarction). Other comparative studies, in which tPA was given for invasive and noninvasive management after myocardial infarction, but in which the number of units of blood transfused was not stated, have not been included.

MAJOR COMPLICATIONS OF PULMONARY ANGIOGRAPHY

In 1111 patients, the major complications of pul-

monary angiography were death (0.45%), respiratory distress requiring cardiopulmonary resuscitation or intubation (0.36%), renal failure requiring dialysis (0.27%), and bleeding at the site of catheter insertion requiring blood transfusion of 2 or more units (0.18%).[12] One or more major complications occurred in 1.3% of patients (CI, 0.6% to 19.9%). These major complications were independent of pulmonary artery pressure, volume of contrast material, and presence of PE.

Statistical Analysis

We performed a decision analysis based on data from other studies. The 95% CI for relative risk was calculated using the method of Woolf,[13] as described more recently by Schlesselman.[14]

RESULTS

The average frequency of major bleeding in patients with acute PE who had pulmonary angiography before the administration of tPA was 18 of 129 (14.0%; CI, 7.9% to 20.1%) (Table 1).[1] Bleeding in patients who received heparin with tPA was not significantly more frequent than in patients in whom heparin was temporarily withheld (9 of 63 [14.3%] compared with 9 of 66 [13.6%], P = 0.9).

The risk of major bleeding with tPA after a noninvasive diagnosis of PE was estimated to be 4.2% (estimated CI, 1.4% to 9.3%), using the risk ratio (derived above) of 3:3 (CI, 1.5% to 9.8%) for major bleeding with tPA associated with invasive management of myocardial infarction compared with noninvasive management of myocardial infarction.[1]

Figure 1 shows the calculated risks for complications from pulmonary angiography plus bleeding from tPA after pulmonary angiography. These risks are based on a frequency of major complications from pulmonary angiography of 1.3% and risks of major bleeding from thrombolytic therapy of 7.9%, 14.0%, and 20.1% in patients in whom an angiographic diagnosis is made. The risk of major bleeding with thrombolytic therapy after angiography is a key consideration in determining whether to do pulmonary angiography in patients who are potential candidates for thrombolytic therapy. If the frequency of major bleeding with thrombolytic therapy is 4.2% after a noninvasive diagnosis and 14% after an invasive diagnosis, noninvasive management with thrombolytic therapy would be associated with fewer complications if the probability of PE exceeds 21%, as shown in Figure 1. Only if the estimated probability of PE is 20% or lower would it be safer to do pulmonary angiography.[1]

Assuming that the frequency of major bleeding with thrombolytic therapy after a noninvasive diagnosis is 9.3% (based on the upper end of the estimated 95% CI) and if the risk of major bleeding after an invasive diagnosis is 14%, noninvasive therapy management is associated with fewer major complications if the estimated probabil-

Table 1
Major Bleeding in Patients with Pulmonary Embolism Treated with Tissue Plasminogen Activator after Pulmonary Angiography

Author (reference)	tPA Dose, mg	tPA with Heparin	Patients with Major Bleeding, n/N(%)	Bleeding Complication
Verstraete et al.[2]	50 to 100	Yes	4/34 (11.7)	Required ≥ 2 units blood
PIOPED*[3]	40 to 80	Yes	1/9 (11.1)	Required ≥ 2 units blood
Dalla-Volta et al.[4]	100	Yes	4/20 (30) or 5/20 (25) +	1 patient, intracerebral; 2 patients, pericardial; 1 patient, retroperitoneal +
Goldhaber et al.[5]	100	No	4/22 (18.2)	≥ 10 point decrease in hematocrit
Goldhaber et al.[6]	100	No	5/44 (11.4)	2 patients, intracerebral; 3 patients required ≥ 2 units blood

* PIOPED = Prospective Investigation of Pulmonary Embolism Diagnosis; tPA = tissue plasminogen activator.
+ There were four or possibly five patients who had major bleeding.
≠ Also melena in one patient, number of units transfused not stated.
Reproduced with permission from Stein PD, et al. Ann Intern Med 1994;121:313–317.[1]

ity of PE is more than 57% (Figure 1). Assuming that the risk of major bleeding with thrombolytic therapy after a noninvasive diagnosis is 1.4% (based on the lower limit of the estimated 95% CI), it would always be safer to treat on the basis of noninvasive diagnosis (see Figure 1).

For sensitivity analysis, the risk of major bleeding with thrombolytic therapy after an angiographic diagnosis was assumed to be 20.1% (the upper end of the 95% CI). Comparisons were made using an assumed risk of 4.2% for major bleeding with thrombolytic therapy after a

noninvasive diagnosis. Total complications (major bleeding plus major complications from angiography) were calculated to be fewer, if therapy were to be administered on the basis of a noninvasive diagnosis if the estimated probability of PE exceeded 14% (see Figure 1).[1]

In another sensitivity analysis, an assumed risk of 7.9% (the lower end of the 95% CI) for major bleeding with thrombolytic therapy, after an angiographic diagnosis was compared with an assumed risk of 4.2% for major bleeding with thrombolytic therapy after a noninvasive

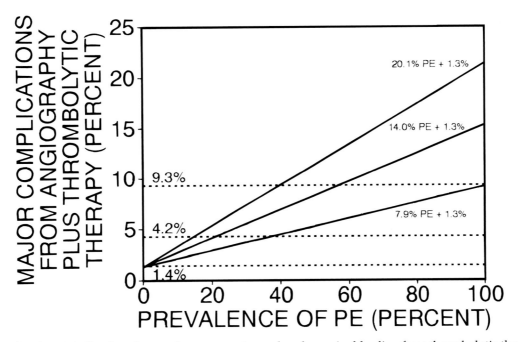

Figure 1. Predicted major complications from pulmonary angiography plus major bleeding from thrombolytic therapy shown as a function of the prevalence of pulmonary embolism. Total major complications were major complications from angiography plus major bleeding from thrombolytic therapy. Predicted complications assume a rate of 1.3% for major complications from angiography and rates of 14.0% (observed value); 7.9%, and 20.1% (lower and upper ends of the 95% CI, respectively) for major bleeding among patients treated with thrombolytic therapy after an angiographic diagnosis. The total predicted complications describe a straight line with the slope = rate of major bleeding after angiography and the intercept = percentage of major complications of angiography. Major bleeding from thrombolytic therapy after a noninvasive diagnosis is shown by horizontal lines at assumed rates of 4.2% (observed value), 1.4%, and 9.3% (lower and upper ends of the 95% CI, respectively). PE = pulmonary embolism. (Reproduced with permission from Stein PD, et al. Ann Int Med. 1994;121:313–317.)[1]

diagnosis. Total complications (major bleeding from thrombolytic therapy plus major complications of angiography) were calculated to be fewer if therapy were to be administered on the basis of a noninvasive diagnosis if the estimated probability of PE exceeded 37% (see Figure 1).[1]

If major bleeding with thrombolytic therapy after pulmonary angiography is only 1.0% more than major bleeding with a noninvasive diagnosis (that is, 5.2% compared with 4.2%), it would be safer to treat patients on a noninvasive basis if the probability of PE exceeded 55% (Figure 1).[1]

DISCUSSION

Thrombolytic therapy for patients with massive acute PE is indicated for patients who are hypotensive, or hypoxic when receiving high levels of oxygen, or clinically stable with echocardiographic evidence of right ventricular failure.[9(I)] Our calculations lead to a conclusion that differs from traditional ideas about the necessity of an angiographically proven diagnosis. We conclude that, in a patient who is unstable from what appears to be massive acute PE, at the appropriate level of probability of PE, it is safer to treat on the basis of a noninvasive diagnosis rather than an angiographically proven diagnosis. The observations of Goldhaber and associates[9(I)] tend to support our conclusion. They found that among the 87% of patients with PE who were treated on the basis of a ventilation-perfusion lung scan, the rate of major bleeding after tPA was relatively low (6.5%). It is unfortunate that if thrombolytic therapy is initiated on the basis of noninvasive diagnosis, some patients who do not have PE will receive thrombolytic drugs and will have bleeding complications. Overall, however, fewer patients will have major complications using the approach identified by these calculations. (We emphasize that we are not suggesting that the indications for thrombolytic therapy be broadened. If thrombolytic therapy is necessary, however, a noninvasive approach in some instances may be associated with fewer complications.)

The risk ratio based on the TIMI-IIA study for bleeding with thrombolytic therapy after invasive compared with noninvasive management of myocardial infarction is conservative. Califf and associates,[15(I)] studied patients who received tPA followed in 90 minutes by coronary arteriography. They reported transfusion of 2 or more units of blood or intracranial hemorrhage in 66 of 302 (21.8%) patients. In noninvasive trials of tPA in myocardial infarction, the frequency was approximately 1% for transfusion of 2 or more units of blood or for intracranial hemorrhage; in trials in which a transfusion of 1 or more units was considered major, the bleeding rate was 1.5%.[16(I),17(I),18(I)] This would result in a risk ratio of 14 : 5 for major bleeding with an invasive compared with a noninvasive diagnosis. Based on such a risk ratio, the estimated risk would be approximately 1% for major bleed-

ing in patients with acute PE after a noninvasive diagnosis. With such a relative risk for major bleeding, it would always be safer to treat patients on the basis of a noninvasive diagnosis.

In the few studies that indicated where bleeding occurred in patients who received a blood transfusion, the groin was a frequent site.[2(I),6(I)] Our estimate of the risk ratio for invasive management of myocardial infarction compared with noninvasive management of myocardial infarction was based on a randomized trial.[11(I)] The groups were similar, the only difference being that one group underwent an invasive procedure. The difference in frequency of bleeding with thrombolytic therapy resulted from this invasive procedure. We are confident, therefore, that the rate of bleeding with thrombolytic therapy after an invasive procedure is higher than with a noninvasive procedure. In patients with PE, the bleeding rate in patients who have had recent surgery or underlying pathological problems, regardless of whether a pulmonary angiogram was done, may be higher than in patients with myocardial infarction. Patients who are at a higher risk for bleeding are readily identified by their medical history and physical examination before therapy.[19(I)]

In pulmonary angiography, the catheter is usually inserted percutaneously through a femoral vein. When thrombolytic therapy is used, perhaps there would be less bleeding if a superficial vein of the arm were used. Many useful suggestions related to the administration of thrombolytic agents and treatment of bleeding were made in a review of the hemorrhagic complications of thrombolytic therapy by Levine and associates.[6]

The risks of bleeding with heparin or warfarin were not considered separately in this analysis. The risk, based on averaged data, was 4.9% (CI, 3.4% to 6.5%) for major hemorrhagic complications from heparin in patients treated for thromboembolic disease, whether heparin was administered via intermittent intravenous, continuous infusion, or subcutaneous routes in doses ranging from 29 180 U to 40 320 U over 24 hours.[20(I),21(I),22(I),23(I)] These risks have been refined for patients at high and low risk of bleeding.[18] Patients at high risk were defined as those who had undergone surgery within the previous 14 days, a history of peptic ulcer disease, gastrointestinal or genitourinary tract bleeding, disorders predisposing to bleeding, thrombotic studies within 14 days, or platelet counts $< 150 \times 10^9/L$. The frequency of major bleeding from heparin in such high-risk patients was 10.8% (CI, 5.0% to 16.6%).[19(I)] In patients at a low risk of bleeding, the frequency of major bleeding with heparin was 1.1% (CI, 0% to 3.3%).[19(I)] The risk, based on averaged data, was 1.7% (CI, 0.3% to 3.0%), for major hemorrhagic complications in patients with thromboembolic disease who were treated with "less intense" warfarin therapy (international normalized ratio, 2 : 3).[19(I),20(I),24(I)]

It would be ideal if, in patients who require thrombolytic therapy, a noninvasive diagnosis of PE could be based on a high-probability ventilation-perfusion lung scan combined with a high-likelihood clinical assessment. In the collaborative study from the Prospective Investigation of Pulmonary Embolism Diagnosis (PIOPED) group, 96% of such patients had PE.[24] Unfortunately, however, only 11% of patients with PE had this concordance of a high-probability ventilation-perfusion lung scan and a high-likelihood clinical assessment.[25(I)] Among all patients with a high-probability ventilation-perfusion lung scan, regardless of the clinical assessment, PE was present in 87%. Only 41% of patients with PE in the PIOPED study, however, had a high-probability ventilation-perfusion lung scan. Because most patients with PE do not have a high-probability ventilation-perfusion lung scan, the physician is often in the uncomfortable position of assessing the probability of PE based on less definitive data. It may be safer to administer thrombolytic therapy on the basis of a noninvasive diagnosis despite some uncertainty in the diagnosis.

The probability of PE can be assessed in several ways. In the PIOPED study,[25(I)] the probability of PE was derived on the basis of a clinical-likelihood estimate and a ventilation-perfusion lung-scan probability as follows: (1) if the ventilation-perfusion lung scan was intermediate-probability (indeterminate-probability) and the clinical assessment indicated a high likelihood of PE, the frequency of PE was 66%; (2) if the ventilation-perfusion lung scan was low-probability and the clinical assessment was high-likelihood, or if the lung scan was intermediate-probability and the clinical assessment was intermediate-probability, the frequency of PE was 28% to 40%; (3) if the ventilation-perfusion lung scan was intermediate-probability and the clinical assessment was low-probability, or vice versa, the frequency of PE was 16%; (4) a ventilation-perfusion lung scan of low probability with a concordant low-likelihood clinical assessment, or a nearly normal lung scan with an intermediate- or low-likelihood clinical assessment, was associated with PE in 6% or fewer patients.

Based on these probabilities, and assuming a 14.0% frequency of major bleeding with tPA after angiography, it would be safer to treat unstable patients on the basis of a noninvasive diagnosis unless they had a ventilation-perfusion lung scan of intermediate probability with a low-probability clinical assessment, or had a low-probability or nearly normal lung scan with an intermediate- or low-probability clinical assessment.

The probability of PE also can be assessed by the number of ventilation-perfusion scan defects found among patients stratified according to previous cardiopulmonary disease and clinical-risk assessment.[26(I),27(I),28(I)] Clinical estimation of the probability of PE may be assisted by neural network logic.[29(I)] If the physician is uncomfortable with his or her assessment of the probability of PE, then he or she must choose one of two alternatives: the traditional approach of angiography, with its attendant high risk for bleeding at the site of catheter insertion; or treatment on the basis of a noninvasive diagnosis, recognizing that some patients who do not have PE will be treated inadvertently.

We recognize that there are uncertainties in assessing the probability of acute PE. Even though physicians may be unable to accurately assess the likelihood of PE, it is useful to know the relative risks for thrombolytic therapy administered on the basis of invasive compared with noninvasive diagnoses. In the future, the calculations in this study may permit a broadening of the indications for thrombolytic therapy in acute PE. This will require prospective testing. Until this is accomplished, we recommend thrombolytic therapy for patients with massive acute PE who are hypotensive, hypoxic when receiving high levels of oxygen, or clinically stable with echocardiographic evidence of right ventricular failure.

REFERENCES

1. Stein PD, Hull RD, Raskob G. Risks for major bleeding from thrombolytic therapy in patients with acute pulmonary embolism: Consideration of noninvasive management. Ann Intern Med 1994;12:313–317.

(I)2. Verstraete M, Miller GA, Bounameaux H, Charbonnier B, Colle JP, et al. Intravenous and intrapulmonary recombinant tissue-type plasminogen activator in the treatment of acute massive pulmonary embolism. Circulation 1988;77:353–360.

(I)3. A collaborative study by the PIOPED investigators. Tissue plasminogen activator for the treatment of acute pulmonary embolism. Chest 1990;97:528–533.

(I)4. Dalla-Volta S, Palla A, Santolicandro A, Giuntini C, Pengo V, et al. PAIMS-2: Alteplase combined with heparin versus heparin in the treatment of acute pulmonary embolism. Plasminogen Activator Italian Multicentre Study 2. J Am Coll Cardiol 1992;20: 520–526.

(I)5. Goldhaber SZ, Kessler CM, Heit J, Markis J, Sharma GV, et al. Randomised controlled trial of recombinant tissue plasminogen activator versus urokinase in the treatment of acute pulmonary embolism. Lancet 1988;2:293–298.

(I)6. Goldhaber SZ, Kessler CM, Heit JA, Elliott CG, Friedenberg WR, et al. Recombinant tissue-type plasminogen activator versus a novel dosing regimen of urokinase in acute pulmonary embolism: a randomized controlled multicenter trial. J Am Coll Caridol 1992:20:24–30.

7. Levine MN, Goldhaber SZ, Califf RM, Gore JM, Hirsh J. Hemorrhagic complications of thrombolytic therapy in the treatment of myocardial infarction and venous thromboembolism. Chest 1992;102(4 Suppl):364S-373S.

(II)8. Marini C, Di Ricco G, Rossi G, Rindi M, Palla R, et al. Fibrinolytic effects of urokinase and heparin in acute pulmonary embolism: a randomized clinical Trial. Respiration 1988;54:162–173.

(I)9. Goldhaber SZ, Haire WD, Feldstein ML, Miller M, Toltzis R, et al. Alteplase versus heparin in acute pulmonary embolism: randomised trial assessing right-ventricular function and pulmonary perfusion. Lancet 1993;341:507–511.

(I)10. Levine M, Hirsh J, Weitz J, Cruickshank M, Neemeh J, et al. A randomized trial of single bolus dosage regimen of recombinant tissue plasminogen activator in patients with acute pulmonary embolism. Chest 1990;98:1473–1479.

(I)11. The TIMI Research Group. Immediate vs. delayed catheterization and angioplasty following thrombolytic therapy for acute myocardial infarction. TIMI IIA results. JAMA 1988;260:2849–2858.

12. Stein PD, Athanasoulis C, Alavi A, Greenspan RH, Hales CA, et al. Complications and validity of pulmonary angiography in acute pulmonary embolism. Circulation 1992;85:462–468.

13. Woolf B. On estimating the relation between blood group and disease. Ann Hum Genet 1955;19:251–253.

14. Schlesselman JJ. Case-Control Studies: Design, Conduct and Analysis. New York, Wiley, 1982: 176–177.

(I)15. Califf RM, Topol EJ, George BS, Boswick JM, Abbottsmith C, et al. Hemorrhagic complications associated with the use of intravenous tissue plasminogen activator in treatment of acute myocardial infarction. Am J Med 1988;85:353–359.

(I)16. Gruppo Italiano per lo Studio della Supravvivenza nell'Infarto Miocardico. GISSI-2: a factorial randomised trial of alteplase versus streptokinase and heparin versus no heparin among 12,490 patients with acute myocardial infarction. Lancet 1990;336:65–71.

(I)17. The GUSTO Investigators. An international randomised trial comparing four thrombolytic strategies for acute myocardial infarction. N Engl J Med 1993;329: 673–682.

(I)18. Third International Study of Infarct Survival Collaborative Group. ISIS-3: a randomised comparison of streptokinase vs tissue plasminogen activator vs anistreplase and of aspirin plus heparin vs aspirin alone among 41,299 cases of suspected acute myocardial infarction. Lancet 1992;339:753–770.

(I)19. Hull RD, Raskob GE, Rosenbloom D, Panju AA, Brill-Edwards P, et al. Heparin for 5 days as compared with 10 days in the initial treatment of proximal venous thrombosis. N Engl J Med 1990;322:1260–1264.

(I)20. Hull RD, Raskob GE, Hirsh J, Jay RM, LeClerc JR, et al. Continuous intravenous heparin compared with in-termittent subcutaneous heparin in the initial treatment of proximal-vein thrombosis. N Engl J Med 1986;315:1109–1114.

(I)21. Doyle DJ, Turpie AG, Hirsh J, Best C, Kinch D, et al. Adjusted subcutaneous heparin or continuous intravenous heparin in patients with acute deep vein thrombosis. A randomized trial. Ann Intern Med 1987;107:441–445.

(I)22. Pini M, Pattachini C, Quintavalla R, Poli T, Megha A, et al. Subcutaneous vs intermittent heparin in the treatment of deep vein thrombosis— a randomized clinical trial. Thromb Haemost 1990;64:222–226.

(I)23. Hull RD, Raskob GE, Pineo GF, Green D, Trowbridge AA, et al. Subcutaneous low-molecular-weight heparin compared with continuous intravenous heparin in the treatment of proximal-vein thrombosis. N Engl J Med 1992;326:975–982.

(I)24. Hull R, Hirsh J, Jay R, Carter C, England C, et al. Different intensities of oral anticoagulant therapy in the treatment of proximal-vein thrombosis. N Engl J Med 1982;307:1676–1681.

(I)25. The PIOPED Investigators. Value of the ventilation/perfusion scan in acute pulmonary embolism. Results of the Prospective Investigation of Pulmonary Embolism Diagnosis (PIOPED). JAMA 1990;263:2753–2759.

(I)26. Stein PD, Gottschalk A, Henry JW, Shivkumar K. Stratification of patients according to poor cardiopulmonary disease and probability assessment based on the number of mismatched segmental equivalent perfusion defects. Approaches to strengthen the diagnostic value of ventilation/perfusion lung scans in acute pulmonary embolism. Chest 1993;104:1461–1467.

(I)27. Stein PD, Henry JW, Gottschalk A. Mismatched vascular defects. An easy alternative to mismatched segmental equivalent defects for the interpretation of ventilation/perfusion lung scans in pulmonary embolism. Chest 1993;104:1468–1472.

(I)28. Stein PD, Henry JW, Gottschalk A. The addition of clinical assessment to stratification according to prior cardiopulmonary disease further optimizes the interpretation of ventilation/perfusion lung scans in pulmonary embolism. Chest 1993;104:1472–1476.

(I)29. Patil S, Henry JW, Rubenfire M, Stein PD. Neural network in the clinical diagnosis of acute pulmonary embolism. Chest 1993;104:1685–1689.

33

Venous Thromboembolism: Vena Caval Filters

C. Gregory Elliott, Bo Eklof

HISTORICAL OVERVIEW

In 1868, Trousseau proposed ligation of the inferior vena cava as a treatment for recurrent pulmonary thromboembolism. This ligation, however, led to chronic venous insufficiency with attendant ulceration. Therefore, surgical techniques to simultaneously filter the vena cava and preserve blood flow were developed. Initially, external suture application and serrated clips (Adams-DeWeese clips) were applied externally to the vena cava. These were soon replaced by transvenous devices such as the Hunter balloon and the Mobin-Uddin umbrella. These early transvenous devices were subsequently discontinued because occlusion of the inferior vena cava caused unacceptable morbidity. In 1973, the Greenfield filter replaced the more primitive early transvenous filters. This stainless steel cone-shaped device had, as its principal advance, a shape which optimized the capture of thrombi and, at the same time, permitted the preservation of blood flow.

CURRENT DEVICES

Through technological advances, a variety of intravascular vena cava filters have been developed (Figure 1). These filters vary in design, filter material, length, diameter, and clot-filtering efficiency. Filter designs include a conical shape (Greenfield or LGM), a tangle with hooks to engage the vena cava wall (Gianturco-Roehm "bird's nest"), a "clover leaf", and a pyramidal structure (Amplatz-Spider or Simon-nitinol). Materials include stainless steel, titanium, eligiloy, and nickel titanium alloy. The thrombogenicity of titanium is similar to that of stainless steel, but it can be compressed into a smaller carrier because of its increased tolerance to flexion stress.[1] The current introducer systems are smaller (9–14 French) than the older devices; this feature decreases the risk of thrombosis at the insertion site.[2,3] Differences in filter diameter are clinically important. The bird's-nest filter can be placed in larger vena cava (up to 40 mm in diameter) than the other filters.[4]

Although differences in clot-filtering efficiency also may be important clinically, there are no adequately controlled direct clinical comparisons. *In vitro* studies suggest that the Greenfield filter is less likely to capture smaller thrombi (2–4 mm × 20–30 mm) than the bird's-nest filter[5] or the clover-leaf filter,[6] and that eccentric positioning of the Greenfield filter markedly diminishes its clot-trapping efficiency. More efficient filters, such as the bird's-nest filter, may increase the risk of obstruction of the inferior vena cava.[7(V)]

TECHNIQUE

At present, the most widely used approach to inferior vena cava filtration is percutaneous venotomy. Because the left iliac vein may be partially compressed by the right iliac artery, and the internal jugular veins pose the risk of air embolism (the latter having occurred in 1% of internal jugular insertions), the preferred site for venous access is the right femoral vein.[8(V)] Because of the potential danger of air embolism, the left common femoral vein should be used when the right common femoral vein is not available, or when severe levoscoliosis is present.[9] The femoral veins offer an additional advantage: the same puncture site can be used for pulmonary angiography and cavography.

A vena cavagram is important for identifying caval size, anatomy, and thrombi between the venotomy site and the proposed point of filter placement. Such vena cavagrams frequently identify: (1) cavae which are too large for standard Greenfield filters, (2) inferior vena cava thrombi, or (3) anatomical variants which influence filter placement.[10,11(V),12]

From *Venous Thromboembolism: An Evidence-Based Atlas* edited by Russell Hull, Gary Raskob, Graham Pineo © 1996, Futura Publishing Co., Armonk, NY.

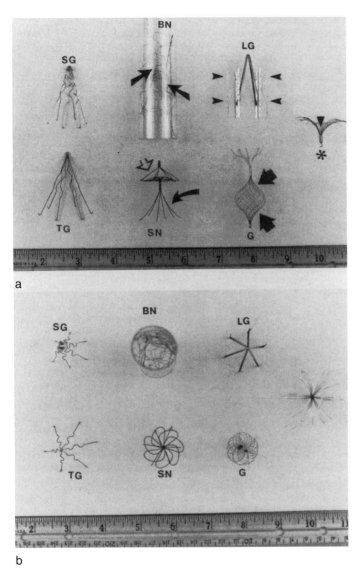

a

b

Figure 1. Longitudinal (a) and short axis (b) views of seven current vena cava filters. The Bird's nest™ (BN) is designed for use in vena cava up to 40 mm in diameter. SG = stainless steel Greenfield; LG = LGM filter; A = Amplatz filter, TG = titanium Greenfield; SN = Simon nitinol; and G = Gunther filter. (Reproduced with permission from Dorfman GS, Radiology, 1990).

INDICATIONS

The purpose of vena cava filtration is to prevent pulmonary embolism (PE). Available data suggest that recurrent PE is unlikely after a vena cava filter has been properly placed. Becker et al, reported recurrent pulmonary emboli in 26 of 1094 patients after vena cava filtration; 8 deaths (0.7%) were attributed to PE.[13] In subsequent studies using a variety of vena cava filters, investigators have reported similar low rates of recurrent thromboembolism and death due to PE.[14] Such data compare favorably with recurrence rates and deaths after anticoagulant treatment of acute proximal deep-vein thrombi[15(I),16(I)] and acute PE.[17] These comparisons, al-

though imperfect, provide the basis for the use of vena cava filters.

Two widely accepted indications for vena cava filtration are: (1) an absolute contraindication to anticoagulation or (2) a complication of anticoagulant therapy (Table 1). Absolute contraindications are active bleeding that cannot be easily controlled and situations in which life-threatening bleeding is likely (such as recent central nervous system trauma). Serious complications of anticoagulant therapy such as major bleeding or heparin-induced thrombocytopenia with thromboses also warrant the use of vena cava filtering.

There may be relative contraindications to anticoagulation, such as recently treated active gastrointestinal ulceration or active inflammatory bowel disease. In these circumstances clinicians must use available clinical information in deciding whether or not to anticoagulate. Vena caval filtration is appropriate when the risk of anticoagulation is excessive.

Another clinical problem requiring vena cava filtering is the need for surgery in a patient with incompletely treated proximal deep-vein thrombosis (DVT). Interruption of anticoagulation therapy increases the risk of recurrent thromboembolism, and prophylactic doses of anticoagulant (e.g., subcutaneous heparin 5000 IU b.i.d.) are insufficient in the setting of active thrombosis. In this case a vena cava filter is necessary, as it is when anticoagulation is contraindicated because of recent major surgery.

Surgery for patients with chronic large-vessel thromboembolic pulmonary hypertension may also be an indication for vena caval filtration. Even if active thrombosis does not exist, Moser et al, advocate placement of vena cava filters before surgical thromboendarterectomy.[18]

Table 1
Indications for Filtration of the Inferior Vena Cava

Absolute contraindication to anticoagulation
   Active bleeding of clinical consequence
   Life threatening or serious bleeding likely e.g., CNS surgery or trauma within two weeks
Complications of anticoagulant therapy
   Major bleeding
   Heparin induced thrombocytopenia with thromboses
Emergency surgery for a patient with incompletely treated proximal deep-vein thrombosis
Thromboendarterectomy with chronic large-vessel thromboembolic pulmonary hypertension
Objectively documented recurrent pulmonary embolism in the presence of adequate anticoagulant therapy
Acute massive thromboembolism treated by thrombectomy or treated by thrombolysis with residual proximal deep-vein thrombi
? Free floating iliofemoral or vena cava thrombi
? Prophylactic placement for high-risk patients prior to orthopedic surgery or following trauma

Filter placement, instead of more conventional prophylactic measures, may be justified by: (1) the risks of anticoagulants after cardiopulmonary bypass, (2) the possibility that recurrent thromboemboli may not dissolve, and (3) the fact that these patients have a demonstrated predisposition to serious venous thromboembolism (VTE).

When recurrent thromboembolism occurs in spite of anticoagulant threatment, the insertion of a vena cava filter may be warranted. However, several caveats apply. Objective proof of recurrent pulmonary thromboembolism is important, but is rare when adequate initial doses of anticoagulants are given.[15(I),16(I)] Symptoms and signs which suggest a recurrence are nonspecific, and may reflect complications of previous PE or anxiety. Furthermore, before anticoagulant therapy is started, up to 50% of patients who present with acute DVT have lung-scan patterns suggestive of occult PE.[19–21] When recurrent PE complicates inadequate initial anticoagulant therapy, the clinician may choose not to place a vena cava filter, particularly if the patient is young, has ample cardiopulmonary reserve and little remaining clot burden, and an adequate anticoagulant effect can be achieved.

Another clinical problem to be considered is acute massive PE. Thrombectomy for this condition justifies vena cava filter placement[22,23] because anticoagulation is contraindicated and the risk of recurrent thromboembolism is high. Vena cava filtration may also be warranted if extensive thrombus remains in the lower extremities and thrombolysis is planned; in this situation, partial lysis of loosely attached venous thrombi can produce fatal thromboemboli.[24]

The presence of unattached tails of adherent thrombi, often referred to as "floating thrombi", presents a controversial indication for vena cava filtration.[25,26] The risks posed by such thrombi remain uncertain (Table 2). Some investigators have reported that most free-floating thrombi do not embolize[27]; others have reported a high rate of PE when thrombi with nonadherent segments are treated with anticoagulants alone.[28,29] When free-floating thrombi are identified, difficulties of diagnosis[30] and co-existing conditions which influence prognosis (such as advanced cancer) complicate the decision to use a vena cava filter. In the absence of compelling data, the decision must be individualized, taking into account the size of the unattached segment, the presence and nature of preexistent cardiopulmonary compromise, the presence of coexisting disease (e.g., advanced malignancy) which limits the prognosis, and the patient's wishes. When unattached thrombus extends into the vena cava and thrombectomy is planned, a filter should be placed proximal to the thrombus.[31]

Prophylactic placement of vena cava filters has been suggested for selected "high-risk" patients: examples include multiorgan trauma victims or patients undergoing hip or knee arthroplasty who have risk factors for VTE.[32] However, there have been no clinical trials examining these indications. Furthermore, the low rates of fatal pulmonary emboli which follow widely accepted prophylactic measures make the use of vena cava filters difficult to justify in these circumstances.

CONTRAINDICATIONS

The few contraindications to the use of vena cava filtering include patients who are uncooperative or unwilling, and patients who cannot have filters inserted percutaneously because they lack suitable venous access. The latter circumstance requires operative filter placement. Under such circumstances coagulopathy or thrombocytopenia contraindicate filter placement.

Although sepsis does not contraindicate the use of a vena cava filter,[33,34(V)] thrombus trapped by a filter can become infected, necessitating treatment with parenteral antibiotics and surgical removal of the filter.[33,35] Therefore, in the presence of sepsis, clear and compelling indications for vena cava filtration are necessary.

COMPLICATIONS

Fatal complications are uncommon.[13] Some reported deaths were associated with massive embolism of throm-

Table 2
The Clinical Significance of Unattached Venous Thrombi

Author, Date	Method	Imaging Technique	N-Total	N-Free-floating Thrombi	Observations
Voet, 1991	Retrospective	Serial duplex ultrasound 2 weeks and 3 months (D)	—	30	4 suffered massive PE ≤4 days after duplex diagnosis (2 were fatal)
Norris, 1985	Retrospective	Venography (L)	78	5	3 of 5 had symptomatic PE in spite of anticoagulation
Berry, 1990	Retrospective	Duplex ultrasound (D)	65	—	17 (26%) developed PE
Baldridge, 1990	Retrospective	Duplex ultrasound (D)	732	73	2 (3%) developed PE

* Inferior vena cava; D = Dynamic Movement; L = Length of tail > 5 cm.

bus attached to a filter,[7] sudden cardiopulmonary collapse,[10] and misplacement of a Greenfield filter.[36(V)] Fatalities have also resulted from recurrent thromboembolism in spite of vena cava filtration[37,38(V),14]; recurrent thromboemboli may arise from the vena cava filter (Figure 2), or they may pass through a malpositioned filter.[39]

Nonfatal complications include: (1) those related to the insertion procedure such as infection, thrombosis, and hematoma, and (2) those which occur later such as filter migration, erosion of a hook through the vena cava, or vena cava obstruction. Thrombosis at the insertion site was a common complication when large-bore introducer systems were used. The use of smaller (12–14 French) delivery systems has reduced the incidence of this complication to approximately 10% to 30%.[40] Infections are uncommon and hematomas are rarely of clinical consequence. Migration of vena cava filters occurs commonly,[41(V)] but is seldom clinically important. Rarely, caudal migration beyond the bifurcation of the inferior vena cava may permit fatal PE from the opposite iliac vein.[11] Erosion of anchoring filter struts can cause chronic neuralgia[8(V),11(V)] or intestinal perforation,[42] but perforation of the vena cava is often asymptomatic and clinically unimportant.[11(V),43]

Vena cava obstruction in the lower extremities is a potentially serious complication. The reported incidence varies from 0% to 21%. The wide variation in reported incidence reflects the different methods used to detect caval obstruction as well as differences in filter design, anticoagulation practice, and the duration of follow-up. Caval obstruction may contribute to chronic venous stasis with swelling, ulceration, and even venous gangrene which necessitates amputation.[11] Acute caval obstruction causes sudden cyanosis of the lower extremities, swelling, and pain; it seems more likely to occur within a few weeks after insertion of a filter.[44] Treatment of acute vena caval obstruction calls for volume replacement to avoid hypotension and thrombolysis to relieve the obstruction whenever possible.

LONG-TERM ANTICOAGULATION

The use of anticoagulants after vena cava filter placement must include an assessment of the risk and benefit for the individual patient. There have been no well designed clinical trials to provide guidance. Risks such as vena caval thrombosis and recurrent thromboemboli favor continued anticoagulation, particularly when the risks for bleeding complications are minimal. Since the filter does not prevent thrombosis, and since the risk of recurrent thromboembolism is substantial without anticoagulation, we recommend anticoagulants in the absence of strong contraindications or bleeding complications. The presence of a vena cava filter does not contraindicate anticoagulant therapy, because clinically important hemorrhage at the site where the filter anchors to the vena cava rarely occurs. Furthermore, contraindications to anticoagulants (such as recent surgery) often resolve within several weeks after vena cava filters are placed, allowing anticoagulant therapy to be resumed.

INFECTIONS

Pyophlebitis involving a vena cava filter may occur.[35] Such infections may present a clinical picture of persistent generalized septicemia after bacteremia. Successful treatment may require both parenteral antibiotics and surgical removal of the filter. Although such infections appear to be exceedingly infrequent, the presence

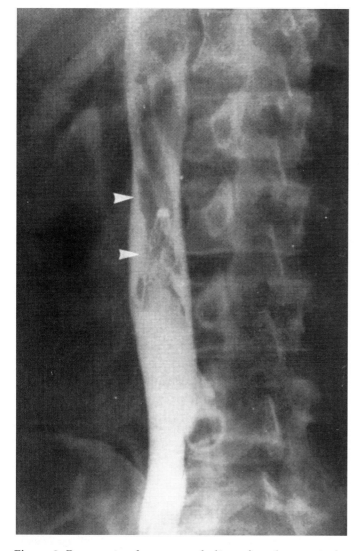

Figure 2. Recurrent pulmonary embolism after placement of a Greenfield filter prompted this vena cava gram which demonstrates extensive thrombus which has propagated above the vena cava filter. (Reproduced with permission Braun et al, Chest, 1985).

of an intravascular foreign body has led some authors to recommend antimicrobial prophylaxis during procedures that may give rise to bacteremia.[33] Furthermore, although sepsis is not an absolute contraindication to the placement of a filter, the risk of pyophlebitis involving the filter must be considered.

UPPER-EXTREMITY THROMBOSIS

The deep veins of the upper extremities must be considered potential sources of VTE. Indwelling catheters increase the incidence of upper-extremity thrombosis. Thrombi involving the subclavian and axillary vena may complicate more than one-fourth of subclavian catheters; a substantial fraction of these may result in pulmonary emboli,[45] some of which have proved to be fatal.[46] Thus, treatment of upper-extremity thrombosis is often necessary, and anticoagulants may be contraindicated. Under such circumstances, a Greenfield filter can be placed in the superior vena cava,[47] although the exact indications for this procedure remain poorly defined.

MAGNETIC RESONANCE IMAGING

Vena cava filters may complicate magnetic resonance images (MRI). The ferromagnetic components of these filters degrade MRI studies.[48] Furthermore, magnetic forces can move ferromagnetic structures. To date, the application of forces up to 1.5 T have not affected patients with Greenfield,[49] Simon-nitinol,[50,51] or bird's-nest filters.[48] However, caution is appropriate within the first several weeks after filter insertion, before fibrin and endothelial proliferation stabilize the filter.

THROMBOLYTIC THERAPY

Severe bleeding is the major risk associated with thrombolytic therapy. Since the hooks or barbs which secure the vena cava filter penetrate the vessel wall, significant retroperitoneal hemorrhage is a potential risk for patients who receive thrombolytic therapy shortly after vena caval filtration. However, major hemorrhage has not been reported for the few patients that have received thrombolytic agents after insertion of filters with hooks or barbs.[44,36] Removable filters have also been used successfully when thrombolytic therapy has been used for DVT.[52(V)]

Suprarenal Placement

Suprarenal placement of the vena cava filter is necessary when thrombus arises at or above the renal veins (Table 3). Thrombus arising from the left ovarian vein can be managed either by suprarenal filter placement or by ligation of the ovarian vein. Thromboemboli following re-

Table 3
Indications for Suprarenal Placement of Vena Cava Filter

Renal-vein thrombosis
Infra-renal vena cava thrombosis
Large patent left ovarian vein (pregnancy *or* childbearing)
Thrombus propagating proximal to a filter below the renal veins

nal transplant may arise from the iliac vein on the grafted side, necessitating placement of vena cava filters above the anastomosis of the renal and iliac veins.

Most patients tolerate suprarenal filter placement.[53(V),54] Greenfield et al, reported that of 60 patients who had filters placed above the renal veins none died from recurrent thromboembolism or renal failure.[53(V)] However, thrombotic obstruction of a suprarenal vena cava filter can precipitate acute renal failure or even the rupture of a renal transplant.[55]

REFERENCES

1. Greenfield LJ, Cho KJ, Procter M, Bonn J, Bookstein JJ, et al. Results of a multicenter study of the modified hook-titanium Greenfield filter. J Vasc Surg 1991;14: 253–257.
2. Mewissen MW, Erickson SJ, Foley WD, Lipchik EO, Oldon DL, et al. Thrombosis at venous insertion sites after inferior vena caval filter placement. Radiology 1989;173:155–157.
3. Dorfman GS, Cronan JJ, Paolella LP, Lamriase RE, Haas RA, et al. Iatrogenic changes at the venotomy site after percutaneous placement of the Greenfield filter. Radiology 1989;173:159–162.
4. Gianturco-Roehm Bird's Nest™ Vena Cava Filter; Suggested Instructions for Placement. Cook Incorporated; Bloomington, Indiana.
5. Katsamouris AA, Waltman AAC, Delichatsios MA, Athanasoulis CA. Inferior vena Cava filters: in vitro comparison of clot trapping and flow dynamics. Radiology 1988;166:361–366.
6. Palestrant AM, Faykus MH. Clover leaf inferior vena cava filter: In vitro evaluation of filter deployment and comparison of emboli—capturing ability. J Vasc Intervent Radiol 1991;2:117–121.
(V)7. Roehm JOF, Johnsrude IS, Barth MH, Gianturco C. The bird's nest inferior vena cava filter: progress report. Radiology 1988;168:745–749.
(V)8. Greenfield LJ, Michna BA. Twelve-year clinical experience with the Greenfield vena caval filter. Surgery 1988;104:706–712.
9. Dorfman GS. Percutaneous inferior vena caval filters. Radiology 1990;174:987–992.
10. Pais SO, Tobin KD, Austin CB, Queral L. Percutaneous insertion of the Greenfield inferior vena cava filter: experience with 96 patients. J Vasc Surg 1988;8:460–464.
(V)11. Carabasi RA, Moritz MJ, Jarrell BE. Complications encountered with the use of the Greenfield filter. Am J Surg 1987;154:163–168.
12. Smith DC, Kohne RE, Taylor FC. Steel coil embolization supplementing filter placement in a patient with a duplicated inferior vena cava. JVIR 1992;3:577–580.

13. Becker DM, Philbrick JT, Selby JB. Inferior vena cava filters: indications, safety, effectiveness. Arch Intern Med 1992;152:1985–1994.
14. Ferris EJ, McCowan TC, Carber DR, Mcfarland DR. Percutaneous inferior vena caval filters: follow up of seven designs in 320 patients. Radiology 1993;188:851–856.
(I)15. Hull RD, Raskob GE, Rosenbloom D, Panju AA, Britt-Edwards P, et al. Heparin for 5 days as compared with 10 days in the initial treatment of proximal venous thrombosis. N Engl J Med 1990;322:1260–1264.
(I)16. Hull RD, Raskob GE, Pineo FT, Green D, Trowbridge AA, et al. Subcutaneous low-molecular-weight heparin compared with continuous intravenous heparin in the treatment of proximal vein thrombosis. N Engl J Med 1992;326:975–982.
17. Carson JL, Kelley MA, Duff A, Weg JG, Fulkerson WL, et al. The clinical course of pulmonary embolism. N Engl J Med 1992;326:1240–1245.
18. Moser KM, Auger WR, Fedullo PF, et al. Chronic thromboembolic pulmonary hypertension: clinical picture and surgical treatment. Eur Respir J 1992;5:334–342.
19. Monreal M, Ruiz J, Olazabal A, et al. Deep venous thrombosis and the risk of pulmonary embolism. Chest 1992;102:677–681.
20. Dorfman GS, Cronan JJ, Tupper TB, et al. Occult pulmonary embolism: a common occurrence in deep vein thrombosis. AJR 1987;148:263–266.
21. Huisman MV, Buller HR, ten Cate JW, et al. Unexpected high prevalence of silent pulmonary embolism in patients with deep venous thrombosis. Chest 1989;95:498–502.
22. Meyns B, Sergeant P, Flameng W, Daenen W. Surgery for massive pulmonary embolism. Acta Cardiologies 1992;XLVII:487–493.
23. Kieny R, Charpentier A, Kieny MT. What is the place of pulmonary embolectomy today? J Cardiovasc Surg 1991;32:549–554.
24. Goldsmith JC, Lollar P, Hoak JC. Massive fatal pulmonary emboli with fibrinolytic therapy. Circulation 1982;64:1068–1069.
25. Page Y, Decourus H, Tardy B, Comlet C, Simitsidis S, et al. Criteria for prophylactyic caval interruption in venous thromboembolism. Am Rev Respir Dis 1993;147(4):A1001.
26. Girard P, Hauuy MP, Musset D, Simonneau G, Petitpretz P. Acute inferior vena cava thrombosis. Chest 1989;95:284–291.
27. Baldridge ED, Martin MA, Welling RE. Clinical significance of free-floating venous thrombi. J Vasc Surg 1990;11:62–67.
28. Norris CS, Greenfield LJ, Barnes RW. Free-floating iliofemoral thrombus: a risk of pulmonary embolism. Arch Surg 1985;120:806–808.
29. Voet DA, Afschrift M. Floating thrombi: diagnosis and follow-up by duplex ultrasound. Brit J Radiol 1991;64:1010–1014.
30. Schmidt JA, Gartenschlager M, Joseph U, von Wichert P, Klose KJ. The diagnosis of floating venous thrombi: a comparison between venography, sonography and so-called phlebo-computer-tomography. Am Rev Respir Dis 1993;147(4):A998.
31. Eklof B, Juhan C. Revival of thrombectomy in the management of acute iliofemoral venous thrombosis. Contemporary Surgery 1992;40:21–30.

32. Vaughn BK, Knezevich S, Lombardi AV, Mallory TH. Use of the Greenfield filter to prevent fatal pulmonary embolism associated with total hip and knee arthroplasty. J Bone and Joint Surg 1989;71:1542–1548.
33. Peyton JWR, Hylemon MB, Greenfield LJ, Crute SL, Sugerman HJ, et al. Comparison of Greenfield filter and vena caval ligation for experimental septic thromboembolism. Surg 1983;93:533–537.
(V)34. Kantor A, Glanz S, Gordon DH, Sclafani SJA. Percutaneous insertion of the Kimray-Greenfield filter: incidence of femoral vein thrombosis. AJR 1987;149:1065–1066.
35. Scott JH, Anderson CL, Shankar PS. Septicemia from infected filter. JAMA 1980;243:1133–1134.
(V)36. Scurr JH, Jarrett PE, Wastell C. The treatment of recurrent pulmonary embolism: Experience with the Kimray-Greenfield vena cava filter. Ann R Coll Surg Engl 1983;65:233–234.
37. Geisinger MA, Zelch MG, Risius B. Recurrent pulmonary embolism after Greenfield filter placement. Radiology 1987;165:383–384.
(V)38. Cohen JR, Grella L, Citron M. Greenfield filter instead of heparin as primary treatment for deep venous thrombosis or pulmonary embolism in patients with cancer. Cancer 1992;70:1993–1996.
39. Greenfield LJ, Peyton R, Crute S, Barnes R. Greenfield vena caval filter experience. Arch Surg 1981;116:1451–1456.
40. Molgaard CP, Yucel EK, Geller SC, Knox TA, Waltman AC. Access site thrombosis after placement of inferior vena cava filters with 12–14-F delivery sheaths. Radiology 1992;185:257–261.
(V)41. Rose BS, Simon DC, Hess ML, Van Aman ME. Percutaneous transfemoral placement of the Kimray-Greenfield vena cava filter. Radiology 1987;165:373–376.
42. Sidawy AN, Menzoian JO. Distal migration and deformation of the Greenfield vena cava filter. Surgery 1986;99:369–372.
43. Long W, Schweiger H, Fietkau R., Hofmann-Preiss K. Spontaneous disruption of two Greenfield vena caval filters. Radiology 1990;174:445–446.
44. Greenfield LJ. Current indications for and results of Greenfield filter placement. J Vasc Surg 1984;1:502–504.
45. Horattas MC, Wright DJ, Fenton AH, Evans DM. Changing concepts of deep venous thrombosis of the upper extremity—report of a series and review of the literature. Surgery 1988;104:561–567.
46. Lindblad B, Tengborn L, Bergqvist D. Deep vein thrombosis of the axillary-subclavian veins: Epidemiologic data, effects of different types of treatment and late sequelae. Eur J of Vasc Surg 1988;2:161–165.
47. Hoffman MJ, Greenfield LJ. Central venous septic thrombosis managed by superior vena cava Greenfield filter and venous thrombectomy: a case report. J Vasc Surg 1986;4:606–611.
48. Watanobe AT, Teitelbaum GP, Gomes AS, Roehm JOF. MR imaging of the bird's nest filter. Radiology 1990;177:578–579.
49. Liebman CE, Messersmith RN, Levin DN, Chien-Tai L. MR imaging of inferior vena cava filters: safety and artifacts. AJR 1988;150:1174–1176.
50. Teitelbaum GP, Bradley WG Jr, Klein BD. MR imaging artifacts, ferromagnetism, and magnetic torque of intravascular filters, stents, and coils. Radiology 1988;166:657–664.

51. Teitelbaum GP, Ortega HV, Vinitski S, Clark RA, Watanabe AT, et al. Optimization of gradient echo imaging parameters for intracaval filters and trapped thromboemboli. Radiology 1990;174: 1013–1019.

(V)52. Thery C, Asseman P, Amrouni N, Becquant J, Pruvost P, et al. Use of a new removable vena cava filter in order to prevent pulmonary embolism in patients submitted to thrombolysis. Eur Heart J 1990;11:334–341.

(V)53. Greenfield JL, Cho KJ, Proctor MC, Sobel M, Shah S, et al. Late results of suprarenal Greenfield vena cava filter placement. Arch Surg 1992;127:969–973.

54. Pasquale MD, Abrams JH, Najarian JS, Cerra FB. Use of Greenfield filters in renal transplant patients—are they safe? Transplantation 1993;55:439–442.

55. Swanson RJ, Carlson RE, Olcott C, et al. Rupture of the left kidney following renosplenic shunt. Surgery 1976;79:710.

SECTION VI

Special Problems

34

The Management of Common Thrombotic Disorders During Pregnancy

Karen A. Valentine, Linda Barbour, Jeffrey Pickard,
Russell D. Hull, Graham F. Pineo

INTRODUCTION

An important cause of obstetric morbidity and mortality is pulmonary embolism (PE). It is the leading cause of maternal mortality in Wales and England,[1] and of death after a live birth in the United States.[2] The risk of venous thrombosis is increased five-fold by pregnancy.[3]

Because the absolute risk is low, there have been very few prospective studies.[4(II)] Current recommendations are based on retrospective studies and case reports. Many of the inferences drawn from these data have led to clinical contradictions. This review should lead to a better understanding of the underlying rationale for current clinical practice, and to awareness of the need for multicenter trials addressing this important complication of pregnancy.

METHODOLOGICAL CONSIDERATIONS

In the nonpregnant patient, most of the uncertainties that a clinician commonly encounters in selecting appropriate management for common thrombotic disorders have been resolved. For example, in the treatment of venous thromboembolism (VTE), it is clear that clinically effective heparin therapy is dependent on the intensity of the heparin anticoagulant effect (as measured by the activated partial thromboplastin time [APTT] or the heparin blood level).[5(I)]

The keystone for making specific recommendations for clinical practice is the strength of evidence from clinical trials.[6] We have used the "levels of evidence" approach[6] of the American College of Chest Physicians for the consensus conference on antithrombotic therapy. Developing evidence-based[6] guidelines for antithrombotic therapy and prophylaxis in pregnant women has been difficult because

of the complete absence of Level I data in the literature. Indeed, to support firm recommendations in the context of pregnancy, it is necessary to incorporate a wealth of literature reporting Level I trials evaluating antithrombotic management of the nonpregnant patient into the decision-making process. An overriding caveat of using these Level I data (from the nonpregnant patient) is the safety of the developing baby (for example warfarin toxicity) as well as the mother's well-being.

EPIDEMIOLOGY

The absolute risk of venous thrombosis in pregnant women is small. In women without a history of VTE, the estimated risk is 0.5–3.0 per thousand.[7,8] Women with a history of VTE are considered to be at high risk for further events during pregnancy.[9(V),10(V)]

Venous thromboembolism may present at any time during pregnancy in addition to the puerperium.[10(V),11,12,13(V),14(V),15] Pulmonary embolism may occur more frequently in the postpartum period, particularly in patients undergoing a cesarean section.[7] Peculiar to pregnancy is the striking predilection for pregnancy-associated deep-vein thrombosis (DVT) to present in the left leg.[10(V),16(I)] Factors that may significantly increase the risk of pregnancy-associated thromboembolism are mode of delivery, age and parity, obesity, prolonged hospitalization, operative procedures, underlying hypercoagulable states (e.g., antiphospholipid antibody syndrome), and prior VTE.[3,14(V),17,18(I)]

DIAGNOSIS

In patients with clinically suspected venous thrombosis the difficulties of clinically differentiating between nonthrombotic disorders and DVT are compounded by

From *Venous Thromboembolism: An Evidence-Based Atlas* edited by Russell Hull, Gary Raskob, Graham Pineo © 1996, Futura Publishing Co., Armonk, NY.

pregnancy.[19] Venography remains the "gold standard" for making the diagnosis of venous thrombosis, even in pregnancy. The quantity of radiation associated with limited venography (using pelvic shielding) is low (< .05 rads).[20] Two noninvasive methods for diagnosing DVT which show promise in the pregnant patient are impedance plethysmography (IPG)[16(I),21,22,23(I),24,25(I)]and duplex ultrasonography. Impedance plethysmography was recently studied prospectively in 152 consecutive pregnant women with clinically suspected DVT.[16(I)] Patients were studied during the third trimester. They were studied in the left lateral decubitus position because of possible external compression of the pelvic vessels by the gravid uterus.[16(I)] Patients with abnormal IPGs had their diagnoses confirmed by venography and were treated with anticoagulation. Those women with negative IPGs initially were retested on days 1, 3, 5 or 7, 10, and 14 after the initial exam. All were followed until 3 months postpartum. Impedance plethysmography was negative in 139 of 152 patients; these patients were not given therapy and were followed as described above. None of these women developed clinical evidence of PE or DVT. The authors concluded that it is safe to withhold therapy in pregnant women who have negative results after serial IPG.

Duplex ultrasonography is a proven noninvasive technique for diagnosing DVT in nonpregnant patients,[22,23(I),24,25(I)] but remains to be evaluated during pregnancy. The ventilation-perfusion lung scan remains the pivotal test for diagnosing PE during pregnancy. The dose of ionizing radiation is low, particularly if the ventilation scan can be avoided in patients who have a normal perfusion scan. The role of pulmonary angiography for diagnosing PE during pregnancy is controversial. The risks and benefits must be weighed in the individual patient.

ANTICOAGULANT THERAPY

Heparin

Classical heparin therapy remains the initial treatment of choice in patients with documented VTE.[26,27(I),28(I),29(I)] Heparin has the advantage that it is unable to cross the placenta. Therefore, on pharmacological evidence, it is very unlikely to affect the fetus. However, retrospective studies have reported conflicting observations about the safety of heparin during pregnancy. One series concluded that heparin adversely affected fetal outcome. However, this study did not control for serious confounding maternal conditions which were known to adversely affect the fetus.[30(V)] A more recent retrospective series did control for confounding variables. The rate of adverse fetal or neonatal outcomes was comparable in pregnant patients treated with heparin to those who were not.[31(IV)]

Because warfarin sodium therapy is contraindicated throughout pregnancy, therapeutic adjusted-dose he-

parin therapy has become the standard long term therapy. Patients suffering VTE during pregnancy are treated with initial heparin therapy for 6 days followed by adjusted-dose subcutaneous heparin every 12 hours.[32] The duration of long-term therapy is mandated by the need to protect the patient during the remainder of pregnancy, and for 4 to 6 weeks postpartum. Subcutaneous therapeutic heparin therapy every 12 hours is monitored by the APTT, the mid-interval APTT being adjusted to the therapeutic range.[33(I)]

Osteoporosis is a special concern arising from the prolonged use of therapeutic doses of heparin. Heparin-induced osteoporosis in pregnancy is poorly documented. The literature contains scattered case reports of women with vertebral fractures associated with heparin therapy.[14(V),34,35] Retrospective studies by Dahlman et al,[36] suggest that approximately 15% to 20% of pregnant women exposed to significant heparin doses may suffer from osteoporosis. A recent prospective series using dual photon bone densitometry was done in 14 pregnant women requiring heparin therapy and 14 pregnant controls matched for age, race, and smoking status.[37(IV)] Proximal femur measurements were taken at entry during pregnancy, immediately postpartum, and at 6 months postpartum. In five of 14 cases (36%), the immediate postpartum values were at least 10% lower than their baseline proximal femur measurements. None of the 14 matched controls showed a decrease. Mean proximal femur bone density also decreased only in the heparin-treated women, and this difference continued to be statistically significant at 6 months postpartum. As in Dahlman's study, no dose-response relationship could be demonstrated. Pregnancy alone does not appear to affect bone density.[38]

Subcutaneous heparin prophylaxis is recommended during pregnancy and 4 to 6 weeks postpartum in women with a history of VTE.[32] The use of subcutaneous heparin prophylaxis is based on extrapolation from the knowledge that low-dose heparin prophylaxis is effective in other moderate-risk patient groups,[39] and that adjusted-dose subcutaneous heparin is effective in high-risk groups.[40(I),41(I)] It is uncertain whether low-dose or adjusted-dose subcutaneous heparin is required for prophylaxis in pregnant patients.[32] By extrapolation from other patient groups at high risk for venous thrombosis, it is well-documented that low-dose heparin is relatively ineffective compared with adjusted doses of heparin in these high-risk patients.[42(I)] Current recommendations assume that pregnant patients with prior VTE are at moderate risk and should receive low-dose heparin prophylaxis throughout pregnancy and the postpartum period.[32]

Warfarin

The use of warfarin therapy is contraindicated throughout pregnancy. Warfarin exposure during the first trimester is associated with embryopathies (e.g., stippled epiphyses, nasal, and limb hypoplasia).[43] Exposure during the second trimester is associated with central nervous system abnormalities, including dorsal midline dysplasia (agenesis of the corpus callosum and Dandy-Walker malformations), midline cerebellar atrophy, and ventral midline dysplasia manifested by optic atrophy and hemorrhage.[44] In the third trimester rates of spontaneous abortions and stillbirths are elevated, probably as a result of hemorrhage.[45(V),46,47(III)] A review of 1,325 pregnancies from 186 different studies reported a 16.9% incidence of adverse outcomes when warfarin was used during pregnancy after exclusion of pregnancies with maternal comorbid conditions and prematurity with normal outcomes.[30(V)] Selection bias may affect the accuracy of this figure.

Warfarin is thought to be safe in women who breastfeed their babies. Studies, although small, have found little or no warfarin activity in breast milk or in the infants' circulation.[48,49]

Other Therapies

Streptokinase and urokinase are relatively contraindicated in pregnancy and within the first 10 days after delivery.[50–55] Although little streptokinase crosses the placenta,[56] placental abruption and excessive blood loss in the puerperium have been noted with its use.[57]

Low-molecular-weight heparin (LMWH) promises several advantages for antithrombotic therapy or prophylaxis during pregnancy. The long half-life of some of the LMWH preparations, and the observation that monitoring is not required, offer the possibility of a once-daily subcutaneous approach without monitoring.[58] Low-molecular-weight heparin does not cross the placenta,[59–62(III)] and one study suggested that there was a lower risk of osteoporosis when it was used in the long-term management of nonpregnant individuals.[63(V)] Low-molecular-weight heparin has been used in a small number of pregnant women who had adverse reactions to heparin.[59–61] Because the molecular weight and activity of LMWH vary widely, depending on the preparation, individual preparations need to be tested independently during pregnancy.

THROMBOEMBOLIC COMPLICATIONS OF PROSTHETIC HEART VALVES

In pregnant women, prosthetic mechanical valves pose major concerns because of the need for continued therapeutic anticoagulation. Although it is the accepted standard of care for preventing valve thrombosis and systemic embolism, oral anticoagulant therapy is contraindicated during pregnancy. At present, the practical alternative is full therapeutic doses of heparin, administered subcutaneously and monitored by the APTT to ensure that the therapeutic range is achieved. The use of subcutaneous heparin therapy in this context is based on extrapolation of heparin use in other patient groups.[40(I),41(I)]

Some information is available from observational studies. A study of 156 women with prosthetic valves who had 223 pregnancies, suggested that antiplatelet agents alone are inadequate prophylaxis against systemic embolism.[64]

Limited data suggest that adjusted-dose heparin to keep the APTT in the therapeutic range at midinterval may be adequate in preventing thromboembolism,[65,66(I),67] but considerable uncertainty persists.

REFERENCES

1. Department of Health, Welsh Office, Scottish Home and Health Department and Department of Health and Social Services, Northern Ireland (1991). Report on confidential enquiries into maternal deaths in the United Kingdom 1985–1987, HMSO, London.
2. Atrash HK, Koonin LM, Lawson HW, et al. Maternal mortality in the United States 1979–1986. Obstet Gynecol 1990;76(6):1055–1060.
3. Bonnar J. Venous thromboembolism in pregnancy. Clin Obstet Gynaecol 1981;8(2):455–473.
(II)4. Howell R, Fidler J, Letsky E, et al. The risks of antenatal subcutaneous heparin prophylaxis: a controlled trial. Br J Obstet Gynaecol 1983;90:1124–1128.
(I)5. Hull RD, Raskob GE, Rosenbloom D, et al. Optimal therapeutic level of heparin therapy in patients with venous thrombosis. Arch Int Med 1992;152:1589–1595.
6. Cook DJ, Guyatt GH, Laupacis A, et al. Rules of evidence and clinical recommendations on the use of antithrombotic agents. Chest 1992;102(4)(Suppl):305S-311S.
7. Rutherford S, Montoro M, McGehee W, et al. Thromboembolic disease associated with pregnancy: an 11 year review. Am J Obstet Gynecol 1991;164(1):286.(Abstract)
8. Dixon JE. Pregnancies complicated by previous thromboembolic disease. Br J Hosp Med 1987:449–452.
(V)9. Badaracco MA, Vessey MP. Recurrence of venous thromboembolic disease and use of oral contraceptives. Br Med J 1974;1:215–217.
(V)10. Tengborn L, Bergqvist D, Mätzsch T, et al. Recurrent thromboembolism in pregnancy and puerperium. Am J Obstet Gynecol 1985;28(1):107–118.
11. DHSS (1980): Report on Confidential Enquiries into Maternal Deaths in England and Wales 1976–1978. HMSO, London.
12. Aaro LA, Juergens JL. Thrombophlebitis associated with pregnancy. Am J Obstet Gynecol 1971;109(8):1128–1133.
(V)13. Bergqvist A, Bergqvist D, Holböök T. Deep-vein thrombosis during pregnancy: A prospective study. Acta Obstet Gynecol Scan 1983;62:443–448.
(V)14. Hellgren M, Nygards EB. Long-term therapy with subcutaneous heparin during pregnancy. Gynecol Obstet Invest 1982;13:76–89.
15. Ginsberg JS, Brill-Edwards P, Burrows RF, et al. Venous thrombosis during pregnancy: leg and trimester of presentation. Thromb Haemost 1992;67(5):519–520.
(I)16. Hull RD, Raskob GE, Carter CJ. Serial impedance plethysmography in pregnant patients with clinically

suspected deep-vein thrombosis. Ann Int Med 1990; 112:663–667.

17. de Swiet M. Thromboembolism. Clin Haematol 1985; 14(3):643–661.

(I)18. Moseley P, Kerstein M. Pregnancy and thrombophlebitis. Surg Gynecol Obstet 1980;150:593–599.

19. Lee RV, McComb LE, Mezzadri FC. Pregnant patients, painful legs: the obstetrician's dilemma. Obstet Gynecol Surv 1990;45:290–298.

20. Ginsberg JS, Hirsh J, Rainbow AJ, Coates G. Risk to the fetus of radiologic procedures used in the diagnosis of maternal thromboembolic disease. Thromb Haemost 1989;61:189–196.

21. Clarke-Pearson DL, Jelovsek FR: Alterations of occlusive cuff impedance plethysmography results in the obstetric patient. Surgery 1981;89:594–598.

22. Cronan JJ, Dorfman GS, Scola FH, et al. Deep venous thrombosis: US assessment using vein compressibility. Radiology 1987;162:191–194.

(I)23. Lensing AWA, Prandoni P, Brandjes D, et al. Detection of deep-vein thrombosis by real-time B-mode ultrasonography. N Engl J Med 1989;320:342–345.

24. Rose ST, Zwiebel WJ, Nelson BD, et al. Symptomatic lower extremity deep venous thrombosis: accuracy, limitations, and role of colour duplex flow imaging in diagnosis. Radiology 1990;175:639–644.

(I)25. Heijboer H, Buller HR, Lensing AWA, Turpie AGG, et al. A comparison of real-time compression ultrasonography with impedance plethysmography for the eiagnosis of deep-vein thrombosis in symptomatic outpatients. New Engl J Med 1993;329(19):1365–1369.

26. Hyers TM, Hull RD, Weg J. Antithrombotic therapy for venous thromboembolic disease. Chest 1992;102:408S–425S.

(I)27. Salzman EW, Deykin D, Shapiro RM, et al. Management of heparin therapy: controlled prospective trial. N Engl J Med 1976;292:1046–1050.

(I)28. Gallus A, Jackaman J, Tillett J, et al. Safety and efficacy of warfarin started early after submassive venous thrombosis or pulmonary embolism. Lancet 1986;2: 1293–1296.

(I)29. Hull RD, Raskob GE, Rosenbloom D, et al. Heparin for 5 days as compared with 10 days in the initial treatment of proximal venous thrombosis. N Engl J Med 1990;322:1260–1264.

(V)30. Ginsberg JS, Hirsh J, Turner DC, et al. Risks to the fetus of anticoagulant therapy during pregnancy. Thrombos Haemost 1989;61(2):197–203.

(IV)31. Ginsberg JS, Kowalchuk G, Hirsh J, et al. Heparin therapy during pregnancy: risks to the fetus and mother. Arch Intern Med 1989;149:2233–36.

32. Ginsberg JS, Hirsh J. Use of antithrombotic agents during pregnancy. Chest 1992;102(4)(Suppl):385S–390S.

(I)33. Hull R, Delmore T, Carter C, et al. Adjusted subcutaneous heparin versus warfarin sodium in the long-term treatment of venous thrombosis. N Engl J Med 1982;306:189–193.

34. Aarskog D, Aksnes L. Low 1,25-dihydroxy vitamin D in heparin-induced osteopenia. Lancet 1980;650–651.

35. Zimran A, Shilo S, Fisher D, et al. Histomorphometric evaluation of reversible heparin-induced osteoporosis in pregnancy. Arch Intern Med 1986;46: 386–388.

36. Dahlman TC, Lindvall N, Hellgren M. Osteopenia in pregnancy during long-term heparin treatment: a radi-

ological study post partum. Br J Obstet Gyneacol 1990;97:221–228.

(IV)37. Barbour LA, Kick SD, Steiner JF, et al. A prospective study of heparin induced osteoporosis in pregnancy using bone densitometry. Am J Obstet Gynecol 1994;170:862–869.

38. Sowers M, Crutchfield M, Jannausch M, et al. A prospective evaluation of bone mineral change in pregnancy. Obstet Gynecol 1991;77(6):841–845.

39. Collins R, Scrimgeour A, Yusuf S, et al. Reduction in fatal pulmonary embolism and venous thrombosis by perioperative administration of subcutaneous heparin. N Engl J Med 1988;318:1162–1173.

(I)40. Leyvraz PF, Richard J, Bachmann F. Adjusted versus fixed-dose subcutaneous heparin in the prevention of deep-vein thrombosis after total hip replacement. N Engl J Med 1983;309:954–958.

(I)41. Hull RD, Delmore TJ, Carter C, et al. Adjusted subcutaneous heparin versus warfarin sodium in the long-term treatment of venous thrombosis. N Engl J Med 1982;306:189–194.

(I)42. Hull RD, Delmore TJ, Genton E, et al. Warfarin sodium versus low-dose heparin in the long-term treatment of venous thrombosis. N Engl J Med 1979;301:855–858.

43. Hall JG, Pauli RM, Wilson KM. Maternal and fetal sequelae of anticoagulation during pregnancy. Am J Med 1980;68:122–140.

44. Stevenson RE, Burton OM, Ferlauto GJ, et al. Hazards of oral anticoagulants during pregnancy. JAMA 1980;243:1549–1551.

(V)45. Chen WWC, Chan CS, Lee PK, et al. Pregnancy in patients with prosthetic heart valves: an experience with 45 pregnancies. Quart J Med 1982;(203):358–65.

46. Chong MKB, Harvey D, deSwiet M: Follow-up study of children whose mothers were treated with warfarin during pregnancy. Br J Obstet Gynaecol 1984;91: 1070–1073.

(III)47. Iturbe-Alesio I, del Carmen Fonseca M, Mutchinik O, et al.: Risks of anticoagulant therapy in pregnant women with artificial heart valves. N Eng J Med 1986;22(315):1390–1393.

48. L'e Orme M, Lewis PJ, deSwiet M, et al. May mothers given warfarin breast-feed their infants? Br Med J 1977;1564–1565.

49. McKenna R, Cole E, Vasan U. Is Warfarin sodium contraindicated in the lactating mother? J Ped 1983;103(2): 325–27.

50. Pfeifer GW. The use of thrombolytic therapy in obstetrics and gynaecology. Australas Ann Med 1970; 19(Suppl):28–31.

51. McTaggart DR, Engram TG: Massive pulmonary embolism during pregnancy treated with streptokinase. Med J Aust 1977;1:18–20.

52. Amias AG. Streptokinase, cerebral vascular disease—and triplets. Br Med J 1977;1:1414–1415.

53. Delclos GL, Davila F. Thrombolytic therapy for pulmonary embolism in pregnancy: a case report. Am J Obstet Gynecol 1986;155:375–376.

54. Hall RJC, Young C, Sutton GC, et al. Treatment of acute massive pulmonary embolism by streptokinase during labor and delivery. Br Med J 1972;4:647–649.

55. Birger F, Mats A, Birger A. Acute massive pulmonary embolism treated with streptokinase during labor and the early puerperium. Acta Obstet Gynecol Scand 1990;69:659–662.

56. Pfeifer GW. Distribution and placental transfer of [131]I

streptokinase. Australas Ann Med 1970;19(Suppl): 17–18.

57. Fagher B, Ahlgren M, Astedt B. Acute massive pulmonary embolism treated with streptokinase during labor and the early puerperium. Acta Obstet Gynecol Scand 1990;69:659–662.

58. Hirsh J, Levine MN. Low molecular weight heparin. Blood 1992;79:1–17.

59. de Boer K, Heyboer H, ten Cate JW, et al. Low molecular weight heparin treatment in a pregnant woman with allergy to standard heparins and heparanoid. Thromb Haemost 1989;61(1):148.

60. Priollet P, Roncato M, Aiach M, et al. Low molecular-weight heparin in venous thrombosis during pregnancy. Br J Haematol 1986;63:605–66.

61. Henny ChP, ten Cate H, ten Cate JW, et al. Thrombosis prophylaxis in an AT-III deficient pregnant woman: application of a low molecular weight heparinoid. Thromb Haemost 1986;55–30.

(III)62. Omri A, Delaloye JF, Anderson H, et al. Low molecular weight heparin Novo (LHN-1) does not cross the placenta during the second trimester of pregnancy. Thromb Haemost 1989;61(1):55–56.

(V)63. Monreal M, Lafoz E, Olive A, et al. Comparison of subcutaneous unfractionated heparin with a low molecular weight heparin (Fragmin) in Patients with Venous Thromboembolism and Contraindications to Coumarin. Thromb Haemost 1994;71:7–11.

64. Salazar E, Zajarias A, Gutierrez N, et al. The problem of cardiac valve prostheses, anticoagulants and pregnancy. Circulation 1984;70(Suppl I):169–177.

65. Levine HJ, Pauker SE, Salzman EW. Antithrombotic therapy in valvular heart disease. Chest 1986;89(Suppl 2):36S-45S.

(I)66. Wang RYC, Lee PK, Chow JSF, et al. Efficacy of low dose, subcutaneously administered heparin in treatment of pregnant women with artificial heart valves. Med J Aust 1983;2:126–128.

67. Chesebro JH, Adams PC, Fuster V. Antithrombotic therapy in patients with valvular heart disease. J Am Coll Cardiol 1986;8(6 Suppl B)41B-56B.

35

Chronic Pulmonary Thromboembolism and Pulmonary Hypertension

Gordon T. Ford, Sidney M. Viner, Brent R. Bagg, William R. Auger

INTRODUCTION

Chronic pulmonary thromboembolism (CPT) involving the major pulmonary vessels is being increasingly recognized as a cause of pulmonary hypertension. There have been recent advances in diagnostic modalities along with an increased awareness of the disorder and a better understanding of the pathophysiology. In the past, patients with this disease received only medical management for the secondary pulmonary hypertension including oxygen, vasodilator, fibrinolytic and anticoagulant therapy and occasionally vena caval interruption or filtering. It is now recognized that chronic thromboembolic pulmonary hypertension is amenable to surgical therapy, with a successful thromboendarterectomy offering the best chance of long term survival.[1–5]

HISTORICAL OVERVIEW

The concept of CPT was suspected at the turn of the century by Hart and Moller.[1] In 1928, Ljungdahl provided the first clinicopathological correlation describing two patients with progressive respiratory insufficiency and cor pulmonale. Both patients died of right ventricular failure. At autopsy, chronic emboli were demonstrated obstructing the proximal pulmonary arteries.[6] In the mid 1900s, there were several case reports of chronic cor pulmonale thought to be secondary to recurrent pulmonary emboli. In 1950, Carroll reported a series of five patients with this condition.[7] He provided the first detailed description of the clinical signs and symptoms and results of diagnostic tests including right ventricular catheterization and pulmonary angiography. One of the patients he described underwent surgical exploration by Blalock in 1948. This patient was found to have a large dilated main pulmonary artery and the completely occluded proximal left pulmonary artery was shown to contain organized thrombus on biopsy. Aspiration of the left pulmonary artery distal to the occlusion revealed bright red, free flowing blood. This observation confirmed earlier hypotheses that blood flow beyond proximally obstructed pulmonary arteries was maintained by bronchial artery collaterals.[1]

In 1908, Trendelenburg described a surgical treatment for acute pulmonary embolism (PE).[8] Subsequent case reports described different surgical approaches for chronic pulmonary thromboembolic disease but it was not until 1956 that Hollister et al, proposed pulmonary thromboendarterectomy as the favored approach.[9] He noted that the introduction of anticoagulant and enzyme therapy made possible some degree of prevention and control of thromboembolic disease. In 1957, Hurwitt et al, was the first to attempt endarterectomy on a patient with chronic PE.[10] Vena caval inflow occlusion and hypothermia were utilized. A large amount of organized embolic material was removed; unfortunately the patient died of an intraoperative cardiac arrest. Pioneering work performed by Snyder et al, in 1961 and Houk et al, in 1963, established that pulmonary endarterectomy was the treatment of choice for chronic PE due to the adherent and endothelialized nature of the organized thrombus.[11,12] The first reported procedure utilizing cardiopulmonary bypass to assist in the surgical approach was in 1964 by Castleman et al.[13] Over the next two decades the surgical procedure was perfected and by 1984 there were 85 patients who had been operated on throughout the world with an overall mortality of 20% to 25%.[1,14–21] Since that time, there have been over 300 more cases of pulmonary endarterectomy reported, with the vast majority coming from the UCSD Medical Center, San Diego, California.[2,22,23] (Figure 1)

From *Venous Thromboembolism: An Evidence-Based Atlas* edited by Russell Hull, Gary Raskob, Graham Pineo © 1996, Futura Publishing Co., Armonk, NY.

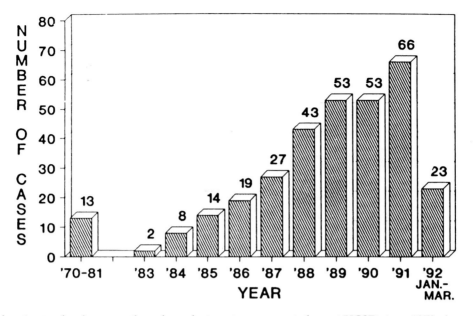

Figure 1. Number of patients of pulmonary thromboendarterectomy operated on at UCSD since 1970. Annualized projection for 1992 is 90 patients. (Reprinted with permission from Jamieson SW, Auger WR, Fedullo PF, et al. Experience and results with 150 pulmonary thromboendarterectomy operations over a 29-month period. J Thorac Cardiovasc Surg 1993;106:116–127.)

INCIDENCE OF RECURRENT UNRESOLVED PULMONARY EMBOLI

In the United States alone some 600,000 patients experience pulmonary embolus each year.[24–26] Approximately 50,000 of these patients die, but the majority of pulmonary emboli resolve spontaneously and result in either minimal or no symptoms or sequelae. Less than 5% of patients receiving anticoagulation have recurrent pulmonary emboli. These are generally patients who are insufficiently anticoagulated.

The fibrinolytic system is responsible for the resolution of large pulmonary emboli. In many instances, by six weeks emboli have been demonstrated to be reduced to vestigial strands. Complete resolution of pulmonary emboli usually occurs by 3 to 6 months, although up to 16% of patients have residual signs of chronic embolization pathologically.[1,27] The true incidence of pulmonary hypertension secondary to unresolved emboli is unknown, with estimates ranging from 0.1% to 2.0%.[2–4,19,20,28] Recently, Jamieson et al, have estimated that some 540 to 1080 patients of the 600,000 who experience pulmonary embolus each year go on to develop chronic thromboembolic pulmonary hypertension.[2]

NATURAL HISTORY OF CHRONIC PULMONARY EMBOLISM AND PULMONARY HYPERTENSION

The majority of patients surviving acute pulmonary embolus resolve both the acute embolus and the venous thrombotic site from which the embolus arose.[19,25] For as yet unexplained reasons, a minority of patients fail to achieve resolution of their emboli, which become organized, fibrotic masses obstructing proximal pulmonary arteries. The masses become endothelialized and part of the vessel wall. Some patients have minor residua, whereas others retain extensive vascular occlusion of the major (main, lobar, and segmental) pulmonary vessels. The pulmonary hypertension that develops as a result of these occlusive chronic thrombi may simply reflect a critical reduction in effective cross-sectional area for blood flow. It has recently been proposed that there is not necessarily such a direct correlation between the observed elevation in pulmonary vascular resistance and the degree of occluded pulmonary arteries. Over an unknown duration, in the nonoccluded pulmonary vascular bed, the relatively high flow of blood may incite secondary hypertension changes in the resistive or precapillary vessels. It may be these changes that play a substantial role in the eventual development of pulmonary hypertension.[4,29]

Depending upon the degree of pulmonary vascular obstruction patients may have no symptoms at rest or be extremely debilitated, dying prematurely as a direct result of their disease. Reidel has demonstrated that there is a strong correlation between survival and the severity of pulmonary hypertension.[30] (Figure 2)

Risk factors for the development of acute PE are also felt to be the predisposing factors for CPT and have been discussed elsewhere in this text. It has been hypothesized that the small number of patients who develop chronic disease may have defective fibrinolytic mechanisms, a hypercoagulable state, embolization of material that is already partially organized and thus less likely to undergo fibrinolysis or a chronic unrecognized source of recurrent embolization.

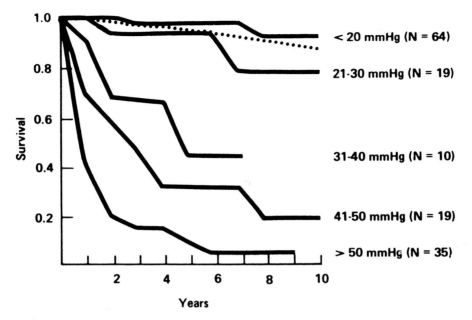

Figure 2. Cumulative survival curves in patients with pulmonary hypertension resulting from chronic pulmonary thromboembolism. Patient groups are compared at different mean pulmonary artery pressures. Dotted line represents predicted survival among men 40–50 years old. (Reprinted with permission as modified from Reidel M, Stanek V, Widinsky J, et al. Long-term follow-up of patients with pulmonary thromboembolism: late prognosis and evaluation of hemodynamic and respiratory data. Chest 1982;81:151–158.)

The pathology of chronic major vessel pulmonary thromboembolism has been well described.[31–33] On gross examination, ectatic main pulmonary arteries and/or lobar vessels may be completely occluded by firmly adherent, rubbery, laminated thrombus. In most patients, partial recanalization occurs resulting in the formation of intra-arterial cords, bands and webs. Organized thrombus becomes endothelialized and may grossly appear to be part of the arterial wall. Organized thrombus typically involves right and left main and lobar pulmonary arteries, often extending into segmental branches and beyond. In many patients both partially-organized and chronic emboli are simultaneously present.

Histologically the chronic thrombus consists of fibrinous organized networks firmly adherent to the vascular intima. Vascular bands and webs generally have an endothelial lining and may also be covered by more recently formed thrombus. Major pulmonary arteries often contain calcification and atherosclerotic intimal plaques. More distal, muscular pulmonary arteries may undergo medial hypertrophy and plexiform changes as seen in patients with primary pulmonary hypertension.[34] Pulmonary capillaries and venules are normal. Bronchial arteries become dilated and hypertrophied, forming collaterals which provide flow to the distal lung.

CLINICAL PRESENTATION

Chronic pulmonary thromboembolism is often misdiagnosed due to the infrequent number of cases and a general lack of awareness of the clinical entity. Symptoms are often of insidious onset and slowly progressive in nature. Less than half of all patients relate a past history of venous thrombosis or acute pulmonary embolus.[2–4] On questioning, patients may retrospectively recall a nonspecific event suggestive of a venous thrombotic event. The venous thrombotic event may have been diagnosed as a muscle strain or cellulitis, and the pulmonary embolic event diagnosed as pneumonia, pleurisy or some other disease entity.[3,4] A negative history of a prior venous thrombotic event cannot be used to exclude the diagnosis of chronic thromboembolic pulmonary hypertension.

Just as there is a wide spectrum in the degree of obstruction among patients, there is also a wide variety in their clinical presentations. Dyspnea is the most common presenting symptom. In the earliest stages of the disease, dyspnea may only occur on exertion and is often attributed to poor physical conditioning. Over time, pulmonary hypertension worsens and dyspnea will occur with minimal exertion and at rest. Patients may be symptomatic during the period of the acute embolic event, then enjoy a "honeymoon period" (a term coined by Moser) during which pulmonary hypertension is present, but symptoms are few. It is believed that during the "honeymoon period," compensatory right ventricular hypertrophy develops, allowing for maintenance of an adequate cardiac output, despite the presence of pulmonary hypertension and increased pulmonary vascular resistance.[4] Since pulmonary vascular resistance is relatively fixed, the increase in cardiac output that normally occurs during exertion results in further increases in pulmonary artery pressure causing symptoms that may not be present at rest.[35] Ultimately, the disease tends to be progressive with limitation of cardiac output producing symptoms of fatigue, presyncope and less commonly, syncope. Chest pain may be present and pleuritic in nature, or may be of the "six dermatome" pain also associated with myocardial ischemia.[36] This pain is thought to be caused by acute dilatation of the pulmonary outflow tract. Hemoptysis is uncommon.

The physical signs at presentation may be minimal or may include signs of overt pulmonary hypertension and cor pulmonale. In the later stages, jugular venous pressure is commonly elevated with a positive hepatojugular reflex. Precordial examination may reveal a right ventricular heave and a palpable pulmonary artery and P2. On auscultation, patients may have an increased P2 and murmurs associated with tricuspid insufficiency. Ejection systolic murmurs related to turbulent flow across the pulmonary valve also occur. There may be signs of right ventricular dysfunction including a right ventricular S3, S4 or summation gallop. With progressive right heart failure, a pulsatile liver and increasing peripheral edema may be present. Often the patients demonstrate peripheral and central cyanosis. Clubbing is uncommon. Characteristic of this disease are flow murmurs or bruits present over the major pulmonary arteries.[37,38] These high pitched and continuous bruits are augmented by respiration, and are believed to be related to flow through pulmonary arteries partially obstructed by organized thrombi. The bruits may be inaudible during respiration and may be only heard by having the patients hold their breath for short periods of time. They are similar to those heard in congenital branch stenosis of pulmonary arteries or with pulmonary AV fistulas. The lower extremities may show evidence of venous stasis including areas of hyperpigmentation.

INVESTIGATIONS

Noninvasive

The findings of the noninvasive investigations depend primarily on when, during the clinical course of the disease, they were obtained. Routine hematologic and blood chemistry studies are usually normal until chronic hypoxemia causes an increase in hematocrit and hemoglobin. Liver function tests may be abnormal in patients with severe right heart failure. Routine coagulation studies are typically unremarkable. Moser's group has identified the presence of a lupus anticoagulant identified in about 10% of patients, while < 1% manifest deficiencies of protein C, protein S or antithrombin III.[4] Patients with abnormalities of coagulation may relate a family history of thrombosis.

The chest roentgenogram can appear surprisingly unremarkable, especially in the early stages of the disease. The radiographic features of CPT were detailed by Fleischner in 1967.[39] Findings include an increased radiolucency of the vascular markings either of the entire lung or of localized areas. Areas of hyperperfusion may be seen and are often interpreted as interstitial fibrosis. Pulmonary hypertension is usually associated with bilateral enlargement of the pulmonary artery trunks at the hilum, which may be misinterpreted as hilar adenopathy. However, in CPT, the presence of organized thrombus in one or both main pulmonary arteries may prevent such enlargement. Therefore, if enlargement is not seen, or if it is asymmetrical in the presence of pulmonary hypertension, CPT should be among the diagnostic considerations. In addition, there may be pleural thickening related to residual or prior pulmonary emboli or infarction. As the course of the disease progresses, there will be evidence of right ventricular and right atrial enlargement. This is best demonstrated on the lateral roentgenogram. (Figure 3)

The resting electrocardiogram may be normal or may show abnormalities including sinus tachycardia, right axis deviation, P pulmonale or findings indicative of right ventricular hypertrophy or strain. Marked T wave inversion across the precordium may be due to right ventricular hypertrophy as opposed to anterior myocardial ischemia.

Pulmonary function tests are commonly ordered, as the presenting complaint of many patients is exertional dyspnea. The results are usually within normal limits. About 20% of patients will have a restrictive pulmonary defect with a reduction in lung volumes below 80% of that which was predicted.[40,41] It is thought that this restrictive defect may be due to a combination of pleural disease and small infarcts throughout the lower lobes. This finding often leads to the erroneous diagnosis of interstitial lung disease. The diffusing capacity for carbon monoxide may be within normal range or reduced secondary to ablation of the pulmonary vascular bed. Even with severe disease, patients may have normal or near normal diffusing capacities for carbon monoxide. It has been speculated that this is related to extensive bronchial artery collateral flow, which may be up to 10% of the cardiac output. This collateral flow may back perfuse into the capillary bed and achieve substantial carbon monoxide transfer.[4] In early disease, arterial blood gas testing at rest is often normal but oxygen desaturation may be demonstrated by exercise testing. With advanced disease resting arterial hypoxemia may be seen, related to ventilation perfusion abnormalities, and exacerbated by a reduction in cardiac output and mixed venous PO_2.[42]

Impedance plethysmography (IPG) or venous compression duplex ultrasound may be normal or may demonstrate evidence of proximal venous obstruction. In patients with severe pulmonary hypertension, the IPG may be bilaterally positive (falsely positive) due to the high central venous pressure.

In patients presenting with symptomatic disease, echocardiography studies will usually demonstrate signs

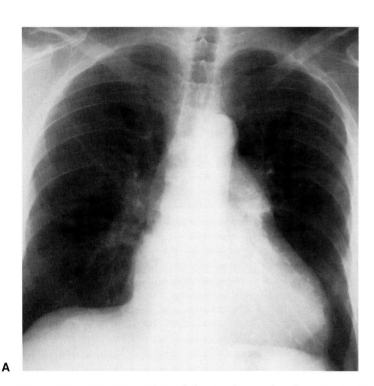
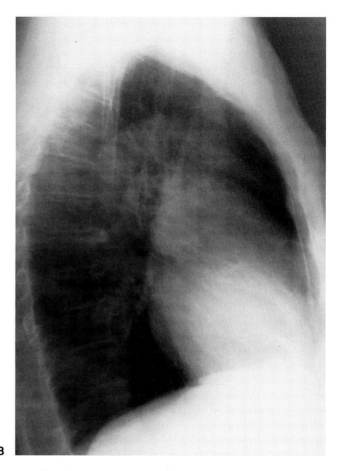

Figure 3A and B. PA and lateral chest radiographs of a patient with chronic thromboembolic pulmonary hypertension. Features include central pulmonary artery enlargement, increased vascular markings to both upper lobes with oligemia of the lower lung fields, cardiomegaly, and a prominent pulmonary outflow tract. The latter finding is best appreciated by "filling" of the retrosternal space on the lateral view.

of right atrial and right ventricular enlargement and right ventricular pressure overload. Tricuspid regurgitation is commonly present and allows for estimation of pulmonary artery systolic pressure. Cardiac echo is also useful to assess for thrombus in the right atrium or ventricle and to rule out other secondary causes of pulmonary hypertension such as occult atrial septal defect, or left atrial myxoma. Transesophageal echocardiography and bubble studies may be particularly useful in this regard.

The most directive noninvasive test for the diagnosis of chronic thromboembolic disease is the ventilation/perfusion lung scan. This has been shown to be a safe study even in the presence of severe pulmonary hypertension.[5] The lung scans of patients with CPT show at least one segmental sized or larger perfusion defect, with most patients showing several segmental or lobar defects bilaterally. (Figure 4) Perfusion defects are typically mismatched and significantly larger than any ventilation abnormalities. Patients with documented pulmonary hypertension and perfusion scans which are normal or show patchy, subsegmental abnormalities are more likely to have primary pulmonary hypertension. Thus the V/Q

scan provides a means of differentiating between these two disorders[43–45] It should be cautioned that the extent of perfusion defects cannot be used reliably to predict the severity of central vessel obstruction. Perfusion scans have been shown to consistently underestimate, often markedly, the degree of severity of large vessel obstruction and pulmonary hypertension.[46] Other conditions such as fibrosing mediastinitis or pulmonary arteritis may mimic the lung scan of CPT, underlining the importance of following up an abnormal lung scan with pulmonary angiography.[47,48]

Invasive Testing

Although noninvasive diagnostic tests are vitally important in the initial evaluation of patients with pulmonary hypertension, a definitive diagnosis of CPT can only be made on the basis of results from more invasive studies. Right heart catheterization is used to confirm the presence of pulmonary hypertension and define its severity. It must also be performed to rule out other causes of pulmonary hypertension such as left to right shunting or

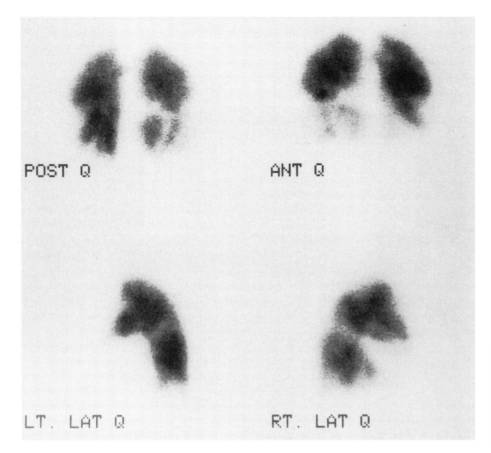

POST Q

ANT Q

LT. LAT Q

RT. LAT Q

Figure 4. Lung perfusion study of the same individual in Figure 3. Multiple segmental and subsegmental defects are apparent, principally involving both lower lobes, the right middle lobe and lingula. The ventilation scan (not shown) was normal.

postcapillary pulmonary hypertension. In the absence of left heart disease, the pulmonary capillary wedge pressure should be normal. However, wedge pressure can be difficult to measure accurately due to wedging of the pulmonary artery catheter in a proximal pulmonary artery partially or totally occluded by thrombus. The cardiac output should be measured and pulmonary vascular resistance calculated, as patients may have a misleadingly low pulmonary artery pressure due to a marked diminution of cardiac output. It has been found useful to exercise patients during right heart catheterization to see how well the right heart can augment cardiac output and the degree to which pulmonary vascular resistance is fixed.[35] It also provides information regarding left ventricular function. The absence of a substantial rise in pulmonary wedge pressure excludes the presence of significant left heart dysfunction.

The most valuable test for the diagnosis of CPT is pulmonary angiography. It not only confirms the diagnosis, but it also defines thrombus extent and location, thus determining the feasibility of thromboendarterectomy. Older reports had indicated high complication rates, including death, with pulmonary angiography in patients with severe pulmonary hypertension, particularly in those patients with right sided cardiac failure and right ventricular end diastolic pressures of > 20 mmHg.[49,50] These reports have caused a reluctance among physicians

to order this test for these patients. Recent studies, however, have shown that the procedure can be performed safely if several simple precautions are taken.[51] Catheterization should be performed via the brachial or internal jugular vein, or the patency of the femoral vein and inferior vena cava should be confirmed prior to advancement of the catheter to prevent inadvertent dislodgment of clot. Patients should be monitored and provided with supplemental oxygen. Finally, single injections of contrast media into the right and left main pulmonary arteries are used and repetitive injections avoided. Several recent studies have shown that even in patients with severe pulmonary hypertension, pulmonary angiography has a low mortality and morbidity risk associated with it. Mills et al, reported a 0.2% mortality and 4.5% complication rate in 1,350 studies done at Duke and in the Primary Pulmonary Hypertension Registry, the only complication in 50 patients undergoing pulmonary angiography was one episode of hypotension.[49,52] Nicod et al, reported minimal complications as a result of pulmonary angiography in 67 patients with primary or thromboembolic pulmonary hypertension even though the right ventricular end diastolic pressure was equal to or exceeded 20 mmHg in 14 of these patients.[51]

In assessing patients with suspected CPT, one injection is made into the right main pulmonary artery in the PA projection and one into the left main pulmonary artery in a slight left anterior oblique projection. These views provide clear visualization of the central pulmonary arteries (main, lobar, segmental) which are critical for determining thrombus accessibility. The smaller pulmonary arteries and the venous phase can often be visualized, but it is not as important to localize obstructions in the more distal arteries, as they are less likely to be amenable to surgical dissection. The use of nonionic contrast media make the injections less uncomfortable for the patient and may help to further reduce the risk.

The interpretation of these pulmonary angiograms can be difficult, particularly for angiographers unfamiliar with this disease. These images are significantly different from those seen in acute embolism, in which sharply bordered, rounded, well defined filling defects and cut-offs are the diagnostic standard.[53] Chronic thrombi appear in highly variable locations and the artery may recanalize in an unpredictable way, producing unusual radiographic images. Chronic thrombi are often incorporated into the arterial wall and often retract the vessel wall.[51,54] Obstructions in CPT present as bands or webs causing narrowed segmental pulmonary arteries, sometimes accompanied by poststenotic dilatation. Irregularities of intima, rounded termination of segmental branches, luminal narrowing of the central vessels and oddly shaped pulmonary arteries are reliable indicators of chronic emboli.[51,54,55] (Figure 5)

Left heart catheterization with evaluation of the coronary arteries may be performed to establish that left ventricular and atrial pressures are normal, and to rule out coexisting coronary artery disease. If significant coronary artery stenosis is found, it is often necessary to perform coronary artery bypass surgery in conjunction with pulmonary thromboendarterectomy in view of the prolonged bypass time and cardioplegia necessary to perform surgical thromboendarterectomy.

In the past, bronchial arteriography had been performed to determine if pulmonary artery branches were open beyond proximal obstructions to ensure operability. This is now felt to be unnecessary.[3]

In specialized centers, pulmonary fiberoptic angioscopy may be performed allowing direct visualization

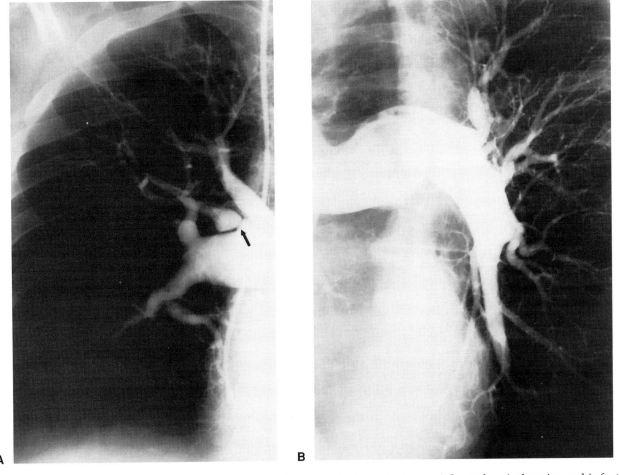

A **B**

Figure 5A and B. Pulmonary angiogram of the patient whose lung scan is shown in Figure 4. Several typical angiographic features of chronic thromboembolic disease include an abrupt narrowing of this patient's left descending pulmonary artery, several occluded right lower lobe vessels, a vascular "web" involving a right upper lobe artery (black arrow), and an irregularly contoured left upper lobar vessel. The main pulmonary arteries are also markedly enlarged.

of the pulmonary vascular bed.[56] This procedure is important prior to surgery where pulmonary angiographic findings do not clearly define the surgical accessibility of the chronic thromboemboli. Other procedures including intravascular ultrasound imaging, ultrafast computed tomographic scanning and magnetic resonance imaging are under investigation as imaging techniques to precisely define thrombus location.

TREATMENTS

Medical Treatment

There are significant limitations in the medical treatment of patients with severe chronic pulmonary thromboembolic hypertension. Medical therapy fails to address the basic underlying problems of fixed pulmonary vasculature obstruction causing increased right ventricular afterload eventuating in right heart failure. Nonetheless, not all patients are candidates for surgical therapy and in all patients it is important to institute measures to prevent further embolization of clot to the lung and to treat cor pulmonale. In patients with CPT, anticoagulation is immediately initiated and usually maintained for life. There is no role for the use of thrombolytic therapy as the clot within the lung is fibrotic and organized and often covered by a layer of endothelium. Insertion of an IVC filter is generally advisable, except in very rare patients where emboli are known to have originated in the upper extremities or right side of the heart or where IVC obstruction is shown to be present with venous return occurring via collaterals.[57] If hypoxemia is present, oxygen should always be administered. Adjuvant therapy for right heart dysfunction includes a low-salt diet and judicious use of loop diuretics and digoxin.

The role of pulmonary vasodilator therapy in patients with chronic pulmonary thromboembolic hypertension has yet to be defined. Vasodilators would not be expected to impact on the proximal, fixed pulmonary vascular obstruction. It is known, however, that if the pulmonary vasculature of "normal lung" is subjected to increased pressure or flow, secondary pulmonary hypertensive changes may develop. These changes include intimal hyperplasia, medial smooth muscle hypertrophy and obliterative fibrosis. They lead to further increases in pulmonary vascular resistance. There is increasing evidence that secondary hypertensive changes are related to endothelial cell dysfunction, accelerated growth of pulmonary vascular smooth muscle cells and vascular remodeling. Recent studies suggest that vasodilators such as prostacyclin, calcium channel blockers and nitric oxide may be of benefit in preventing and treating these secondary changes.[35,58–60] As in patients with primary pulmonary hypertension, if patients with secondary pulmonary hypertension due to CPT are given a trial of vasodilators, it should only be done with invasive

monitoring of pulmonary artery pressure and cardiac output. Pulmonary vasodilators would be considered to be of possible benefit if it was demonstrated that there was a fall in the pulmonary artery pressure with no significant fall in systemic blood pressure and no change or an increase in cardiac output. Experience in patients with primary pulmonary hypertension has shown that prostacyclin and nitric oxide are ideal agents for assessing acute vasodilator responses while orally administered calcium channel blockers are more suitable for long term therapy.[61,62] It should be emphasized that surgical thromboendarterectomy is the first line treatment for CPT. Medical therapy may play an adjunctive role, but must not delay surgical assessment and therapy.

Surgical Treatment

Pulmonary thromboendarterectomy is now established as the treatment of choice for selected patients with CPT. Criteria for selecting patients who are candidates to undergo pulmonary thromboendarterectomy are summarized in Table 1. Most patients referred for surgery have NYHA class III or IV dyspnea. Younger patients with a pulmonary vascular resistance < 300 dynes × sec × cm^{-5} and significant symptoms may also be taken for surgery. Thrombi must be accessible as defined by angiography or angioscopy, as current surgical techniques allow removal of chronic thrombi residing in main, lobar or segmental arteries. Severe right ventricular dysfunction is not a contraindication to surgery. If pulmonary vascular obstruction can be relieved successfully, right ventricular function improves dramatically.[63]

The surgical procedure has been well described elsewhere.[62] Most patients with CPT have significant disease involving both pulmonary arteries, only rarely will a patient present with total unilateral occlusion. Therefore, surgery is performed by median sternotomy to obtain bilateral exposure. The surgery has been done by thoracotomy, but bronchial collateral flow through the pleura and suboptimal exposure makes this approach more difficult. Surgery involves the use of cardiopulmonary bypass and periods of cardioplegia and deep hypothermia. This allows periods of circulatory arrest, permitting optimum visualization of the distal lobar and segmental ves-

Table 1
Selection Criteria for Thrombendarterectomy

1. Chronic thrombi judged to be surgically accessible
2. The absence of significant co-morbid disease
3. Pulmonary vascular resistance > 300 dynes × sec × cm^{-5}
4. Symptmatic, high dead space ventilation in the presence of surgically accessible chronic thrombi
5. A willingness of the patient and his family to accept the significant risks of surgery

sels. Care is taken to ensure cardiac cooling to 20° C while avoiding hypothermic injury to the phrenic nerves. The surgical technique involves removing the organized thrombus along with its lining of neointima while leaving the media and most of the original intima intact. (Figure 6) (See color figure on p. 298A) At present, the surgery is performed at a limited number of centers due to the complexities involved. In inexperienced hands, incomplete thromboendarterectomies have been performed leading to an inadequate postoperative pulmonary hemodynamic outcome. Chronic organized thrombus may be lined by a neointima that grossly appears very similar to the native intima; thus patients may be mistakenly thought to have less thrombus than is actually present. With experience, the "pits and ridges" characteristic of organized thrombus can be recognized. Careful dissection down to the native intima is imperative for an optimal surgical outcome.

The postoperative management of these patients can be difficult and complex. These patients are subject to the usual problems associated with open heart surgery including hemodynamic instability, cardiac arrhythmias, bleeding, electrolyte disturbance, infection, pericarditis, and pericardial effusion. They are also subject to unique problems specific to thromboendarterectomy, the most serious being reperfusion pulmonary edema. The major complications are listed in Table 2. Investigations into the cause of this edema are ongoing, but it seems to involve similar mediators implicated in other types of high-permeability lung injury.[64,65] The edema has been shown radiographically to involve lung areas distal to where organized thrombi have been dissected. Reports indicate that the edema may appear at any time after surgery, though typically within 72 hours postoperatively. Manifestations range in severity from acute hemorrhage with fatal consequences to mild edema associated with mild hypoxemia. As documented on lung scans, perfusion of the edematous areas continues, resulting in significant shunting and hypoxemia. Mechanical ventilation and increased oxygen concentrations for periods from a few days to a few weeks may be required to manage this lung injury. Corticosteroids have been used with observed clinical benefit.[4]

At the University of California, San Diego, anticoagulant therapy is started in the immediate postoperative period unless there are major bleeding problems. Almost all patients have an inferior vena caval filter inserted prior to surgery. Most patients are weaned and extubated within 3 days, discharged from ICU at 5 days and from hospital at 14 days following surgery.[4]

OUTCOMES

The vast majority of pulmonary thromboendarterectomies have been done at the University of California, San Diego. The largest published series on outcome are from this center. With increased experience and refinements in surgical techniques and perioperative management, operative mortality has dropped from 17% to 8.7%.[2] Although this mortality rate is relatively high, it reflects the critical status of many of these patients at the time they are referred for surgery. Many of the patients undergoing the operation are severely limited with New York Heart Association functional class IV dyspnea. Because patients with CPT and severe pulmonary hypertension have an extremely poor prognosis without surgery, few patients have been turned down on the basis of age or significant collateral disease. The presence of concomitant coronary artery disease, obstructive lung disease, renal or liver disease, or hematological abnormalities will influence perioperative mortality and long term outcome. Several patients with extreme hemodynamic instability have undergone surgery with a good outcome. Over the past several years, the two major causes of perioperative mortality are unrelenting reperfusion edema and persistent pulmonary hypertension, due to an inability to remove an adequate amount of thrombotic material.

Among survivors, substantial improvement is seen postoperatively. Hemodynamic results demonstrate a significant reduction in pulmonary vascular resistance, a decline in pulmonary artery pressure and an increase in cardiac output (Table 3).[2,4] This degree of hemodynamic improvement is sustained or improved long-term.[2,4] (Table 4) Postoperative echocardiograms reflect these he-

Table 2
Postoperative Complications

Delerium
Reperfusion pulmonary edema
Persistent pulmonary hypertension from the inability to remove sufficient thrombotic material at the time of surgery
Bleeding
Cardiac supraventricular arrythmias
Pleuro-pericarditis
Pericardial effusions

Table 3
Hemodynamic Results in 128 of 150 Patients in Whom Postoperative Values Were Obtained 48–72 Hours After Intensive Care Unit Admission (off all vasoactive agents)

	Preoperative	Postoperative
PA mean (mmHg)	47 ± 12	28 ± 9*
PA systolic (mmHg)	76 ± 21	47 ± 16*
CO (L/min)	3.7 ± 1.1	5.7 ± 1.2*
PVR (dynes × sec × cm^{-5})	901 ± 467	261 ± 163*

PA: pulmonary artery; CO: cardiac output; PVR: pulmonary vascular resistance. Values are mean ± SD. *: p < 0.0001 vs preoperative value. (Data from University of California, San Diego Medical Center. Reprinted with permission from Moser KM, Auger WR, Fedullo PF, Jamieson SW. Chronic thromboembolic pulmonary hypertension: clinical picture and surgical treatment. Eur Respir J 1992;5:334–342.)

Table 4
Hemodynamic Values Obtained in 47 of the First 150 Patients Who Returned For Follow-Up
Cardiac Catheterization at 6–24 Months After Surgery

	Preoperative	Postoperative	Follow-up
PA mean (mmHg)	48 ± 12	27 ± 8*	24 ± 10
PA systolic (mmHg)	80 ± 21	44 ± 15*	39 ± 17**
CO (L/min)	3.7 ± 1.17	6.0 ± 1.1*	4.8 ± 1.0†
PVR (dynes × sec × cm^{-5})	971 ± 551	232 ± 111*	282 ± 251

For abbreviations see table 3. *: p < 0.001 *vs* preoperative value; **: p < 0.0015 *vs* postoperative value; †: p < 0.0001 *vs* postoperative value. (Data from University of California, San Diego Medical Center. Reprinted with permission from Moser KM, Auger WR, Fedullo PF, Jamieson SW. Chronic thromboembolic pulmonary hypertension: clinical picture and surgical treatment. Eur Respir J 1992;5:334–342.)

modynamic changes. There is a reduction in right atrial and right ventricular size, a return of the interventricular septum to a normal position with loss of paradoxical motion and minimal or no tricuspid regurgitation.[63,66] On physical examination, signs of pulmonary hypertension and right heart failure quickly regress. Functionally, patients show significant improvement typically within a few weeks after surgery with continued improvement occurring over the ensuing 9 to 12 months. This further improvement is thought to be related to resolution of postoperative edema, anemia and the deconditioned state. At 12 months, 95% of patients are in NYHA Class I or II (Table 5).[4] Not unexpectedly, postoperative lung perfusion scans and angiography show marked improvements in perfusion. In a study of 34 postendarterectomy patients, cardiac catheterization and angiography results were either normal or showed minimal residual distal obstruction in one or more segmental artery.[3] In that group, only one patient failed to show significant restoration of vascular patency.

As previously noted, patients are maintained on lifelong anticoagulation therapy. Long-term follow-up of these patients (up to 18 years) has revealed only three patients who have suffered recurrent venous thrombosis, and in each case the patient had discontinued warfarin

therapy.[4] There have been no instances of thrombosis of the IVC filter during postdischarge follow-up.[3]

CPT can be quite silent until severe pulmonary hypertension and frank right heart failure occur, therefore, early diagnosis and subsequent management presents an ongoing challenge to clinicians. It is anticipated that with earlier recognition of this disease, followed by timely intervention, the surgical result and functional outcome of these patients can be further improved. Even as more is learned about this disease, many questions related to causation, pathogenesis, and therapy remain to be answered.

REFERENCES

1. Chitwood WR, Sabiston DC, Wechsler AS. Surgical treatment of chronic unresolved pulmonary embolism. Clin Chest Med 1984;5:507–536.
2. Jamieson SW, Auger WR, Fedullo PF, et al. Experience and results with 150 pulmonary thromboendarterectomy operations over a 29-month period. J Thorac Cardiovasc Surg 1993;106:116–127.
3. Moser KM, Auger WR, Fedullo PF. Chronic major vessel thromboembolic pulmonary hypertension. Circulation 1990;81:1735–1743.
4. Moser KM, Auger WR, Fedullo PF, et al. Chronic thromboembolic pulmonary hypertension: clinical picture and surgical treatment. Eur Respir J 1992;5:334–342.
5. Rich S, Sevitsky S, Brundage BH. Pulmonary hypertension from chronic pulmonary thromboembolism. Ann Intern Med 1988;108:425–434.
6. Ljungdahl M. Gibt es eine chronische embolistierung der lungen arterie? Dtsch Arch Klin Med 1928;102:1–23.
7. Carroll D. Chronic obstruction of major pulmonary arteries. Am J Med 1950;9:175–185.
8. Trendelenburg F. Ueber die operative behandlung der embolie der lungenarterie. Arch Klin Chir 1908;24:687–700.
9. Hollister LE, Cull VL. The syndrome of chronic thrombosis of the major pulmonary arteries. Am J Med 1956;21:312–320.
10. Hurwitt ES, Schein CJ, Rifkin H, et al. A surgical approach to the problem of chronic pulmonary artery obstruction due to thrombosis or stenosis. Ann Surg 1958;147:157–165.
11. Snyder WH, Kent DC, Baisch BF. Successful endarterectomy of chronically occluded pulmonary artery: clinical report and physiologic studies. J Thorac Cardiovasc Surg 1964;45:482–489.
12. Houk VN, Hufnagel CA, McClenathan JE, Moser KM. Chronic thrombosis obstruction of major pulmonary arter-

Table 5
New York Heart Association Functional Classification of 117 Patients of the First 150 Who Were Evaluated At One Year Following Surgery

Class	Preoperative	Follow-up
IV	63	0
III	49	6
II	5	26
I	0	85
Total	117	117

(Data from University of California, San Diego Medical Center. Reprinted with permission from Moser KM, Auger WR, Fedullo PF, Jamieson SW. Chronic thromboembolic pulmonary hypertension: clinical picture and surgical treatment. Eur Respir J 1992;5:334–342.)

ies. Report of a case successfully treated by thromboendarterectomy and review of the literature. Am J Med 1963;35:269–282.

13. Castleman B, McNeely BU, Scannell G. Case records of the Massachusetts General Hospital. Case 32–1964. N Engl J Med 1964;271:40–50.

14. Moser KM, Houk VN, Jones RC, Hufnagel CA. Chronic massive thrombotic obstruction of the pulmonary arteries: analysis of four operated cases. Circulation 1965;32:377–385.

15. Moser KM, Rhodes PG, Hufnagel CA. Chronic unilateral pulmonary-artery thrombosis: successful thromboendarterectomy with thirty-month follow-up. N Engl J Med 1965;272:1195–1199.

16. Moser KM, Braunwald NS. Successful surgical intervention in severe chronic thromboembolic pulmonary hypertension. Chest 1973;64:29–35.

17. Daily PO, Johnson GG, Simmons CJ, Moser KM. Surgical management of chronic pulmonary embolism: surgical treatment and late results. J Thorac Cardiovasc Surg 1980;79:523–531.

18. Utley JR, Spragg RG, Long WB 3rd, et al. Pulmonary endarterectomy for chronic thromboembolic obstruction: patient surgical experience. Surgery 1982;92:1096–1102.

19. Cabrol C, Cabrol A, Acar J, et al. Surgical correction of chronic postembolic obstruction of the pulmonary arteries. J Thorac Cardiovasc Surg 1978;76:620–628.

20. Dor V, Jourdan J, Schmitt R, Sabatier M, Arnulf JJ, et al. Delayed pulmonary thrombectomy via a peripheral approach in the treatment of pulmonary embolism and sequelae. Thorac Cardiovasc Surg 1981;29:227–232.

21. Sabiston DC, Wolfe WG, Oldham HN Jr, et al. Surgical management of chronic pulmonary embolism. Ann Surg 1977;185:699–712.

22. Lang SJ, Mulder DG. Thromboembolic obstruction of the pulmonary artery treated by endarterectomy. Ann Thorac Surg 1986;42:557–559.

23. Bengtsson L, Henze A, Homgren A, Bjork VO. Thromboendartectomy in chronic pulmonary embolism: Report of 3 cases. Scan J Thor Cardiovasc Surg 1986;20:67–70.

24. Moser KM. Venous thromboembolism. Am Rev Resp Dis 1990;141:235–249.

25. Benotti JR, Dalen JE. The natural history of pulmonary embolism. Clin Chest Med 1984;5:403–410.

26. Anderson FA, Wheeler HB, Goldberg RJ, et al. A population-based perspective of the hospital incidence and case-fatality rates of deep vein thrombosis and pulmonary embolism. Arch Intern Med 1991;151:933–938.

27. Freiman DG, Suyemoto J, Wessler S. Frequency of pulmonary thromboembolism in man. N Engl J Med 1965;272:1278–1280.

28. Presti B, Berthrong M, Sherwin M. Chronic thrombosis of major pulmonary arteries. Hum Pathol 1990;21:601–606.

29. Moser KM, Bloor CM. Pulmonary vascular lesions occuring in patients with chronic major vessel thromboembolic pulmonary hypertension. Chest 1993; 103:685–692.

30. Riedel M, Stanek V, Widinsky J, Prevosky I. Long-term follow-up of patients with pulmonary thromboembolism: late prognosis and evaluation of hemodynamic and respiratory data. Chest 1982;81:151–158.

31. Korn D, Gore I, Blenke A, Collins DP. Pulmonary arterial bands and webs: an unrecognized manifestation of organized pulmonary emboli. Am J Pathol 1962;40:129–151.

32. Scully RE, Mark EJ, McNeely BU. Case records of the Massachusetts General Hospital. N Engl J Med 1981;305:685–793.

33. Wagenvoort CA, Wagenvoort N. Pathology of Pulmonary Hypertension. New York, John Wiley and Sons, 1977.

34. Moser KM, Bloor CM. Pulmonary vascular lesions occurring in patients with chronic major vessel thromboembolic pulmonary hypertension. Chest 1993;103:685–692.

35. Fedullo PF, Auger WR, Moser KM, Watt CN, Buchbinder M, et al. Hemodynamic response to exercise in patients with chronic, major vessel thromboembolic pulmonary hypertension. Am Rev Resp Dis 1990;141:A890.(Abstract)

36. DeGowin EL, DeGowin RL. Bedside Diagnostic Examination. New York, Macmillan Pub Co., Inc., pp. 235, 1981.

37. Auger WR, Moser KM. Pulmonary flow murmurs: A distinctive physical sign found in chronic pulmonary thromboembolic disease. Clin Res 1989;37:145A.(Abstract)

38. Perloff JK. Ausculatory and phonocardiographic manifestations of pulmonary hypertension. Prog Cardiovasc Dis 1967;9(4):303–340.

39. Fleischner FG. Recurrent pulmonary embolism and cor pulmonale. N Engl J Med 1967;276:1213–1220.

40. Horn M, Ries AL, Neveu C, Moser KM. Restrictive ventilatory pattern in precapillary pulmonary hypertension. Am Rev Resp Dis 1983;128:163–165.

41. Ryan KL, Fedullo PF, Clausen J, Moser KM. Pulmonary function in chronic thromboembolic pulmonary hypertension. Am Rev Resp Dis 1986;84:679–683.

42. Kapitan KS, Buchbinder M, Wagner PD, Moser KM, Mechanism of hypoxemia in chronic thromboembolic pulmonary hypertension. Am Rev Resp Dis 1989;139:1149–1154.

43. Hull RD, Hirsh J, Carter CJ, et al. Pulmonary angiography, ventilation lung scanning, and venography for clinically suspected pulmonary embolism with abnormal perfusion lung scan. Ann Intern Med 1983;98:891–899.

44. D'Alonzo GE, Bower JS, Dantzker DR. Differentiation of patients with primary and thromboembolic pulmonary hypertension. Chest 1984;85:457–461.

45. Fishman AJ, Moser KM, Fedullo PF. Perfusion lung scans versus pulmonary angiography in evaluation of suspected primary pulmonary hypertension. Chest 1983;84:679–683.

46. Ryan KL, Fedullo PF, David GB, Vasquez TE, Moser KM. Perfusion scans underestimate the severity of angiographic and hemodynamic compromise in chronic thromboembolic pulmonary hypertension. Chest 1988;93:1180–1185.

47. Berry DF, Buccigrossi D, Peabody J, et al. Pulmonary vascular occlusion and fibrosing mediastinitis. Chest 1986;89:296–301.

48. Lupi E, Sanchez G, Horwitz S, Gutierrez E. Pulmonary arteritis involvement in Takayasu's arteritis. Chest 1975;67:69–74.

49. Mills SR, Jackson DC, Older RA, et al. The incidence, etiologies and avoidence of complications of pulmonary angiography in a large series. Radiology 1980;136:295–299.

50. Perlmutt LM, Braum SD, Newman GE, et al. Pulmonary arteriography in the high-risk patient. Radiology 1987;162:187–189.

51. Nicod P, Moser KM, Peterson KL, et al. Pulmonary angiography in severe pulmonary hypertension. Ann Intern Med 1987;107:565–568.

52. Rich S, Dantzker DR, Ayers SM, et al. Primary pulmonary hypertension: A natural prospective study. Ann Int Med 1987;107:216–223.

53. Greenspan RH. Angiography in pulmonary embolism. In Abrams HL, (ed.) Angiography: vascular and interventional radiology. 3rd ed. Boston, Little Brown, pp. 803–816, 1983.

54. Owen WR, Thomas WA, Castleman B, et al. Unrecognized emboli to the lungs associated with subsequent cor pulmonale. N Engl J Med 1953;249:919–926.

55. Auger WR, Fedullo PF, Moser KM, Buchbinder M, Peterson KL. Chronic major-vessel thromboembolic pulmonary artery obstruction: appearance at angiography. Radiology 1992; 182:393–398.

56. Shure D, Gregoratos G, Moser KM. Fiberoptic angioscopy: Role in the diagnosis of chronic pulmonary arterial obstruction. Ann Intern Med 1985;103:844–850.

57. Greenfield LJ, Scher LA, Elkins RC. KMA-Greenfield filter placement for chronic pulmonary hypertension. Ann Surg 1979;93:170–175.

58. Adnot S, Kouyoumdjian C, Eddahibi S, et al. Continuous inhalation of nitric oxide protects against developments of pulmonary hypertension in chronically hypoxic rats. Am Rev Resp Dis 1993;147:A494.(Abstract)

59. Serraf A, Labat C, Herve P, et al. Surgical model of pulmonary hypertension in the neonatal piglet: hemodynamic, morphological and endothelial features. Am Rev Resp Dis 1993;147:A496.(Abstract)

60. Schiller L, Ward H, Archer S, et al. Endothelial dysfuntion in a canine model of high flow pulmonary hypertension. Am Rev Resp Dis 1993;147:A497.(Abstract)

61. Rich S, Brundage BH. High-dose calcium channel blocking therapy for primary pulmonary hypertension: evidence for long-term reduction in pulmonary arterial pressure and regression of right ventricular hypertrophy. Circulation 1987;76:135–141.

62. Pepke-Zaba J, Higenbottam TW, Dinh-Xuan AT, et al. Inhaled nitric oxide as a cause of selective pulmonary vasodilation in pulmonary hypertension. Lancet 1991;338: 1173–1174.

63. Chow LC, Dittrich HC, Hoit BO, et al. Doppler assessment of changes in right-sided cardiac hemodynamics after pulmonary thromboendarterectomy. Am J Cardiol 1988;61: 1092–1097.

64. Levinson RM, Shure D, Moser KM. Reperfusion pulmonary edema following pulmonary artery thromboendarterectomy. Am Rev Res Dis 1986;134:1241–1245.

65. Auger WR, Smith RM, Spragg, RG. Protease release and antiprotease inactivation in a clinical model of acute high permeability lung injury. Am Rev Resp Dis 1988;137:A146.(Abstract)

66. Dittrich HC, Nicod PH, Chow LC, et al. Early changes of right heart geometery after pulmonary thromboendarterectomy. J Am Coll Cardiol 1988;11:937–943.

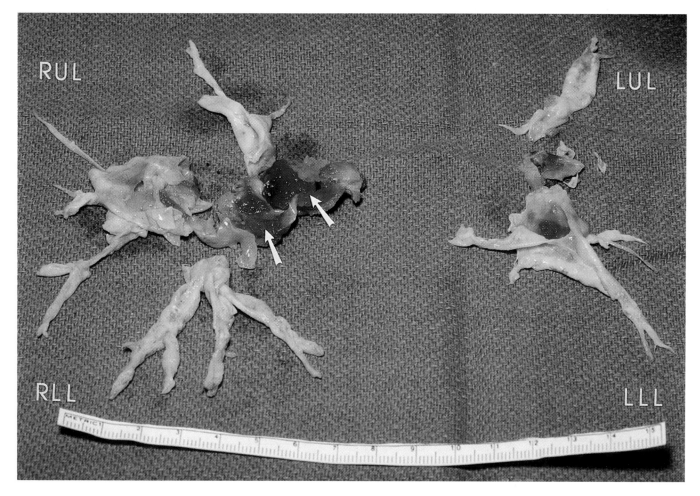

Figure 6. Chronic thrombi removed by surgical endarterectomy in the patient. A small amount of partially-organized thrombus (arrows) lines the fibrotic, organized material which involved the right main pulmonary artery.

36

Congenital and Acquired Hypercoagulable States

Philip C. Comp

INTRODUCTION

A variety of patients suffer from recurrent venous thromboembolic disease. Some of these patients not only have a personal history of thrombophlebitis and pulmonary embolism (PE), but also have a family history of these conditions. In these patients it is increasingly possible to identify biochemical abnormalities in the blood coagulation system associated with the development of thrombosis.

Other patients develop thromboembolism in particular high-risk clinical settings, such as the postoperative surgical period. While no specific coagulation marker can specifically identify these patients before developing the blood clots, a variety of changes in the coagulation system do occur in these settings. These subtle alterations in the balance between hemorrhage and thrombosis may be involved in triggering clot formation. Unlike the hereditary hypercoagulable states, these acquired conditions combine not just a single coagulation abnormality but encompass a variety of physical changes as well. These include immobility and local vein trauma, which can create additional predisposition to blood clot formation.

The biochemistry of the clotting factors involved in hereditary and acquired hypercoagulable states has been the subject of frequent excellent reviews and will not be reiterated here, other than to outline basic principles of the relevant coagulation mechanisms.[1–5]

Advances in our understanding of blood clotting now allow the identification of an underlying hereditary cause of thrombosis in a minimum of 10% of patients with recurring thromboembolic disease. As will be discussed, the recent identification of an inherited defect characterized by an insensitivity to the anticoagulant effect of activated protein C may explain the propensity to thrombosis in an even higher percentage of such patients. Besides these abnormalities, other abnormalities of the blood clot

lysis system also contribute to inherited venous thrombosis.

As a complicating factor, a variety of acquired clinical conditions can result in acquired deficiencies of the plasma proteins involved in hereditary thrombosis. Therefore, while providing assurance in certain cases to the physician and patient that an explanation exists for recurrent thrombosis, the use of newly developed laboratory tests to screen for these inherited abnormalities presents a new set of clinical problems. Specifically, a variety of medical conditions result in acquired abnormalities of these clinical parameters. This can lead to the overdiagnosis of inherited disease in acutely ill individuals. Secondly, the proper clinical use of these test results has yet to be demonstrated, especially in the proper treatment of asymptomatic deficient individuals and the optimal duration of treatment of affected individuals with a single episode of venous thrombosis.

Other acquired coagulation associated abnormalities are found in patients with venous thrombosis. These are the lupus anticoagulant and anticardiolipin antibodies. Both these conditions are characterized by antibodies in the blood which interfere with blood clotting tests or bind to negatively charged phospholipids. The need for prospective demonstration of the thrombotic risk imposed by these antibodies remains a major area of interest in clinical coagulation.

HEREDITARY DEFECTS ASSOCIATED WITH RECURRENT VENOUS THROMBOSIS

The blood clotting system in the body may be divided into three sets of plasma proteins. First are the blood clotting factors that by way of both the intrinsic and extrinsic clotting pathway produce blood clots. The second system consists of natural anticoagulant proteins

From *Venous Thromboembolism: An Evidence-Based Atlas* edited by Russell Hull, Gary Raskob, Graham Pineo © 1996, Futura Publishing Co., Armonk, NY.

which prevent blood clot formation and hold the clotting system in check. The third system consists of the fibrinolytic proteins which dissolve clots once they are formed. The hereditary absence of a blood clotting protein, such as factor VIII, results in a bleeding diathesis, whereas a deficiency for the natural anticoagulant proteins predisposes to uncontrolled blood clot formation. Unfortunately, deficiencies of anticoagulant proteins do not affect routinely used coagulation tests. This significantly delayed the discovery of these abnormalities.

The best characterized deficiencies of the natural anticoagulant proteins are antithrombin III (ATIII), protein C and protein S. The most recent abnormality predisposing to thrombosis involves abnormal factor V molecules. Factor V plays not only a critical role in blood clot formation, but, as does protein S, serves as a cofactor for the anticoagulant effects of activated protein C. In the thrombophiliacs who inherit this abnormality, the clotting promoting function of factor V functions correctly but the ability to potentiate the anticoagulant activity of activated protein C is missing.

Antithrombin III Deficiency

Antithrombin III deficiency was the first abnormality identified with recurrent venous and arterial thrombosis.[6–9] Antithrombin III functions in concert with heparin to inhibit the vitamin K-dependent clotting factors when they are in the enzymatically active forms (e.g., Factor Xa). The frequency with which thromboembolic events occur in deficient patients varies with the baseline level of ATIII. The lower the level of ATIII, the higher the frequency of thromboembolic events. Antithrombin III deficiency frequently present with their first thromboembolic event between puberty and middle age with median age of onset of 27 years. Approximately half of the thromboembolic events appear spontaneously, while the remainder are associated with conditions of increased risks such as pregnancy and surgery. Antithrombin III deficiency is more common than previously supposed. Recent studies have demonstrated that ATIII levels <50% are present in approximately one in 200 to one in 500 individuals in the normal population.[10,11] The vast majority of these deficient individuals do not have venous thrombosis.

Protein C Deficiency

Protein C is a vitamin K-dependent plasma protein. On the endothelial cell surface, the clotting enzyme thrombin binds to a receptor protein thrombomodulin and the bound thrombin then converts protein C to activated protein C.[3,12] Activated protein C functions as an anticoagulant, by inhibiting the clotting cascade at the levels of factor V and factor VII.

Hereditary protein C deficiency is associated with recurrent venous thrombosis. The majority of deficient individuals have a heterozygous deficiency state with protein C levels of between 50% and 65% in normal individuals. Homozygous deficient infants with essentially no detectable protein C develop a severe thrombotic condition termed purpura fulminans neonatalis.[13,14] This condition occurs shortly after birth and is characterized by extensive thrombosis in the small veins of the skin. This results in large necrotic areas of the skin and underlying fatty tissue. The heterozygous deficient individuals have much milder thrombotic complications, primarily venous thrombosis.

Two distinct types of protein C heterozygous-deficient kindreds exist. The majority of protein C-deficient kindreds do not exhibit venous thrombosis.[15] Affected families may be relatively common because the frequency of protein C deficiency is relatively high and may be present in as many as one out of every 250 people in the normal population. The latter figure is conservative since it is based on antigenic measurements of protein C alone and does not account for other individuals in the population who may have functionally abnormal protein C molecules or who may already be on chronic oral anticoagulation and therefore cannot be tested.

The second, or symptomatic, type of protein C-deficient families have a high incidence of thromboembolic complications, typically venous thrombosis of the leg veins. There is to date no biochemical or genetic difference between these two types of families. The reason one type of family develops venous thrombosis while the other does not, is not clear. The coinheritance of another trait predisposing to thrombosis may play a role. However, the autosomal dominant nature of the inheritance pattern indicated that the two coinherited traits would need to be very tightly linked.

Coumarin induced skin (or tissue) necrosis has been associated with protein C deficiency,[16] as well as deficiencies of protein S[17] and ATIII.[18] Coumarin necrosis is a rare condition characterized by necrosis of the skin and underlying fatty tissue shortly after the initiation of oral anticoagulant therapy.[19] The association with deficiencies of the natural anticoagulant proteins is thought to occur due to the rapid decrease in protein C following the initiation of such therapy. During this initial 12 to 18-hour period, the antithrombotic effects of the protein C system are lost before the patient is fully anticoagulated, and blood clot formation occurs in the small venules of the skin. Such a drop in protein C occurs in all individuals undergoing oral anticoagulation, but the hypercoagulable state may be exaggerated in protein C deficient individuals, as is the case with purpura fulminans neonatalis associated with homozygous protein C deficiency. Why the skin is the target organ for this intravascular clot formation is unknown. Coumarin necrosis occurs most frequently in the setting of acute deep-vein thrombosis (DVT).[20] The majority of patients who develop coumarin necrosis do not have a demonstrable underlying abnormality of the natural anticoagulant proteins. An association with hereditary activated protein C resistance has not yet been demonstrated.

Measurement of Protein C Levels

Laboratory measurement of protein C is relatively straightforward. However, care must be taken in interpretation of results obtained from patients on oral anticoagulation. Protein C is a vitamin K-dependent plasma protein; therefore, the levels of protein C normally drop during oral anticoagulation. This makes the measurement of protein C in such patients difficult and, while various measures have been proposed to estimate the baseline protein C data of such individuals, the results must be regarded as an estimate of baseline protein C status. Obtaining protein C levels at a time when the patient is no longer on oral anticoagulation is the useful approach, as is measuring protein C levels of other family members who are not on chronic anticoagulation.

Care must be taken not to overinterrupt the protein C levels that are obtained in critically ill individuals.[21] Low protein C levels have been found in conditions such as sepsis or extensive trauma, and do not indicate an underlying hereditary deficiency. Acquired protein C deficiency has been well documented in bacterial sepsis[22] and this has resulted in the therapeutic use of protein C concentrate in these settings. The acquired protein C deficiency is associated with purpuric skin lesions which respond rapidly to administration of the protein C concentrate.

Protein S Deficiency

Protein S is a vitamin K-dependent plasma protein which serves as a cofactor for anticoagulant effects of activated protein C.[23] Patients deficient in protein S appear very similar to those with a deficiency in protein C and are at risk of recurrent venous thrombosis and PE.[24,25] Unlike protein C deficiency, no protein S deficient kindreds have been identified who are completely free of thromboembolic complications.

Protein S differs from the other vitamin K-dependent plasma proteins in that two forms of protein S are found in normal plasma.[26] Free protein S serves as the cofactor for activated protein C, an inhibitor of the classic complement pathway. The protein S which is bound to C4b-binding protein is functionally inactive. Heterozygous protein S deficiency can result in approximately 50% of protein S is bound to C4b-binding protein, an inhibitor of the classic complement pathway. The protein S which is bound to C4b-binding protein is functionally inactive. Heterozygous protein S deficiency can result in approximately 50% of the normal level of total protein S and a corresponding reduction of free protein S levels, but a disproportionate amount of protein S is bound to C4b-binding protein with a resulting low level of free protein S.[27]

C4b-binding protein is an acute phase protein and abrupt shifts in the level of protein S from the free (active) to the bound (inactive) form can occur during an inflammatory events as the level of C4b-binding protein rises. Whether this transient shift in protein S results in thrombotic complications is unknown. However, this shift does cause difficulty in the diagnosis of protein S in the acutely ill individuals, since free protein S levels may be transiently reduced. Caution must be employed in making a diagnosis of hereditary protein S deficiency based on simple plasma determinations. Again, as with protein C deficiency, measuring the protein S levels of other family members not receiving oral anticoagulation may be useful.

Two other plasma protein disorders have been associated with recurrent venous thrombosis: plasminogen deficiency and abnormal fibrinogen molecules. Plasminogen is converted to the active enzyme plasmin by tissue plasminogen activator and the resulting plasmin enzymatically degrades fibrin clots. If the plasminogen molecules are abnormal or missing, inadequate clot lysis occurs and thrombophlebitis results since the body cannot eliminate growing clots. Structurally abnormal fibrinogen molecules can also result in blood clot accumulation. The abnormal fibrinogen is converted to structurally abnormal fibrin clot which is not subject to normal fibrinolysis. This resistance to fibrinolysis is thought to result in clot propagation.

Plasminogen abnormalities can be detected by laboratory testing. Fibrinogen abnormalities are more difficult to detect and involve testing for fibrinogen which does not clot at the normal rate (i.e., the thrombin clotting time is prolonged). This test obviously may miss potential fibrinogen abnormalities which affect the rate of fibrinolysis but not the rate of clot formation.

Hereditary Resistance to Activated Protein C

A new inherited coagulation defect which is associated with the development of venous thrombosis has recently been identified[28]. The plasma of affected individuals is not anticoagulated by activated protein C, although protein S is functioning properly. This resistance to the anticoagulant effects of activated protein C is inherited as an autosomal dominant trait. The inherited defect involves coagulation factor V.[29] In addition to the role of factor V as a vital component of the clotting cascade, Factor V also serves as a potent cofactor for the anticoagulant effect of activated protein C in plasma clotting assays. In patients resistant to activated protein C, adding purified factor V corrects the lack of responsiveness to activated protein C. While binding of activated protein C to factor V has been recognized in the past,[30] it is not known if this molecular event correlates with the enhancement of activated protein C anticoagulant activity. Protein S also serves as a cofactor for activated protein C, but is normal in the activated protein C resistant individuals. This defect in the protein C system was initially identified in 33% of patients with recurrent and/or familial venous thrombosis.[31] In a cohort of 301 unselected consecutive patients under 70 years of age presenting with their first episode of documented DVT, resistance to activated protein C was found in 21%.[32] A small series of highly selected thrombophilic patients demonstrated the abnormality in half the patients studies[33] as well as in two of 22 patients with concomitant protein C or protein S deficiency. Approximately 5% to 7% of the normal population also carry this trait,[31,32] suggesting that factors other than this trait alone are necessary for the development of thrombosis. The finding of resistance to activated protein C in patients with systemic lupus erythematosus who have thrombosis[34] has prompted speculation that autoantibodies may arise in lupus patients to induce an acquired resistance to activated protein C.[33]

This newly postulated role for factor V as not only a procoagulant but also as a potent participant in the protein C anticoagulant pathway, may explain why a significant number of patients with severe plasma factor V deficiency do not bleed.[35] In such patients, the bleeding tendencies induced by low levels of factor V could be balanced by the clot forming tendencies resulting from the factor V-dependent activated protein C resistance. Disseminated intravascular coagulation has been reported in association with acquired antibodies directed against factor V[36]; this intravascular coagulation may reflect the loss of regulation of the coagulation cascade by the protein C system, as has been reported in protein C deficiency states.[37–39] Future considerations of the treatment of disseminated intravascular coagulation should involve increased emphasis on replenishing factor V, which may have a major effect on restoring hemostatic balance.

At present, laboratory tests to measure resistance to activated protein C are not licensed for clinical use in the United States. However, the assay is technically easy to perform and is available in an increasing number of research reference laboratories.

ACQUIRED DEFICIENCIES OF THE NATURAL ANTICOAGULANT PROTEINS

Acquired deficiencies of the natural anticoagulant proteins can occur. Since protein C, protein S and ATIII are all produced in the liver, severe liver disease can decrease the levels of these proteins. Both protein C and protein S are vitamin K-dependent plasma proteins and are decreased in vitamin K deficiency and during the administration of oral anticoagulants. During disseminated intravascular coagulation, the levels of protein C, protein S and ATIII drop, presumably because they are consumed in the intravascular clotting process.

Table 1
Frequency of Natural Anticoagulant Deficiencies

	Thrombophiliacs	Normals
Antithrombin III	2%	0.2%
Protein C	4%	0.5%
Protein S	5%	?
ACP Resistance	20–30%	5–7%
Total	31–41%	6–8%

* The relative percentage of a given abnormality will increase as the number of patients with a strong family history of recurrent thrombosis increases. (Modified from 82).

Acquired Protein S Deficiencies

The best characterized acquired deficiency of protein S is that seen during normal pregnancy.[40–42] Both the total and free levels of protein S decrease significantly during pregnancy and can drop to as low as 40% of the normal level. This decrease in protein S may represent a protective mechanism to help insure that hemorrhage does not occur during pregnancy. The decrease in this natural anticoagulant protein is accompanied by an elevation of plasminogen activator inhibitor II, which results in inhibition of the fibrinolytic system, with a resulting decrease in the body's ability to dissolve blood clots. To determine whether or not the relative protein S deficiency is a risk factor for thrombophlebitis, which occurs as frequently as 1:1200 pregnancies, would require an extensive prospective study. The predictable decrease in protein S during pregnancy makes measurement of this natural anticoagulant difficult during pregnancy. At present there are no standard criteria for making the diagnosis of hereditary protein S deficiency during pregnancy. Decreased levels of protein S have been reported in diabetes mellitus[43–47] in the majority of studies. Decreased levels of free protein S have been observed in sickle cell disease,[48] as well as in a variety of severely ill hospitalized patients.[21] Decreased protein S levels are found in patients with the acquired immune deficiency syndrome.[49,50] The mechanism responsible for decreased protein S levels in these conditions is not known, but may include decreased hepatic synthesis of protein S, as well as a shift of protein S from the free to the bound form due to an elevation of C4b-binding protein. The contribution low protein S levels make to the thrombotic complications associated with these conditions is also unknown and will require prospective examination.

Free protein S deficiency is found in patients with acute stroke.[51–62] Evidence for the transient nature of free protein S deficiency has been provided in a study which examined stroke patients at times well after the acute event. Free protein S levels were not significantly decreased, compared to other hospitalized patients.[63] This suggests that the acute changes seen in the protein S sta-

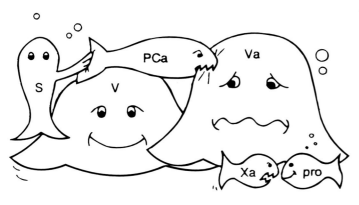

Figure 1. A fanciful marine depiction of the final step in blood coagulation. Activated factor V (V_a) is positioning factor X_a so that factor X_a can convert prothrombin (pro) to thrombin, which will then convert fibrinogen to fibrin to form a clot. Factor V_a is disturbed because activated protein C (PCa) is about to take a bite out of factor V_a and make it drop prothrombin and factor X_a. Thus anticoagulation will occur and a clot will not form. Activated protein C cannot do this difficult job alone and must stand on the back of another factor V molecular and must receive a helping shove from protein S in order to bite factor V_a. If protein S is absent (protein S deficiency) or the factor V has an abnormal back preventing activated protein C from gaining a foothold (activated protein C resistance), activated protein C cannot bite factor V_a. Anticoagulation does not take place, and unwanted blood clots form.

tus revert to normal as the acute inflammatory effects of the stroke resolve. Also, a high incidence of stroke is not reported in families with hereditary protein S deficiency, again suggesting that the changes seen following stroke are acquired. The possibility that acutely decreased free protein S levels may contribute to further extension of the stroke needs further examination.

ANTIBODIES AGAINST PHOSPHOLIPID

Antibodies directed against phospholipid are present in the plasma of certain patients with a history of thrombosis. There are two distinct types of these antibodies—the lupus anticoagulant and antiphospholipid antibodies. The antibodies are defined by the laboratory tests used to detect them. The lupus anticoagulant is an immunoglobulin which binds to the phospholipid used in clotting assays. As a result of this binding the phospholipid is no longer able to catalyze the clotting reaction and the clotting time is prolonged. For example, the activated partial thromboplastin time is prolonged from a normal of 29 seconds to 58 seconds. Antiphospholipid antibodies are identified by their ability to bind to immobilized negatively changed phospholipids (for example, cardiolipin and phosphatidylserine) in an enzyme-linked immunoassay.

In patients there is a significant overlap in these anti-

bodies. Approximately one-third of patients will have lupus anticoagulant only, one-third will have both lupus anticoagulant and antiphospholipid antibodies, and the remaining third will have antiphospholipid antibody alone.[64] These antibodies are seen in patients with systemic lupus erythematosus, acute infections including HIV,[65] malignancy,[66] in association with various medications including cardiac medications and major tranquillizer, in normal individuals, as well as in individuals with a history of arterial and venous thrombosis.[67,68] An association between anticardiolipin antibodies and spontaneous abortions is recognized.[69]

The association between the presence of the lupus anticoagulant and venous and arterial thrombosis has been observed.[67,68,70] Unfortunately, these observations have been based on a limited number of cases reviewed retrospectively; the lupus anticoagulant has been detected after the thrombotic complication occurred. Antiphospholipid antibodies have also been detected in patients with venous thrombosis and in patients with stroke. However, again these antibodies are detected after the clinical event. Given the high frequency in which the lupus anticoagulant and antiphospholipid antibodies are observed in systemic lupus erythematosus patients (an average prevalence of 34% and 44%, respectively[62]), if the antibodies carry a high risk for the development of thrombotic complications, such events should be more common in this population than is currently observed clinically. This does not appear to be the case. Similarly, both antibodies are detected in other disease groups, as well as in normal individuals. A markedly increased risk of thrombotic complications is not clinically apparent in these individuals. The absence of thrombotic complications in patients who develop antiphospholipid antibodies in response to medication or acute infection, further brings into question a causal relationship between these antibodies and the development of thrombosis. Clinical definition of the risk imposed by the lupus anticoagulant and antiphospholipid antibodies will require prospective study, preferably in a large nonselected population. Such a study would help determine if the lupus anticoagulant and antiphospholipid antibodies have a causal relationship to thrombosis or are epiphenomena with thrombotic complications.

CANCER AND VENOUS THROMBOSIS

Cancer patients are prone to the development of thromboembolism and a variety of procoagulant mechanisms may be at work in cancer patients which predispose to blood clot formation.[71-73] The occurrence of DVT in middle aged or older individuals should raise the clinical suspicion of a possible underlying malignancy.[74-78] At present there is no consensus of how extensive the search for a hidden cancer should be in such patients. At a minimum, a chest x-ray, stool guaiac, and thorough pelvic examination for female patients should be carried out in addition to a comprehensive physical examination.

TESTING FOR UNDERLYING CAUSES OF THROMBOSIS

An initial work-up for an underlying abnormality should include determination of protein S, protein C, ATIII, and soon, activated protein C resistance.[79,80] Ideally, a plasma sample should be obtained from a patient presenting with venous thrombosis prior to the initiation of heparin and oral anticoagulation. On this sample, a baseline activated partial thromboplastin time should be obtained. This will detect the possibility of a lupus anticoagulant and will prevent basing heparin therapy on a prolonged, preheparin, APTT. If a patient has an undetected baseline activated partial thromboplastin time of 80 seconds, the administration of intravenous heparin with a resulting clotting time of 80 seconds would represent an inadequate level of anticoagulation.

Protein C and protein S levels will drop once oral anticoagulation is started and activated protein C resistance is no longer measurable. Antithrombin III levels are also affected by anticoagulant administration.

If a patient is already receiving oral anticoagulation, the measurement of these factors may wait until several weeks after this therapy is discontinued. Measuring the ratio of protein C antigen to prothrombin antigen while patients are on oral anticoagulation has been proposed,[81] but is dependent on very stable oral anticoagulation therapy.

Although many physicians will only see a limited number of patients with venous thrombosis, a number of issues should be considered regarding the testing for hereditary and acquired abnormalities associated with thrombosis. Clearly, a patient with a third episode of DVT will require long-term oral anticoagulation, regardless of any test results. For a patient with the first episode of DVT, there is no conclusive evidence that patients with an identifiable coagulation abnormality should be treated differently than those without such an abnormality. The possible benefits of preventing some future recurrence of thrombosis may or may not outweigh the risks of bleeding associated with lifetime oral anticoagulation.

Measurement of these coagulation parameters is useful in detecting other affected family members. There is no firm evidence that asymptomatic carriers of these abnormalities should be treated prophylactically for prolonged periods of time. Again, the possible benefits of remaining thrombosis-free versus the risks associated with long-term oral anticoagulation is unknown in this group. Consideration should be given to the possibility that asymptomatic carriers will be labelled as such and that this may affect their future insurability and eligibility for military service. Asymptomatic individuals who are

identified can be treated with maximal clot preventive measures at times of particular high risk, for example, following orthopedic surgery. However, considering all that we do not know about the development of thrombosis, this is wise in the case of the other, ostensibly normal, family members as well. Long-term oral anticoagulation carries significant risk in women of childbearing potential. There is no information on the advisability of prophylactic heparin administration during pregnancy in asymptomatic women with an underlying coagulation abnormality.

MANAGEMENT OF THROMBOPHILIACS

The presence of an identifiable coagulation abnormality predisposing to thrombosis does not alter the clinical management of these patients. All suspected thromboembolic events must be documented by objective means, both in patients with previous thrombotic episodes and in previously asymptomatic individuals. As with any chronic illness, patient education remains of paramount importance both in therapy and recognition of the signs and symptoms of disease.

REFERENCES

1. Davies MG, Hagen PO. The vascular endothelium. A new horizon. Ann Surg 1993;218:593–609.
2. Esmon CT. Cell mediated events that control blood coagulation and vascular injury. Ann Rev Cell Biol 1993;9:1–26.
3. Esmon CT. Molecular events that control the protein C anticoagulant pathway. Thromb Haemost 1993;70:29–35.
4. Miletich JP, Prescott SM, White R, et al. Inherited predisposition to thrombosis. Cell 1993;72:477–480.
5. Sala N, Fontcuberta J, Rutllant ML. New biological concepts on coagulation inhibitors. Intensive Care Med 1993;19(1):S3-S7.
6. Sas G. The Biology of Antithrombins. Boca Raton, CRC Press, 1989.
7. Hirsk J, Piovella F, Pini M. Congenital antithrombin III deficiency. Incidence and clinical features. Am J Med 1989;87:34S-38S.
8. Meade TW, Cooper J, Miller GJ, et al. Antithrombin III and arterial disease. Lancet 1991;338:850–851.
9. Hathaway WE. Clinical aspects of antithrombin III deficiency. Semin Hematol 1991;28:19–23.
10. Tait RC, Walker ID, Davidson JF, et al. Antithrombin III activity in healthy blood donors: age and sex related changes and prevalence of asymptomatic deficiency. Br J Haematol 1990;75:141–142.
11. Meade TW, Dyer S, Howarth DJ, et al. Antithrombin III and procoagulant activity: sex differences and effects of the menopause. Br J Haematol 1990;74:77–81.
12. Esmon CT. The protein C anticoagulant pathway. Arterioscler Thromb 1992;12:135–145.
13. Marlar RA, Neumann A. Neonatal purpura fulminans due to homozygous protein C or protein S deficiencies. Semin Thromb Hemost 1990;16:299–309.
14. Marlar RA, Montgomery RR, Broekmans AW. Diagnosis and treatment of homozygous protein C deficiency. Report of the Working Party on Homozygous Protein C Deficiency

of the Subcommittee on Protein C and Protein S, International Committee on Thrombosis and Haemostasis. J Pediatr 1989;114:528–534.

15. Miletich J, Sherman L, Broze G, Jr. Absence of thrombosis in subjects with heterozygous protein deficiency. N Engl J Med 1987;317:991–996.

16. McGehee WG, Klotz TA, Epstein DJ, et al. Coumarin necrosis associated with hereditary protein C deficiency. Ann Intern Med 1984;101:59–60.

17. Grimaudo V, Gueissaz F, Hauert J, et al. Necrosis of skin induced by coumarin in a patient deficient in protein S. BMJ 1989;298:233–234.

18. Scheffler P, Kiehl R, Braun B, et al. Thromboembolism complications and coumarin necrosis in a patient with congenital antithrombin III deficiency. Internist (Berl) 1988;29: 54–57.

19. Comp PC, Elrod JP, Karzenski S. Warfarin-induced skin necrosis. Semin Thromb Hemost 1990;16:293–298.

20. Comp PC. Coumarin-induced skin necrosis. Incidence, mechanisms, management and avoidance. Drug Saf 1993;8: 128–135.

21. Sheth SB, Carvalho AC. Protein S and C alterations in acutely ill patients. Am J Hematol 1991;36:14–19.

22. Powars D, Larsen R, Johnson J, et al. Epidemic meningococcemia and purpura fulminans with induced protein C deficiency. Clin Infect Dis 1993;17:254–261.

23. Clouse LH, Comp PC. The regulation of hemostasis: the protein C system. N Engl J Med 1986;314:1298–1304.

24. Comp PC, Nixon RR, Cooper MR, et al. Familial protein S deficiency is associated with recurrent thrombosis. J Clin Invest 1984;74:2082–2088.

25. Comp PC, Esmon CT. Recurrent venous thromboembolism in patients with a partial deficiency of protein S. N Engl J Med 1984;311:1525–1528.

26. Dahlback B. Protein S and C4b-binding protein: components involved in the regulation of the protein C anticoagulant system. Thromb Haemost 1991;66(1):49–61.

27. Comp PC, Doray D, Patton D, et al. An abnormal plasma distribution of protein S occurs in functional protein S deficiency. Blood 1986;67:504–508.

28. Dahlback B, Carlsson M, Svensson PJ. Familial thrombophilia due to a previously unrecognized mechanism characterized by poor anticoagulant response to activated protein C: prediction of a co-factor to activated protein C. Proc Natl Acad Sci USA 1993;90:1004–1008.

29. Dahlback B, Hildebrand B. Inherited resistance to activated protein C is corrected by anticoagulant co-factor activity found to be a property of factor V. Proc Natl Scad Sci USA 1994;91:1396–1400.

30. Walker FJ, Scandella D, Fay PJ. Identification of the binding site for activated protein C on the light chain of factor V and VIII. J Biol Chem 1990;265:1484–1489.

31. Svensson PJ, Dahlback B. Resistance to activated protein C as a basis for venous thrombosis. N Engl J Med 1994;330: 517–522.

32. Koster T, Rosendaal FR, de Ronde H, et al. Venous thrombosis due to poor anticoagulant response to activated protein C: Leiden Thrombophilia Study. Lancet 1993;342: 1503–1506.

33. Griffin JH, Evatt B, Wideman C, et al. Anticoagulant protein C pathway defective in majority of thrombophilic patients. Blood 1993;82:1989–1993.

34. Potzsch B, Kawamura H, Preissner KT, et al. Thrombophilia in patients with lupus anticoagulant correlates with the impaired anticoagulant activity of activated protein C but not with decreased activation of protein C. Blood 1992;80: 267.(Abstract)

35. Nesheim ME, Nichols WL, Cole TL, et al. Isolation and study of an acquired inhibitor of human coagulation factor V. J Clin Invest 1986;77:405–415.

36. Lane TA, Shapiro SS, Burka ER. Factor V antibody and disseminated intravascular coagulation. Ann Intern Med 1978;89:182–185.

37. Deguchi K, Tsukada T, Iwasaki E, et al. Late-onset homozygous protein C deficiency manifesting cerebral infarction as the first symptom at age 27. Intern Med 1992;31:922–925.

38. Pescatore P, Horellou HM, Conard J, et al. Problems of oral anticoagulation in an adult with homozygous protein C deficiency and late onset of thrombosis. Thromb Haemost 1993;69:311–315.

39. Gerson WT, Dickerman JD, Bovill EG, et al. Severe acquired protein C deficiency in purpura fulminans associated with disseminated intravascular coagulation: treatment with protein C concentrate. Pediatrics 1993;91:418–422.

40. Comp PC, Thurnau GR, Welsh J, et al. Functional and immunologic protein S levels are decreased during pregnancy. Blood 1986;68:881–885.

41. Malm J, Laurell M, Dahlback B. Changes in the plasma levels of vitamin K-dependent proteins C and S and of C4b-binding protein during pregnancy and oral contraception; General Hospital, Sweden. Br J Haematol 1988;68:437–443.

42. Warwick R, Hutton RA, Goff L, et al. Changes in protein C and free protein S during pregnancy and following hysterectomy. J R Soc Med 1989;82:591–594.

43. Schwarz HP, Schernthaner G, Griffin JH. Decreased plasma levels of protein S in well-controlled type I diabetes mellitus. Thromb Haemost 1987;57:240.

44. Saito M, Kumabashiri I, Jokaji H, et al. The levels of protein C and protein S in plasma in patients with type II diabetes mellitus. Thromb Res 1988;52:479–486.

45. Ceriello A, Giugliano D, Quatraro A, et al. Possible role for increased C4b-binding protein level in acquired protein S deficiency in type I diabetes. Diabetes 1990;39:447–449.

46. Takahashi H, Tatewaki W, Wada K, et al. Plasma protein S in disseminated intravascular coagulation, liver disease, collagen disease, diabetes mellitus, and under oral anticoagulant therapy. Clin Chim Acta 1989;182:195–208.

47. Lee P, Jenkins A, Bourke C, et al. Prothrombotic and antithrombotic factors are elevated in patients with type I diabetes complicated by microalbuminuria. Diabet Med 1993;10:122–128.

48. Francis RB, Jr. Protein S deficiency in sickle cell anemia. J Lab Clin Med 1988;111:571–576.

49. Bissuel F, Berruyer M, Causse X, et al. Acquired protein S deficiency: correlation with advanced disease in HIV-1-infected patients. J Acquir Immune Defic Syndr 192;5: 484–489.

50. Stahl CP, Wideman CS, Spira TJ, et al. Protein S deficiency in men with long-term human immunodeficiency virus infection. Blood 1993;81:1801–1807.

51. Israels SJ, Seshia SS. Childhood stroke associated with protein C or S deficiency. J Pediat 1987;111:562–564.

52. Wallis DE, Godwin J. Mitral valve prolapse, cerebral ischemia, and protein S deficiency. Am J Med 1988;84:974.

53. Sacco RL, Own J, Tatemichi TK, et al. Protein S deficiency and intracranial vascular occlusion. Ann Neurol 1987;22: 115.(Abstract)

54. Allaart CF, Aronson DC, Ruys T, et al. Hereditary protein S deficiency in young adults with arterial occlusive disease. Thromb Haemost 1990;64:206–210.

55. Sacco RL, Own J, Mohr JP, et al. Free protein S deficiency: a possible association with cerebrovascular occlusion. Stroke 1989;20:1657–1661.

56. Girolami A, Simioni P, Lazzaro AR, et al. Severe arterial

cerebral thrombosis in a patient with protein S deficiency (moderately reduced total and markedly reduced free protein S): a family study. Thromb Haemost 1989;61:144–147.

57. Green D, Otoya J, Oriba H, et al. Protein S deficiency in middle-aged women with stroke. Neurol 1992;42:1029–1033.

58. Comp PC. The natural anticoagulant proteins and cardiovascular disease. In: Francis RB Jr., (ed.). Atherosclerotic Cardiovascular Disease, Hemostasis, and Endothelial Function, New York: Marcel Decker, Inc., 1992, pp. 87–106.

59. Barinagarrementeria F, Cantu-Brito C, De La Pena A, et al. Prothrombotic states in young people with idiopathic stroke. A prospective study. Stroke 1994;25:287–290.

60. Carr ME, Jr., Zekert SL. Protein S and C4b-binding protein levels in patients with stroke: implications for protein S regulation. Haemostasis 1993;23:159–167.

61. Brown DC, Livingston JH, Minns RA, et al. Protein C and S deficiency causing childhood stroke. Scott Med J 1993;38: 114–115.

62. Coull BM, Clark WM. Abnormalities of hemostasis in ischemic stroke. Med Clin North Am 1993;77:77–94.

63. Mayer SA, Sacco RL, Hurlet-Jensen A, et al. Free protein S deficiency in acute ischemic stroke. A case-control study. Stroke 1993;24:224–227.

64. Triplett DA, Brandt J. Laboratory identification of the lupus anticoagulant. Br J Haematol 1989;73:139–142.

65. Doweiko JP. Management of the hematologic manifestations of HIV disease. Blood Rev 1993;7:121–126.

66. Kunkel LA. Acquired circulating anticoagulants in malignancy. Semin Thromb Hemost 1992;18:416–423.

67. Kunket LA. Acquired circulating anticoagulants. Hematol Oncol Clin North Am 1992;6:1341–1357.

68. Creagh MD, Greaves M. Lupus anticoagulant. Blood Rev 1991;5:162–167.

69. Sammaritano LA, Gharavi AE, Lockshin MD. Pregnancy and a PL. Bull Rheum Dis 1991;40:3–6.

70. Tobelem G, Cariou R, Camez A. The lupus anticoagulant and its role in thrombosis. Blood Rev 1987;1:21–24.

71. Dhami MS, Bona RD. Thrombosis in patients with cancer. Postgrad Med 93 1993;131–3:137–140.

72. Edwards RL, Silver J, Rickles FR. Human tumor procoagulants: registry of the Subcommittee on Haemostasis and Malignancy of the Scientific and Standardization Committee, International Society on Thrombosis and Haemostasis. Thromb Haemost 1993;69:205–213.

73. Bick RL. Coagulation abnormalities in malignancy: a review. Semin Thromb Haemost 1992;18:353–372.

74. Gore JM, Appelbaum JS, Greene HL, et al. Occult cancer in patients with acute pulmonary embolism. Ann Intern Med 1982;96:556–560.

75. Griffin MR, Stanson AW, Brown ML, et al. Deep venous thrombosis and pulmonary embolism. Risk of subsequent malignant neoplasms. Arch Intern Med 1987;147:1907–1911.

76. Goldberg RJ, Seneff M, Gore JM, et al. Occult malignant neoplasm in patients with deep venous thrombosis. Arch Intern Med 1987;147:251–253.

77. Prandoni P, Lensing AWA, Buller HR, et al. Deep-vein thrombosis and the incidence of subsequent symptomatic cancer. N Engl J Med 1992;327:1128–1133.

78. Prandoni P. Deep vein thrombosis and occult cancer. Ann Med 1993;25:447–450.

79. Comp PC. Laboratory evaluation of protein S status. Semin Thromb Hemost 1990;16:177–181.

80. Comp PC. Measurement of the natural anticoagulant protein S. How and when. Am J Clin Pathol 1990;94:242–243.

81. Griffin JH, Evatt B, Zimmerman TS, et al. Deficiency of protein C in congenital thrombotic disease. J Clin Invest 1981;68:1370–1373.

82. Kolodziej M, Comp PC. Hypercoagulable states due to natural anticoagulant deficiencies. Curr Opinion Hemat 1993: 301–307.

37

Calf-Vein Thrombosis

Gary E. Raskob

INTRODUCTION

During the past 15 years, there have been major advances in the diagnosis, treatment, and prevention of venous thromboembolism (VTE).[1,2] An example is the concept that proximal-vein thrombosis (popliteal, femoral, or iliac vein thrombosis) is a prognostic category distinct from deep-vein thrombosis (DVT) confined to the calf veins.[1-7]

Proximal-vein thrombosis is a serious and potentially lethal disorder. Inadequately treated proximal-vein thrombosis is associated with a 20% to 50% risk of clinically important recurrent venous thromboembolic events.[8(I),9(I),10(I),11(I)] There is a strong association between proximal-vein thrombosis and fatal pulmonary embolism (PE), an association documented in studies on patients having major orthopedic surgery (such as hip or knee replacement) without preventive measures. These studies have revealed a rate of proximal-vein thrombosis of 20% to 30%,[12,13] and a rate of fatal PE of 2% to 3%.[14(III),15] The data, therefore, support a 10% rate of fatal PE associated with untreated proximal-vein thrombosis. In contrast, data from clinical trials supports the inference that thrombosis which remains confined to the calf veins is associated with a low risk of clinically important PE.[3,4,16(I),17(I),18(I),19(I),20(I)] In the context of this chapter, "clinically important" PE refers to either fatal PE or nonfatal symptomatic PE.

The management of patients with calf-vein thrombosis continues to receive attention.[5,6,21(V),22] The literature is potentially confusing, and contains divergent, contradictory recommendations for several reasons: (1) the low risk of important PE in patients with thrombosis that remains confined to the calf veins may incorrectly lead to the conclusion that "no further management" is required, (2) case-reports[22] and autopsy studies[23,24] which attribute PE to a source in the calf veins create doubt about the validity of the concept that isolated calf-vein thrombosis has a low risk of important PE, and (3) the observation that pa-

tients with calf-vein thrombosis may develop extension into the proximal veins has led to the suggestion that all patients with calf-vein thrombosis should be treated with anticoagulant therapy.[21(V)]

This chapter reviews the available data on the clinical course of untreated calf-vein thrombosis. It also covers the evidence supporting three alternative management strategies: (1) no further intervention, (2) antithrombotic therapy with heparin and oral anticoagulants, and (3) serial noninvasive leg testing to monitor for proximal extension.

SCOPE OF THE PROBLEM

The incidence of calf-vein thrombosis in symptomatic patients is well-documented. Prospective studies in which venography was performed in consecutive patients presenting with symptoms or signs suggesting DVT[25(I),26,27(I),28(I),29(V)] have shown that 4% to 13% of such patients have DVT confined to the calf, about 30% have proximal-vein thrombosis (popliteal, femoral, or iliac thrombosis), and 57% to 66% of patients have normal venograms. These studies show that most patients with confirmed thrombosis have proximal-vein thrombosis (with or without associated calf thrombosis), and a minority of patients have thrombosis confined to the calf veins.

Since the mid-1980s, noninvasive testing has replaced venography in most centers as the first-line test for evaluating patients who present with symptoms or signs of venous thrombosis.[16(I),17(I),18(I),19(I),20(I)] The most commonly used noninvasive tests are B-mode or duplex ultrasound, or impedance plethysmography (IPG). These tests fail to detect most cases of DVT confined to the calf.[30,31] Consequently, the patient with symptomatic calf-vein thrombosis is less commonly encountered by physicians than in the past when venography was used as the first-line objective test. In centers where noninvasive tests are not available, or where there is a preference for venography, thrombosis confined to the calf is more commonly identified.

In recent years, the incidence of asymptomatic calf-vein thrombosis in high-risk patients has been well-documented by clinical trials performed to evaluate preventive approaches. In these trials, venography was used routinely as the diagnostic endpoint. For example, in patients undergoing hip or knee replacement who received prophylaxis with either warfarin or low-molecular-weight heparin (LMWH), thrombosis confined to the calf-veins was present in 10% to 40%.[32(I),33(I),34] In patients over the age of 40 years undergoing abdominal or thoracic surgery, neurosurgery, or urologic surgery without prophylaxis, it was present in 10% to 30%.[13,15] In patients with stroke causing paralysis it was present in up to 50%.[15] Most of these patients are asymptomatic and, therefore, remain undetected in most centers unless case-finding with venography is performed as part of routine care or as part of a clinical trial. The asymptomatic calf-vein thrombi are usually clinically unimportant as long as they remain confined to the calf veins. However, in some patients, these thrombi may extend proximally, as discussed below, and lead to important and even fatal PE.

Recent data indicate that most patients with symptomatic proximal-vein thrombosis or PE are outpatients at the time of presentation,[16(I),35] and most of these patients have a history of surgery or hospital admission for medical illness during the previous 6 months.[36,37(I)] It is likely that many of these patients had asymptomatic calf-vein thrombosis at the time of discharge from hospital and that during the subsequent weeks to months, these thrombi evolved leading to symptomatic proximal-vein thrombosis or PE. This inference is further supported by the findings of a study in which venography was performed preoperatively and then serially after surgery in patients undergoing knee replacement.[38] The results indicate that in 90% of patients with thrombosis, the thrombus is present within 24 hours after surgery, and is present when the patient is discharged several days later. Because the length of hospital stay has decreased markedly for most surgical procedures, including major procedures such as hip or knee replacement which are high risk for VTE, many patients who in the past would have presented with symptomatic VTE during the hospital stay are now presenting as outpatients or during their convalescence at rehabilitation hospitals. The result is a shift in the burden of illness of VTE from the acute hospital setting to the community and nonacute-care setting.

CLINICAL COURSE OF UNTREATED CALF-VEIN THROMBOSIS

In this section the available data on the clinical course of untreated calf-vein thrombosis are summarized. Two outcomes are presented: (1) the extension of thrombosis into the proximal veins, and (2) the incidence of clinically important PE.

The postphlebitic syndrome is a potentially important long-term outcome. The incidence of the postphlebitic syndrome in patients with calf-vein thrombosis is currently uncertain.[7] It is also not clear whether thrombi which remain confined to the calf lead to postphlebitic symptoms, or whether calf thrombi must first extend into the proximal veins to be associated with subsequent postphlebitic problems. Postphlebitic symptoms are a common sequelae in patients with symptomatic proximal-vein thrombosis.[7] Because untreated calf-vein thrombosis may extend proximally and lead to symptomatic proximal-vein thrombosis, at least some patients with calf-vein thrombosis subsequently develop the postphlebitic syndrome due to proximal progression of thrombosis. However, it is possible that thrombosis confined to the calf also contributes to postphlebitic symptoms. Further studies are required to resolve these issues.

Proximal Extension of Calf-vein Thrombosis

Extension of thrombosis into the popliteal vein or more proximally occurs in 15% to 25% of patients with calf-vein thrombosis.[3,21(V),39(I)] This rate applies to patients with either symptomatic or asymptomatic calf-vein thrombosis. These data come from two types of studies: (1) studies including a series of consecutive patients with untreated calf-vein thrombosis who were monitored for proximal extension using objective tests (^{125}I-fibrinogen leg scanning, IPG, duplex ultrasound, or venography),[3,4,21(V)] and (2) a randomized trial (level I) evaluating alternative regimens for the treatment of calf-vein thrombosis.[39(I)] The studies evaluating the clinical course of untreated calf-vein thrombosis are summarized in Table 1.

In a randomized trial by Lagerstedt et al,[39(I)] patients were treated with an initial course of intravenous heparin for 5 days. They were then randomly allocated to receive either continued long-term treatment with warfarin or no long-term anticoagulant treatment. Of the 28 patients who did not receive warfarin, five (18%) had proximal extension confirmed by venography. Two additional patients had "recurrence of" but the venographic findings were not described in detail. In contrast, none of the 23 patients treated with warfarin had proximal extension of thrombosis or recurrent thromboembolism. These results indicate that calf-vein thrombosis may extend proximally, even when it is treated with initial heparin but not followed by oral anticoagulant therapy. The results have important implications for patients in whom a decision is made to treat with anticoagulants (see below under "Antithrombotic Therapy").

Incidence of Clinically Important Pulmonary Embolism

The incidence of clinically important PE is low (1% or less) in patients in whom thrombosis remains confined to the calf veins. This inference is supported by two lines of

Table 1
Studies Evaluating Extension of Calf-Vein Thrombosis

Study and Year	No. of Patients	Patient Status	Test Used To Detect Extension	No. (%) With Extension Into Proximal Veins
Kakkar et al. 1969[3]	40	Asymptomatic Postoperative elective surgery	^{125}I-fibrinogen scan and venography	9 (22.5%)
Moser and LeMoine 1981[4]	21	Mixed symptomatic and asymptomatic high-risk	^{125}I-fibrinogen scan, IPG, venography	0
Lagerstedt et al. 1985[39]	28	Symptomatic	Venography	5 (18%)*
Lohr et al. 1991[21]	75	Symptomatic (62) & asymptomatic (13), 36 outpatients, 39 inpatients	Duplex ultrasound	11 (15%)

* 2 additional patients had "recurrence" but the venographic findings were not described; if these 2 patients are included, the rate is 7/28 (25%).

evidence: (1) studies in relatively small numbers of consecutive patients with untreated calf-vein thrombosis who were followed to document the incidence of PE,[3,4] and (2) five large prospective studies[16(I),17(I),18(I),19(I),20(I)] in patients with symptoms or signs suggestive of DVT whose management was based on noninvasive tests which are insensitive for calf-vein thrombosis, and in whom anticoagulant therapy was withheld if these tests remained negative. In the studies by Kakkar et al,[3] and by Moser and LeMoine,[4] no patient in whom thrombosis remained confined to the calf developed clinically evident PE (rates of 0/31 and 0/21, respectively). In the trial by Lagerstedt et al,[39(I)] one of the 28 patients presented with symptomatic PE confirmed by ventilation-perfusion lung scanning, but the lung-scan criteria for this diagnosis were not described. In this study, the patients were not monitored for proximal extension using objective testing, and so it is unknown if the patient developed proximal extension of thrombosis before PE occurred. In the study by Lohr et al,[21(V)] there is no report on whether patients developed PE or on the objective tests used to confirm or exclude this diagnosis.

The large prospective studies evaluating noninvasive testing in patients with clinically suspected venous thrombosis provide data on the incidence of important PE.[16(I),17(I),18(I),19(I),20(I)] These data are summarized in Table 2. The results are relevant to the issue of calf-vein thrombosis because each of these studies evaluated the safety of withholding anticoagulant therapy in patients in whom noninvasive tests which are sensitive for proximal-vein thrombosis but insensitive for calf-vein thrombosis remained negative. None of the more than 1600 patients evaluated died from PE (95% confidence interval 0% to 0.2%), and only three patients (0.3%) had symptomatic nonfatal PE. These data support the strategy of serial test-

ing for proximal extension as one approach for managing patients with DVT confined to the calf.

The question remains of how the above data can be reconciled with case reports or autopsy studies which report important PE associated with calf-vein thrombosis.[22–24] This issue has been clarified by the findings of recent prospective studies in patients with clinically suspected PE who underwent routine objective testing for DVT.[37(I),40(I),41(I)] In these studies, objective testing was done using venography or IPG. Impedance plethysmography is sensitive for proximal-vein thrombosis in patients with suspected PE.[40(I)] The results indicated that proximal-vein thrombosis was absent in about 50% of patients with confirmed PE.[40(I),41(I)] A possible explanation is that all or most of the thrombus embolized; little or no residual thrombosis would be left in the legs to be detected by objective testing at the time the patient presented with clinical symptoms or signs of PE. This explanation is strongly supported by the findings of a recent large prospective study which evaluated serial noninvasive testing for proximal-vein thrombosis, in patients who had suspected PE and nondiagnostic lung scans.[35(I),37(I)] The findings indicated that anticoagulant therapy can be safely withheld in such patients if they have adequate cardiorespiratory reserve at presentation, providing the results of objective testing for proximal-vein thrombosis are negative, and remain negative on serial testing for 10 to 14 days. Of 627 patients with nondiagnostic lung scans, adequate cardiorespiratory reserve, and serially negative results by noninvasive leg testing, only four patients (0.6%) returned with clinically important PE during 3 months of follow-up. Because the noninvasive test used in this study is insensitive for calf-vein thrombosis, the findings support the inference that isolated calf-vein thrombosis is associated with a low risk of clinically important PE, and

Table 2
Incidence of Clinically Important Pulmonary Embolism in Patients with Suspected Venous Thrombosis and Negative Results by Serial Noninvasive Testing: Prospective Studies

Study and Year	Diagnostic Test	No. of Patients With Negative Results	Fatal PE No. of Patients (%)	Symptomatic Non-fatal PE No. of Patients (%)
Hull et al. 1985[16]	0	311	0	0
Huisman et al. 1986[17]	0	289	0	0
Huisman et al. 1989[18]	0	131	0	0
Hull et al. 1990[19]	0	139	0	0
Heijboer et al. 1993[20]	IPG	361	0	2 (0.6%)
	C-UD	390	0	1 (0.3%)
Total		1621	0*	3 (0.2%)*

IPG = impedance plethysmography C-US = compression ultrasound.
* 95% confidence intervals: 0/1621, 0% to 0.2% and 3/1621, 0.07% to 0.4%.

that serial testing with IPG can be used to identify patients with proximal extension of calf-vein thrombosis who require treatment with anticoagulants.

The accumulated evidence from patients with suspected venous thrombosis[16(I),17(I),18(I),19(I),20(I)] and those with clinically suspected PE[35(I),37(I),40(I),41(I)] supports the inference that proximal-vein thrombosis is the key prognostic marker for clinically important PE. If thrombosis remains confined to the calf, the risk of clinically important PE is low.[16(I),17(I),18(I),19(I),20(I),35(I),37(I)] The finding of isolated calf-vein thrombosis in a patient with confirmed PE does not establish that the embolus originated directly from deep veins in the calf. All the available data[3,4,16(I),17(I),18(I),19(I),20(I),35(I),37(I)] support the explanation that such calf thrombi represent the residua of larger proximal-vein thrombosis which embolized

MANAGEMENT OF CALF-VEIN THROMBOSIS

No Further Intervention

The outcomes for a "no intervention" strategy can be predicted from data on the rates of proximal extension[3,4,21(V)] and randomized trial data (level I) for inadequately managed proximal-vein thrombosis.[8(I),9(I),10(I),11(I)] Of 100 patients with calf-vein thrombosis who are managed using "no further intervention," extension into the proximal-veins would be expected in 20 of these patients.[3,4,21(V)] Since inadequately treated or untreated proximal-vein thrombosis is associated with a 20% to 50% rate of recurrent venous thromboembolic events[8(I),9(I),10(I),11(I)] and a 10% risk of fatal PE, the outcomes in the 20 patients with proximal-vein thrombosis can be predicted: two patients would be expected to die from PE, and five to ten patients would be expected to return with either symptomatic PE or symptomatic recurrent DVT. Thus, of 100 patients with untreated calf-vein thrombosis, the expected mortality rate from PE would be 2%, and the ex-

pected frequency of nonfatal symptomatic PE would be approximately 5%.

Antithrombotic Therapy

Anticoagulant therapy with intravenous heparin followed by oral warfarin is effective in preventing extension and/or recurrence of thromboembolism in patients with calf-vein thrombosis.[39(I)] The trial by Lagerstedt et al,[39(I)] establishes the need for long-term treatment following the initial course of heparin. In this trial, extension and/or recurrence of VTE occurred in eight of 28 patients (29%) who did not receive long-term warfarin, compared with none of the 23 patients given long-term therapy (p<0.01). All of these thrombosis extension/recurrences occurred within the first 3 months, and 5 of 8 occurred in the first 6 weeks.

Certain LMWH preparations given subcutaneously once or twice daily have been shown to be as effective as intravenous unfractionated heparin in the initial treatment of patients with proximal-vein thrombosis.[42(I),43(I)] These LMWH preparations should also be effective in treating patients with calf-vein thrombosis (a lower-risk group than proximal-vein thrombosis). If LMWH is available, data from clinical trials in patients with proximal-vein thrombosis indicate that it could be used for initial treatment of calf-vein thrombosis.

Treatment with oral anticoagulants alone is not recommended for patients with documented calf-vein thrombosis. Although convenient, the effectiveness of using only oral anticoagulant therapy for preventing extension of calf-vein thrombosis remains uncertain. Further, treatment with oral anticoagulants alone is less effective than treatment with initial heparin and oral anticoagulants in patients with proximal-vein thrombosis.[10(I)] This observation suggests that oral anticoagulant treatment alone may not be effective in preventing extension in patients with documented calf-vein thrombosis.

The available data from clinical trials indicates that oral anticoagulant therapy should be continued for at least 6 weeks in patients with calf-vein thrombosis.[8,39(I)] Hull et al, reported that none of 32 patients with calf-vein thrombosis who received anticoagulant therapy for 6 weeks developed symptomatic VTE during the subsequent year (0/32, 95% confidence interval 0 to 11%). In the trial by Lagerstedt, only one of 23 patients (4%) with calf-vein thrombosis treated for 3 months developed recurrent VTE during the subsequent year (1/23, 95% confidence interval 0 to 15%). These data indicate that patients with calf-vein thrombosis should be treated for 6 weeks to 3 months and, in many patients, 6 weeks is probably sufficient. It may be prudent to continue treatment for longer than 6 weeks in selected patients with continuing risk factors. Moderate doses of subcutaneous heparin provide an effective and safe alternative to warfarin for long-term treatment in patients in whom warfarin is contraindicated or for whom prothrombin time monitoring is not feasible.[44(I)]

The risk of major bleeding during treatment with initial intravenous heparin is about 5%.[9(I),10(I),42(I),43(I)] However, there is a marked difference in the risk of major bleeding among patients without risk factors (1%) compared with patients who have had recent surgery or have other risk factors; in such patients the risk for major bleeding is 11%.[45(I)] The risk of major bleeding during long-term treatment with warfarin (INR 2.0 to 3.0) is about 2% during the initial 3 months.[46(I)] Multiple randomized trials in large numbers of patients with venous thrombosis indicate that the risk of fatal bleeding during either initial heparin or long-term warfarin therapy is low (<1%).[47] These risks of bleeding with current anticoagulant therapy are outweighed by the estimated risk of fatal PE (2%) and the risk of nonfatal symptomatic PE (5%) if patients with calf-vein thrombosis receive no further intervention.

The availability of LMWH for the initial treatment of DVT will probably shift the risk/benefit calculation markedly in favor of treating patients with calf-vein thrombosis because certain LMWH preparations are associated with a markedly lower risk of major bleeding than intravenous unfractionated heparin.[42(I),43(I)] In a trial by Hull et al,[43(I)] 11 of 219 patients (5.0%) who received continuous intravenous heparin had major bleeding, compared with only one of 213 patients (0.5%) who were given the LMWH tinzaparin (a risk reduction of 90%, p<0.01). This trial included a substantial number of patients at high risk of bleeding because of risk factors such as recent surgery, a history of gastrointestinal or genitourinary bleeding, thrombocytopenia, or other disorders predisposing to bleeding. Low-molecular-weight heparin can be given subcutaneously once or twice daily without the need for laboratory monitoring and dose adjustment.[42(I),43(I)] This simplified therapy will enable patients to be managed as outpatients and is likely to be more cost-effective than treatment in hospital with intravenous heparin for 4 to 5 days. These factors are likely to shift future practice towards treating most patients with documented calf-vein thrombosis.

Monitoring for Proximal Extension

Repeated testing with IPG or B-mode ultrasound is effective for detecting extension of calf-vein thrombosis into the popliteal or more proximal veins. The use of monitoring for proximal extension is supported by the findings of several prospective studies[16(I),17(I),18(I),19(I),20(I),35(I),37(I)] which document the safety of withholding anticoagulant therapy in patients in whom repeated noninvasive testing remains negative. These studies used repeated testing over a 10- to 14-day period.

The potential advantage of monitoring for proximal extension, rather than treating all patients with anticoagulant therapy, is that treatment can be confined to patients who develop proximal-vein thrombosis; in patients in whom thrombosis remains confined to the calf, the risk of bleeding with anticoagulant therapy can be avoided, since these thrombi are associated with a low risk of subsequent clinically important venous thromboembolic events.

At present, serial testing for proximal extension may be preferred in selected patients with calf-vein thrombosis who are at very high risk for bleeding (e.g., surgery within the previous week). If serial testing is used, the test should be repeated every 2 to 3 days for at least a 10- to 14-day period. This may not be practical in some patients who live far from the hospital or clinic.

RECOMMENDATIONS

1. Patients with thrombosis confined to the calf should either be treated with anticoagulant therapy to prevent extension, or undergo monitoring for proximal extension using serial noninvasive testing. Such testing would use either IPG or compression ultrasound imaging.
2. The choice between anticoagulant treatment or monitoring for extension depends on the risk of bleeding, and on the availability and feasibility of performing serial noninvasive testing.
3. The strategy of "no further intervention" (i.e., no treatment or serial noninvasive testing) is not recommended. This approach exposes patients to an unacceptable risk of clinically important PE.
4. If the decision to treat with anticoagulant therapy is made, at the present time this should consist of intravenous heparin for 4 to 5 days followed by oral warfarin sodium for 6 weeks to 3 months. If available, certain LMWH preparations given subcutaneously could be used in place of intravenous unfractionated heparin, depending upon their established effectiveness in patients with proximal-vein thrombosis.

REFERENCES

1. Weinmann E, Salzman EW. Deep-vein thrombosis. N Engl J Med 1994;331:1630–1641.

2. Moser KM. Venous thromboembolism. Am Rev Respir Dis 1990;141:235–249.

3. Kakker VV, Howe CT, Flanc C, Clarke MB. Natural history of postoperative deep-vein thrombosis. Lancet 1969;2:230–233.

4. Moser KM, LeMoine JR. Is embolic risk conditioned by location of postoperative deep-vein thrombosis? Ann Intern Med 1981;94:439–444.

5. Philbrick JT, Becker DM. Calf deep venous thrombosis. A wolf in sheep's clothing? Arch Intern Med 1988;148:2131–2138.

6. Powers LR. Distal deep vein thrombosis. What's the best treatment? J Gen Intern Med 1988;3:288–292.

7. Hirsh J, Lensing AWA. Natural history of minimal calf deep-vein thrombosis. In: Berstein EF. Vascular Diagnosis, 4th ed., St. Louis, Mosby 1993, pp. 779–781.

(I)8. Hull R, Delmore T, Genton E, et al. Warfarin sodium versus low-dose heparin in the long-term treatment of venous thrombosis. N Engl J Med 1979;301:855–858.

(I)9. Hull R, Raskob G, Hirsh J, et al. Continuous intravenous heparin compared with intermittent subcutaneous heparin in the initial treatment of proximal-vein thrombosis. N Engl J Med 1986;315:1109–1114.

(I)10. Brandjes DPM, Heijboer H, Buller HR, et al. Acenocoumarol and heparin compared with acenocoumarol alone in the initial treatment of proximal-vein thrombosis. N Engl J Med 1992;327:1485–1489.

(I)11. Raschke RA, Reilly BM, Guidry JR, Fontana JR, Srinivas S. The weight-based heparin dosing nomogram compared with a "standard care" nomogram. A randomized controlled trial. Ann Intern Med 1993;119:874–881.

12. Imperiale TF, Speroff T. A meta-analysis of methods to prevent venous thromboembolism following total hip replacement. JAMA 1994;271:1780–1785.

13. Gallus AS, Salzman EW, Hirsh J. Prevention of venous thormboembolism. In: Coleman RW, Hirsh J, Marder V, Salzman EW. Hemostasis and Thrombosis: Basic Principles and Clinical Practice. 3rd ed. Philadelphia, J.B. Lippincott 1994, pp. 1331–1345.

(III)14. Coventry MB, Nolan DR, Beckenbaugh RD. "Delayed" prophylactic anticoagulation: a study of results and complications in 2,012 total hip arthroplasties. J Bone Joint Surg [Am] 1973;55:1487–1492.

15. Clagett GP, Anderson FA, Levine MN, Salzman EW, Wheeler HB. Prevention of venous thromboembolism. CHEST 1992;102:Oct Supplement:391S-407S.

(I)16. Hull R, Hirsh J, Carter C, et al. Diagnostic efficacy of impedance plethysmography for clinically suspected deep-vein thrombosis: a randomized trial. Ann Intern Med 1985;102:21–28.

(I)17. Huisman MV, Buller HR, ten Cate JW, Vreeken J. Serial impedance plethysmography for suspected deep venous thrombosis in outpatients. The Amsterdam General Practitioner Study. N Engl J Med 1986;314:823–828.

(I)18. Huisman MV, Buller HR, ten Cate JW, Heijermans HSF, van der Laan J, et al. Management of clinically suspected acute venous thrombosis in outpatients with serial impedance plethysmography in a community hospital setting. Arch Intern Med 1989;149:511–513.

(I)19. Hull R, Raskob G, Carter CJ. Serial impedance plethysmography in pregnant patients with clinically suspected deep-vein thrombosis. Clinical validity of negative findings. Ann Intern Med 1990;112:663–667.

(I)20. Heijboer H, Buller HR, Lensing AWA, Turpie AGG, Colly LP, et al. A comparison of real-time compression ultrasonography with impedance plethysmography for the diagnosis of deep-vein thrombosis in symptomatic outpatients. 1993;329:1365–1369.

(V)21. Lohr JM, Kerr TM, Lutter KS, Cranley RD, Spirtoff K, et al. Lower extremity calf thrombosis: to treat or not to treat? J Vasc Surg 1991;14:618–623.

22. Chapman WHH, Lee MYT, Foley KT. Pulmonary embolism from a venous thrombosis distal to the popliteal vein. Military Medicine 1991;156:252–254.

23. Havig GO. Source of pulmonary emboli. Acta Chir Scan 1977;478:(Suppl):42–47.

24. Giachino A. Relationship between deep-vein thrombosis in the calf and fatal pulmonary embolism. Can J Surg 1988;31:129–130.

(I)25. Hull R, Hirsh J, Sackett DL, Powers P, Turpie AG, et al. Combined use of leg scanning and impedance plethysmography in suspected venous thrombosis. An alternative to venography. N Engl J. Med 1977;296:1497–1500.

26. O'Donnell TF, Abbott WM, Athanasoulis CA, Millan VC, Callow AD. Diagnosis of deep venous thormbosis in the outpatient by venography. Surg Gyn Obstet 1980;150:69–74.

(I)27. Hull R, Hirsh J, Sackett DL, et al. Replacement of venography in suspected venous thrombosis by impedance plethysmography and ^{125}I-fibrinogen leg scanning. A less invasive approach. Ann Intern Med 1981;94:12–15.

(I)28. Lensing AWA, Prandoni P, Brandjes D, et al. Detection of deep-vein thrombosis by real-time B-mode ultrasonography. N Eng J Med 1989;320:342–345.

(V)29. Cogo A, Lensing AWA, Prandoni P, Hirsh J. Distribution of thrombosis in patients with symptomatic deep vein thrombosis. Arch Intern Med 1993;153:2777–2780.

30. Wheeler HB, Hirsh J, Wells P, Anderson FA. Diagnostic tests for deep-vein thrombosis. Clinical usefulness depends on probability of disease. Arch Intern Med 1994;154:1921–1928.

31. White RW, McGahan J, Daschbach M, Hartling RP. Diagnosis of deep-vein thrombosis using Duplex ultrasound. Ann Intern Med 1989;111:297–304.

(I)32. Hull R, Raskob G, Pineo G, et al. A comparison of subcutaneous low-molecular weight heparin with warfarin sodium for prophylaxis against deep-vein thrombosis after hip or knee implantation. N Engl J Med 1993;329:1370–1376.

(I)33. RD Heparin Arthroplasty Group. RD heparin compared with warfarin for prevention of venous thromboembolic disease following total hip or knee arthroplasty. J Bone Joint Surg 1994;76-A:1174–1185.

34. Leclerc JR, Geerts WH, Desjardins L, et al. Prevention of venous thromboembolism (VTE) after knee arthroplasty—a randomized double-blind trial comparing a low-molecular-weight heparin fragment (enoxaparin) to warfarin. Blood 1994;84:(Suppl 1):246a.

(I)35. Hull R, Raskob G, Ginsberg J, et al. A noninvasive strategy for the treatment of patients with suspected pulmonary embolism. Arch Intern Med 1994;154:289–297.

36. Anderson FA, Wheeler HB, Goldberg RJ, et al. A population-based perspective of the hospital incidence and case-fatality rates of DVT and pulmonary embolism. The Worcester deep-vein thrombosis Study. Arch Intern Med 1991;151:933–938.

(I)37. Hull R, Raskob G, Coates G, Panju A, Gill GJ. A new noninvasive management strategy for patients with suspected pulmonary embolism. Arch Intern Med

1989;149:2549–2555.

38. Maynard M, Sculco TP, Ghelman B. Progression and regression of DVT after total knee arthroplasty. Clinical Orthopedics and Related Research 1991;273:125–130.

(I)39. Lagerstedt CI, Olsson CG, Fagher BO, Oqvist BW, Albrechtsson U. The need for long-term anticoagulant treatment in symptomatic calf-vein thrombosis. Lancet 1985;2:515–518.

(I)40. Hull R, Hirsh J, Carter C, et al. Pulmonary angiography, ventilation lung scanning and venography for clinically suspected pulmonary embolism with abnormal perfusion lung scan. Ann Intern Med 1983;98:891–899.

(I)41. Hull R, Hirsh J, Carter C, et al. Diagnostic value of ventilation-perfusion lung scanning in patients with suspected pulmonary embolism. CHEST 1985;88:819–828.

(I)42. Prandoni P, Lensing AWA, Buller HR, et al. Comparison of subcutaneous low molecular weight heparin with intravenous standard heparin in proximal deep-vein thrombosis. Lancet 1992;339:441–445.

(I)43. Hull R, Raskob G, Pineo G, et al. Subcutaneous low molecular weight heparin compared with continuous intravenous heparin in the treatment of proximal vein thrombosis. N Engl J Med 1992;326:975–982.

(I)44. Hull R, Delmore T, Carter C, et al. Adjusted subcutaneous heparin versus warfarin sodium in the long-term treatment of venous thrombosis. N Engl J Med 1982;306:189–194.

(I)45. Hull RD, Raskob GE, Rosenbloom D, et al. Heparin for 5 days as compared with 10 days in the initial treatment of proximal venous thrombosis. N Engl J Med 1990;322:1260–1264.

(I)46. Hull R, Hirsh J, Jay R, et al. Different intensities of oral anticoagulant therapy in the treatment of proximal-vein thrombosis. N Engl J Med 1982;307:1676–1681.

47. Levine M, Raskob G, Landefeld S, Hirsh J. Hemorrhagic complications of anticoagulant treatment. CHEST 1995;108:276S–290S.

38

Venous Thromboembolism in the Cancer Patient

Sherri S. Durica

INTRODUCTION

Venous thromboembolism (VTE) is a common problem in patients with cancer. Not only are patients with known malignancy at increased risk of deep-vein thrombosis (DVT) and pulmonary embolism (PE), but clinical trials suggest that recurrent idiopathic DVT may herald the development of clinically evident cancer. Clinical and laboratory observations suggest that patients with malignancies are more susceptible to thromboembolic diseases because of immobility, surgery, and chemotherapy, and the cancer itself may play an integral role in the development of a prothrombotic state. The diagnosis and treatment of venous thromboembolism is often challenging in cancer patients. Interpretation of noninvasive tests for PE and DVT may be difficult in symptomatic patients who have lung tumors or large intra-abdominal masses. Patients with cancer who develop VTE may be at increased risk of bleeding due to a variety of reasons including recent surgery, vascular invasion by tumor and intracerebral masses. Therefore, making a definitive diagnosis of VTE is imperative and clinical care planning may be more complicated.

This chapter will discuss the relationship between malignancy and thromboembolic disease, exploring both clinical and basic science observations. Special considerations regarding the diagnosis, management, and prophylaxis of PE, DVT, and catheter-related central vein thrombosis will be presented. Therapeutic recommendations will be based on the best available evidence from clinical trials. Finally, this chapter will discuss the role of extensive screening for occult malignancy in the patient with idiopathic venous thromboembolic disease.

THE ASSOCIATION BETWEEN MALIGNANCY AND VENOUS THROMBOEMBOLISM

The relationship between cancer and DVT or PE is appreciated by most clinicians. The reported clinical incidence of DVT and/or PE in patients with cancer ranges from 1% to 15% and this incidence is even higher in autopsy series.[1–4] Retrospective studies indicate that patients with objectively documented symptomatic DVT or PE are at increased risk of developing clinically overt malignancy, compared to patients whose symptoms are caused by conditions other than thrombosis.[5,6] Goldberg et al, reviewed the records of 1443 hospitalized patients who presented with signs and symptoms of DVT. Three hundred and seventy patients had objectively documented DVT while 1073 patients had other causes of a sore leg. Patients were followed for up to 5 years after hospital discharge. The cumulative rates of cancer after discharge were 6.3% for patients who had DVT and 2.4% for patients without thrombosis, a relative risk of 2.4 (95% confidence interval 1.5 to 4.7). The risk of developing cancer was highest in patients under the age of 50.[5] Another retrospective study examined the risk of subsequent cancer in patients who undergo angiography for suspected PE.[6] The authors identified 128 patients with documented PE. Patients were matched on the basis of sex, age, and date of angiography to patients who had negative angiograms. Follow-up data were available for 88 of the patients with PE and 82 patients without PE. In the 2 years after pulmonary angiography, cancer was documented in 13 (14.7%) of 88 patients with PE in contrast to none of the patients with negative angiograms.[6] The results of these two studies support the hypothesis that patients who have VTE are at increased risk of the subsequent development of cancer.

The incidence of subsequent cancer appears to be higher in patients with idiopathic thrombosis compared to patients that have known risk factors for VTE. Although two retrospective studies did not detect any difference in the incidence of subsequent malignancy between patients with idiopathic versus secondary DVT,[7,8] two small prospective studies noted a trend toward an in-

From *Venous Thromboembolism: An Evidence-Based Atlas* edited by Russell Hull, Gary Raskob, Graham Pineo © 1996, Futura Publishing Co., Armonk, NY.

creased incidence of malignancy in patients with idiopathic DVT or PE.[9,10] A recently published prospective study indicates that patients who present with recurrent idiopathic VTE are at especially high risk of developing clinically evident cancer.[11] Prandoni et al, followed 250 patients with symptomatic, venographically proven DVT for a 2-year period in order to determine the rate of recurrent VTE as well as the development of clinically apparent malignancy. One hundred and five patients had documented risk factors for the development of thrombosis while 145 were considered to have idiopathic DVT. The incidence of cancer in patients with secondary thrombosis was 1.9% while for patients with idiopathic thrombosis it was 6.1% (odds ratio 2.3; 95% confidence interval; 1.0 to 5.2). Recurrent episodes of thromboembolic disease were documented in five (4.8%) of 105 patients with secondary DVT; none of these patients developed malignancy. Of the 145 patients with idiopathic DVT, 35 (24.1%) had recurrent venous thromboembolic events. Six (17.1%) of these patients developed symptomatic cancer. Therefore, the risk of developing cancer is significantly higher for patients with recurrent idiopathic thromboembolism compared to patients with secondary DVT (odds ratio 9.8; 95% confidence interval, 1.8 to 52.2).

RISK FACTORS FOR VENOUS THROMBOEMBOLISM IN THE CANCER PATIENT

The susceptibility of cancer patients to thrombosis is likely due to many factors. First, increased activation of the coagulation system has been observed in many cancer patients.[12-15] This activation, which may be subclinical or overtly manifested as disseminated intravascular coagulation, occurs by a variety of mechanisms.[2,12,13,16] Platelet aggregation or adhesion may be tumor-cell mediated. Malignant cells elaborate procoagulation factors, including tissue factor[16] and direct activators of factor X.[17-19] In addition, indirect elaboration of procoagulants by tumor-associated macrophages and monocytes has been observed. These procoagulants include tissue factor, prothrombin activators, and activators of factor X.[20] The zymogen forms of factors I, V, VII, VIII:C, IX, and XI have been found to be elevated in patients with malignancy.[12] These factors, if activated by tumor-associated procoagulants may predispose patients to thrombosis. In addition, patients with liver failure due to massive involvement by tumor may have impaired clearance of these activated coagulation factors as well as decreased synthesis of the natural anticoagulants ATIII, protein C, and protein S.

Second, cancer patients are often quite debilitated in the latter weeks to months of their illnesses and may become bed-ridden, increasing the risk of DVT. Patients who undergo surgical procedures for removal or debulking of tumor masses are at risk of VTE in the perioperative period. Vascular structures may be compromised by ex-

trinsic compression or by direct tumor invasion as has been reported with malignancies such as renal cell cancer, germ cell cancer, hepatocellular carcinoma, gastric carcinoma, lung cancer, and adrenocortical carcinoma.[2]

Third, the administration of antineoplastic agents is associated with various thrombotic events including pulmonary veno-occlusive disease, hepatic veno-occlusive disease, myocardial infarction and ischemia, as well as venous thromboembolic disease.[25-37] Numerous cases of DVT and PE have been reported in patients with malignancies such as Hodgkins disease, nonHodgkins lymphoma, germ cell tumors, and breast cancer. Often these thrombotic events occur during the administration of chemotherapeutic or hormonal agents.[25-37] Treatment regimens involving cisplatinum, cyclophosphamide, methotrexate, 5-fluorouracil, or tamoxifen are reported to be associated with an incidence of venous thromboembolic events of 5% to 7%. Most of these studies are retrospective and many are limited by the lack of objective documentation of DVT and PE as well as lack of control groups. However, there is reasonable evidence that the administration of chemotherapy and/or hormonal therapy does place patients at increased risk of thrombosis.

In a prospective study, Levine et al, compared the rate of thrombotic events in 205 patients randomized to receive either 12 weeks or 36 weeks of adjuvant chemotherapy for node-positive breast cancer.[29] All patients were evaluated for evidence of thrombotic disease upon entry to the study and at fixed intervals throughout the trial. Fourteen of the 205 patients (6.8%) developed some type of thrombosis. Nine of these 205 (4.4%) had proximal-vein thrombosis and/or PE. One patient developed symptomatic subclavian vein thrombosis, and brachial artery thrombosis occurred in one subject. An additional three patients developed extensive superficial thrombophlebitis of the long saphenous vein. During the first 12 weeks of the study, five patients randomized to receive 12 weeks of therapy and four patients in the 36-week group had thrombosis. During the next 24 weeks of the trial, five of the patients randomized to receive 36 weeks of chemotherapy developed thrombi. Patients who received only 12 weeks of chemotherapy had no events during the subsequent 24 weeks of the study. Thus, all of these thrombotic events occurred during the 949 patient-months of chemotherapy. In contrast, there were no events during the 2413 patient-months without chemotherapy.[29] Saphner et al, reported a review of the records of 2673 patients who participated in various randomized trials comparing adjuvant therapies for Stage II, node-positive breast cancer.[37] Patients were randomized to observation (12%), tamoxifen (3.2%), chemotherapy (22.6%), or a combination of chemotherapy and tamoxifen (62.2%). The odds ratios of objectively documented VTE compared to the observation group were 5.5, 8.9, and 21.1 for the tamoxifen group, chemotherapy only group, and the combined therapy group, respectively. The results of both of these studies support the hypothesis that the administration of chemotherapy and or hormonal therapy increases the risk of VTE in patients with cancer.

The etiology of chemotherapy-related thrombosis is uncertain. Two studies have documented a decrease in serum levels of protein C in patients with breast cancer who received either adjuvant or palliative chemotherapy.[38,39] Protein C levels decreased during treatment and returned to normal or near-normal within a few weeks after therapy. There were no thrombotic events reported, and levels of proteins C and S were not studied in breast cancer patients not receiving chemotherapy so a direct causal effect cannot be established.[38,39] Similarly levels of antithrombin III may be lower in patients receiving tamoxifen.[40–42] Two studies compared antithrombin III levels in patients receiving tamoxifen for breast cancer to levels in patients on no hormonal therapy.[40,41] There was a trend toward lower levels in patients taking tamoxifen. No thromboembolic events were reported. Powles et al, studied antithrombin III levels in patients receiving tamoxifen for breast cancer prophylaxis and in patients receiving placebo. Levels were measured before and during treatment.[42] Again, there was a nonsignificant trend toward lower levels of antithrombin III when tamoxifen was begun.

Finally, the placement of central venous catheters for chemotherapy, blood product support, and parenteral nutrition is associated with thrombosis of the cannulated veins. This is discussed further below. (see "Central Venous Catheters and the Risk of Venous Thromboembolism")

THE ROLE OF COAGULATION IN CANCER GROWTH

It has been suggested that the activation of the coagulation system plays an integral role in the growth and spread of malignant neoplasms. Fibrin is found at the site of tumor masses and metastatic nodules where it is thought to provide a suitable stroma for tumor cell growth and invasion, stimulate neovascularization, facilitate attachment of tumor cells to endothelial cells, and provide protection from host defense mechanisms and chemotherapeutic agents.[16] Some tumor types (i.e., colon) can activate plasminogen, leading to collagenase activity and dissolution of basement membranes, an important step in the metastatic process.[39–41] It has been recently demonstrated that human and rat tissues which are preferred sites of metastatic spread have a higher tissue procoagulant activity as measured by the ability to activate factor X.[42] This procoagulant activity was significantly reduced by the administration of warfarin. The observation that the coagulation cascade is involved in the metastatic process has led to studies in which anticoagulants have been used to alter the natural history of various malig-

nancies.[13] A discussion of these studies is beyond the scope of this chapter.

DIAGNOSIS OF DEEP-VEIN THROMBOSIS AND PULMONARY EMBOLISM

In general, the diagnosis of DVT and/or PE is made by the same diagnostic tests discussed elsewhere in this book. There are some situations however, when the use of noninvasive tests may be misleading. When vascular or lymphatic structures in the abdomen are involved, as in patients with large pelvic masses, lower extremity swelling may occur, leading to the suspicion of DVT. Impedance plethysmography may be used to screen symptomatic patients but may be unreliable in the differentiation of venous outflow obstruction due to thrombosis from that due to extrinsic compression or vascular invasion, and false-positive tests may occur. Compression ultrasound may be unreliable in patients with tumor infiltration in the inguinal nodes or thigh regions due to difficulty in visualization and compression of the vessels. Therefore, venography should be considered in this group of patients who have positive noninvasive testing. Lung tumors, either primary or metastatic may cause extrinsic compression of the pulmonary vasculature and can mimic PE on perfusion scanning.[43] Pulmonary angiography should be considered in patients who are thought to be at significant risk of bleeding with anticoagulant therapy when noninvasive testing is inconclusive. The combination of lung scanning and noninvasive leg testing as discussed elsewhere in this text should be used when making therapeutic decisions for most cancer patients who present with signs and symptoms of PE.

TREATMENT OF VENOUS THROMBOEMBOLISM IN THE PATIENT WITH CANCER

The treatment of deep venous thrombosis and PE in patients with cancer should parallel that of patients without malignant neoplasms. This therapy, which is discussed in detail elsewhere in this book, consists of initial heparin administration followed by long-term anticoagulation with warfarin or adjusted-dose subcutaneous heparin. Vena caval filters should be considered in patients who have a contraindication to anticoagulant therapy. Of interest is the observation from two randomized treatment studies that the use of low-molecular-weight heparin (LMWH) may decrease the risk of cancer-related death.[44,45] These two trials randomized patients with DVT to initial therapy with either LMWH or unfractionated heparin. The cancer-related death rate was determined for those patients who had malignancy at study entry. Combined results of these two trials showed a cancer-related death rate of 21/67 (31%) for patients receiving standard heparin and 7/62 (11%) for patients on LMWH (p = 0.005), a relative risk reduction of 65%.[46] This difference in death rate cannot be attributed to a difference in thromboembobolic or bleeding deaths.[46]

Two questions remain unresolved when considering treatment of VTE in patients with malignancy: the duration of therapy and the safety of anticoagulant therapy in patients with primary or secondary central nervous system neoplasms. There have been no randomized studies comparing standard length with extended length anticoagulation therapy in patients with extensive malignancy. However, since the presence of malignancy and various treatment regimens for cancer are known to place patients at a higher risk of venous thromboembolic events, it is reasonable to consider these patients as having continuing risk factors for DVT and PE. It may be prudent to continue anticoagulation therapy indefinitely in this group of patients unless there is a contraindication to do so.

A major concern when treating VTE in the cancer patient is the potential for serious bleeding at tumor sites, particularly intracranial lesions. There have been reports of intracerebral hemorrhage in patients with primary or metastatic tumors of the brain who have been treated with anticoagulants for DVT or PE.[47–49] Some authors have suggested the placement of vena caval filters in such patients. There are many other case series in which patients with objectively documented VTE have been treated with conventional heparin/warfarin regimens without symptomatic intracranial hemorrhage.[50–53] At present, there are no randomized trials that directly assess the risk of bleeding during anticoagulation in patients with known central nervous system lesions. However, indirect evidence of the safety of such therapy is available upon review of seven randomized trials of various anticoagulation regimens.[44,45,54–58] A total of 1186 patients were treated for DVT. Of these, 183 had clinically apparent malignancy at the time of presentation. It is reasonable to presume that some of these patients had occult brain metastases, yet no patient had an intracranial hemorrhage (0 of 183, 95% CI 0% to 2%). This observation suggests that conventional anticoagulation therapy is safe in patients with malignancy as well as being effective in reducing the risk of recurrent deep venous thrombosis. The presence of an intracranial malignancy per se, should not be considered an absolute contraindication to anticoagulation. Vena caval filters do not prevent recurrent venous thrombosis, and they are not completely effective in preventing recurrent PE[50,59] and are associated with clinical sequelae such as lower extremity edema and perforation of the vena cava. These complications may not be particularly significant in the patient with widely metastatic cancer but would be of major importance in the patient being given curative therapy for their malignancy. Therefore, careful consideration of each patient's clinical status and prognosis should be considered before using a caval filter in place of anticoagulation for VTE.

PREVENTION OF VENOUS THROMBOEMBOLISM IN THE CANCER PATIENT

At the present time, there are no data to suggest that all patients with malignancy should be placed on routine prophylaxis against DVT or PE. Certainly, patients with cancer who undergo surgical procedures should receive the standard prophylactic regimens as outlined in another section of this book. In addition, a recent clinical trial demonstrates the safety and efficacy of very-low-dose warfarin (mean INR = 1.52) in the prevention of VTE in women receiving chemotherapy for metastatic breast cancer.[60] Three hundred and eleven patients with metastatic breast cancer were randomized to placebo or low-intensity warfarin. Patients were given 1 mg of warfarin daily for the first 6 weeks. The warfarin dose was then adjusted to maintain the INR between 1.3 to 1.9. The average warfarin dose was 2.6 mg per day and the mean INR was 1.52. Seven of 159 (4.4%) patients in the placebo group had thromboembolism compared to one of 152 in the warfarin group. Major bleeding occurred in two placebo and one warfarin patient and there was no difference in survival between the two groups. Warfarin should be considered in patients receiving chemotherapy for metastatic breast cancer. It is possible that lower doses of warfarin would be effective and would eliminate the need for laboratory monitoring. In addition, patients receiving chemotherapy for other malignancies may benefit from low-dose warfarin administration. However, both of these questions should be addressed in controlled clinical trials. Prevention of central venous catheter thrombosis is discussed below.

CENTRAL VENOUS CATHETERS AND THE RISK OF VENOUS THROMBOEMBOLISM

The placement of central venous catheters for chemotherapy, blood product support, and parenteral nutrition is associated with thrombosis of the cannulated vein. The incidence is uncertain due to limited prospective studies, but is estimated to occur in 17% to 35% of patients with central lines. Patients present with pain, redness, swelling, and venous distention in the arm and/or face.[61–67] Venography is the diagnostic procedure of choice. Patients with subclavian vein thrombosis are at risk of PE with an estimated incidence of 10%.[61,62] While many of these pulmonary emboli are asymptomatic, fatal PE has been reported in patients with catheter-related thrombosis.[61–63] Currently there are no definitive recommendations regarding the therapy of subclavian vein thrombosis. However, standard anticoagulation with heparin and warfarin may relieve the acute symptoms and lower the risk of postphlebitic problems and should be considered in patients with catheter-related thrombosis.

It is uncertain if it is necessary to remove the catheter, although it may be advisable to do so when it is no longer needed or no longer functioning.

Two prospective studies document the efficacy and safety of low-dose warfarin therapy in the prevention of thrombosis in patients with central venous catheters.[66,67] In a nonrandomized study, patients with central venous catheters for administration of total parenteral nutrition were given low doses of warfarin that did not prolong the prothrombin time.[66] The thrombosis rate in patients given warfarin was less than that of the patients who were not treated. One untreated patient had a minor bleeding event. Two bleeding events occurred in the warfarin group. One was a minor bleed from a ureteral stone and one patient had a major retroperitoneal bleed during an episode of bacterial sepsis.

Bern et al, randomized 82 cancer patients with central lines for chemotherapy administration to placebo or 1 mg of warfarin.[67] The warfarin was started 3 days prior to insertion of the catheter and continued for 90 days. Venography was done at ninety days or sooner if symptoms developed. Four of 42 patients on warfarin had thrombosis as documented by venography compared to 15 of 40 patients who were given placebo (P<0.0001). The majority of the patients with venogram-proven thrombosis had symptoms. There were no bleeding events in either the warfarin-treated or the control group. Therefore, warfarin at a dose of 1 mg per day should be considered in patients with chronic indwelling central venous catheters.

SEARCHING FOR OCCULT MALIGNANCY IN THE PATIENT WITH IDIOPATHIC VENOUS THROMBOEMBOLISM

The observed relationship between venous thromboembolic disease and cancer raises the question of whether or not patients who present with idiopathic DVT should undergo screening for occult malignancy. Patients who would potentially benefit from screening are those in whom early diagnosis and treatment of malignancy would result in prolonged survival. The types of malignant disease in patients with DVT or PE is similar to that of patients in the general population.[5–10,68,69] Although many studies indicate that patients with VTE have an increased incidence of cancer, most do not document the stage of malignancy at the time of presentation with thrombosis.[5–10] Monreal et al, performed a prospective study in 113 patients who presented with DVT. Extensive screening was performed including blood counts, chemistry, CEA levels, chest radiograph, and abdominal ultrasound and CT scanning. Twelve cases of malignancy were discovered. Seven of these occurred in patients with idiopathic DVT while five were in patients who had known risk factors for thrombosis. Of these 12 patients

with malignancy, six had symptoms at the time of presentation that suggested the presence of cancer. The remaining six cases were identified through the elaborate screening process. These six cases included two cases of chronic lymphocytic leukemia (CLL), two superficial transitional cell carcinomas of the urinary bladder, and one case each of lung and colon cancer. The stage of the lung and colon tumors was not specified so it is difficult to ascertain whether their diagnosis at an asymptomatic stage impacted significantly on patient outcome. It is also uncertain that the cases of bladder cancer would not have been detected while still curable since it is quite likely that these patients may have presented with hematuria once anticoagulant therapy was started. In addition, the CLL is easily diagnosed by examination of the blood cell counts and/or peripheral smear and is generally left untreated unless there are other hematologic abnormalities. Therefore, at the present time, it is unclear as to what proportion of patients with idiopathic VTE have malignancies that can be identified and treated while at an early stage. Likewise, it is unclear whether or not early detection will significantly impact patient outcome. Routine screening is expensive and often uncomfortable both physically and emotionally for the patient. Therefore, extensive screening cannot be recommended as a routine process in patients who present with idiopathic VTE. Currently a randomized clinical trial that includes cost analysis and quality-of-life outcome measures is being planned.[69]

REFERENCES

1. Dhami MS, Bona RD. Thrombosis in patients with cancer. Postgraduate Med 1993:93:131–140.
2. Scates, SM. Diagnosis and treatment of cancer-related thrombosis. Hem Onc Clin North Amer 1992;6:1329–1339.
3. Luzatto G, Schaffer AI. The prothrombotic state in cancer. Sem Onc 1990;17:147–159.
4. Shen VS, Pollak EW. Fatal pulmonary embolism in cancer patients—is heparin prophylaxis justified? South Med J 1980;73:841–843.
5. Goldberg RJ, Seneff M, Gore JM, et al. Occult malignant neoplasm in patients with deep venous thrombosis. Arch Intern Med 1987:147:251–253.
6. Gore JM, Appelbaum JS, Greene HL, Dexter L, Dalen JE. Occult cancer in patients with acute pulmonary embolism. Ann Int Med 1982;96:556–560.
7. Griffin MN, Stanson AW, Brown ML, et al. Deep vein thrombosis and pulmonary embolism: risk subsequent malignant neoplasms. Arch Int Med 1987;147:1907–1911.
8. O'Conner NJT, Fletcher EW, Cederhold-Williams SA, Allington M, Sharp AA. Significance of idiopathic deep vein thrombosis. Post Grad Med J 1984;60:275–277.
9. Monreal M, Casals A, Lafoz E, Angles A. Pulmonary embolism and occult cancer; a prospective study. Thromb Haemost 1991;65:1174.(Abstract)
10. Monreal M, Salvador R, Soriano V, Sabria M. Cancer and deep vein thrombosis. Arch Intern Med 1988;148;485.
11. Prandoni P, Lensing Anthonie WA, Buller HR, et al. Deep-vein thrombosis and the incidence of subsequent symptomatic cancer. N Engl J Med 1992:327:1128–1133.

12. Bick RL. Coagulation abnormalities in malignancy: a review. Sem in Thromb and Hemost 1992;18:353–372.

13. Rickles FR, Hancock WW, Edwards Rl, Zacharski LR. Antimetastatic agents. A. Role of cellular procoagulants in the pathogenesis of fibrin deposition in cancer and the use of anticoagulants and/or antiplatelet drugs in cancer treatment. Sem Thromb Hem 1988;14:88–94.

14. Patterson WP, Ringenberg QS. The pathophysiology of thrombosis in cancer. Sem Onc 1990;2:140–146.

15. Callander N, Rapaport SI. Trousseau's syndrome. West Med J 1993;158:364–371.

16. Donati MB, Semeraro N. Cancer cell procoagulants and their pharmacological modulation. Haemostasis 1984;14: 422–429.

17. Pineo GF, Brain MC, Gallus AS, Hirsh J, Hatton MWC, Regoeczi E. Tumor, mucus production, and hypercoagulability. Ann NY Acad Sci 1974;230:262–270.

18. Gordon SG, Cross BA. A factor X-activating cysteine protease from malignant tissue. J Clin Invest 1981;67:1665–1671.

19. Falanga A, Gordon SG. Isolation and characterization of cancer procoagulant. A cysteine proteinase from malignant tissue. Biochem 1985:24:5558–5567.

20. Edwards RL, Rickles FR. Macrophage procoagulants. Prog Hem Thromb 1984;7:183–209.

21. Doll DC, Yarbor JW. Vascular toxicity associated with antineoplastic agents. Sem Onc 1992;19:580–596.

22. Clahsen PC, van de Velde CJ. Thromboembolic complications after perioperative chemotherapy in women with early breast cancer: A European organization for research and treatment of cancer breast cancer cooperative group study. J Clin Onc 1994;12:1266–1271.

23. Weiss RB, Tormey DC. Venous thrombosis during multi-modal treatment of primary breast carcinoma. Can Treat Rep 1981;65:677–679.

24. Lipton A, Harver HA, Hamilton RW. Venous thrombosis as a side effect of tamoxifen treatment. Can Treat Rep 1984;68: 887–889.

25. Levine MN, Gent M, Hirsh J, et al. The thrombogenic effect of anticancer drug therapy in women with stage II breast cancer. N Engl J Med 1988;318:404–407.

26. Nevasaari K, Heikkinen M, Taskinen PJ. Tamoxifen and thrombosis. Lancet 1978;2:947.

27. Hendrick A, Subramanian VP. Tamoxifen and thromboembolism. JAMA 1980;243:514–515.

28. Goodnough LT, Hedehiko S, Saito H, Manni A, Jones PK, et al. Increased incidence of thromboembolism in stage IV breast cancer patients treated with a five-drug chemotherapy regimen. Cancer 1984;54:1264–1268.

29. Cantwell MJ, Carmichael J, Ghani SE, Harris AL. Thrombosis and thromboemboli in patients with lymphoma during cytotoxic chemotherapy. Br Med J 1988;297:179–180.

30. Lederman GS, Garnick MB. Pulmonary emboli as a complication of germ cell cancer treatment. J Urol 1987;137: 1236–1237.

31. Seifter EJ, Young RC, Longo DL. Deep venous thrombosis during therapy for Hodgkins's disease. Cancer Treat Rep 1985;69:1011–1013.

32. Cantwell BMJ, Mannix KA, Roberts JT, Ghani SE, Harris AI. Thromboembolic events during combination chemotherapy for germ cell malignancy. Lancet 1988;2:1086–1087.

33. Saphner T, Tormey DC, Gray R. Venous and arterial thrombosis in patients who received adjuvant therapy for breast cancer. J Clin Oncol 1991;9:286–294.

34. Rogers JS, Murgo AJ, Fontana JA, Raich PC. Chemotherapy for breast cancer decreases plasma protein C and protein S. J Clin Onc 1988;6:276–281.

35. Feffer SE, Carmosino S, Fox RI. Acquired protein C deficiency in patients with breast cancer receiving cyclophosphamide, methotrexate, and 5-fluorouracil. Cancer 1989;63: 1303–1307.

36. Jordan VC, Fritz NF, Tormey DC. Long-term adjuvant therapy with tamoxifen: effects on sex hormone binding globulin and antithrombin III. Canc Res 1987;47:4517–4519.

37. Enck RE, Rios CN. Tamoxifen treatment of metastatic breast cancer and antithrombin III levels. Cancer 1984;53: 2607–2609.

38. Powles TJ, Hardy JR. A pilot trial to evaluate the acute toxicity and feasibility of tamoxifen for prevention of breast cancer. Br J Canc 1989;60:126–131.

39. Burtin P, Fondaneche M. Receptor for plasmin on human carcinoma cells. J Nat Canc Inst 1988;80:762–765.

40. Reich R, Thompson EW. Effects of inhibitors of plasminogen activator, serine proteinases, and collagenase IV on the invasion of basement membranes by metastatic cells. Canc Res 1988;48:3307–3312.

41. Wojtukiewicz MZ, Zarchaski LR, Memoli VA, et al. Indirect activation of blood coagulation in colon cancer. Thromb Haemost 1989;62:1062–1066.

42. Carty NJ, Talyor I, Roath OS, El-Baruni K, Francis JL. Tissue procoagulant activity may be important in sustaining metastatic tumor growth. Clin Exp Metastasis 1992;10: 175–181.

43. Levine M, Hirsh J. the diagnosis and treatment of thrombosis in the cancer patient. Sem Oncol 1990;17:160–171

44. Prandoni P, Lensing AWA, Buller HR, et al. Comparison of subcutaneous low-molecular-weight heparin with intravenous standard heparin in proximal deep-vein thrombosis. Lancet 1992;339:441–445.

45. Hull RD, Raskob GE, Pineo GF, et al. Subcutaneous low-molecular-weight heparin compared with continuous intravenous heparin in the treatment of proximal-vein thrombosis. 1992;326:975–982.[ep[el1]

46. Green D, Hull RD, Brant R, Pineo GF. Lower mortality in cancer patients treated with low molecular weight heparin versus standard heparin. Lancet 1992;339:1476.

47. Swann KW, Black P, Baker MF. Management of symptomatic deep venous thrombosis and pulmonary embolism on a neurosurgical service. J Neurosurg 1986;64:563–567.

48. So W, Hugenholtz H, Richard MT. Complications of anticoagulant therapy in patients with known central nervous system lesions. Can J Surg 1983;26:181–183.

49. Moore FD, Osteen RT, Karp DD, Steele G, Wilson RE. Anticoagulants, venous thromboembolism, and the cancer patient. Arch Surg 1981;116:405–407.

50. Olin JW, Young JR, Graor RA, Ruschhaupt Wf, Beven EF, et al. Treatment of deep vein thrombosis and pulmonary emboli in patients with primary and metastatic brain tumors. Arch Intern Med 1987;147:2177–2199.

51. DiRicco G, Marini C, Rindi M, et al. Pulmonary embolism in neurosurgical patients; diagnosis and treatment. J Neurosurg 1984;60:972–975.

52. Dhami MS, Bona RD, Calogero JA, Hellman RM. Venous thromboembolism and high grade gliomas. Thromb Haemost 1993;70:393–396.

53. Altschuler E, Moosa H, Selker RG, Vertosick FT. The risk and efficacy of anticoagulant therapy in the treatment of thromboembolic complications in patients with primary malignant brain tumors. Neurosurg 1990;27:74–77.

54. Hull RD, Delmore T, Carter C, et al. Adjusted subcutaneous heparin versus warfarin sodium in the long-term treatment of venous thrombosis. N Engl J Med 1982;306:189–194.

55. Hull R, Delmore T, Genton E, et al. Warfarin sodium versus low-dose heparin in the long-term treatment of venous thrombosis. N Engl J Med 1979;301:855–858.

56. Hull R, Hirsh J, Carter C, et al. Different intensities of oral anticoagulant therapy in the treatment of proximal-vein thrombosis. N Engl J Med 1982;307:1676–1681.

57. Hull RD, Raskob GE, Rosenbloom D, et al. Heparin for 5 days as compared with 10 days in the initial treatment of proximal venous thrombosis. N Engl J Med 1990;322:1260–1264.

58. Hull RD, Raskob GE, Hirsh J, et al. Continuous intravenous heparin compared with intermittent subcutaneous heparin in the initial treatment of proximal-vein thrombosis. N Engl J Med 1986;315:1109–1114.

59. Cohen JR, Grella L, Citron M. Greenfield filter instead of heparin as primary treatment of deep venous thrombosis or pulmonary embolism in patients with cancer. Cancer 1992;70:1993–1996.

60. Levine M, Hirsh J, Gent M, et al. Double-blind randomized trial of a very-low-dose warfarin for prevention of thromboembolism in stage IV breast cancer. Lancet 1994;343(8902):886–889.

61. Monreal M, Lafoz E, Ruiz J, Valls R, Alastrue A. Upper-extremity deep venous thrombosis and pulmonary embolism, a prospective study. Chest 1991;99:280–283.

62. Becker DM, Philbrick JT, Walker FB. Axillary and subclavian vein thrombosis. Prognosis and treatment. Arch Intern Med 1991;151:1934–1943.

63. Anderson AJ, Krasnow SH, Boyer MW, et al. Thrombosis: the major hickman catheter complication in patients with solid tumor. Chest 1989;85:71–75.

64. Lokich JJ, Becker B. Subclavian vein thrombosis in patients treated with infusion chemotherapy for advanced malignancy. Cancer. 1983:52:1586–1589.

65. Raad II, Luna M, Khalil SM, Costerton JW, Lam C, et al. The relationship between the thrombotic and infectious complications of central venous catheters. JAMA 1994:271:1014–1016.

66. Bern MM, Bothe A, Bistrian B, Champagne CD, Keane MS, et al. Prophylaxis against central vein thrombosis with low-dose warfarin. Surgery 1984;99:216–221.

67. Bern MM, Lokich JJ, Wallach SR, et al. Very low doses of warfarin can prevent thrombosis in central venous catheters: A randomized prospective trial. Ann Int Med 1990;112:423–428.

68. Monreal M, Lafoz E, Casals A, et al. Occult cancer in patients with venous thrombosis: a systematic approach. Cancer 1991;67:541–545.

69. Prins MH. Lensing WA, Hirsh J. Idiopathic deep venous thrombosis. Is a search for malignant disease justified? Arch Intern Med 1994;154:1310–1312.

39

Complications of Heparin

Gary E. Raskob, Sherri S. Durica, James N. George

INTRODUCTION

The complications of heparin include bleeding,[1–12] thrombocytopenia,[13–24] osteoporosis,[25–28] elevations of serum transaminase levels,[29–32] and a variety of less common side-effects including hypoaldosteronism,[33–38] hyperkalemia,[39–44] skin reactions and hypersensitivity,[45–64] and priapism.[65,66] Bleeding is the most common complication of heparin therapy. Thrombocytopenia is less common but can be devastating when it is associated with arterial thromboembolism or recurrent venous thromboembolism (VTE). Osteoporosis is a potential complication of long-term heparin administration. Elevation of serum transaminase levels is not uncommon, but the clinical importance of this laboratory abnormality is uncertain. These elevations in transaminase levels usually return to normal after heparin is discontinued. The other side-effects of heparin listed above are rare.

This chapter reviews the complications of heparin treatment in the context of heparin use for the treatment and prevention of VTE.

BLEEDING

The rates of bleeding complications are well documented from contemporary clinical trials evaluating intravenous heparin treatment for VTE. Bleeding occurs in 2% to 12% of patients during heparin treatment by continuous intravenous infusion.[1–12] The risk of bleeding is greater in patients who receive intravenous heparin by intermittent injection than in those who receive continuous infusion.[2–5]

The severity of bleeding is classified as either major or minor. Major bleeding is defined as clinically overt bleeding that is associated with a decline in hemoglobin of 2 gm/dl or more, requires transfusion of two or more units, or is retroperitoneal, intracranial, or occurs into a major joint.[6,8,10–12] Minor bleeding refers to clinically overt bleeding which does not meet the other criteria for major bleeding. The recent clinical trials evaluating continuous intravenous heparin treatment for VTE report rates of major bleeding ranging from 2% to 7%.[6–12] A recent large multicenter trial,[10] which entered a broad spectrum of patients, reported major bleeding in 5% of patients given continuous intravenous heparin infusion. Most major bleeding episodes occur early during heparin therapy (within the first 2 to 3 days).

Patients can be classified as either high risk or low risk for major bleeding based on the presence or absence of identifiable clinical risk factors. A recent clinical trial has clarified the relation between risk factors for bleeding, heparin dose, and the rate of major bleeding complications.[8,11] Before commencing heparin, patients were classified according to the presence or absence of one or more risk factors for bleeding:

1. Surgery or trauma within the previous 14 days.
2. A history of peptic ulcer disease, gastrointestinal bleeding or genitourinary bleeding.
3. The presence of clinical disorders or conditions predisposing the patient to bleeding (e.g., liver disease, multiple invasive lines, etc.)
4. Stroke within the previous 14 days.
5. Thrombocytopenia (platelet count less than 150,000).

Patients were classified as high risk for bleeding if one or more of the above risk factors were present. If none were present, the patient was classified as low risk for bleeding. All patients received an initial intravenous bolus of 5,000 units. In low-risk patients, the heparin infusion was begun at a dose of 40,000 units per 24 hours (1,660 units per hour). In high-risk patients, the heparin infusion was begun at a dose of 30,000 units per 24 hours (1,250 units per hour).[8,11] Major bleeding occurred in 12 of 111 (11%) high-risk patients, compared with only 1 of 88

(1%) low-risk patients (p = 0.007).[8] The striking difference in the incidence of major bleeding between the predefined low risk and high-risk groups occurred even though the low-risk patients received a higher initial heparin infusion dose. In six of the 13 patients with major bleeding, the bleeding occurred while the activated partial thromboplastin time (APTT) was within the predefined therapeutic range (APTT ratio 1.5 to 2.5).[8] Many patients without bleeding complications had APTT values more than 2.5 times control for 24 hours or more throughout the course of therapy.[8,11] Taken together, the above findings suggest that the risk of bleeding is determined mainly by the presence or absence of identifiable clinical risk factors, rather than the initial heparin infusion dose or APTT response. In the absence of readily identifiable clinical risk factors (defined above), the risk of major bleeding is low (1%) even when these patients receive relatively high initial heparin infusion doses (1,660 units per hour or 40,000 units per 24 hours). To date, an association between an excessively prolonged APTT response (e.g., more than 2.5 times control) and an increased risk of bleeding has not been established in patients with VTE.[11]

Bleeding and Low-Molecular-Weight Heparin

Low-molecular-weight heparin (LWMH) has undergone extensive evaluation by clinical trials for the prevention and treatment of venous thrombosis.

For the prevention of VTE, LMWH given once or twice daily by subcutaneous injection is associated with a similar risk of bleeding as the conventional low dose regimen of unfractionated heparin (5,000 units every 8 hours subcutaneously).[1] However, when the same 24-hour dose is given as two divided doses (7,500 units every 12 hours) to patients undergoing hip replacement, a regimen of LMWH (enoxaparin 30 mg every 12 hours) was associated with a reduced risk of overall bleeding (from 9.3% to 5.1%, risk reduction, 45%).[67] Major bleeding occurs in 3% to 5% of patients given LMWH prophylaxis after hip or knee replacement surgery.[1]

Clinical trials of LMWH in the treatment of established venous thrombosis indicate that certain LMWH preparations are associated with less bleeding than continuous intravenous unfractionated heparin. In a randomized double-blind trial[10] comparing LMWH (tinzaparin) with continuous intravenous unfractionated heparin, major bleeding occurred in 11 of 219 patients (5.0%) given unfractionated heparin, compared with 1 of 213 patients (0.5%) who received the once daily LMWH regimen, a risk reduction of 91% (p = 0.006). A similar risk reduction in the incidence of major bleeding was observed in the trial by Prandoni et al,[9] using the LMWH nadroparin (Fraxiparine), but this was a smaller clinical trial and the difference did not achieve statistical significance.

THROMBOCYTOPENIA

Thrombocytopenia is now a well-documented complication of heparin treatment.[13–24] The clinical manifestations of heparin-associated thrombocytopenia range from common, minimal and transient decreases of the platelet count to severe thrombocytopenia that may be accompanied by arterial thromboembolism and/or disseminated intravascular coagulation (DIC). The mild form of thrombocytopenia, with platelet counts not less than 50,000/ul, usually has its onset soon after heparin treatment and may continue throughout treatment, although commonly the platelet count recovers despite continued heparin treatment. The mechanism of this mild thrombocytopenia is probably the result of a direct effect of heparin to induce platelet aggregation.[68–72] The more severe form of thrombocytopenia usually appears after several days of heparin treatment, although it can occur earlier. The mechanism of more severe heparin-associated thrombocytopenia involves heparin-dependent antiplatelet antibodies.[73,74] The role of heparin appears to involve alteration of the platelet surface, facilitating the binding of antibody to platelet antigens and antigen-antibody complexes to platelet Fc receptors.[75–80] The major target antigen appears to be a heparin-platelet-factor 4 complex[81–84] which localizes the IgG on the platelet surface although other surface antigens may also be involved.[75,85] The IgG from patients with heparin-associated thrombocytopenia may also bind to endothelial cells in the presence of heparin,[83–84,86] an observation that could have relevance to the occurrence of DIC and thromboembolic complications. The mechanisms of heparin-associated thrombocytopenia are reviewed in more detail elsewhere.[87]

The actual incidence of thrombocytopenia during heparin treatment is unclear, in part because of variability of the definition of thrombocytopenia used in prospective studies.[87] Some define thrombocytopenia as the occurrence of any platelet count less than normal (150,000/ul), whereas others require the occurrence of platelet counts less than 100,000/ul for at least 2 consecutive days. The early prospective studies reported frequencies of thrombocytopenia of 11% to 24%, but in contemporary studies since 1986, the incidence of thrombocytopenia has been about 2% to 3%,[1,6–12] and in most of these studies, the criteria for thrombocytopenia was only an isolated platelet count of less than 150,000/ul. The apparent decrease in the incidence of heparin-associated thrombocytopenia between 1976 to present is probably the result of two factors. First, a change in the composition of commercial heparin occurred. In many of the earlier studies, heparin prepared from bovine lung was used. Bovine lung heparin appears to be associated with a greater risk for thrombocytopenia than heparin prepared from porcine intestinal mucosa.[87] Current commercial heparin preparations are essentially all isolated from porcine intestinal mucosa. Second, current clinical practice and the more recent clinical trials have used shorter durations of heparin treatment for VTE. In the earlier studies, heparin was given for 7 to 10 days and the typical time for the onset of thrombocytopenia was 5 to 7 days after starting heparin. In current practice, heparin is discontinued on the fourth or fifth day in most patients. The recent studies evaluating this shorter course of heparin treatment report an incidence of any thrombocytopenia (platelet count less than 150,000/ul) of about 3%.[8,10,87]

Thrombocytopenia can occur with any heparin preparation, dose and route of administration.[87] Thrombocytopenia has been reported during treatment with unfractionated heparin, LMWH, condroitin sulfate-like glycosaminoglycan agents, heparin-like compounds such as pentosan, polysulfate, and with the heparinoid glycosaminoglycan, Danaparoid (previously known as Org 10172). Thrombocytopenia has occurred even when heparin was used only to flush indwelling intravenous catheters in doses as low as 100 units per day and with use of heparin-coated pulmonary catheters.[87]

Thromboembolism is the most important sequela of heparin-associated thrombocytopenia. Most case-series have emphasized the association with arterial thrombosis ("white clot syndrome"), but heparin-associated thrombocytopenia may also be associated with venous thromboembolic events.[87,88] The incidence of thromboembolism complicating heparin-associated thrombocytopenia is unknown. With current practice of heparin therapy for 5 days, the incidence is probably less than 1%. The incidence of thromboembolic complications associated with thrombocytopenia has probably been reduced by two factors in recent years. First, with increased awareness of the syndrome by clinicians, and the availability of automated platelet counts, patients receiving heparin can be monitored for thrombocytopenia and heparin discontinued if thrombocytopenia occurs before thromboembolism develops. Second, shortening the duration of heparin treatment for venous thrombosis has probably helped to reduce the incidence of heparin-associated thrombocytopenia with thrombosis.

Diagnosis and Management

Awareness of the potential for thrombocytopenia, with frequent monitoring of platelet counts, is the most important measure for preventing serious sequelae from heparin-associated thrombocytopenia. Patients receiving heparin therapy for venous thrombosis should have a daily platelet count. The diagnosis is made on the basis of a significant decline in platelet count in the absence of other etiologic factors, usually to a platelet count of less than 100,000/ul. However, there is no specific cut-off for the platelet count which establishes the diagnosis. Importantly, heparin-associated thrombocytopenia with thrombosis may be foreshadowed by a large rapid decline in platelet count without overt thrombocytopenia (for ex-

ample, a decline in platelet count from the high-end of normal such as 400,000 to between 100,000 to 150,000). A significant decline in platelet count over 2 to 3 days should raise the suspicion of heparin-associated thrombocytopenia.

Heparin should be stopped as soon as the diagnosis of heparin-associated thrombocytopenia is made. Heparin should be stopped because it is not possible to predict which patients will develop thromboembolic complications, and these complications can be devastating. In most patients receiving heparin treatment for venous thrombosis, by the time heparin-associated thrombocytopenia becomes evident, warfarin therapy has been established and these patients can stop heparin and be continued on warfarin treatment. The thrombocytopenia should resolve within several days of stopping heparin. If laboratory assays for heparin-dependent antibodies are available, they may provide supportive data for the diagnosis, but do not alter clinical management decisions.

If alternative antithrombotic treatment is required, two agents have been evaluated in descriptive studies (level V). These are the heparinoid, Danaparoid sodium,[89] and the defibrinogenating snake venom ancrod (Arvin).[90,91] An immediate onset of anticoagulation is achieved with Danaparoid following intravenous bolus administration. With ancrod, there is a delay of about 12 hours before effective defibrinogenation is achieved. Unfortunately neither Danaparoid or ancrod are currently approved for use in the United States, and there may be difficulty obtaining them by compassionate release quickly. Hirudin or other direct thrombin inhibitors appear promising, but these agents are also not approved for use in North America and further studies are needed. Additional treatment options have included the use of intravenous dextran, intravenous IgG, and plasma pheresis.[87]

OSTEOPOROSIS

Osteoporosis is a potential complication of long-term heparin administration. The earliest clinical manifestation is usually the onset of nonspecific low back pain primarily involving the vertebrae or ribs; patients may present with spontaneous fracture in these areas.

The incidence of heparin-associated osteoporosis is uncertain because most of the reports have been either case-series or individual case reports.[25–27,92–100] There appears to be a relation between the dose and duration of heparin treatment, and the development of osteoporosis. In all but one report,[27] the daily dose of heparin was 15,000 units or more and the duration of treatment was longer than 3 months. The concept of a "threshold" for osteoporosis developing with treatment with large doses of heparin for longer than 3 months is supported by two additional pieces of evidence from randomized trials: (1) Hull et al, reported no episodes of clinically evident osteoporosis among 53 patients treated with 20,000 units of subcutaneous heparin daily for 3 months,[101] and (2) Monreal et al,[102] reported spinal fractures in 6 of 40 patients treated with 20,000 units of heparin daily for 3 to 6 months. In this latter trial, spinal fracture developed in only 1 of 40 patients in the comparison group who were treated with LMWH in a dose of 10,000 international factor Xa units daily (p = 0.054).[102]

The long-term clinical outcome in patients who develop heparin-associated osteoporosis is uncertain. Recovery of bone may occur after heparin treatment is stopped, but the extent and time course of recovery remains uncertain.

The optimal management of patients with heparin-associated osteoporosis is uncertain. The patient should maintain an adequate intake of calcium and vitamin D. Beyond these measures, the role of specific interventions such as treatment with calcitonin or biphosphonate is unknown. The decision to use these or additional therapies depends on the physician's judgment of the risk and potential benefit in the individual patient. The problem of heparin effects on bone has been reviewed in more detail recently.[103] (See Chapter 40.)

EFFECTS ON SERUM TRANSAMINASE

Heparin treatment may be associated with elevation of the serum transaminases.[29–32] There may be elevated levels of SGPT and SGOT which usually occurs within 5 days after initiating heparin, remain elevated for the duration of therapy and gradually return to normal several days after stopping heparin.[29–32] To date, no significant clinical sequelae have been reported in association with the elevated serum transaminase levels. However, studies incorporating long-term follow-up are lacking.

The clinician should be aware that heparin treatment may cause elevations of serum transaminase to avoid unnecessary interruption of heparin treatment for liver biopsy or other investigations in these patients.

SKIN REACTIONS

Two types of skin reactions have been associated with heparin treatment: delayed hypersensitivity (type IV) and skin necrosis.

The delayed hypersensitivity is usually seen only at the injection site and is not associated with skin necrosis.[45–55] The hypersensitivity usually occurs 3 to 21 days after starting heparin treatment. The lesion has the appearance of an indurated, erythematous lesion with a variable amount of vesicle and bullae formation. Biopsies of these areas show changes consistent with an acute dermatitis with a mononuclear infiltrate composed largely of helper T-cells. This type IV skin reaction is seen with both unfractionated heparin and LMWH.[47,53] Sensitivity to one preparation does not necessarily predict sensitivity to

others. Sensitivity testing may be helpful to select an appropriate formulation in patients with a history of heparin-associated type IV hypersensitivity who require subcutaneous heparin treatment. Patch or prick testing are not reliable indicators of heparin sensitivity and subcutaneous testing should be performed.

The heparin-associated skin lesions usually respond to topical treatment with corticosteroids. New plaques may continue to appear for a few days after stopping the heparin injections, and it may be necessary to continue corticosteroids during this time.

Skin necrosis is a well-documented but uncommon complication of heparin therapy. It is usually seen after 5 to 6 days of heparin treatment although may occur earlier in patients who have had prior exposure to heparin. Skin necrosis is usually seen at the site of subcutaneous injections, but has been reported to occur at sites distant from the injection site or with intravenous administration.[56,57,61] Skin necrosis may be seen with unfractionated heparin as well as LMWH,[62,63] and has been reported with both sources of heparin (porcine and bovine).

The clinical presentation is usually an initial area of painful erythema followed by the evolution of a central necrotic spot. Biopsy of the area reveals necrosis of the dermis and subcutaneous fat with thrombosis of dermal vessels. Grossly and histopathologically, the lesions of heparin skin necrosis appear very similar to those of warfarin-induced skin necrosis. The etiology of heparin-associated skin necrosis is uncertain but may be related to heparin-induced thrombocytopenia and may involve local platelet aggregation and microvascular thrombosis. Patients who develop skin necrosis with subcutaneous injection of heparin may be at risk for the development of heparin-associated thrombosis of either the venous or arterial systems.[58,59,60,64]

Heparin should be discontinued in patients who develop skin necrosis, and alternative approaches for the prevention and treatment of VTE should be used in these patients. The skin lesions may resolve spontaneously after heparin is stopped but may require debridement and/or skin grafting.

HYPOALDOSTERONISM AND HYPERKALEMIA

Heparin may inhibit the production of aldosterone.[33–38] Measurable decreases in serum aldosterone levels can be identified within 2 to 4 days of starting heparin treatment.[36] This suppression of aldosterone production does not appear to be dose-dependent and may occur with a variety of heparin dosing schedules. Both unfractionated heparin and LMWH preparations may suppress aldosterone production.[37,38] The mechanism by which heparin inhibits the synthesis of aldosterone is unknown.

Most patients do not develop clinically important sequelae associated with decreased aldosterone production. However, patients who have a pre-existing disturbance of the renin-angiotensin-aldosterone pathway may experience hyperkalemia, hyponatremia and hypotension.[40–44] Diabetics who may have juxtaglomerular sclerosis and low plasma renin levels may be particularly prone to the effects of hypoaldosteronism. It is prudent to monitor electrolytes closely during heparin treatment in patients who may be prone to the effects of hypoaldosteronism, such as those with diabetic nephropathy, or other causes of renal impairment, and those taking medications which may interfere with aldosterone metabolism or action, such as angiotensin converting enzyme inhibitors or potassium-sparing diuretics. The effects of heparin on aldosterone are usually transient and subside within a few days after stopping heparin.

REFERENCES

1. Levine M, Raskob G, Landefeld S, Hirsh J. Hemorrhagic complications of anticoagulant treatment. CHEST 1995;108:276s-290s.
2. Salzman EW, Deykin D, Shapiro RM, Rosenberg R. Management of heparin therapy: controlled prospective trial. N Engl J Med 1975;292:1046–1050.
3. Glazier RL, Crowell EB. Randomized prospective trial of continuous vs. intermittent heparin therapy. JAMA 1976;236:1365–1367.
4. Mant MJ, O'Brien BD, Thong KL, Hammond GW, Birtwhistle RV, et al. Haemorrhagic complications of heparin therapy. Lancet 1977;1:1133–1135.
5. Wilson JR, Lampman J. Heparin therapy: a randomized prospective study. Am Heart J 1979;97:155–158.
6. Hull RD, Raskob GE, Hirsh J, et al. Continuous intravenous heparin compared with intermittent subcutaneous heparin in the initial treatment of proximal-vein thrombosis. N Engl J Med 1986;315:1109–1114.
7. Gallus AS, Jackaman J, Tillett J, Mills W, Wycherley A. Safety and efficacy of warfarin started early after submassive venous thrombosis or pulmonary embolism. Lancet 1986;2:1293–1296.
8. Hull RD, Raskob GE, Rosenbloom D, et al. Heparin for 5 days as compared with 10 days in the initial treatment of proximal venous thrombosis. N Engl J Med 1990;322:1260–1264.
9. Prandoni P, Lensing AW, Buller HR, et al. Comparison of subcutaneous low-molecular-weight heparin with intravenous standard heparin in proximal deep vein thrombosis. Lancet 1992;339:441–445.
10. Hull R, Raskob G, Pineo G, et al. Subcutaneous low-molecular-weight heparin compared with continuous intravenous heparin in the treatment of proximal-vein thrombosis. N Engl J Med 1992;326:975–982.
11. Hull R, Raskob G, Rosenbloom D, et al. Optimal therapeutic level of heparin therapy in patients with venous thrombosis. Arch Intern Med 1992;152:1589–1595.
12. Raschke RA, Reilly BM, Guidry J, et al. The weight-based heparin nomogram compared with a standard care nomogram: a randomized controlled trial. Ann Intern Med 1993;119:874–881.
13. Natelson EA, Lynch EC, Alfrey CP, Gross JB. Heparin-induced thrombocytopenia. An unexpected response to treatment of consumption coagulopathy. Ann Intern Med 1969;71:1121–1125.
14. Rhodes GR, Dixon RH, Silver D. Heparin induced thrombocytopenia with thrombotic and hemorrhagic manifestations. Surg Gynecol Obstet 1973;136:409–416.
15. Klein HG, Bell WR. Disseminated intravascular coagulation during heparin therapy. Ann Intern Med 1974;80:477–481.
16. Bell WR. Thrombocytopenia occurring during heparin therapy. N Engl J Med 1976;295:276–277.
17. Bell WR, Tomasulo PA, Alving BA, Duffy TP. Thrombocytopenia occurring during the administration of heparin. A prospective study of 52 patients. Ann Intern Med 1976;85:155–160.
18. Babcock RB, Dumper CW, Scharfman WB. Heparin-induced immune thrombocytopenia. N Engl J Med 1976;295:237–241.
19. Nelson JC, Lerner RG, Goldstein R, Cagin NA. Heparin-induced thrombocytopenia. Arch Intern Med 1978;138:548–552.
20. Cimo PL, Moake JL, Weinger RS, et al. Heparin-induced thrombocytopenia: Association with a platelet aggregating factor and arterial thromboses. Am J Hematol 1979;6:125–133.
21. Weismann RE, Tobin RW. Arterial embolism occurring during systemic heparin therapy. Arch Surg 1958;76:219–227.
22. Roberts B, Rosata FE, Rosato EF. Heparin—a cause of arterial emboli? Surgery 1964;55:803–808.
23. Cines DB, Kaywin P, Bina M, et al. Heparin-associated thrombocytopenia. N Engl J Med 1980;303:788–795.
24. Bell WR. Heparin-associated thrombocytopenia and thrombosis. J Lab Clin Med 1988;111:600–604.
25. Griffith GC, Nichols G Jr, Asher JD, et al. Heparin osteoporosis. JAMA 1965;193:91–94.
26. Wise PH, Hall AJ. Heparin-induced osteoporosis in pregnancy. Br Med J 1980;281:110–111.
27. Griffith HT, Liu DTY. Severe heparin osteoporosis in pregnancy. Postgrad Med J 1984;60:424–425.
28. deSwiet M, Dorrington Ward P, Fidler J, et al. Prolonged heparin therapy in pregnancy causes bone demineralization. Br J Obstet Gynaecol 1983;90:1129–1134.
29. Olsson R, Korsan-Bengtsen BM, Korsan-Bengtsen K, et al. Serum aminotransferases after low-dose heparin treatment. Acta Med Scand 1978; 204:229–230.
30. Saffle JR, Russo J JR, Dukes GE JR, et al. The effect of low-dose heparin therapy on serum platelet and transaminase levels. J Surg Res 1980;28:297–305.
31. Nielsen HK, Husted SE, Koopman HD, et al. Heparin-induced increase in serum levels of aminotransferases. A controlled clinical trial. Acta Med Scand 1984;215:231–233.
32. Dukes GE Jr, Sanders SW, Russo J Jr. et al. Transaminase elevations in patients receiving bovine or porcine heparin. Ann Intern Med 1984;100:646–650.
33. Wilson D, Goeta FC. Selective hypoaldosteronism after prolonged heparin administration. Amer J Med 1964;36:635–540.
34. Conn JW, Rovner DR, Cohen EL, et al. Inhibition by heparinoid of aldosterone biosynthesis in man. J Clin Endocr 1966;26:527–532.
35. Lechey D, Gantt D, Lim V. Heparin-induced hypoaldosteronism. JAMA 1981;246:2189–2190.
36. O'Kelley R, Magee F, McKenna TJ. Routine heparin therapy inhibits adrenal aldosterone production. J Clin Endo and Metab 1983;56:108–112.
37. Levesque H, Verdier S, Cailleux N, et al. Low molecular weight heparin and hypoaldosteronism. Br Med J 1990;300:1437–1438.
38. Seibles M, Andrassy K, Vecesi P, et al. Dose dependent

suppression of mineralocorticoid metabolism by different heparin fractions. Thrombosis Res 1992;66:467–473.

39. Phelps KR, Oh MS, Carroll HJ. Heparin-induced hyperkalemia: report of a case. Nephron 1980;25:254–258.

40. Edes TE, Sunderrajan EV. Heparin-induced hyperkalemia. Arch Intern Med 1985;145:1070–1072.

41. Busch EH, Ventura HO, Lavie CJ. Heparin-induced hyperkalemia. So Med J 1987;80:1450–1451.

42. Durand D, Ader JL, Rey JP, et al. Inducing hyperkalemia by converting enzyme inhibitors and heparin. Kidney Int 1988;34:(Suppl)25:S-196–S-197.

43. Aull L, Chao H, Coy K. Heparin-induced hyperkalemia. DICP, The Annals of Pharmacotherapy 1990;24:244–246.

44. Gonzalez-Martin G, Diez-Molinas MS, Martinez AM, et al. Heparin-induced hyperkalemia: a prospective study. Int J Clin Pharm Therapy Toxicol 1991;29:446–450.

45. Young E. Allergy to subcutaneous heparin. Contact Dermatitis 1988;19:152–153.

46. Korstanje MJ, Bessems MJ, Hardy E, et al. Delayed-type hypersensitivity reaction to heparin. Contact Dermatitis 1989;20:383–384.

47. Schey S. Hypersensitivity reactions to heparin and the use of new low molecular weight heparins. Eur J Haem 1989;42:107.(Letter)

48. Guillet G, Delarie P, Plantin P, et al. Eczema as a complication of heparin therapy. J Amer Acad Derm 1989;20:1130–1132.

49. Klein GF, Kofler H, Wolf H, et al. Eczema-like, erythematous, infiltrated plaques: a common side effect of subcutaneous heparin therapy. J Amer Acad Derm 1989;21:703–707.

50. Bircher AJ, Fluckiger R, Buchner SA. Eczematous infiltrated plaques to subcutaneous heparin: a type IV allergic reaction. Br J Derm 1990;123:507–514.

51. Rivers JK, Gianoutsis MP. Delayed hypersensitivity reaction to subcutaneous heparin. Aust NZ J Surg 1991;61:865–868.

52. Valsecchi R, Rozzoni M, Cainelli T. Allergy to subcutaneous heparin. Contact Dermatitis 1992;26:129–130.

53. Odeh M, Oliven A. Urticaria and angioedema induced by low-molecular-weight heparin. Lancet 1992;340:972–973.

54. O'Donnell BF, Tan Cy. Delayed hypersensitivity reaction to heparin. Br J Derm 1993;129:634–636.

55. Bircher A, Itin PH, Stanislaw AB. Skin lesions, hypereosinophilia, and subcutaneous heparin. Lancet 1994;343:861.

56. Kelly RA, Gelfand MD, Pincus SH. Cutaneous necrosis caused by systemically administered heparin. JAMA 1981;246:1582–1583.

57. Jackson AM, Pollock AV. Skin necrosis after heparin injection. Brit Med J 1981;283;1087–1088.

58. Levine LE, Bernstein JE, Soltani K, et al. Heparin-induced cutaneous necrosis unrelated to injection sites. A sign of potentially lethal complications. Arch Dermaol 1983;119:400–403.

59. Rongioletti F, Pisani M, Rebora A. Skin necrosis due to intravenous heparin. Dermatologica 1989;178:47–50.

60. Fowlie J, Stanton PD, Anderson JR. Heparin-associated skin necrosis. Postgrad Med J 1990;66:573–575.

61. Ritchie AJ, Hart NV. Massive tissue necrosis can be induced by heparin. Acta Haematol 1992;87:69–70.

62. Ojeda E, Perez MC, Mataix R, et al. Skin necrosis with a low molecular weight heparin. Br J Haem 1992; 82:620.

63. Manoharan A. Heparin-induced skin reaction with low molecular-weight heparin. Eur J Haem 1992;48:234.(Letter)

64. Yates P, Jones S. Heparin skin necrosis—an important indicator of potentially fatal heparin hypersensitivity. Clin Exp Derm 1993;18:138–141.

65. Duggan ML, Morgan C. Heparin: a cause of priapism? South Med J 1970;63:1131–1134.

66. Klein LA, Hall RL, Smith RB. Surgical treatment of priapism: with a note on heparin-induced priapism. J Urol 1972;108:104–108.

67. Levine MN, Hirsh J, Gent M, et al. Prevention of deep-vein thrombosis after elective hip surgery: a randomized trial comparing low molecular weight heparin with standard unfractionated heparin. Ann Intern Med 1991;114:545–551.

68. Salzman EW, Rosenberg RD, Smith MH, et al. Effect of heparin and heparin fractions on platelet aggregation. J Clin Invest 1980;65:64–73.

69. Saba HI, Saba SR, Morelli GA. Effect of heparin on platelet aggregation. Am J Hematol 1984;17:295–306.

70. Westwick J, Scully MF, Poll C, Kakkar VV. Comparison of the effects of low molecular weight heparin and unfractionated heparin on activation of human platelets in vitro. Thromb Res 1986;42:435–447.

71. Brace LD, Fareed J. An objective assessment of the interaction of heparin and its fractions with human platelets. Semin Thromb Hemost 1985;11:190–198.

72. Chen J, Karlberg K-E, Sylven C. Heparin enhances platelet aggregation irrespective of anticoagulation with citrate or with hirudin. Thromb Res 1992;67:253–262.

73. Green D, Harris K, Reynolds N, et al. Heparin immune thrombocytopenia: evidence for a heparin-platelet complex as the antigenic determinant. J Lab Clin Med 1978;91:167–175.

74. Chong BH, Pitney WR, Castaldi PA. Heparin-induced thrombocytopenia: association of thrombotic complications with heparin-dependent IgG antibody that induces thromboxane synthesis and platelet aggregation. Lancet 1982;2:1246–1248.

75. Anderson GP. Insights into heparin-induced thrombocytopenia. Br J Haematol 1992;80:504–508.

76. Kelton JG, Sheridan D, Santos A, et al. Heparin-induced thrombocytopenia: laboratory studies. Blood 1988;72:925–930.

77. Isenhart CE, Brandt JT. Platelet aggregation studies for the diagnosis of heparin-induced thrombocytopenia. Am J Clin Pathol 1993;99:324–330.

78. Adelman B, Sobel M, Fujimura Y, et al. Heparin-associated thrombocytopenia: observations on the mechanism of platelet aggregation. J Lab Clin Med 1989;113:204–210.

79. Chong BH, Castaldi PA, Berndt MC. Heparin-induced thrombocytopenia: effects of rabbit IgG, and its Fab and Fc fragments on antibody-heparin-platelet interaction. Thromb Res 1989;55:291–295.

80. Chong BH, Fawaz I, Chesterman CN, et al. Heparin-induced thrombocytopenia: mechanism of interaction of the heparin-dependent antibody with platelets. Br J Haematol 1989;73:235–240.

81. Amiral J, Bridey F, Dreyfus M, et al. Platelet factor 4 complexed to heparin is the target for antibodies generated in heparin-induced thrombocytopenia [letter]. Thromb Haemost 1992;68:95–96.

82. Kelton JG, Smith JW, Warkentin TE, et al. Immunoglobulin G from patients with heparin-induced thrombocytopenia binds to a complex of heparin and platelet factor 4. Blood 1994;83:3232–3239.

83. Visentin GP, Ford SE, Scott JP, et al. Antibodies from patients with heparin-induced thrombocytopenia/thrombo-

sis are specific for platelet factor 4 complexed with heparin or bound to endothelial cells. J Clin Invest 1994;93:81–88.

84. Greinacher A, Pötzsch B, Amiral J, et al. Heparin-associated thrombocytopenia: isolation of the antibody and characterization of a multimolecular PF4-heparin complex as the major antigen. Thromb Haemost 1994;71:247–51.

85. Lynch DM, Howe SE. Heparin-associated thrombocytopenia: antibody binding specificity to platelet antigens. Blood 1985;66:1176–1181.

86. Cines DB, Tomaski A, Tannenbaum S. Immune endothelial-cell injury in heparin-associated thrombocytopenia. N Engl J Med 1987;316:581–590.

87. George J. Heparin-associated thrombocytopenia. In: Hull R, Pineo G. Disorders of Thrombosis. Philadelphia: W.B. Saunders 1996;359–373.

88. Warkentin TE, Levine MN, Hirsh J, et al. Heparin-induced thrombocytopenia in patients treated with low-molecular-weight heparin or unfractionated heparin. N Engl J Med 1995;332:1330–1335.

89. Magnani HN. Heparin-induced thrombocytopenia (HIT): an overview of 230 patients treated with Orgaran (Org 10172). Thromb Haemost 1993;70:554–561.

90. Cole CW, Bormanis J. Ancrod: a practical alternative to heparin. J Vasc Surg 1988;8:59–63.

91. Demers C, Ginsberg JS, Brill-Edwards P, et al. Rapid anticoagulation using ancrod for heparin-induced thrombocytopenia. Blood 1991;78:2194–2197.

92. Jaffe MD, Willis PW. Multiple fractures associated with long-term sodium heparin therapy. JAMA 1965;193:152–154.

93. Buchwald H, Rhode TD, Schneider PD, et al. Long-term, continuous intravenous heparin administration by an implantable infusion pump in ambulatory patients with recurrent venous thrombosis. Surgery 1980;88:507–516.

94. Rupp WM, McCarthy HB, RohdeTD, et al. Risk of osteoporosis in patients treated with long-term intravenous heparin. Curr Surg 1982;39:419–422.

95. Sackler JP, Liu L. Heparin-induced osteoporosis. Br J Radiol 1973;46:548–550.

96. Miller WE, DeWolfe VG. Osteoporosis resulting from heparin therapy. Cleve Clin Q 1966;33:31–34.

97. Aarskog D, Aksnes L, Lehmann L. Low 1,23-dihydroxyvitamen D in heparin-induced osteopenia. Lancet 1980;2:650–651.

98. Hellgren M, Nygards CB. Long-term therapy with subcutaneous heparin during pregnancy. Gynecol Obstet Invest 1982;13:76–89.

99. Megard M, Cuche M, Grapeloux A, et al. Osteoporose de l'heparinotherapie analyse histonophometrique de la biopsie osseuse. Nouv Presse Med 1982;11:261–264.

100. Squires JW, Pinch LWC. Heparin-induced spinal fractures. JAMA 1979;241:2417–2418.

101. Hull RD, Delmore T, Carter C, et al. Adjusted subcutaneous heparin versus warfarin sodium in the long-term treatment of venous thrombosis. N Engl J Med 1982;306:189–194.

102. Monreal M, Lafoz E, Olive A, et al. Comparison of subcutaneous unfractionated heparin with a low molecular weight heparin (fragmin) in patients with venous thromboembolism and contraindications to coumarin. Thromb Haemost 1994;71:7–11.

103. Hanley D, Anderson M. Anticoagulants and bone demineralization. In: Hull R, Pineo G. Disorders of Thrombosis. Philadelphia: W.B. Saunders 1996;353–358.

40

Anticoagulants and Bone

David A. Hanley, Melvin A. Andersen

INTRODUCTION

Heparin and the coumarin derivatives, the two major classes of drugs used for long-term anticoagulant therapy in clinical medicine, may both have significant effects on bone. As the clinical indications for their use expand, it becomes increasingly important to understand their potential interactions with bone. The potential for development of metabolic bone disease (specifically, osteopenia) must be examined if long-term use of these drugs is planned. This chapter includes a brief look at normal bone physiology, a review of some of the experimental data on anticoagulants and bone, and a discussion of clinical bone disorders which may be related to the use of anticoagulants.

NORMAL BONE PHYSIOLOGY

The main component of bone tissue is the extracellular matrix; the cellular component is very small. The bone matrix primarily consists of Type I collagen which is uniquely layered so that the collagen fibrils overlap each other with spaces left where the inorganic matrix mineral crystal is incorporated into the structure. The mineral of bone is predominantly a complex calcium phosphate crystal, similar to hydroxyapatite, but also containing small amounts of Na, Mg, K, Zn, citrate, and carbonate. About 10% of the matrix is made up of several noncollagen proteins, some of which are thought to play significant roles in the regulation of mineralization of bone. Vitamin K is required for normal synthesis of at least two of these proteins, osteocalcin (OC) and matrix GLA protein (MPG). These proteins may, therefore, be affected by the use of Coumarin anticoagulants.

Collagen and most of the other matrix proteins of bone are synthesized by the **osteoblast**, a cell of mesenchymal origin. As these cells lay down the normal bone matrix, they eventually become surrounded by matrix. The cells are then termed osteocytes. They appear to maintain communication with the bone forming surface through the extracellular fluid in canaliculi. The osteocyte may serve the function of rapidly mobilizing calcium from bone adjacent to the osteocyte into the extracellular fluid and the circulation. It has been speculated that the osteocyte may be the cell which senses physical strains within bone tissue and modulates bone modeling and remodeling in response to biomechanical factors.[1]

The other major cell of bone is the **osteoclast**. Multinucleated and of probable monocyte/macrophage origin, these migratory cells are stimulated to enter small localized areas of bone and begin the process of resorption of bone. Resorption involves the release of acid, acid hydrolase, and acid phosphatase into the underlying bone matrix. It is presumed that osteoclasts are recruited to the area for bone resorption in response to a signal from osteoblasts in the same area. Recruitment involves differentiation of the osteoclast from precursor cells, and activation of the bone resorption function of the cells. When the osteoclasts have resorbed bone down to a preset depth, then osteoblastic activity takes over. New bone matrix is synthesized, mineralized, and approximately the same amount of bone which was removed is restored. The packet of bone which undergoes this cycle is often referred to as a basic structural unit or basic multicellular unit of bone. In the adult skeleton, this process is termed remodeling. This sequence of resorption followed by formation is followed in normal bone, and even in many abnormal states of bone physiology, such as Paget's Disease of Bone. Bone resorption and formation are said to be "coupled." If bone resorption exceeds formation, abnormal loss of bone occurs. Loss of bone occurs if the processes become uncoupled so that bone resorption proceeds without subsequent bone formation; this may occur in heparin-induced osteoporosis.

From *Venous Thromboembolism: An Evidence-Based Atlas* edited by Russell Hull, Gary Raskob, Graham Pineo © 1996, Futura Publishing Co., Armonk, NY.

On a macroscopic level, there are two major forms of bone: trabecular (also called cancellous or spongy bone) and cortical bone. Trabecular bone also contains marrow, is more actively remodeled, and is found primarily in the axial skeleton (vertebral bodies) and ends of long bones. Cortical bone is the extremely dense thick outer layer of long bones. It provides major structural support and protection against fracture from bending forces. Cortical bone remodels much more gradually than trabecular bone. Trabecular bone can be turned over at a rate of >5% per year in some parts of the skeleton. A good review of normal bone physiology is available.[2]

HEPARIN EFFECTS ON BONE

Several studies, both *in vitro* and *in vivo*, have indicated that heparin increases osteoclast activity and bone resorption.[3,4,5] Earlier suggestions that heparin might do this through potentiating the effects of parathyroid hormone (PTH) on bone,[6] have not been pursued. Heparin may certainly amplify the effect of factors which may be found in serum, such as PTH or osteoclast resorption stimulating activity (ORSA).[8] However, an independent effect of heparin has been suggested by Chowdhury et al,[4] in a recent study. In chick and rat osteoclasts, heparin increased the number of differentiated (multinucleated) osteoclasts, and increased the resorption activity of osteoclasts, as measured by resorption pits per osteoclast number in bone slices. How heparin actually stimulates differentiation of the osteoclasts or increases activity is not known, but its acidic nature, and its structural similarity to heparan sulphate,[9] suggest that it may create a favorable environment for osteoclast adhesion to bone surfaces and subsequent bone resorption.

As noted above, bone resorption is normally coupled with subsequent bone formation. However, *in vitro* evidence shows that heparin reduces collagen synthesis and bone formation in cultures of fetal rat calvaria[10,11]; this combination of increased bone resorption and reduced bone formation would be particularly hazardous to skeletal health.

Because of the association between heparin therapy and bone disease, there has been an interest in whether the newer low-molecular-weight heparins (LMWHs) affect bone. Simmons and Raisz,[12] recently examined the effect of LMWH on bone resorption induced by acid and by basic fibroblast growth factor, two growth factors which are known to bind heparin. In the presence of LMWH, these growth factors stimulated ^{45}Ca release from cultured fetal rat long bone, suggesting that LMWH, like standard preparations of heparin, is also associated with increased bone resorption. Similarly, Hurley et al,[11] demonstrated that several LMWHs and standard heparin preparations had similar inhibitory effects on collagen synthesis, suggesting that LMWH are unlikely to offer a bone-sparing advantage over standard heparin. Mätzsch et al, found that when the dose of unfragmented heparin was matched with LMWH so that Factor Xa inhibitory activity was the same in each, the two forms of heparin were equipotent in causing osteoporosis on a rat model of heparin-induced osteoporosis.[13] This study also found reduced Zn content in bone ash from heparin-treated rats.

VITAMIN K and BONE

Vitamin K metabolism and the effects of the coumarin derivatives on γ-carboxylation of glutamic acid-containing proteins are reviewed elsewhere in this volume. A recent review of the role of vitamin K in skeletal metabolism is available.[14] Vitamin K deficiency (or the use of coumarin derivatives) results in a reduction in γ-carboxylation of glutamic acid residues in a variety of vitamin K-dependent proteins; γ-carboxylation is probably a key to the function of these molecules. It is likely that the effects of this deficiency would be seen in two of the major noncollagen proteins of bone, OC and MGP, both of which are γ carboxylated. Much more is known about OC than MGP in this regard. Recently, a third vitamin K-dependent protein, Protein-S, has been shown to be synthesized and secreted by osteoblast cell lines, and has been extracted from human bone matrix[15]; however, the significance of its presence in bone is not known.

Delmas and coworkers have called attention to the finding of incompletely carboxylated OC in patients with osteoporosis[16,17]; this observation might be a consequence of either vitamin K deficiency or a resistance to vitamin K-mediated gamma carboxylation of OC. In addition, several studies have demonstrated reduced blood levels of vitamin K in patients with osteoporosis.[18,19] In postmenopausal women with low levels of circulating OC and elevated urinary calcium excretion (suggesting reduced bone formation and increased bone resorption), vitamin K corrected these abnormalities[20]; preliminary studies suggest that vitamin K may have use as an osteoporosis therapy.[21] *In vitro* studies of osteoblasts in culture indicate vitamin K_2 has a stimulatory effect on osteoblast proliferation and function.[22] Hara and coworkers have recently demonstrated that the vitamin K metabolite menatetrenone inhibits interleukin-1-induced bone resorption in mouse calvaria.[23] These findings suggest that vitamin K may have a role in stimulating bone formation and reducing bone resorption; this would obviously imply a beneficial effect of vitamin K on the maintenance of bone mass.

CLINICAL BONE DISORDERS RELATED TO ANTICOAGULANTS

Heparin

Chronic subcutaneous heparin therapy was widely used in the treatment and secondary prevention of ischemic cardiac and cerebrovascular disease in the late

1950s and early 1960s. Because of a more recent resurgence of interest in a role for anticoagulants in the prevention of these disorders, a better understanding of anticoagulant-associated osteopenia is of great clinical importance. The first systematic documentation of a link between heparin and osteoporosis was published in 1965.[24] Griffith and coworkers reviewed their experience with patients who received self-administered chronic subcutaneous heparin for recurrent thrombophlebitis, as well as for coronary artery disease and cerebrovascular disease. This paper is the origin of the generally-held view that daily doses of heparin under 15,000 units are not associated with heparin-induced osteoporosis. Of 117 patients, the authors identified 10 who were treated with 15,000 units of heparin or more per day. In this group (which, interestingly, included six physicians and one nurse), six patients suffered spontaneous vertebral and/or rib fractures. The other four were treated prophylactically with calcium supplements and "anabolic steroids." None of the 107 patients who received less than 15,000 units per day experienced fractures. Because no measures of bone density were available to the authors, it cannot be ascertained that bone was not compromised at the lower heparin doses.

In recent years, most individuals receiving long-term subcutaneous heparin have been pregnant women who have had deep-vein thrombosis and pulmonary embolism. There are many case reports of a significant degree of fracturing osteoporosis,[25,26,27] including one report of osteoporotic fractures in a patient receiving 10,000 units of heparin daily during pregnancy.[28] More recently, larger series of patients have been reported,[29,30] including two prospective case-controlled studies in pregnancy.[31,32] The latter two reports include the use of bone-density measurements, rather than osteoporotic fracture, as an end-point. In the first of these two studies, Barbour et al,[31] assessed 14 women who were started on heparin therapy (mean dose 12,000 to 21,000 units daily) at 20 weeks gestation because of a prior history of venous thromboembolism. A comparable group of control subjects was also studied. The authors measured proximal femur bone density by dual energy x-ray absorptiometry at the time of recruitment into the study, at 30 to 34 weeks gestation, immediately postpartum, and at 6 months postpartum. Mean proximal femur bone density decreased in the treated patients compared to control subjects ($p < 0.01$), and this difference remained significant 6 months postpartum ($p < 0.03$). Five of the 14 heparin-treated patients showed a 10% or greater decline in bone density during heparin therapy, compared to none of the control subjects ($p < 0.04$). This study raises the possibility that recovery of bone after treatment with heparin may not be complete.

In the second study, Dahlman et al,[32] measured single photon bone densitometry of the distal (cortical bone) and ultradistal (trabecular bone) radius in 39 consecutive women treated with heparin (average dose 17,300 units daily) for a mean of 28 weeks during pregnancy and 6 weeks postpartum. A control group of 34 women matched for age, height, weight, parity, and smoking habits was also studied. In the heparin group, there was a significant 5% decline in trabecular bone during heparin therapy ($p < 0.01$), and a there was tendency to recover the bone loss after therapy was stopped.

The mechanism of bone loss in heparin-induced osteoporosis has not been well established. However, an imbalance of bone remodeling, with increased bone resorption and a concomitant decrease in bone formation resulting in accelerated bone loss, could account for the findings of the animal and bone cell culture studies outlined above. Interestingly, heparin may also affect vitamin D metabolism. Aarskog et al, found reduced levels of 1,25-dihydroxy-vitamin D in heparin-treated patients.[25,33] If there is reduced formation of 1,25–dihydroxy-vitamin D, reduced calcium absorption and increased parathyroid hormone synthesis and subsequent secretion might be expected,[34] further increasing the likelihood of bone resorption.

The issue of whether there is a specific dose-relationship for heparin-induced osteoporosis has not been settled, although it appears dose and duration of heparin therapy are important variables in the development of osteoporosis. As noted above, most clinical studies seem to suggest that the daily "threshold dose" for the risk of development of fractures is about 10,000 to 15,000 units of heparin, with therapy lasting more than 3 months. Although several studies have been unable to establish a clear dose-relationship for the effect of heparin on bone,[31,35] it would seem that the weight of available evidence suggests that with higher doses, especially more than 15,000 units per day for more than 1 month, the risk of osteoporosis is increased. It is hoped that the use of LMWH may allow lower doses of actual heparin activity and perhaps prevent the bone (and other) risks of chronic heparin therapy. One study of chronic LMWH use in pregnancy (from very early pregnancy to at least 12 weeks postpartum) suggested that the drug could be used safely from the standpoint of fetal development, and that bone density measured after therapy was not significantly different from that of matched control subjects.[36] However, this trial was not designed to examine changes in bone density during therapy, and as noted above, there are animal and *in vitro* data to suggest that LMWH may have deleterious effects on bone.[11,13]

Better assessment of the clinical effects of heparin dose on bone are now possible due to the more recent development of sensitive measurements of bone-related variables, such as bone density and biochemical markers of bone turnover. The studies of bone density mentioned above have demonstrated a significant effect of heparin even though no fractures occurred.[31,32,35] In a short-term study of the effects of 5,000 units of heparin twice daily for 10 days in six normal male adult volunteers, there was no effect on urinary hydroxyproline or serum Type I collagen cross-link C-terminal telopeptide, two biochemical markers of bone resorption. However, there was a small but significant fall in alkaline phosphatase, a marker of bone formation.[37]

To summarize, almost all the osteoporotic fractures associated with heparin use have been reported in uncontrolled retrospective studies or isolated case reports. Prospective studies of heparin effects on bone are starting to appear (e.g.,[31,32]) but these studies must rely on matching the treatment group with similar untreated control subjects. There has been one randomized controlled trial of heparin prophylaxis in 40 pregnant women.[38] In this study, there was one case of symptomatic osteoporosis in the 20 patients who received 20,000 units of heparin daily. The number of patients in this study is too small to predict the incidence of heparin-induced osteoporosis, and present clinical guidelines for anticoagulant use in pregnancy make a randomized placebo-controlled trial of heparin in pregnancy unethical. Today, the only way to perform a randomized prospective controlled trial examining heparin osteopenia would be to compare heparin therapy with an anticoagulant that does not have a significant effect on bone. As discussed above and below, the coumarin derivatives probably do not meet this criterion, and because of the close ties between proteins involved in coagulation and the noncollagen matrix proteins of bone, it is unlikely that a new anticoagulant without bone effects will be available in the near future.

Why is the prospect of heparin-induced osteopenia important? The answer lies in the increasing indications for chronic heparin therapy, and the effects of age on bone mass. It is believed a peak bone mass is attained between 25 and 35 years of age. After that, a gradual age-related decline in measured bone density occurs because, after a certain age, it does not seem to be possible to fully replace bone which has been resorbed as part of the normal remodeling process.[2] Age-related loss of bone (and risk of osteoporotic fracture) is greater in those individuals who have a higher overall rate of bone turnover, or who have had times of increased bone turnover, such as menopause, or courses of bone-depleting drugs such as corticosteroids. Patients over the age of attainment of peak bone mass who lose bone due to heparin therapy may not restore this loss, and prolonged heparin therapy may therefore increase the risk of later symptomatic osteoporosis even if it does not cause serious problems while it is being administered. Although in some studies it appears that recovery of bone does occur after completion of heparin treatment,[27,31,32] the extent of recovery is not certain; one study of heparin use in pregnancy showed persistent cortical bone loss 24 weeks after the heparin was stopped.[30]

At present, no specific therapy of heparin-induced osteoporosis can be recommended. General measures, such as assurance of adequate calcium and vitamin D intake, are appropriate. One small randomized study of heparin use in pregnancy (6 months of treatment) found preservation of bone mass in nine women receiving a unique calcium supplement, Ossein-hydroxyapatite (available in Europe); 11 patients who did not receive the supplement had a significant loss of bone mass.[39] Because heparin bone disease is primarily associated with increased bone resorption, a case might be made for treatment or prevention with an antiresorptive therapy such as a bisphosphonate or calcitonin.[40] However, the bisphosphonates are contraindicated in pregnancy, and even if calcitonin was approved for use in pregnancy, its usual route of administration (injection) would be a deterrent in patients receiving anticoagulants.

In summary, it seems clear that prolonged heparin therapy for more than 3 months, using dose levels often required for effective anticoagulant effect, is likely to cause some degree of osteopenia and, in rare cases, patients may develop fractures. Clinicians must be aware of this potential, serious problem, and more research is needed in several key areas: pathogenesis, dose-relationship, prediction of risk for individual patients, and development of prevention and treatment strategies.

Coumarin Derivatives

There is considerable recent evidence for a role for vitamin K in normal skeletal physiology. Also, there is a serious fetal bone developmental abnormality caused by warfarin.[41] Therefore, there is a significant potential for coumarin derivatives to have deleterious effects on the skeleton. In spite of this, there are few studies indicating that the use of coumarin derivatives for anticoagulant therapy may be associated with bone disease. Fiore et al, in a study of 56 women receiving acenocoumarol as an anticoagulant after aortic valve surgery, found that they had significantly reduced bone density compared to 61 similar patients not taking oral anticoagulants.[42] They found no difference between the groups in serum levels of the vitamin K-dependent protein, OC, but they did not have access to techniques to examine whether there was decreased γ-carboxylation of OC in the coumarin-treated group. Other investigators have found low OC levels in phenprocoumon-treated patients, as well as a reduction in proportional carboxylation of OC in the treated group.[43] However, no evidence of clinical bone disease was present in these patients. Warfarin has also been shown to impair carboxylation of OC in humans.[44] Plantalech et al, found that young patients on chronic warfarin therapy had similar levels of under-carboxylated OC to those found in elderly osteoporotic women.[17] At present, there is a need for large, well-designed studies to address the issue of whether coumarins can be implicated in the development of bone disease, because of the renewed interest in long-term anticoagulant therapy.

REFERENCES

1. Lanyon LE. Biomechanical properties of bone and response of bone to mechanical stimuli: Functional strain as a controlling influence on bone modelling and re-modelling behaviour. In: Hall BK, (ed.) Bone Vol. 3: Bone Matrix and Bone Specific Products. Boca Raton, CRC Press, Inc., 1991, pp. 79–108.

2. Aurbach GD, Marx SJ, Spiegel AM. Metabolic Bone disease. In: Wilson, JD, Foster, DW, (ed.) Williams Textbook of Endocrinology. 8th ed. Philadelphia,: W.B. Saunders Company, 1992, pp. 1477–1516.

3. Glowacki J. The effects of heparin and protamine on resorption of bone particles. Life Sci 1983;33:1019–1024.

4. Chowdhury MH, Hamada C, Dempster DW. Effects of heparin on osteoclast activity. J Bone Min Res 1992;7:771–777.

5. Mätzch T, Bergqvist D, Hedner U, Nilsson B, Østergaard P. Heparin-induced osteoporosis in rats. Thromb Haemostas 1986;56:293–294.

6. Goldhaber P. Heparin enhancement of factors stimulating bone resorption in tissue culture. Science 1965;147:407–408.

7. Wolinsky I, Cohn DV. The stimulation by heparin and parathyroid hormone of bone resorption in tissue culture. Israel J Med Sci 1970;6:691–696.

8. Fuller K, Chambers TJ, Gallagher AC. Heparin augments osteoclast resorption-stimulating activity in serum. J Cell Physiol 1991;147:208–214.

9. Gallagher JT, Lyon M, Steward WP. Structure and function of heparan sulfate proteoglycans. Biochem J 1986;236: 313–325.

10. Hurley MM, Gronowicz G, Kream BE, Raisz LG. Effect of heparin on bone formation in cultured fetal rat calvaria. Calcif Tiss Int 1990;46:183–188.

11. Hurley MM, Kream BE, Raisz LG. Structural determinants of the capacity of heparin to inhibit collagen synthesis in 21 day fetal rat calvariae. J Bone Min Res 1990;5:1127–1133.

12. Simmons HA, Raisz LG. Effects of acid and basic fibroblast growth factor and heparin on resorption of cultural fetal rat long bones. J Bone Min Res 1991;6:1301–1305.

13. Mätzch T, Bergqvist D, Hedner U, Nilsson B, Østergaard P. Effects of low molecular weight heparin and unfragmented heparin on induction of osteoporosis in rats. Thromb Haemostas 1990;63:505–509.

14. Rosen HN, Maitland LA, Suttie JW, et al. Vitamin K and maintenance of skeletal integrity in adults. Am J Med 1993;94:62–68.

15. Maillard C, Berruyer M, Serre CM, Dechavanne M, Delmas PD. Protein-S, a vitamin K-dependent protein, is a bone matrix component synthesized and secreted by osteoclasts. Endocrinology 1992;130:1599–1604.

16. Szulc P, Chapuy MC, Meunier PJ, Delmas PD. Serum undercarboxylated osteocalcin as a marker of the risk of hip fracture in elderly women. J Clin Invest 1993;91: 1769–1774.

17. Plantalech L, Guillaumont M, Leclerq M, Delmas PD. Impaired carboxylation of serum osteocalcin in elderly women. J Bone Min Res 1991;6:1211–1216.

18. Hart JP, Catterall A, Dodds RA, et al. Circulating vitamin K_1 levels in fractured neck of the femur. Lancet 1984;(11):283.

19. Hodges SJ, Pilkington MJ, Stamp TCB, et al. Depressed levels of circulating menaquinones in patients with osteoporotic fractures of the spine and femoral neck. Bone 1991;387–389.

20. Knapen MHJ, Hamulyak K, Vermeer L. The effect of vitamin K supplementation on circulating osteocalcin (bone Gla protein) and urinary calcium excretion. Ann Int Med 1989;111:1001–1005.

21. Orimo H, Fujita T, Onomura T, et al. Clinical evaluation of vitamin K in the treatment of involutional osteoporosis In: Christiansen C, Riis B, (eds.) Proceedings of the Fourth International Symposium on Osteoporosis, Hong Kong 1993 Handelstrykkeriet Aalborg Aps, Aalborg, Denmark, 1993;148–149.

22. Akedo Y, Hosoi T, Inoue S, et al. Vitamin K_2 modulates proliferation and function of osteoblastic cells in vitro. Biochem Biophys Res Comm 1992;187,2:814–820.

23. Hara K, Akiyama Y, Tajima T, Shiraki M. Menatetrenone inhibits bone resorption partly through inhibition of PGE_2 synthesis in vitro. J Bone Min Res 1993;8:535–542.

24. Griffith GC, Nichols G, Jr, Asher JD, Flanagan B. Heparin osteoporosis. JAMA 1965;193:91–94 (see also editorial p. 152, same issue).

25. Aarskog D, Aksnes L, Lehmann V. Low 1,25-dihydroxyvitamin D in heparin-induced osteoporosis. Lancet 1980;2: 650–651.

26. Wise PH, Hall AJ. Heparin-induced osteoporosis in pregnancy. Br Med J 1980;281:110–111.

27. Zimran A, Shilo S, Fisher D, Bab I. Histomorphometric evaluation of reversible heparin-induced osteoporosis in pregnancy. Arch Intern Med 1976;146:386–388.

28. Griffith HT, Liu DTY. Severe heparin osteoporosis in pregnancy. Postgrad Med J 1984;60:424–425.

29. Rupp WM, McCarthy HB, Rohde TD, et al. Risk of osteoporosis in patients treated with long-term intravenous heparin therapy. Curr Surg 1982;39:419–422.

30. deSwiet M, Dorrington Ward P, Fidler J, et al. Prolonged heparin therapy in pregnancy causes bone demineralization. Br J Obstet Gynaecol 1983;90:1129–1134.

31. Barbour LA, Kick SD, Steiner JF, et al. A prospective study of heparin-induced osteoporosis in pregnancy using bone densitometry. Am J Obstet Gynecol 1994;170:862–869.

32. Dahlman TC, Sjöberg HE, Ringertz H. Bone mineral density during long-term prophylaxis with heparin in pregnancy. Am J Obstet Gynecol 1994;170:1315–1320.

33. Aarskog D, Aksnes L, Markestad T, et al. Heparin-induced inhibition of 1,25-dihydroxyvitamin D formation. Am J Obstet Gynecol 1984;148:1141–1142.

34. Watson PH, Hanley DA. Parathyroid hormone: regulation of synthesis and secretion. Clin Invest Med 1993;16: 58–77.

35. Ginsberg JS, Kowalchuk G, Hirsh J, et al. Heparin effect on bone density. Thromb Haemostas 1990;64:286–289.

36. Melissari E, Parker CJ, Wilson NV, et al. Use of low molecular weight heparin in pregnancy. Thromb Haemostas 1992;68:652–656.

37. van der Wiel HE, Lips P, Huijgens PC, Netelenbos JC. Effects of short-term low-dose heparin administration on biochemical parameters of bone turnover. Bone Miner 1993;22:27–32.

38. Howell R, Fidler J, Letsky E, de Swiet M. The risk of antenatal subcutaneous heparin prophylaxis: a controlled trial. Br J Obstet Gynaecol 1983;90:1124–1128.

39. Ringe JD, Keller A. Risk of osteoporosis in long-term heparin therapy of thromboembolic diseases in pregnancy: at-

tempted prevention with ossein-hydroxyapatite. Geburt-shilfe Frauenheilkd 1992;52:426–429.

40. Riggs BL, Melton LJ. Drug therapy: the prevention and treatment of osteoporosis. N Engl J Med 1992;327:620–627.

41. Hall JG, Pauli RM, Wilson KM. Maternal and fetal sequelae of anticoagulation during pregnancy. Am J Med 1980;68: 122–140.

42. Fiore CE, Tamburino C, Foti R, Grimaldi D. Reduced axial bone mineral content in patients taking an oral anticoagulant. South Med J 1990;83:538–542.

43. Pietschmann P, Woloszczuk W, Panzer S, et al. Decreased serum osteocalcin levels in phenprocoumon-treated patients. J Clin Endocrinol Metab 1988;66:1071–1074.

44. Menon RK, Gill DS, Thomas M, Kernoff PB, Dandona P. Impaired carboxylation of osteocalcin in warfarin-treated patients. J Clin Endocrinol Metab 1987;64:59–61.

SECTION VII

Patient Case Studies

PATIENT STUDIES
Graham F. Pineo, Gary E. Raskob, Russell D. Hull

Introduction

The case studies presented in this chapter are derived from a database of over 600 patients presenting with venous thromboembolism to the Thromboembolism Consultation Service at McMaster University between 1980 and 1984. The case studies demonstrate specific features of the clinical presentation, diagnosis and treatment of venous thromboembolism. Each case is presented in a similar fashion with a brief description of the clinical presentation, investigations, treatment, and outcome, and the main teaching point(s) of the case. The relevant investigations are then presented: chest x-ray, ventilation/perfusion lung scan, pulmonary angiography and venography.

The technique for performing ventilation scans changed during the course of these studies. In the earlier ventilation scans, Xenon 133 (^{133}Xe) was used, and therefore only one posterior view was available. With the use of Xenon 127 (^{127}Xe) the best view on the perfusion scan was obtained on the ventilation scan. Later, the use of aerosol technetium 99 (99mTc) permitted presentation of the ventilation scan in the traditional six views. For future comparison, a normal ventilation and perfusion lung scan is demonstrated in Figures 1 and 2 respectively. In all subsequent ventilation/perfusion lung scans, we have demonstrated the various views according to our current practice, i.e., posterior, right posterior oblique and right lateral views above, and anterior, left lateral and left posterior oblique views below.

Reproduction of the pulmonary angiograms does not always do justice to the original films, which in some cases have deteriorated with time. The best views available have been selected for presentation.

For ease of interpretation of ventilation/perfusion lung scans, we add a lung map of the segments visualized on the various projections of the lung scans (Figure 3: page 341). This lung map has been used to decrease inter-observer variability in the interpretation of lung scans with particular reference to the identification of segmental or subsegmental defects.

It is our hope that this series of patient studies will help consolidate a number of the points made in preceding chapters with respect to the diagnosis and treatment of venous thromboembolism. These studies demonstrate the protean nature of venous thromboembolism and the need for a systematic and objective approach to the diagnosis of both deep-vein thrombosis and pulmonary embolism. The comment is still made by experienced clinicians that they dislike seeing patients with suspected pulmonary embolism, because they never quite know how to make a correct diagnosis. We hope the case studies in Venous Thromboembolism makes their task easier.

Graham F. Pineo
Gary E. Raskob
Russell D. Hull

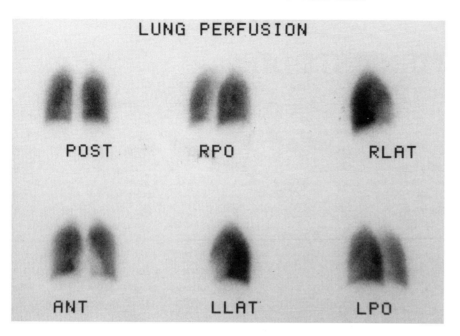

Figure 1. Technetium 99 mAA perfusion scan showing a normal perfusion scan.

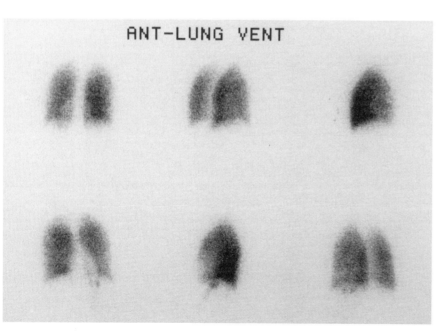

Figure 2. Technetium 99 aerosol ventilation scan (Technigas) showing normal ventilation scan.

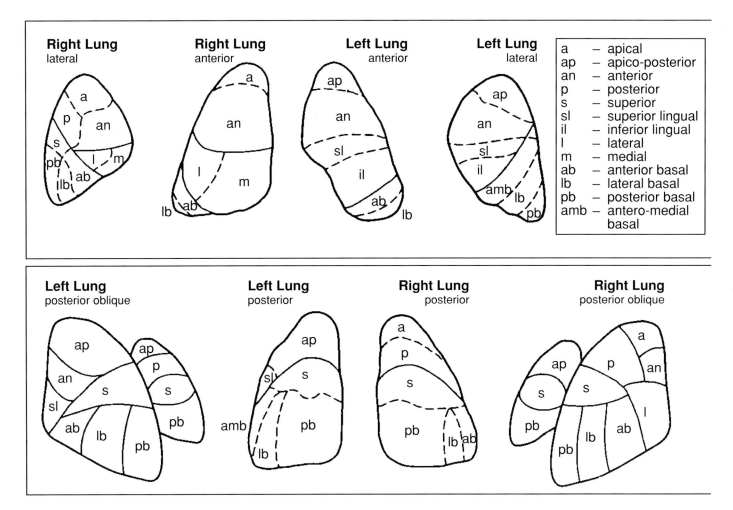

Figure 3. The lung map showing the segments of both lungs.

CASE 1: Clinical Presentation – Pleuritic Chest Pain

CLINICAL PRESENTATION

This 47-year-old man experienced the sudden onset of chest pain one evening while watching television. The pain persisted through the night and was worsened by deep breathing or coughing. It was mainly localized to the right lower chest. There were no other symptoms. Four years ago, he had had a venographically proven deep-vein thrombosis in the right leg with no recurrence.

EXAMINATION

Examination revealed a blood pressure of 180/90, a pulse rate of 75, a respiratory rate of 28, and normal jugular venous pressure. There was decreased entry at both lung bases with crepitations but no friction rub. Cardiovascular examination was normal. There was tenderness in both calves.

INVESTIGATIONS

The chest x-ray showed bilateral pleural effusions, worse on the left. Both diaphragms were elevated. The IPG was normal bilaterally. A V/Q scan on the following day showed multiple segmental perfusion defects with ventilation mismatch (high probability). Angiography revealed a large embolus on the right and venography showed a nonocclusive thrombus in the popliteal vein of the right leg.

TREATMENT

Treatment consisted of intravenous heparin with warfarin which was continued for 3 months. His course was uneventful.

TEACHING POINT

This patient had a large perfusion defect in the right upper lung zone with a normal chest x-ray in this area. The IPG was negative. A pulmonary embolus was confirmed by pulmonary angiography and venography revealed proximal deep-vein thrombosis. Pulmonary angiography is an optional investigation in the context of this patient because of the finding of a high probability scan.

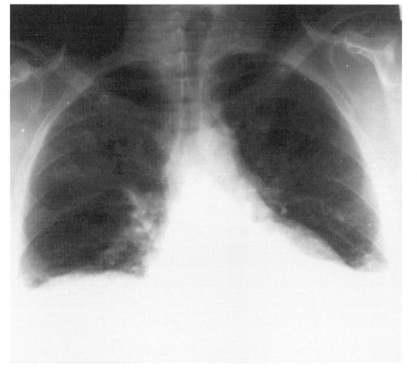

Figure 1. Chest x-ray showing bilateral pleural effusions.

From *Venous Thromboembolism: An Evidence-Based Atlas* by Russell Hull, Gary Raskob, Graham Pineo © 1996, Futura Publishing Co., Armonk, NY.

POST　　　　**RPO**　　　　**R.L.**

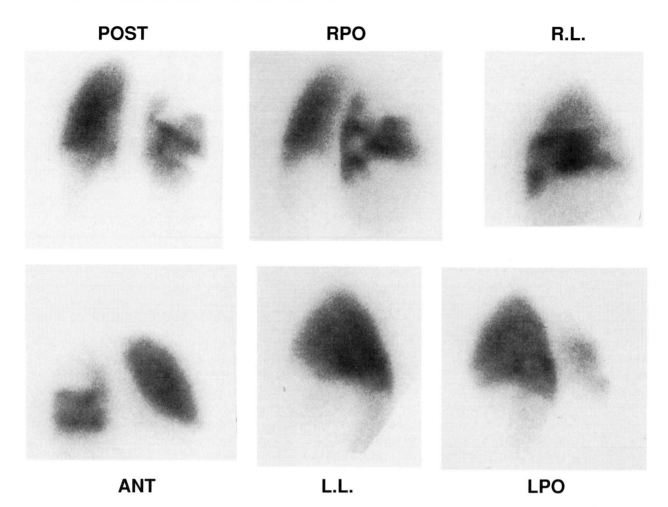

ANT　　　　**L.L.**　　　　**LPO**

Figure 2. Technetium 99 mAA perfusion scan showing multiple lobar and segmental perfusion defects (ventilation scan not available).

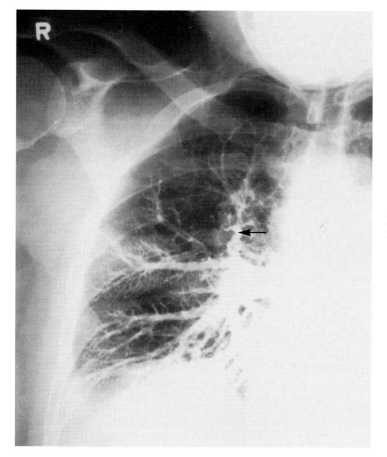

Figure 3. Pulmonary angiogram showing large intraluminal filling defect.

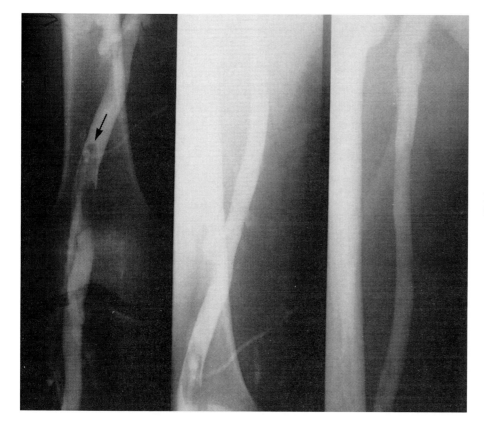

Figure 4. Venogram showing a thrombus in the popliteal vein.

CASE 2: Clinical Presentation – Unexplained Dyspnea

CLINICAL PRESENTATION

A 30-year-old woman was admitted directly to the Intensive Care Unit. On arising that morning, she noticed shortness of breath and palpitations. She had no pain or other symptoms. She was brought directly to hospital. She had given birth to a normal baby 1 week prior to admission. This was a vaginal delivery complicated by a vaginal tear and hematoma formation. She was discharged 2 days before this admission feeling a bit weak and light-headed, but otherwise normal. She had had a previous delivery 11 years earlier without complications.

EXAMINATION

Examination revealed a blood pressure of 120/70, a pulse rate of 150, and a respiratory rate of 16. Chest examination was negative. Heart sounds were normal, with no extra sounds. Jugular venous pressure was normal. Leg examination was negative.

INVESTIGATIONS

The chest x-ray showed prominence of the left pulmonary artery segment. A V/Q scan revealed multiple segmental perfusion defects in the left lung with ventilation mismatch (high probability). Angiography documented large emboli involving both lungs. Both the IPG and venography were normal.

TREATMENT

With the diagnosis of pulmonary embolism, the patient was heparinized and placed on warfarin.

TEACHING POINT

This young woman presented with a massive pulmonary embolus 1 week after a normal delivery. The diagnosis was confirmed by a high probability lung scan and positive pulmonary angiogram in this patient who was potentially at high risk for bleeding.

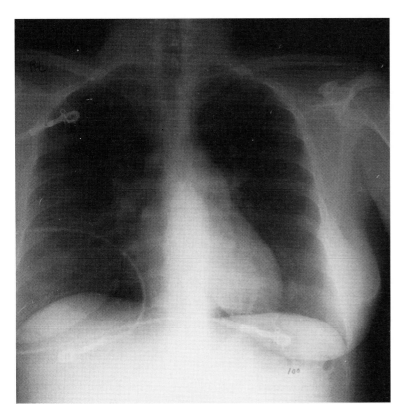

Figure 1. Chest x-ray showing prominence of the left pulmonary artery segment.

POST **RPO** **R.L.**

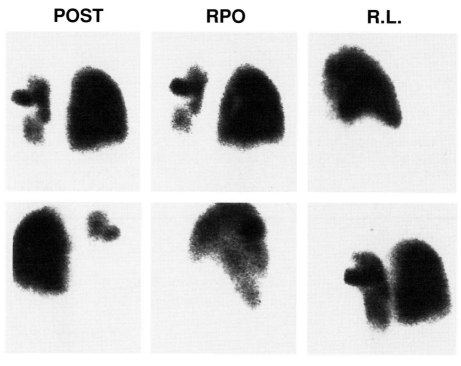

ANT **L.L.** **LPO**

Figure 2. Technetium 99 mAA perfusion scan showing multiple perfusion defects in the left lung.

MAA **WASH IN** **EQUIL 1**

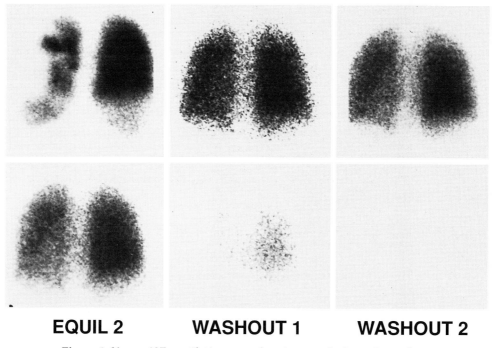

EQUIL 2 **WASHOUT 1** **WASHOUT 2**

Figure 3. Xenon 127 ventilation scan showing ventilation mismatch.

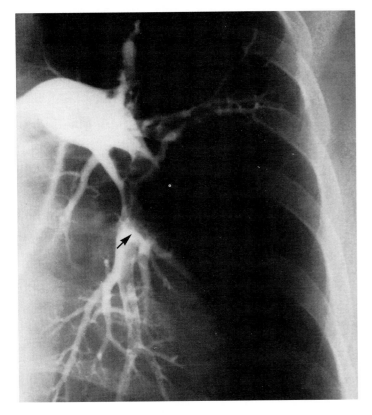

Figure 4. Pulmonary angiogram showing multiple large emboli in the left lung.

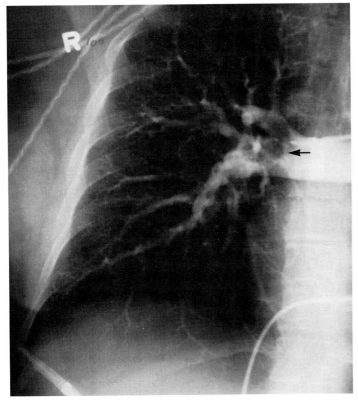

Figure 5. Pulmonary angiogram showing multiple large emboli in the right lung.

CASE 3: Clinical Presentation – Syncope

CLINICAL PRESENTATION

This 75-year-old woman experienced a dizzy spell while sitting on the toilet. She had also complained of left calf pain which developed eight days following a partial gastrectomy for carcinoma of the stomach. Her operation was complicated by a short bout of tachyarrhythmia, but her procedure and recovery were otherwise uneventful.

EXAMINATION

On examination, the blood pressure was 118/60, the pulse rate was 104, and the respiratory rate was normal. Jugular venous pressure was normal. Examination of the chest and cardiovascular systems revealed nothing specific. Leg examination was negative.

INVESTIGATIONS

The chest x-ray showed a slight increase in heart size and a linear opacity in the right mid-zone. The IPG was abnormal in the left leg. Venography revealed a proximal deep-vein thrombosis on the left. The V/Q scan showed multiple segmental perfusion defects with a ventilation mismatch (high probability). The pulmonary angiogram was negative.

TREATMENT

This patient was treated with anticoagulants based on the findings of the leg tests and she made an uneventful recovery.

TEACHING POINT

This elderly patient undergoing surgery for carcinoma of the stomach presented a high risk for venous thromboembolism and in fact developed significant deep-vein thrombosis despite heparin prophylaxis. Pulmonary angiography may have been falsely negative. Because of the presence of proximal venous thrombosis, if untreated, she was at high risk of massive or fatal pulmonary embolism.

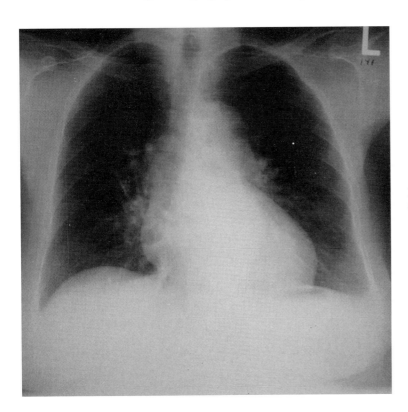

Figure 1. Chest x-ray showing slight increase in heart size and a linear opacity in the right midzone.

POST   **RPO**   **R.L.**

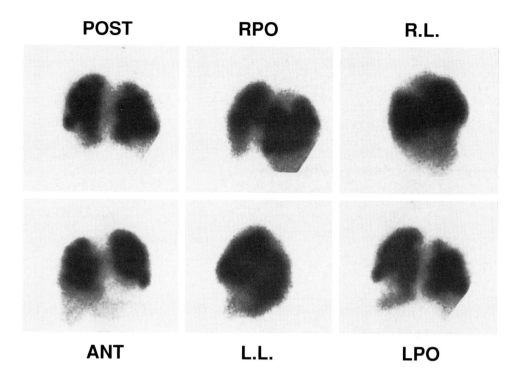

ANT   **L.L.**   **LPO**

Figure 2. Technetium 99 mAA perfusion lung scan showing multiple large segmental perfusion defects.

POST   **RPO**   **R.L.**

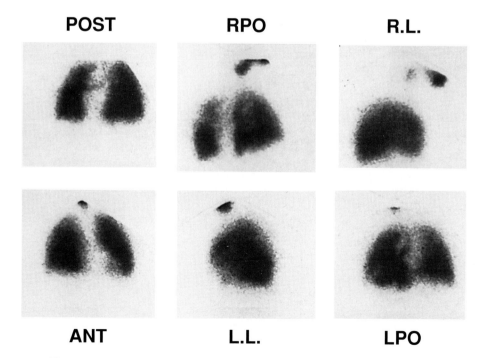

ANT   **L.L.**   **LPO**

Figure 3. Technetium 99 ventilation scan showing a ventilation mismatch.

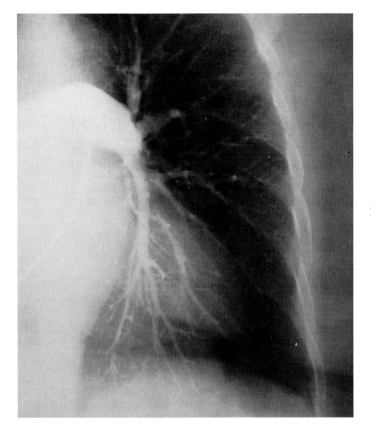

Figure 4. Negative pulmonary angiogram.

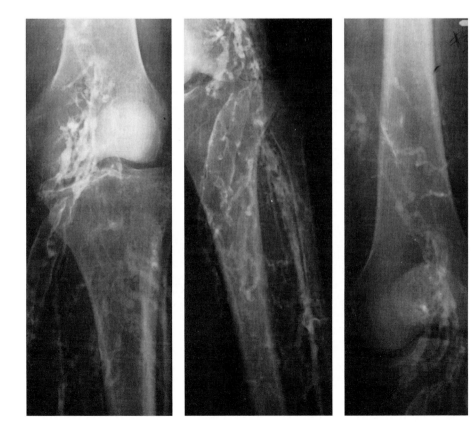

Figure 5. Venogram of left leg showing intraluminal filling defects in the distal and proximal deep veins.

CASE 4: Clinical Presentation – Dyspnea, Orthopnea, and Chest Pain

CLINICAL PRESENTATION

A 63-year-old woman was admitted to the hospital complaining of shortness of breath and nonpleuritic left-sided chest pain. She had a history of moderately severe chronic obstructive pulmonary disease, but a recent onset of increasing shortness of breath for 2 months accompanied by orthopnea, recent swelling of the ankles, and weight gain. She had a cough productive of copious amounts of white sputum but no blood. The left-side chest discomfort was relieved by nitroglycerin, but her dyspnea persisted and required hospital admission.

EXAMINATION

On examination, she was dyspneic at rest; blood pressure was 138/78, the pulse rate was 80, and the respiratory rate was 26. Chest examination revealed decreased air entry and a prolonged expiratory phase but no adventitious sounds. The jugular venous pressure was elevated 10 cm above the sternal angle, and there were no extra heart sounds or murmurs. There was ankle edema.

INVESTIGATIONS

The chest x-ray showed a small pleural effusion with atelectasis and density at the left base. The IPG was normal. The lung scan revealed multiple segmental perfusion defects with ventilation match (low probability). Pulmonary angiography confirmed the diagnosis of multiple pulmonary emboli. The venogram revealed proximal venous thrombosis on the left (popliteal vein).

TREATMENT

With confirmation of the diagnosis, the patient was treated with heparin and warfarin. Her symptoms improved along with treatment with oxygen and bronchodilators and her follow-up was uneventful.

TEACHING POINT

The clinical presentation was complicated by her chronic obstructive pulmonary disease and evidence of right heart failure (poor cardiorespiratory reserve). The lung scan was low probability and the IPG was normal. Pulmonary angiography, however, confirmed the diagnosis. In a patient with poor cardiorespiratory reserve, a low probability lung scan, and negative leg tests, pulmonary angiography is required to make a diagnosis.

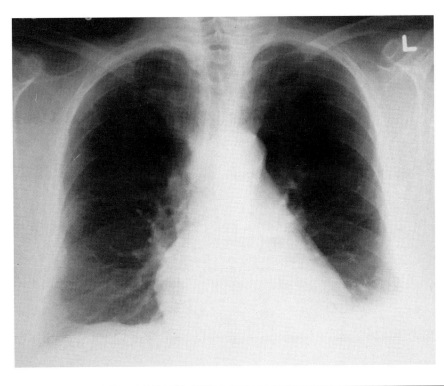

Figure 1. Chest x-ray showing a pleural effusion with atelectasis and density at the left lung base.

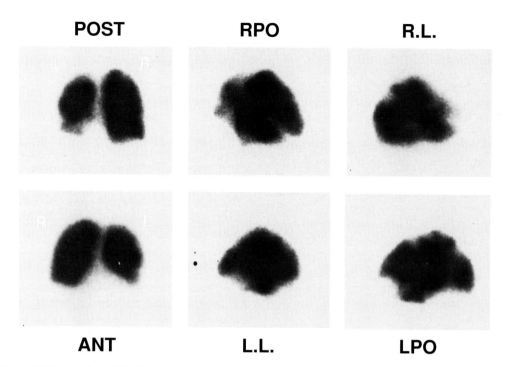

Figure 2. Technetium 99 mAA perfusion lung scan showing multiple segmental perfusion defects.

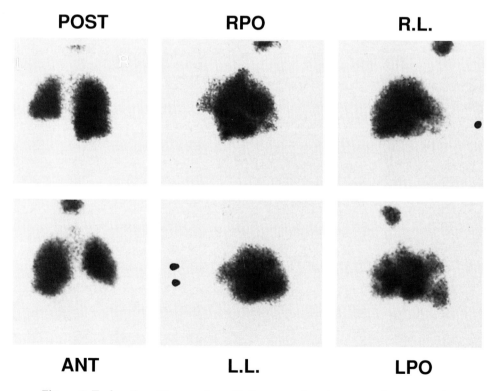

Figure 3. Technetium 99 aerosol ventilation scan showing a ventilation match.

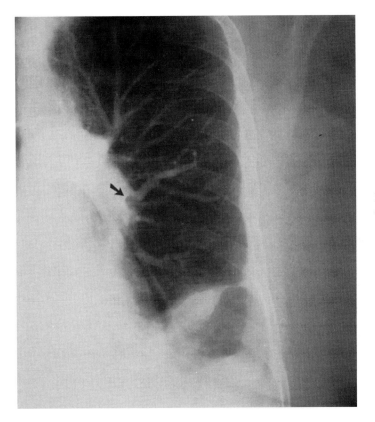

Figure 4. Pulmonary angiogram showing intraluminal filling defect in second order vessels (note density at left lung base.)

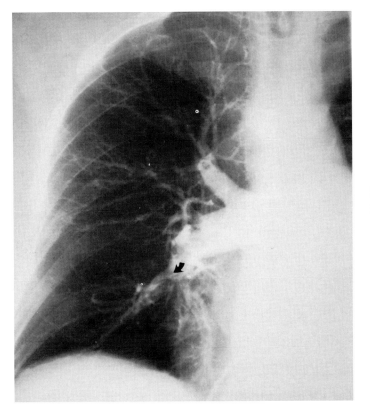

Figure 5. Pulmonary angiogram showing multiple pulmonary emboli on the right side.

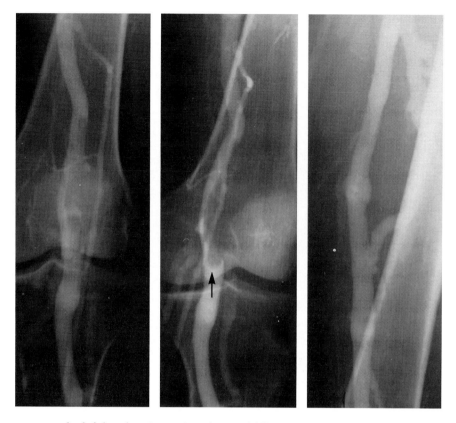

Figure 6. Venogram on the left leg showing an intraluminal filling defect in the proximal deep venous system.

CASE 5: Clinical Presentation – Epigastric Pain Increased on Inspiration

CLINICAL PRESENTATION

This 58-year-old woman presented with a two-day history of epigastric pain, which was increased on inspiration. She also complained of pain in the medial aspect of the right thigh. She had no shortness of breath, cough, or hemoptysis. She had a history of a bilateral aortofemoral bypass for intermittent claudication approximately 20 days before this admission. She had a history of deep vein thrombosis following a cesarean section approximately 20 years previously, and she had a history of superficial phlebitis.

EXAMINATION

Blood pressure was 100/60, the pulse rate was 96, and the respiratory rate was 20. Heart sounds were normal. Chest examination revealed good expansion, normal percussion, and normal breath sounds. Femoral pulses were reduced with a bruit over the right femoral artery. Examination of the extremities revealed superficial varicosities in both legs with slight edema. The medial aspect of the right thigh and the back of the right calf were warm and tender to touch.

INVESTIGATIONS

The chest x-ray on admission was normal. The IPG was initially negative but became positive 2 days later.

A V/Q scan showed a single subsegmental perfusion defect in the left apex with ventilation match (low probability). Pulmonary angiography revealed an embolus in the left lung, and venography the following day showed an intraluminal filling defect in the right thigh.

TREATMENT

The patient was treated with intravenous heparin followed by warfarin and recovered uneventfully.

TEACHING POINT

The clinical presentation was not typical for pulmonary embolism, but she did have a significant risk factor (previous surgery). The lung scan was interpreted as low probability, but the pulmonary angiogram revealed the presence of a pulmonary embolus. A low probability lung scan is a misnomer. The IPGs that were initially negative became positive and venography 2 days later revealed a proximal deep vein thrombosis. Serial testing with IPG or ultrasound is effective in detecting symptomatic patients with proximal deep-vein thrombosis who are at risk of recurrent pulmonary embolism.

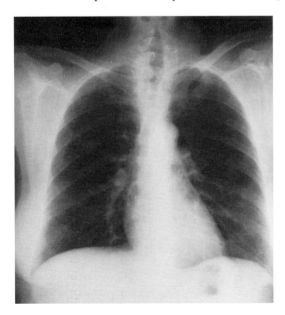

Figure 1. Normal chest x-ray.

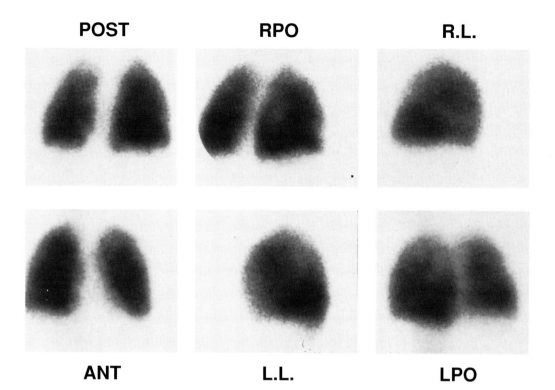

Figure 2. Technetium 99 mAA perfusion lung scan showing a single subsegmental perfusion defect in the left apex.

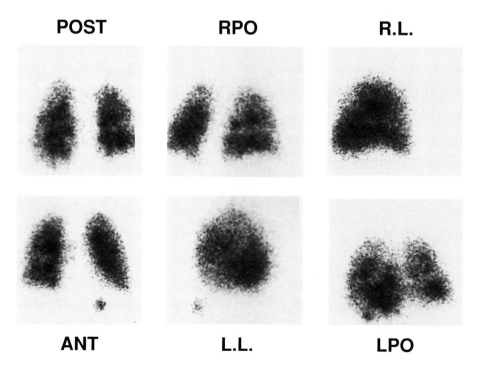

Figure 3. Technetium 99 aerosol ventilation scan showing a ventilation match.

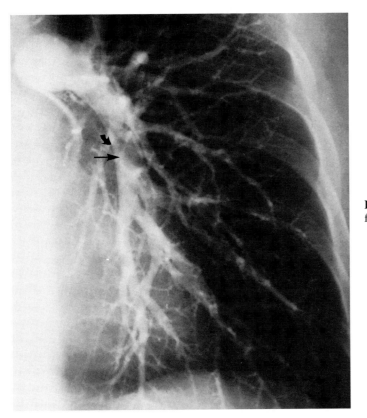

Figure 4. Pulmonary angiogram showing an intraluminal filling defect in second order vessels in the left lung.

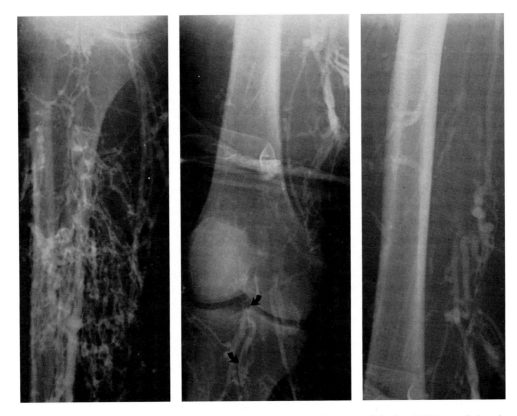

Figure 5. Venogram showing intraluminal filling defects in the popliteal vein and lack of filling of the deep venous system proximally.

CASE 6: Clinical Presentation – Subscapular Pain – Atypical Features of Pneumonia

CLINICAL PRESENTATION

This 66-year-old woman complained of a sharp, constant left subscapular pain that was worse when lying down. It was not accompanied by any other symptom. She had been discharged from hospital 4 days earlier following a laparotomy which revealed metastatic carcinoma of the ovary. Carcinoma of the breast had been diagnosed 3 years earlier, but there was no evidence of recurrence.

EXAMINATION

Examination revealed a blood pressure of 110/70, a pulse of 116, and a respiratory rate of 16. Chest examination showed good air entry but with elevation of the right diaphragm. There was evidence of consolidation over the right middle and lower lobes, and tenderness in the ribs in the overlying area. The cardiovascular system examination was negative. Examination of the legs was negative.

INVESTIGATIONS

The chest x-ray showed a large density involving the right middle and lower lobes. The V/Q scan revealed multiple segmental perfusion defects with ventilation match (low probability). Angiography revealed an embolus in the left and right main pulmonary arteries. Venography revealed proximal deep-vein thrombosis of the left and distal deep-vein thrombosis of the right leg.

TREATMENT

This patient was treated with intravenous heparin on admission. She was then treated long term with an adjusted dose of subcutaneous heparin in view of the fact that she would be receiving chemotherapy for her carcinoma.

TEACHING POINT

The clinical presentation was that of consolidation in the right middle and lower lobes, but objective testing showed evidence of pulmonary embolism. Investigations revealed a low probability lung scan but a positive pulmonary angiogram. This patient probably had infection superimposed on pulmonary infarction.

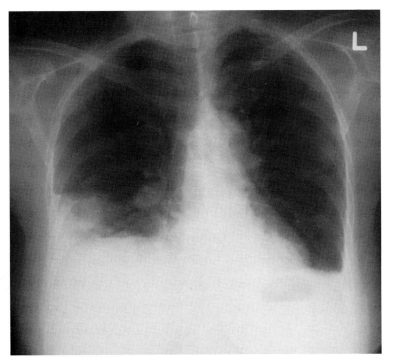

Figure 1. Chest x-ray showing a large density involving the right middle and lower lobes.

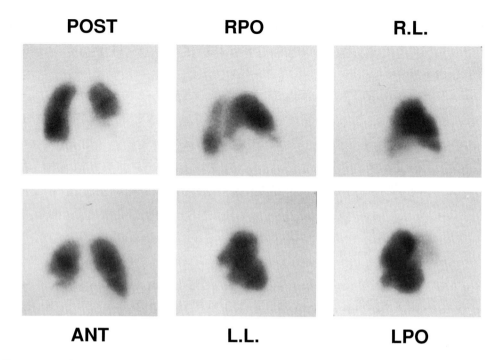

Figure 2. Technetium 99 mAA perfusion scan showing multiple segmental perfusion defects.

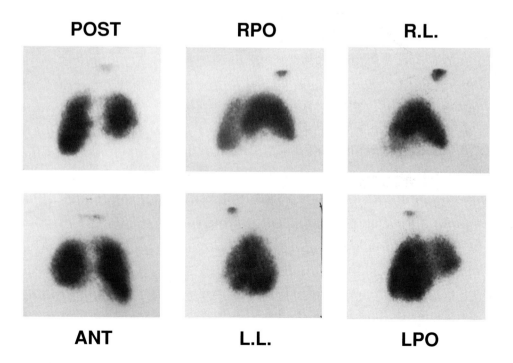

Figure 3. Technetium 99 aerosol ventilation scan showing a ventilation match.

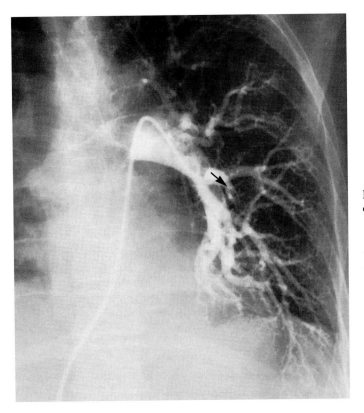

Figure 4. Pulmonary angiogram revealing intraluminal filling defect on the left.

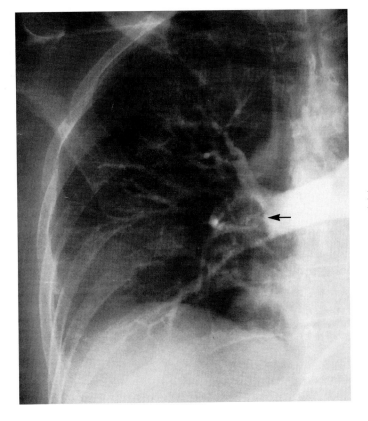

Figure 5. Pulmonary angiogram revealing a saddle embolus in the mainstem of the right middle and right lower lobe vessels.

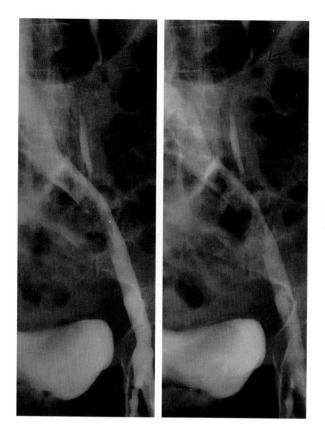

Figure 6. Venogram of the left leg showing a large intraluminal filling defect in the iliac vessels.

CASE 7: Clinical Presentation – Pleuritic Chest Pain and Dyspnea

CLINICAL PRESENTATION

This 73-year-old man came in complaining of pleuritic left sided chest pain and shortness of breath. The symptoms started suddenly and awoke him from his sleep. He likened the pain to that of a pulmonary embolus he had had approximately 20 years before. He had no symptoms of deep vein thrombosis and in fact no other symptoms. His initial pulmonary embolism had occurred following appendectomy, but there were no other risk factors present this time.

EXAMINATION

Examination revealed a blood pressure of 140/80, a pulse rate of 98, a respiratory rate of 26, and normal jugular venous pressure. He was experiencing chest pain. The chest examination showed reduced air entry at the left base and some tenderness over the overlying ribs. There were no adventitious sounds. The cardiovascular system examination was negative. He had pitting edema at both ankles and increased skin temperature on the right, but no tenderness.

INVESTIGATIONS

The chest x-ray showed bilateral pleural effusions and increased pulmonary vascular markings with an enlarged heart in keeping with left ventricular failure. An IPG was negative. The V/Q scan showed multiple segmental defects corresponding to the abnormalities in the chest x-ray (indeterminate scan). Pulmonary angiography revealed the presence of pulmonary emboli on the left.

TREATMENT

This patient was treated with intravenous heparin and then warfarin along with measures to treat his left heart failure. He was discharged on anticoagulants and had an uneventful follow-up.

TEACHING POINT

The clinical presentation was suggestive of both pulmonary embolism and heart failure. The chest x-ray was compatible with the findings of heart failure, the leg tests were negative, and the lung scan was indeterminate. The diagnosis was finally made by pulmonary angiography. Pulmonary angiography is required in such patients who have poor cardiorespiratory reserve.

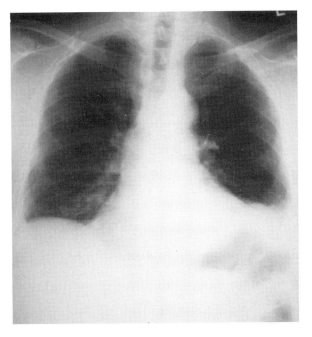

Figure 1. Chest x-ray showing bilateral pleural effusions, increased pulmonary vascular markings and an enlarged heart, in keeping with left ventricular failure.

From *Venous Thromboembolism: An Evidence-Based Atlas* by Russell Hull, Gary Raskob, Graham Pineo © 1996, Futura Publishing Co., Armonk, NY.

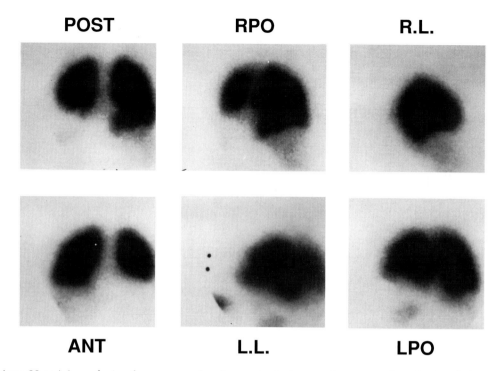

Figure 2. Technetium 99 mAA perfusion lung scans showing a single large subsegmental perfusion defect on the right, corresponding with the abnormality on the chest x-ray.

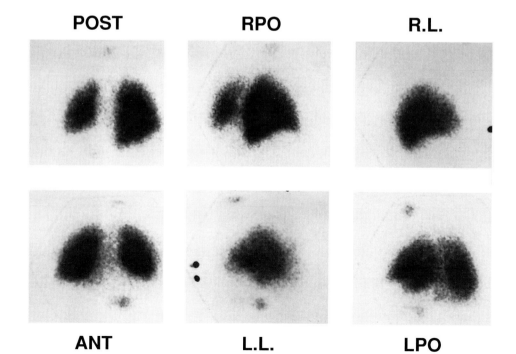

Figure 3. Technetium 99 aerosol ventilation scan showing a ventilation match.

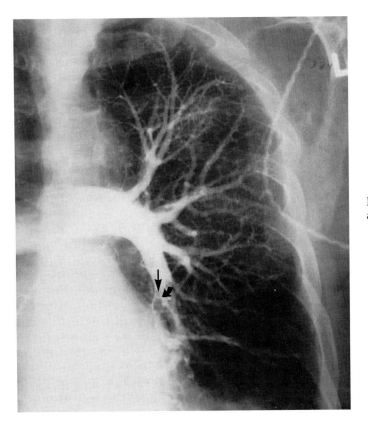

Figure 4. Angiogram showing intraluminal filling defect in first, and second order vessels on the left.

CASE 8: Case Presentation – Pneumonia and Supraventricular Arrhythmia

CLINICAL PRESENTATION

This 59-year-old man initially presented at the hospital with dyspnea, hemoptysis, left pleuritic chest pain, and atrial flutter with 2:1 block and a rate of 150. The initial chest x-ray suggested pneumonia and he was treated with penicillin. Because of persistence of the atrial flutter along with the hemoptysis and chest pain, he was referred to another hospital for further investigations. Further history revealed the presence of chronic bronchitis and cigarette smoking.

EXAMINATION

Following cardioversion, the pulse rate was 72 with normal sinus rhythm. Blood pressure was 110/70. The chest examination and cardiovascular examination were normal. A leg examination was negative.

INVESTIGATIONS

A chest x-ray revealed a density in the left lower lobe compatible with pulmonary infarction. The lung scan showed a large single subsegmental perfusion defect cor-responding to the area of abnormality on chest x-ray (indeterminate). The IPG was abnormal in the right leg. Venography revealed a filling defect in the right femoral vein. Pulmonary angiography was negative.

TREATMENT

Heparin treatment was started with the suspicion of pulmonary embolism and continued when the venogram proved to be positive. He required repeat cardioversion because of his atrial flutter and this was eventually controlled on digoxin and quinidine.

TEACHING POINT

This patient was mistakenly thought to have pneumonia although the chest x-ray pattern in retrospect was suggestive of pulmonary infarction. The persistence of atrial flutter precipitated transfer to a teaching hospital and further studies. Supraventricular arrhythmias may accompany pulmonary embolism, but in this case pulmonary angiography was negative. However, a proximal venous thrombosis was adequate grounds for anticoagulation. The atrial flutter responded to electrical and pharmacological treatment.

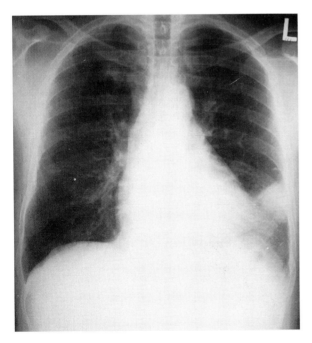

Figure 1. Chest x-ray showing a density in the left lower lobe compatible with pulmonary infarction.

POST **RPO** **R.L.**

ANT **L.L.** **LPO**

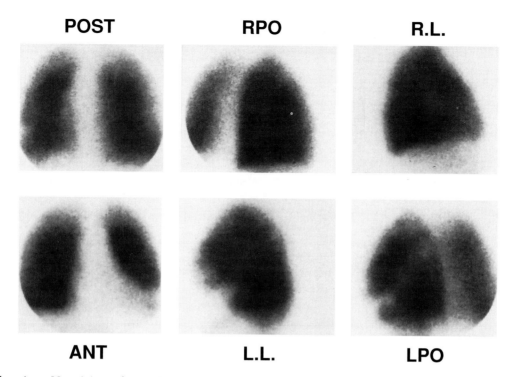

Figure 2. Technetium 99 mAA perfusion lung scan showing a large subsegmental defect corresponding to the area of the abnormality on the chest x-ray.

POST **RPO** **R.L.**

ANT **L.L.** **LPO**

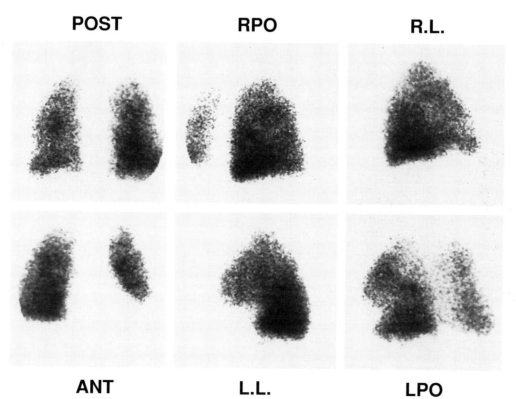

Figure 3. Technetium 99 aerosol ventilation scan showing a matching defect.

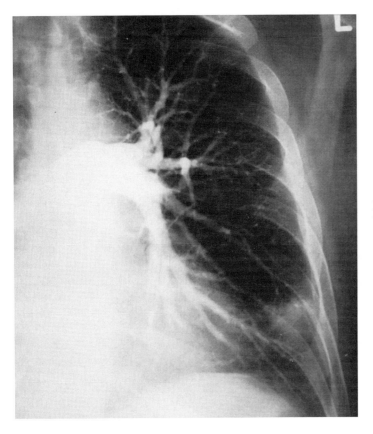

Figure 4. Pulmonary angiogram showing no abnormality on the left (right side negative as well).

CASE 9: Clinical Presentation – Dyspnea, and Pleuritic Chest Pain

CLINICAL PRESENTATION

This 29-year-old man was admitted to the hospital complaining of cough, shortness of breath, and chest pain. In the week prior to admission, he had a cough productive of increasing amounts of greenish sputum at times speckled with blood. He also noticed shortness of breath on exertion and was becoming dyspneic even at rest. Coughing or deep breathing caused a sharp retrosternal pain. He had a past history of systemic lupus erythematosus over the previous 5 years, and he was on prednisone 15 mg daily, Naprosyn 250 mg twice daily, and aspirin as needed. There was a history of pneumonia and septicemia a year prior to admission.

EXAMINATION

Examination revealed a blood pressure of 120/80 and a pulse rate of 100. Breath sounds were normal with inspiratory rales at both bases, being more prominent on the left. There was no friction rub. The cardiovascular system examination revealed elevated jugular venous pressure, a palpable P2, and wide splitting of the second sound on inspiration. A soft third heart sound was noted. There was moderate hepatomegaly. Leg exam revealed no abnormality.

INVESTIGATIONS

The chest x-ray on admission showed some linear atelectasis in the right mid-lung zone. A perfusion lung scan showed a subsegmental defect in the right lung corresponding to the area of atelectasis on the chest x-ray (indeterminate). Pulmonary angiography on the same day revealed high pulmonary pressure, but no evidence of pulmonary embolism. An IPG the following day was negative.

TREATMENT

The patient was not anticoagulated. Treatment consisted of plasmapheresis and high-dose corticosteroids which resulted in resolution of the chest pain and improvement of the right-heart strain.

TEACHING POINT

The perfusion scan was considered indeterminate and pulmonary angiography was negative, thus excluding clinically important pulmonary embolism. Symptoms therefore were attributed to pleuritis and pericarditis secondary to systemic lupus erythematosus. The pulmonary hypertension may have been secondary to lupus.

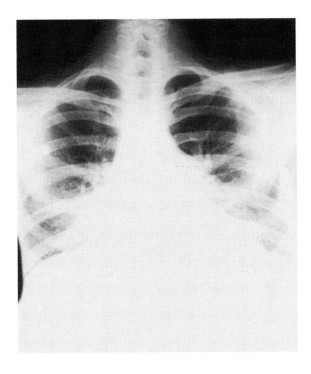

Figure 1. Chest x-ray showing some linear atelectasis in the right mid-lung zone.

POST   **RPO**   **R.L.**

ANT   **L.L.**   **LPO**

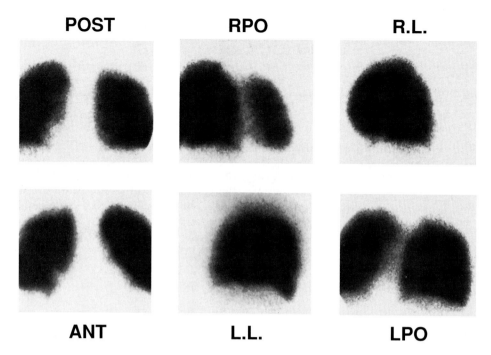

Figure 2. Technetium 99 mAA perfusion scan showing a subsegmental defect in the right lung corresponding with the area of atelectasis.

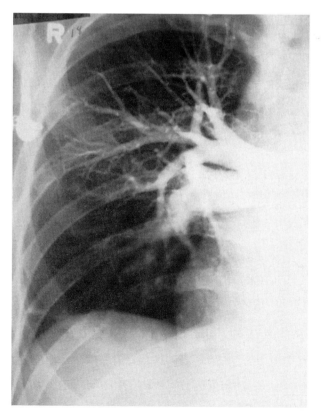

Figure 3. Negative pulmonary angiogram.

CASE 10: Clinical Presentation – Central Chest Pain and Hemoptysis

CLINICAL PRESENTATION

This 39-year-old man presented with central chest pain, numbness in both arms and hands as well as the jaw, extensive diaphoresis, and slight nausea. The central chest pain developed suddenly and was described to be like a "rope tightening" around his chest. The discomfort had come on while he was driving a truck on a long distance haul. He noticed that the pain was worsened by deep breathing or coughing which on a couple of occasions was associated with blood-tinged frothy sputum. He experienced a feeling of suffocation. The pain persisted through the night and he went to the emergency room the following morning. He claimed that he had had a similar bout of chest pain 3 months earlier, and that he had also had some chest pain on exertion from time to time. He had a past history of tuberculosis. He also had a history of peptic ulcer disease with bleeding and perforation, which was relieved by surgery, and a history of alcohol abuse. He had smoked from one to three packs of cigarettes daily for about 25 years.

EXAMINATION

Examination revealed a blood pressure of 108/70, a pulse rate of 58 per minute, and a respiratory rate 14 per minute. The chest examination was normal. Leg examination was negative.

INVESTIGATIONS

The chest x-ray on admission showed linear densities and scattered calcifications, probably due to his previous tuberculosis. The IPG was normal bilaterally. A V/Q scan revealed multiple segmental matched defects (low probability). Pulmonary angiography on the same day was negative and venography also was negative.

TREATMENT

Heparin was started on admission but was discontinued when venous thromboembolism was excluded. His chest pain subsided with nitroglycerin and further investigations were undertaken to rule out cardiovascular disease or an abnormality of esophageal motility.

TEACHING POINT

The clinical presentation was compatible with myocardial infarction or massive pulmonary embolism, but neither was substantiated on his investigations. With the exclusion of thromboembolism, anticoagulants were withdrawn.

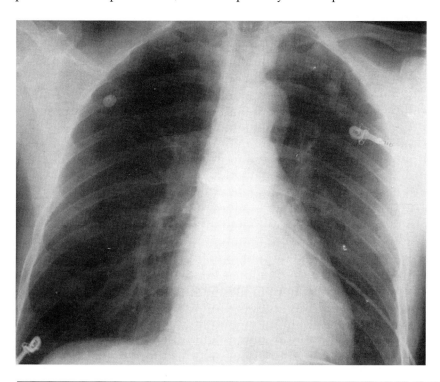

Figure 1. Chest x-ray showing linear densities and scattered calcifications probably due to old tuberculosis.

From *Venous Thromboembolism: An Evidence-Based Atlas* by Russell Hull, Gary Raskob, Graham Pineo © 1996, Futura Publishing Co., Armonk, NY.

POST **RPO** **R.L.**

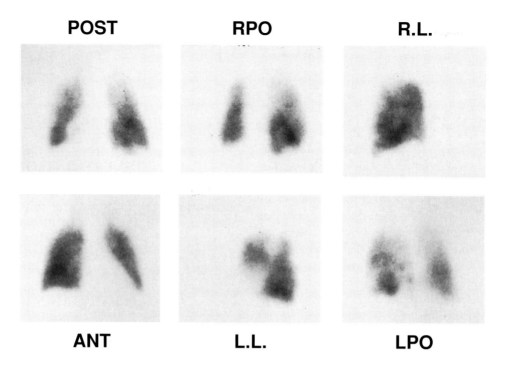

ANT **L.L.** **LPO**

Figure 2. Technetium 99 mAA perfusion scan showing multiple segmental perfusion.

POST **RPO** **R.L.**

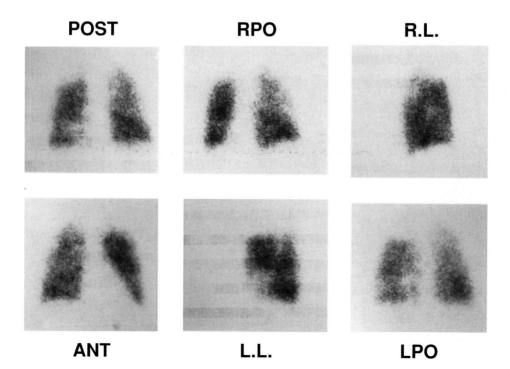

ANT **L.L.** **LPO**

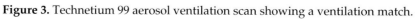

Figure 3. Technetium 99 aerosol ventilation scan showing a ventilation match.

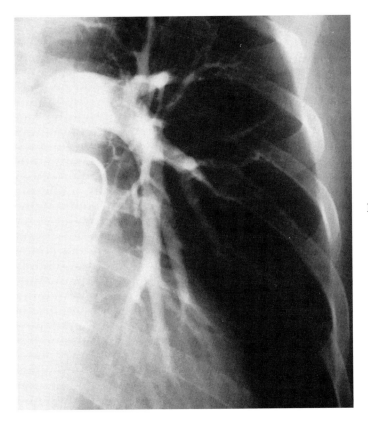

Figure 4. Negative pulmonary angiogram on the left.

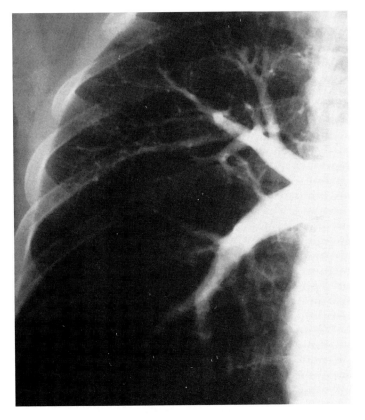

Figure 5. Negative pulmonary angiogram on the right.

CASE 11: Clinical Presentation – Pneumonia

CLINICAL PRESENTATION

This 53-year-old man developed shortness of breath and hemoptysis approximately 2 1/2 weeks after he developed a left cerebrovascular accident thought to be embolic in origin. A CT scan showed extensive involvement of the left temporal lobe with punctate hemorrhages. His past history indicated that he had had an anterolateral myocardial infarction 3 months before this admission.

EXAMINATION

On examination, the pulse rate was 100 per minute and regular. His temperature was 37.9°C. A chest examination revealed dullness to percussion at the right base with decreased air entry and bronchial breathing. The cardiovascular system examination was negative as was examination of the legs.

INVESTIGATIONS

A chest x-ray revealed consolidation of the right lower lobe consistent with pneumonia. The IPG was nor-

mal. A V/Q lung scan revealed multiple subsegmental defects with ventilation match (low probability). Pulmonary angiography revealed a pulmonary embolus in the second-order vessels of the right lung.

TREATMENT

The patient was treated with antibiotics and intravenous heparin followed by warfarin for 3 months. He was transferred to the rehabilitation unit.

TEACHING POINT

The clinical presentation and chest x-ray suggested the diagnosis of pneumonia. The IPG was normal. The angiogram revealed a pulmonary embolus in a patient with a clinical picture of pneumonia. The patient probably had a pulmonary infarct that became infected. He had no complications from his anticoagulant therapy.

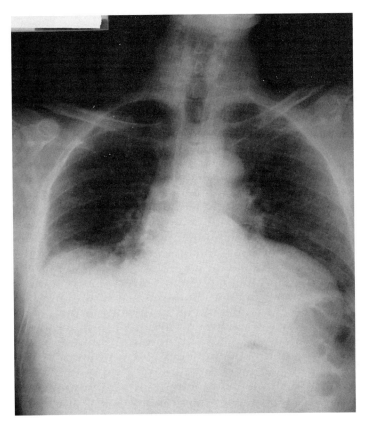

Figure 1. Chest x-ray showing an area of consolidation in the right lower lobe.

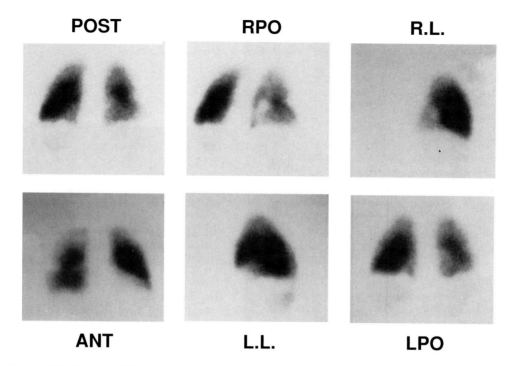

Figure 2. Technetium 99 mAA perfusion scan showing multiple subsegmental perfusion defects.

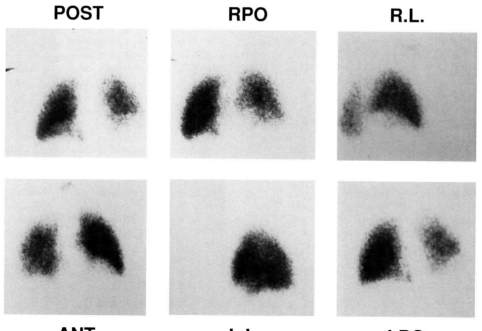

Figure 3. Technetium 99 aerosol ventilation scan revealing a ventilation match.

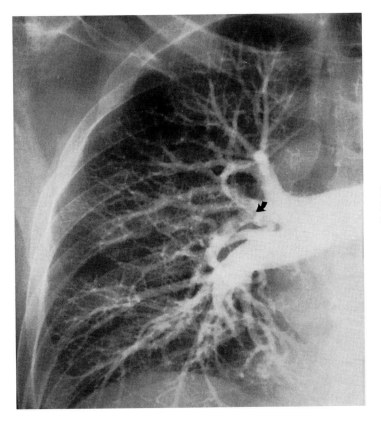

Figure 4. Pulmonary angiogram revealing intraluminal filling defect in the second order vessels in the right lung (see arrow).

CASE 12: Clinical Presentation – Dyspnea and Pleuritic Chest Pain

CLINICAL PRESENTATION

This 61-year-old woman was admitted to the emergency room complaining of a 3-week history of increasing shortness of breath. This was initially noticed after walking a few steps. She denied orthopnea, paroxysmal nocturnal dyspnea, or other symptoms of congestive heart failure. She complained of a sharp, right, pleuritic anterior chest pain that started 1 week before admission. Her pain had worsened 2 days before admission and in fact this is what brought her to the hospital. She had a 36 pack/year history of cigarette smoking. Her medications included Premarin.

EXAMINATION

Blood pressure was 160/90, the pulse rate was 80, the respiratory rate was 28, and the jugular venous pressure was normal. Chest examination revealed slightly decreased air entry on the right side with no adventitious sounds. There was slight tenderness on palpation over the right ribs anteriorly. There was no friction rub. The cardiovascular examination was normal. Examination of the extremities revealed tenderness in the right thigh.

INVESTIGATIONS

The chest x-ray on admission was normal. A V/Q scan revealed multiple segmental defects with ventilation mismatch (high probability). A subsequent pulmonary angiogram showed emboli in both lungs. Both the IPG and the venogram were normal.

TREATMENT

This patient was treated with intravenous heparin and subsequent warfarin therapy and all symptoms resolved. She was discharged to continue warfarin for 3 months. Her Premarin was discontinued.

TEACHING POINT

The presenting symptom in this patient was persistent shortness of breath with a more recent onset of chest pain. The V/Q scan showed a high probability for pulmonary embolism that was confirmed by pulmonary angiography. Both the IPG and the venogram were negative. The only identifiable risk factor in this case was the use of Premarin. Pulmonary angiography was optional in the context of this patient with a high probability scan.

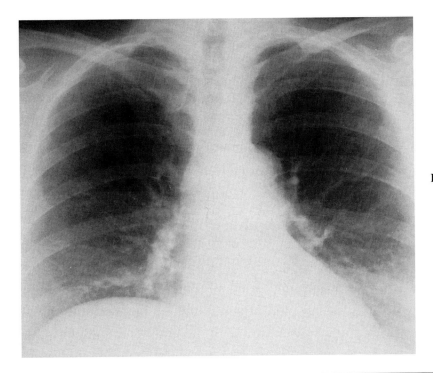

Figure 1. Normal chest x-ray.

POST RPO R.L.

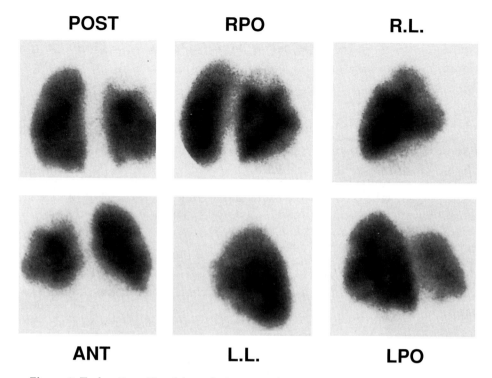

ANT L.L. LPO

Figure 2. Technetium 99 mAA perfusion scan showing multiple segmental defects.

POST RPO R.L.

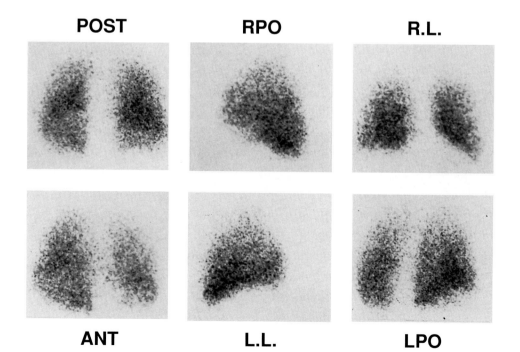

ANT L.L. LPO

Figure 3. Technetium 99 aerosol ventilation scan showing a ventilation mismatch.

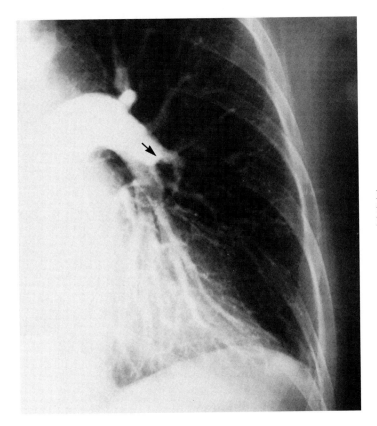

Figure 4. Pulmonary angiogram of the left lung showing intraluminal filling defects in second order vessels in the lower lobe.

CASE 13: Clinical Presentation – Pleuritic Chest Pain

CLINICAL PRESENTATION

This 74-year-old man presented to Emergency complaining of pleuritic chest pain. On further review he had swelling, warmth, and tenderness in the left leg. This was accompanied by left-sided pleuritic chest pain. Five weeks previously he had been in the hospital for amputation of the left foot due to vascular insufficiency. During that admission, extensive deep vein thrombosis was detected by venography in the right leg (the nonoperated leg) and he had been discharged on warfarin.

EXAMINATION

Examination revealed a blood pressure of 140/90, a pulse rate of 96, a respiratory rate of 30, and normal jugular venous pressure. Reduced breath sounds were noted at the left base along with inspiratory crepitations. The cardiovascular system examination was negative. There was swelling of the left leg to the level of the thigh with tenderness on deep palpation. There was evidence of infection at the operative site.

INVESTIGATIONS

The chest x-ray was negative. The IPG was positive on the left but uninterpretable due to the vascular insufficiency. The V/Q scan showed multiple large segmental perfusion defects with matching ventilation defects (low probability). Pulmonary angiography revealed emboli on both sides.

TREATMENT

The patient was treated with intravenous heparin followed by warfarin.

TEACHING POINT

Although the V/Q scan was interpreted to be low probability, angiography revealed multiple pulmonary emboli, again confirming the danger of using this nomenclature. Prospective studies show that 15-40% of patients with low probability lung scan patterns actually have pulmonary emboli on angiography.

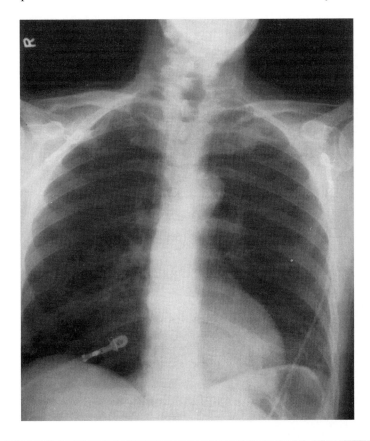

Figure 1. Negative chest x-ray.

From *Venous Thromboembolism: An Evidence-Based Atlas* by Russell Hull, Gary Raskob, Graham Pineo © 1996, Futura Publishing Co., Armonk, NY.

POST   **R.L.**

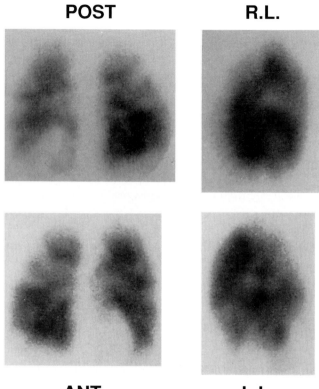

ANT   **L.L.**

Figure 2. Technetium 99 mAA perfusion scan showing multiple large segmental perfusion defect; ventilation scan unavailable but showed a ventilation match (low probability).

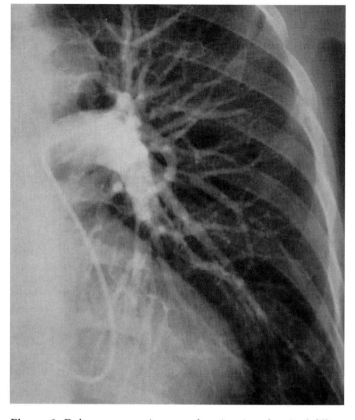

Figure 3. Pulmonary angiogram showing intraluminal filling defect in the second order vessels on the left.

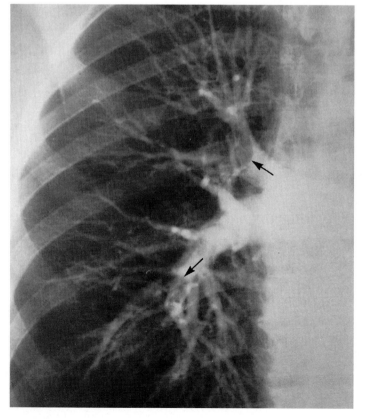

Figure 4. Pulmonary angiogram showing multiple pulmonary emboli in first, second, third order vessels in the right.

CASE 14: Clinical Presentation – Unexplained Dyspnea

CLINICAL PRESENTATION

A 73-year-old woman presented to the emergency room complaining of shortness of breath which commenced the day before admission. It had persisted throughout the day, but was not accompanied by any other chest symptoms. There was nothing else of significance in the history.

EXAMINATION

Examination revealed a blood pressure of 140/80 with a pulsus paradoxus of 15 mm Hg, a pulse rate of 90, and a respiratory rate of 30. Heart sounds were normal as was the rest of the cardiovascular system. Air entry was decreased bilaterally and the expiratory phase was prolonged. Coarse rales were heard in both lung bases and anteriorly as well. She had no clinical evidence of deep-vein thrombosis.

INVESTIGATIONS

The chest x-ray showed hyperinflation and distended pulmonary arteries. The lung fields were clear. A V/Q scan revealed multiple lobar perfusion defects with ventilation match (low probability). Pulmonary angiography showed emboli in both lungs. The IPGs were normal bilaterally.

TREATMENT

The patient was started on heparin on presentation and this was followed by warfarin.

TEACHING POINT

This patient presented with a history of shortness of breath, but had no other pulmonary symptoms. The V/Q scan showed a low probability for pulmonary embolism, but pulmonary angiography was positive. This patient had objective evidence on chest x-ray of chronic obstructive pulmonary disease. Her symptoms could have been falsely attributed to an exacerbation of her pulmonary disease if definitive studies had not been performed. Again, the low probability reading could have been misleading.

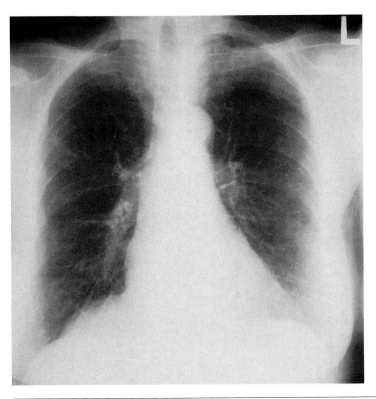

Figure 1. Chest x-ray showing hyperinflation and distended pulmonary arteries.

POST   **RPO**   **R.L.**

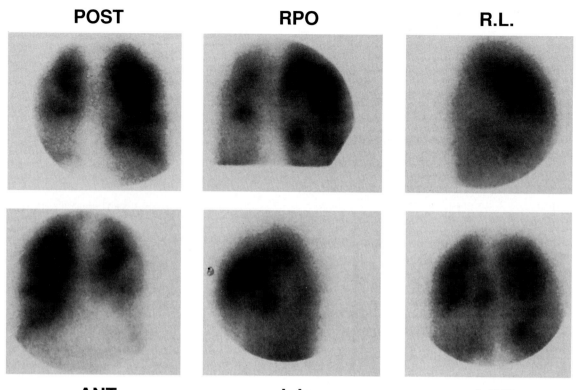

ANT   **L.L.**   **LPO**

Figure 2. Technetium 99 mAA perfusion scan showing lobar perfusion defects.

EQUIL 1   **WASH IN**   **MAA**

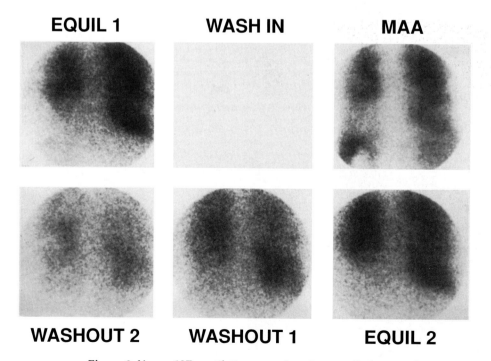

WASHOUT 2   **WASHOUT 1**   **EQUIL 2**

Figure 3. Xenon 127 ventilation scan showing ventilation match.

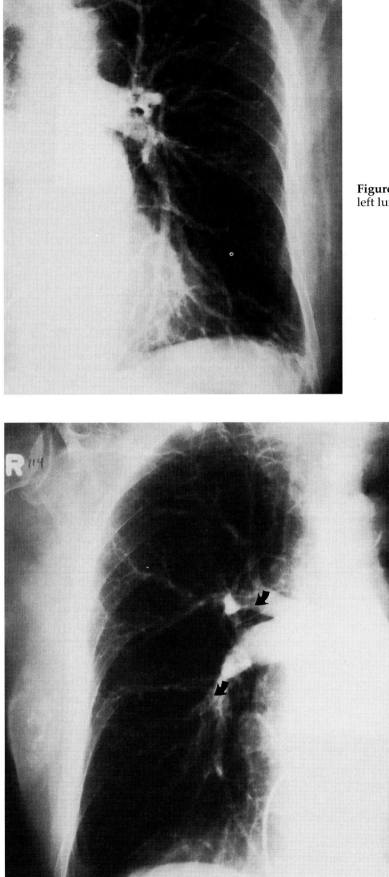

Figure 4. Pulmonary angiogram showing large embolus in the left lung.

Figure 5. Pulmonary angiogram showing emboli in right lung.

CASE 15: Clinical Presentation – Syncope

CLINICAL PRESENTATION

This 77-year-old woman suddenly developed syncope while in hospital recovering from a hip operation. She had suffered a fractured hip approximately 2 months previously and had undergone pinning and was discharged. Unfortunately, the hip fractured again 2 months later and she underwent a subsequent procedure. This, however, was complicated by a dislocation requiring a leg cast. She had a history of hypertension and angina.

EXAMINATION

Examination revealed a blood pressure of 188/100, a pulse rate of 98, a respiratory rate of 18, and normal jugular venous pressure. She was cyanotic, breathing with difficulty, and was expectorating clear, frothy sputum. Physical examination otherwise was unremarkable.

INVESTIGATIONS

The chest x-ray was normal. The venogram revealed bilateral proximal vein thrombosis. An urgent pulmonary angiogram was negative. Lung scans completed over the subsequent 24 hours revealed lobar perfusion defects with ventilation mismatch (high probability).

TREATMENT

The patient was treated with heparin followed by warfarin to be continued for 3 months.

TEACHING POINT

This patient presented a complex problem because of the requirement for repeated operations on her hip. Hip surgery represents a high risk for deep-vein thrombosis under the best of circumstances, and with repeated operations in this elderly lady, she represented a very high risk. While on low dose heparin prophylaxis, she developed a syncopal attack, but pulmonary angiography at the time was negative. A lung scan subsequently showed high probability for pulmonary embolism, suggesting that pulmonary angiography was falsely negative.

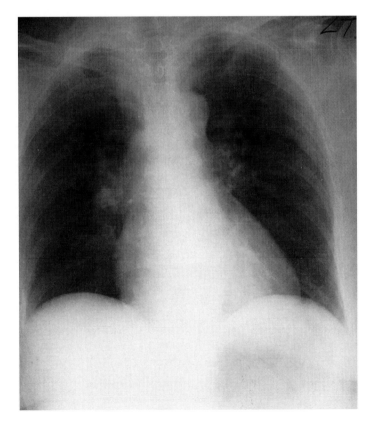

Figure 1. Normal chest x-ray.

POST

R.L.

ANT

L.L.

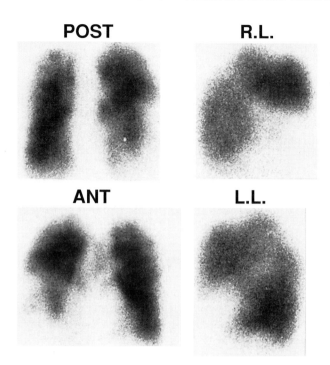

Figure 2. Technetium 99 mAA perfusion scan showing multiple lobar perfusion defects.

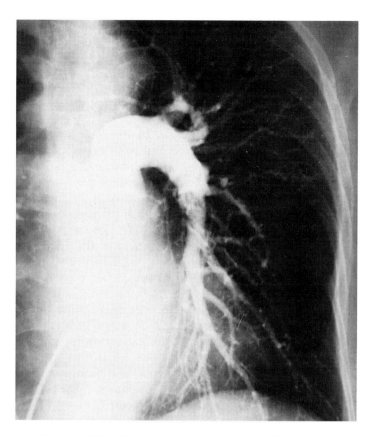

Figure 3. Negative pulmonary angiogram of left lung.

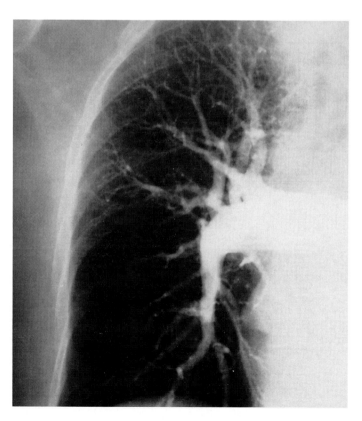

Figure 4. Negative pulmonary angiogram of right lung.

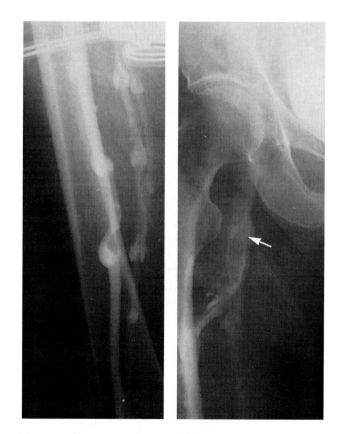

Figure 5. Large intraluminal filling defect in the deep venous system on the right leg.

CASE 16: Clinical Presentation – Pleuritic Chest Pain and Atypical Symptoms of Pneumonia

CLINICAL PRESENTATION

This 17-year-old woman had a 2-week history of flank pain, frequency, nocturia, and proteinuria consistent with a nephrotic syndrome. Two days before this admission, she developed leftsided chest pain initially thought to be pneumonia and was started on antibiotics. The pain recurred and was accompanied by hemoptysis and precipitated her admission to hospital. She had been perfectly healthy up to this time.

EXAMINATION

On admission, the heart rate was 128, blood pressure 90/60, respiratory rate 34. Chest examination revealed dullness to percussion at the left base, with decreased air entry in the same area. Jugular venous pressure was elevated 5 cm but the cardiac examination was otherwise negative. She had slight ankle edema bilaterally.

INVESTIGATIONS

The chest x-ray showed a large left pleural effusion and a large proximal right pulmonary artery. The IPG was normal. The V/Q scan showed multiple large segmental perfusion defects with ventilation mismatch (high probability). The pulmonary angiogram showed a saddle embolus in the main trunk of the right pulmonary artery as well as second-order vessel occlusion of the lower lobe on the left. As part of the procedure, a Valsalva maneuver was performed so that dye refluxed down the inferior vena cava. This showed a large thrombus in the right renal vein extending into the inferior vena cava. There was evidence of thrombus in the left renal vein as well.

TREATMENT

The patient was treated with intravenous streptokinase. A repeat pulmonary angiogram after 15 hours of treatment showed increased flow to the right upper lobe. She was placed on intravenous heparin and subsequently warfarin.

TEACHING POINT

This patient suffered from massive pulmonary embolism documented by lung scan and pulmonary angiography. Leg tests were negative. Inferior vena cavagram revealed thrombosis of the right renal vein with extension into the inferior vena cava with a smaller thrombus noted in the left renal vein. This was the presumed site of the origin for the pulmonary embolus. Her renal vein thrombosis was thought to be due to underlying renal disease (nephrotic syndrome).

POST **RPO** **R.L.**

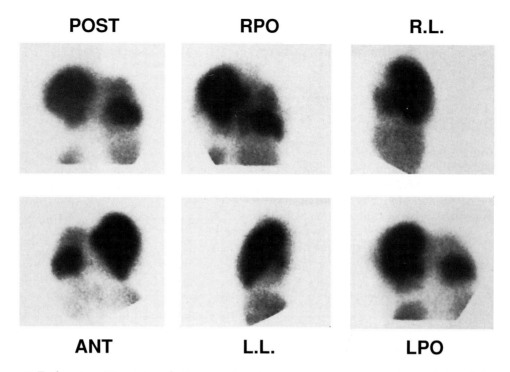

ANT **L.L.** **LPO**

Figure 1. Technetium 99 mAA perfusion scan showing multiple large segmental perfusion defects.

POST **RPO** **R.L.**

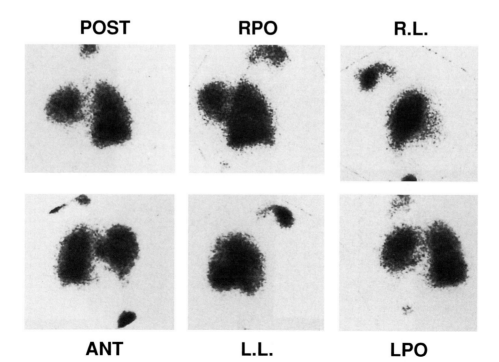

ANT **L.L.** **LPO**

Figure 2. Technetium 99 aerosol ventilation scan showing ventilation mismatch.

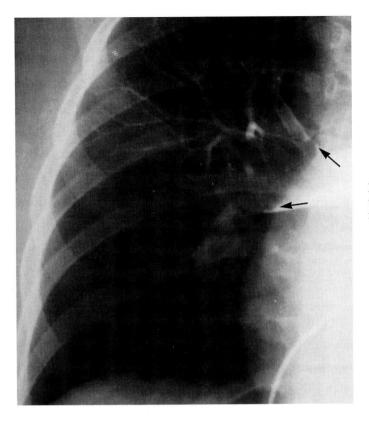

Figure 3. Pulmonary angiogram showing a saddle embolus in the main trunk of the right pulmonary artery, and filling defects in second order vessels.

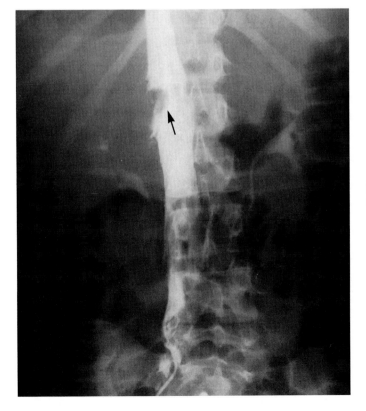

Figure 4. Inferior vena cavagram showing a filling defect in the region of the right renal vein.

CASE 17: Clinical Presentation – Supraventricular Arrhythmia

CLINICAL PRESENTATION

This 56-year-old woman presented with new-onset atrial fibrillation 2 days following hysterectomy. She had no pulmonary symptoms or evidence of deep-vein thrombosis. She had been started on digoxin, which converted her rhythm to sinus. She described a 6-month history of occasional dyspnea and palpitations, particularly on climbing stairs, but she had no history of angina, paroxysmal nocturnal dyspnea, or orthopnea. She was on no medications.

EXAMINATION

Blood pressure was 160/90, the initial pulse rate was 100 with atrial fibrillation, and the respiratory rate was normal. The chest examination was entirely clear as was the remainder of the cardiovascular system. There was no clinical evidence of deep vein thrombosis.

INVESTIGATIONS

The chest x-ray showed possible right lower lobe atelectasis. The IPG was normal. A V/Q scan showed multiple segmental mismatched defects (high probability), and pulmonary angiography confirmed the evidence of pulmonary embolism.

TREATMENT

With confirmation of the pulmonary embolus, the patient was treated with heparin followed by warfarin for 3 months.

TEACHING POINT

This patient presented with the sudden onset of atrial fibrillation 2 days following surgery with no other signs or symptoms of thromboembolism. New-onset atrial fibrillation, particularly in the postoperative setting, should raise the suspicion of pulmonary embolism. The pulmonary investigations confirmed the diagnosis of pulmonary embolism with a high probability scan and positive angiography. With the finding of a high probability scan, pulmonary angiography is optional in this context.

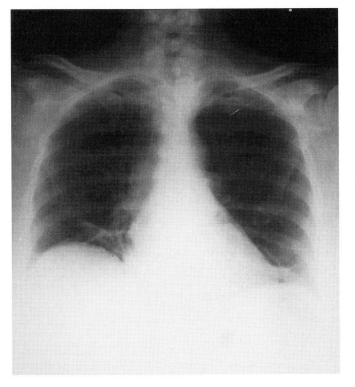

Figure 1. Chest x-ray showing atelectasis in the right lower lobe.

POST **RPO** **R.L.**

ANT **L.L.** **LPO**

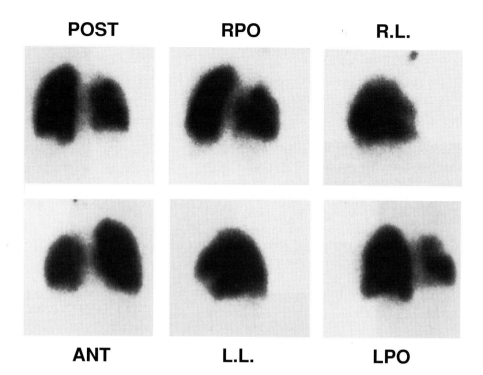

Figure 2. Technetium 99 mAA perfusion scan showing multiple segmental perfusion defects.

POST **RPO** **R.L.**

ANT **L.L.** **LPO**

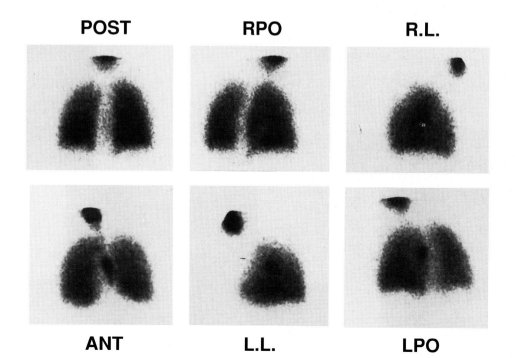

Figure 3. Technetium 99 aerosol ventilation scan showing ventilation mismatch.

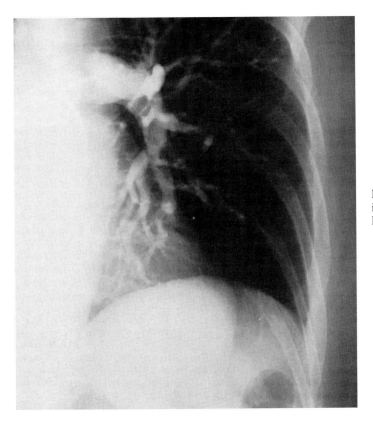

Figure 4. Pulmonary angiogram of the left lung showing intraluminal filling defects in the second order vessels in the lower lobes.

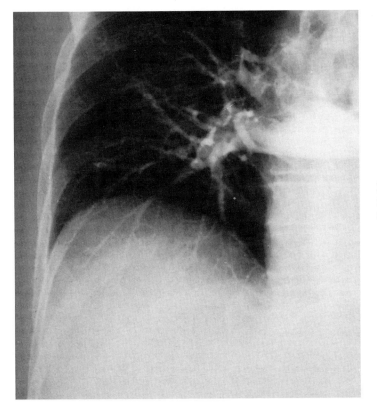

Figure 5. Pulmonary angiogram of the right lung showing intraluminal filling defects in the second order vessels of the upper and lower lobes.

CASE 18: Clinical Presentation – Hemoptysis and Dyspnea

CLINICAL PRESENTATION

A 74-year-old man presented to the emergency room complaining of chest pain, hemoptysis, and shortness of breath. He described retrosternal heaviness with radiation down the left arm, increasing in severity over the previous few weeks. The episode bringing him to the hospital had lasted for 3 hours. It was unrelieved by nitroglycerin and was associated with palpitations and sweating. In the past, he had a myocardial infarction and chronic obstructive pulmonary disease. He had also experienced hemoptysis prior to admission. He smoked cigarettes.

EXAMINATION

On examination, blood pressure was 110/70, the pulse rate was 90, and the respiratory rate was 30. The chest examination demonstrated reduced air entry at both lung bases, expiratory wheezes, and a prolonged expiratory phase. The jugular venous pressure was elevated and there was positive hepatojugular reflux. Otherwise, the cardiovascular examination was negative. There was peripheral edema.

INVESTIGATIONS

The chest x-ray showed chronic fibrotic changes and hyperinflation, but no acute changes. The IPG was normal. A V/Q scan showed multiple large subsegmental perfusion defects with ventilation mismatch (high probability). A pulmonary angiogram was negative. It was not possible to perform a venogram.

TREATMENT

The intravenous heparin that was initially started was discontinued with the negative angiogram. Further investigations revealed the diagnosis of squamous cell carcinoma of the lung. He was discharged without anti-coagulant treatment.

TEACHING POINT

The lung scan was high probability but angiography was negative. The new diagnosis of squamous cell carcinoma of the lung could explain his hemoptysis and the high probability lung scan.

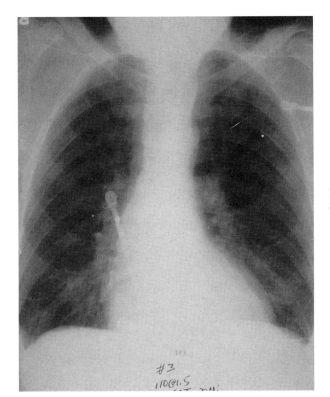

Figure 1. Chest x-ray showing hyperinflation and chronic fibrotic changes.

From *Venous Thromboembolism: An Evidence-Based Atlas* by Russell Hull, Gary Raskob, Graham Pineo © 1996, Futura Publishing Co., Armonk, NY.

POST   **RPO**   **R.L.**

ANT   **L.L.**   **LPO**

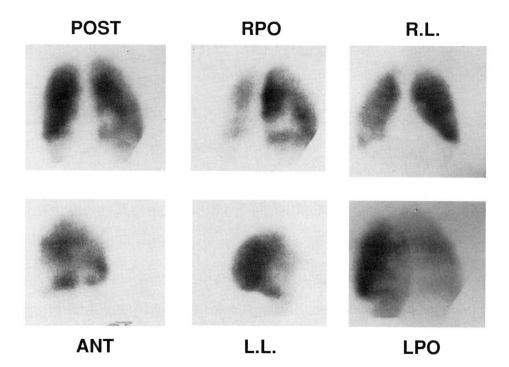

Figure 2. Technetium 99 mAA perfusion scan showing multiple large subsegmental perfusion defects.

MAA   **WASH IN**   **EQUIL 1**

EQUIL 2   **WASHOUT 1**   **WASHOUT 2**

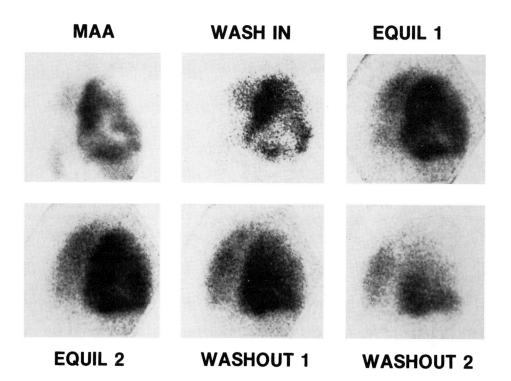

Figure 3. Xenon 127 gas ventilation scan showing ventilation mismatch.

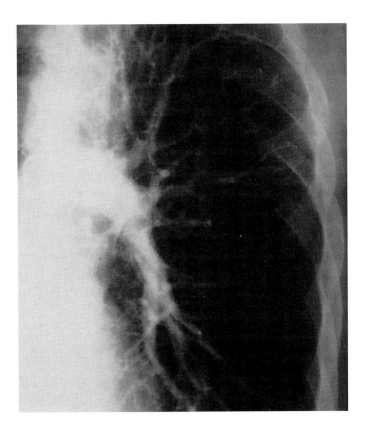

Figure 4. Negative pulmonary angiogram of the left lung.

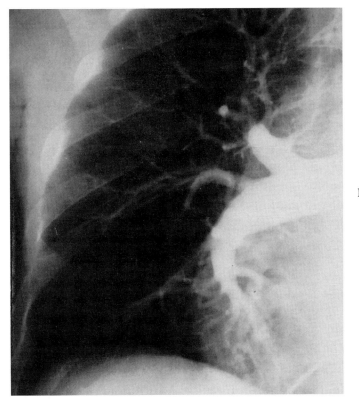

Figure 5. Negative pulmonary angiogram of the right lung.

CASE 19: Clinical Presentation – Pleuritic Chest Pain and Dyspnea on Exertion

CLINICAL PRESENTATION

This 23-year-old woman was admitted to the emergency room complaining of severe, stabbing left anterior chest pain and tingling in the left arm. She had some shortness of breath on exertion. The pain was worsened by deep inspiration. She had no cough and sputum production and no leg symptoms. Risk factors included a 10-hour motorcycle ride 2 days before admission and she had been on birth control pills for about 6 months.

EXAMINATION

On examination she was in no distress. Blood pressure was 120/80, the pulse rate was 80, and the respiratory rate was 16. Examinations of the chest and cardiovascular system were negative and extremities revealed no clinical evidence of deep vein thrombosis.

INVESTIGATIONS

The chest x-ray was negative as was the bilateral IPG. The V/Q scan revealed multiple segmental mismatched defects (high probability). Pulmonary angiography showed a large pulmonary embolus on the left and venography was negative.

TREATMENT

This patient was treated with heparin and warfarin. Birth control pills were discontinued.

TEACHING POINT

This young woman had a large pulmonary embolus. The only risk factors were the 10-hour motorcycle ride and the birth control pills. The high probability lung scan was substantiated by pulmonary angiography. In this young woman, the risk of pulmonary angiography was very low and was outweighed by the need to establish a definitive diagnosis. This case illustrates that a negative venogram does not exclude the diagnosis of pulmonary embolism.

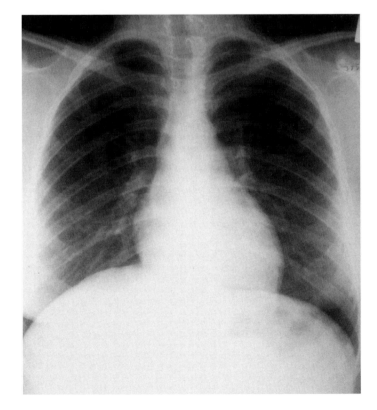

Figure 1. Negative chest x-ray.

From *Venous Thromboembolism: An Evidence-Based Atlas* by Russell Hull, Gary Raskob, Graham Pineo © 1996, Futura Publishing Co., Armonk, NY.

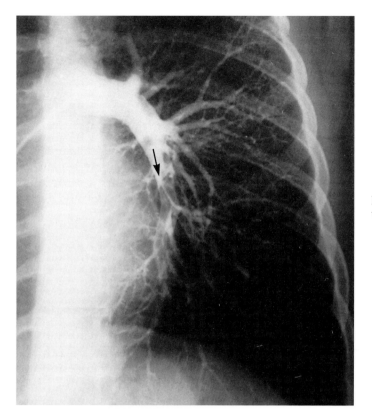

Figure 2. Pulmonary angiogram showing a large embolus in vessels in the left lower lobe.

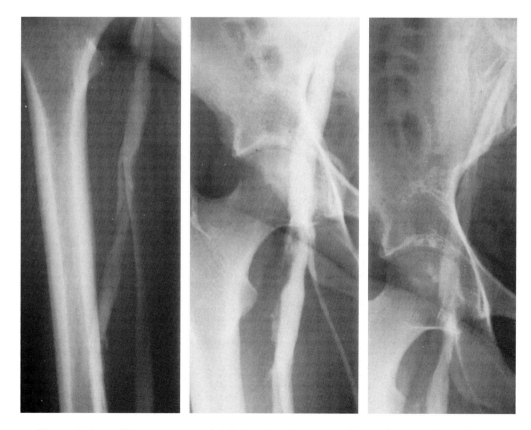

Figure 3. Ascending venogram of right leg showing no evidence of venous thrombosis.

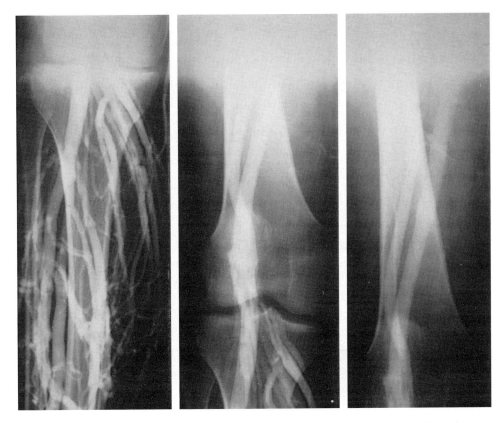

Figure 4. Ascending venogram of right leg showing no evidence of venous thrombosis

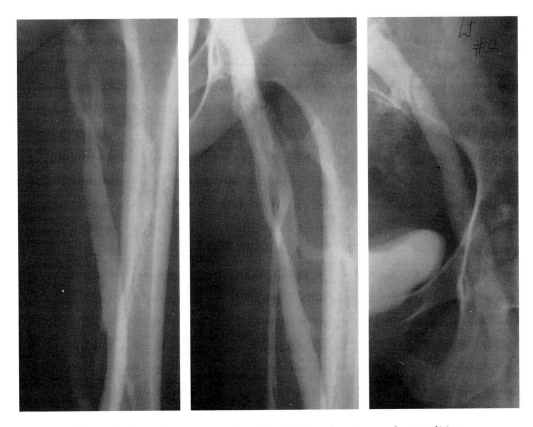

Figure 5. Ascending venography of the left leg showing no abnormalities.

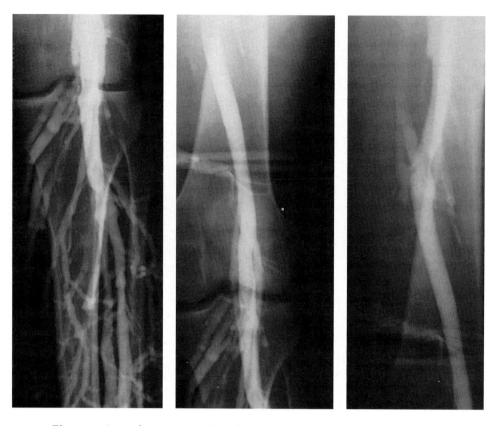

Figure 6. Ascending venography of the left leg showing no abnormalities.

CASE 20: Clinical Presentation – Pleuritic Chest Pain, Dyspnea at Rest

CLINICAL PRESENTATION

This 58-year-old woman was admitted with the acute onset of left-sided chest pain and shortness of breath at rest. The pain was sharp and felt in the lateral chest wall with posterior radiation. It had lasted several hours before admission and was increased by breathing. She had undergone reconstructive surgery on her left great toe 13 days before this admission and had been in a lower leg cast from that time.

EXAMINATION

Examination revealed a blood pressure of 112/80, a pulse rate of 108, and a respiratory rate of 34. The chest examination showed decreased respiratory excursion on the left side and soft crepitations in the lower left lung field. There was tenderness over the left lower chest wall in the region of her pain. The cardiovascular system examination was negative. There was a plaster cast on her left lower leg.

INVESTIGATIONS

The chest x-ray showed minimal blunting of the left costophrenic angle, but the lung fields were clear. A V/Q scan revealed multiple large subsegmental perfusion defects with ventilation mismatch (high probability). Pulmonary angiography demonstrated emboli in the second- and third-order vessels of the left lung. The plaster cast precluded performing studies in the left leg.

TREATMENT

She was treated with intravenous heparin and warfarin to be continued out of hospital. Her course was uneventful.

TEACHING POINT

There was a high clinical suspicion of pulmonary embolism. The lung scan pattern showed high probability, and pulmonary embolism was confirmed by angiography. This patient suffered a serious complication of a relatively minor orthopedic procedure. Pulmonary angiography was an option in this patient with a high probability scan.

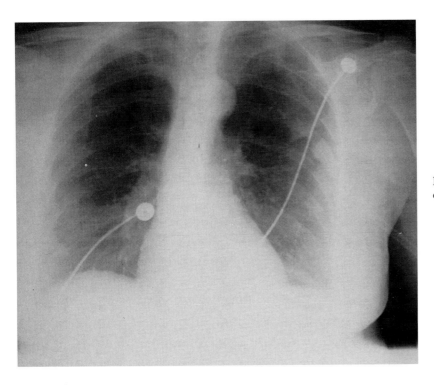

Figure 1. Chest x-ray showing blunting of the left costophrenic angle.

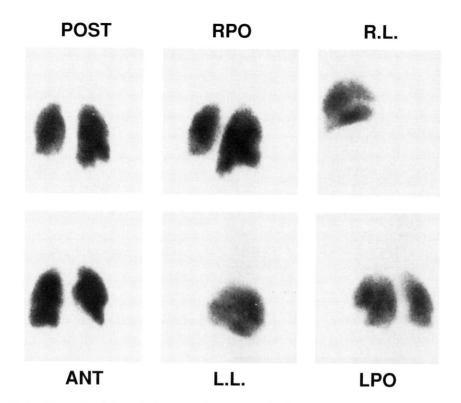

POST   **RPO**   **R.L.**

ANT   **L.L.**   **LPO**

Figure 2. Technetium 99 mAA perfusion scan showing multiple large subsegmental perfusion defects.

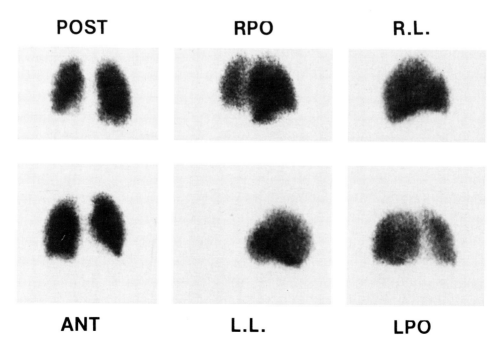

POST   **RPO**   **R.L.**

ANT   **L.L.**   **LPO**

Figure 3. Technetium 99 aerosol ventilation scan showing ventilation mismatch.

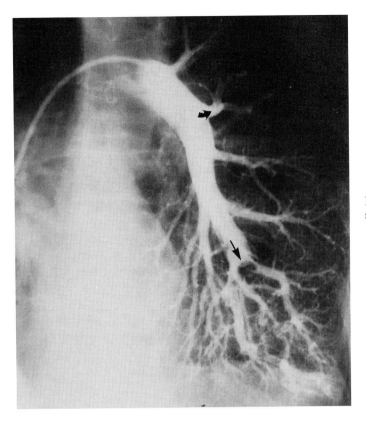

Figure 4. Pulmonary angiogram demonstrating filling defects in second and third order vessels on the left.

CASE 21: Clinical Presentation – Pleuritic Chest Pain

CLINICAL PRESENTATION

This 55-year-old man was admitted complaining of left-sided pleuritic pain associated with a nonproductive cough. He also had a 3-day history of right calf pain with swelling and inflammation. Three weeks earlier, he had been discharged following an acute myocardial infarction. In hospital, he had been on subcutaneous heparin prophylactically.

EXAMINATION

Blood pressure was 120/70, the pulse rate was 74, and the respiratory rate was 16. The chest examination revealed coarse rales at the left base. There was no chest wall pain and no friction rub. Cardiovascular examination was normal. There was some pain in the right calf medially but no swelling or warmth. Pulses were strong.

INVESTIGATIONS

The chest x-ray showed a left pleural effusion. The IPG was normal bilaterally. The lung scan revealed multiple small subsegmental perfusion defects with ventilation mismatch (low probability). Pulmonary angiography showed emboli in the second and third-order vessels in the right lung. A bilateral venogram was normal.

TREATMENT

The patient was treated with intravenous heparin and oral warfarin.

TEACHING POINT

Despite receiving prophylactic subcutaneous heparin, this patient developed venous thromboembolism. The lung scan pattern was low probability but the pulmonary angiogram showed pulmonary embolism.

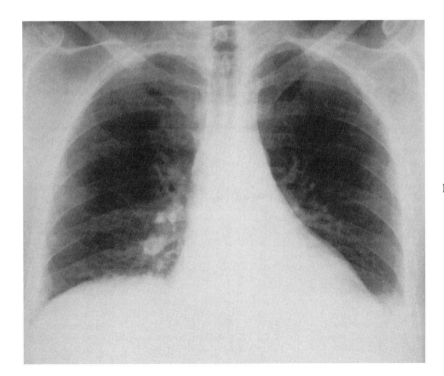

Figure 1. Chest x-ray showing left pleural effusion.

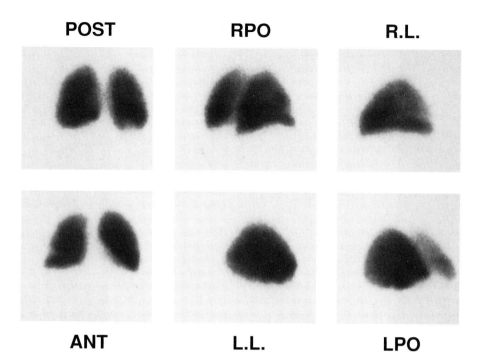

Figure 2. Technetium 99 mAA perfusion scan showing multiple small subsegmental perfusion defects.

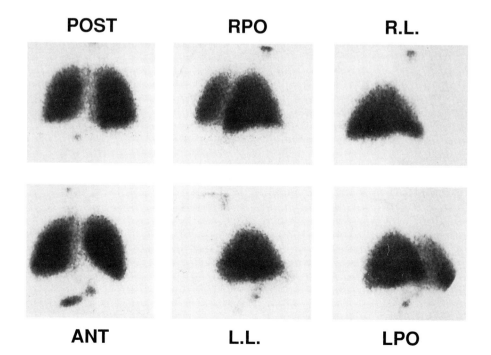

Figure 3. Technetium 99 aerosol ventilation scan showing ventilation mismatch.

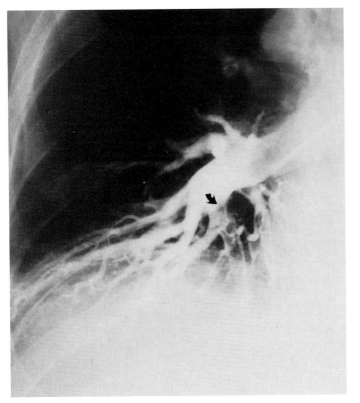

Figure 4. Pulmonary angiogram showing emboli in second and third-order vessels in the right lung.

CASE 22: Clinical Presentation – Leg Pain and Pleuritic Chest Pain

CLINICAL PRESENTATION

This patient was a 67-year-old woman who experienced the sudden onset of left-sided pleuritic chest pain while being investigated for right leg pain. There was a 2-week history of swelling and pain in the right leg, making it increasingly difficult for her to walk. There were no known predisposing factors for deep-vein thrombosis. She had been a one pack per day cigarette smoker for years.

EXAMINATION

On admission, her blood pressure was 140/70, the pulse rate was 90 per minute, the respiratory rate was 24 per minute, and the jugular venous pressure was normal. A chest examination revealed reduced air entry at the left base but no other abnormalities. The cardiovascular system examination was normal.

INVESTIGATIONS

The chest x-ray showed a raised left diaphragm and some obliteration of the costophrenic angle. The admission IPG was abnormal on the right but the following day it had normalized. A V/Q scan showed multiple segmental perfusion defects with ventilation match (low probability). Angiography subsequently revealed an embolus in the third-order vessels on the left.

TREATMENT

Heparin was started on the basis of the positive IPG. On the following day, she experienced further left-sided pleuritic chest pain at the time the IPG had normalized. Venography showed deep-vein thrombosis on the right and pulmonary angiography demonstrated pulmonary embolism. Just prior to discharge, she developed right upper quadrant pain and investigations revealed filling defects in the liver. A liver biopsy revealed metastatic adenocarcinoma from which she ultimately died.

TEACHING POINT

The presentation was that of a deep-vein thrombosis and pulmonary embolism. She developed further symptoms of pulmonary embolism while being investigated. The lung scan was low probability but pulmonary embolism was confirmed at angiography.

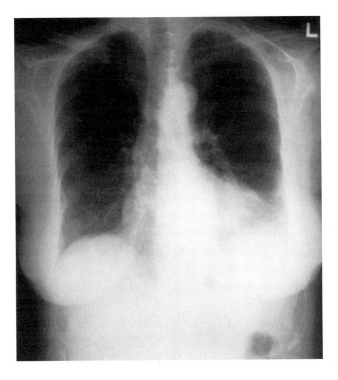

Figure 1. Chest x-ray showed a raised left diaphragm and obliteration of the left costophrenic angle.

POST   **RPO**   **R.L.**

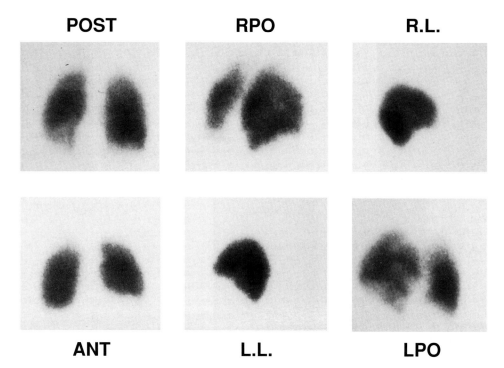

ANT   **L.L.**   **LPO**

Figure 2. Technetium 99 mAA perfusion scan showing multiple segmental perfusion defects.

POST   **RPO**   **R.L.**

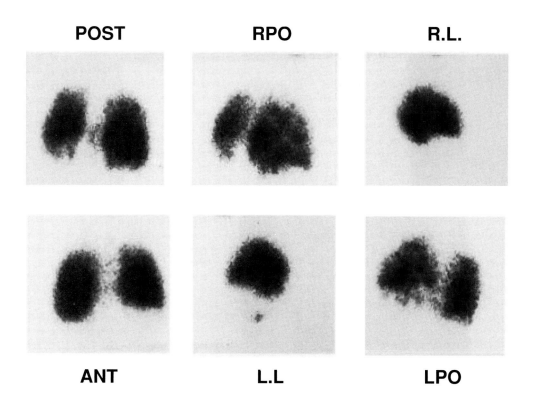

ANT   **L.L**   **LPO**

Figure 3. Technetium 99 aerosol ventilation scan showing ventilation match.

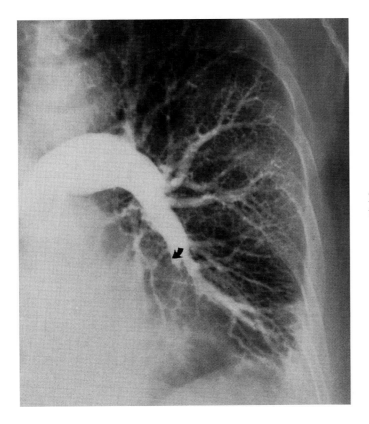

Figure 4. Pulmonary angiogram showing a filling defect in third-order vessel in the left lung.

CASE 23: Clinical Presentation – Pleuritic Chest Pain and Dyspnea

CLINICAL PRESENTATION

This 65-year-old man experienced the sudden onset of right pleuritic chest pain accompanied by shortness of breath. He had a low-grade fever but no chills. There was no cough or sputum production. He had no leg symptoms. He had a past history of a cystoscopy and bladder biopsy 2 weeks before admission. No other risk factors were evident.

EXAMINATION

Examination revealed a blood pressure of 160/90, a pulse rate of 84, and a respiratory rate of 24. Chest examination revealed a pleural friction rub at the right base. The cardiovascular system examination was negative as was examination of the legs.

INVESTIGATIONS

On admission, the chest x-ray was negative. A V/Q scan revealed multiple small, subsegmental perfusion defects with ventilation mismatch (low probability). Angiography, however, revealed an embolus in the second- and third-order vessels in the right lower lobe. Venography was negative.

TREATMENT

The patient was treated with intravenous heparin and warfarin and his course was uneventful.

TEACHING POINT

This patient had symptoms and signs of pulmonary embolism without any major risk factors other than the previous cystoscopy and bladder biopsy. A low probability pattern was seen on the lung scan but the angiogram was positive.

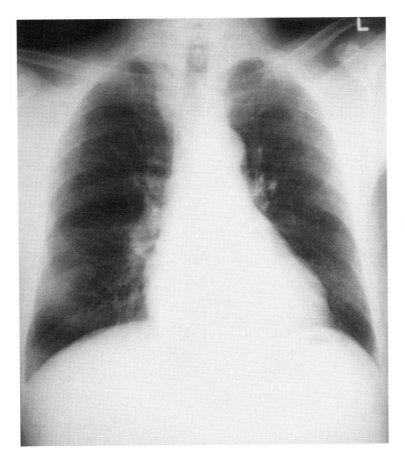

Figure 1. Negative chest x-ray.

POST   **RP**   **R.L.**

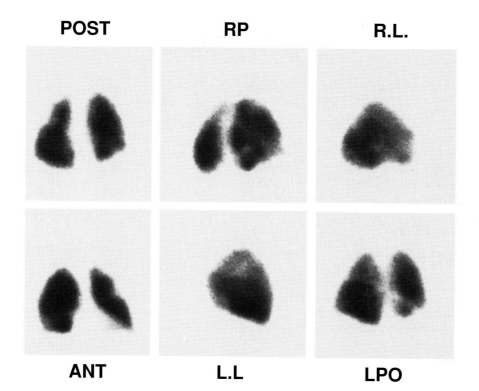

ANT   **L.L**   **LPO**

Figure 2. Technetium 99 mAA perfusion scan showing multiple small subsegmental perfusion defects.

POST   **RPO**   **R.L.**

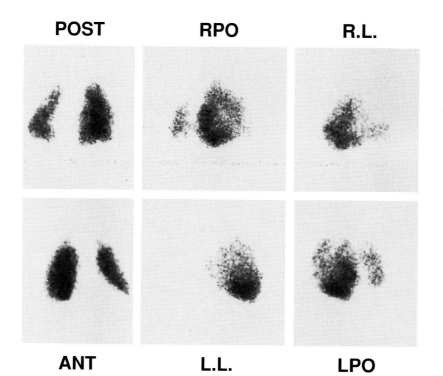

ANT   **L.L.**   **LPO**

Figure 3. Technetium 99 aerosol ventilation scan showing ventilation mismatch.

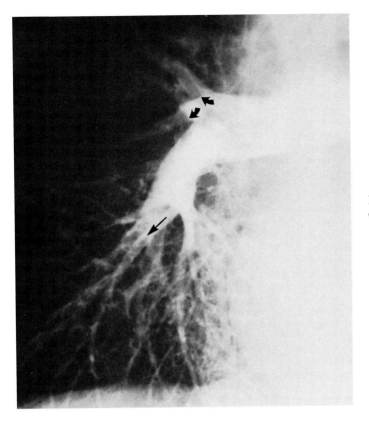

Figure 4. Pulmonary angiogram revealing filling defects in second and third-order vessels in the right lung.

CASE 24: Clinical Presentation – Chest Pain and Dyspnea

CLINICAL PRESENTATION

A 59-year-old man developed right chest pain and shortness of breath 2 weeks following surgery for repair of the medial collateral ligament of his right knee. He had been in a full leg cast since that time. The pain started as a burning retrosternal discomfort, but later became localized to the right side and was pleuritic in nature. He had a history of asthma treated with bronchodilator and previously had been a cigarette smoker.

EXAMINATION

Examination revealed a blood pressure of 150/90 with no pulsus paradoxus, the heart rate was 70 and regular, and the respiratory rate was 20. He had good air entry throughout both lung fields, but there was splinting due to pain. There were no adventitious sounds. The cardiovascular system examination was normal. There was a cast on the right leg.

INVESTIGATIONS

The chest x-ray showed cardiomegaly, right-sided pleural effusion, and a patchy density at the left base. The V/Q scan showed multiple segmental perfusion defects with ventilation mismatch (high probability), and pulmonary angiography confirmed the presence of multiple emboli. Venography revealed thrombi in the peroneal and popliteal veins on the right.

TREATMENT

This patient was treated with heparin and warfarin and recovered uneventfully.

TEACHING POINT

Surgery or trauma involving the knee represents a high risk for deep vein thrombosis even with prophylaxis with either warfarin or low-molecular-weight heparin. This patient suffered a submassive pulmonary embolus, but with appropriate treatment had no further problems. Pulmonary angiography is optional in the context of this patient because of the high probability scan.

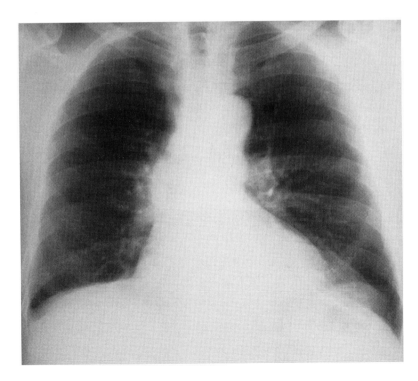

Figure 1. Chest x-ray showed cardiomegaly, right-sided pleural effusion, and a patchy density at the left base.

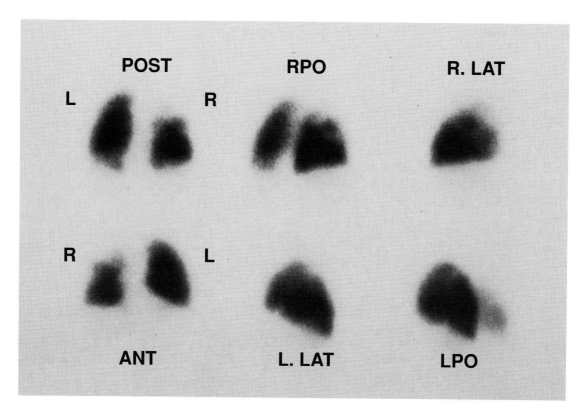

Figure 2. Technetium 99 mAA perfusion scan showing multiple segmental perfusion defects.

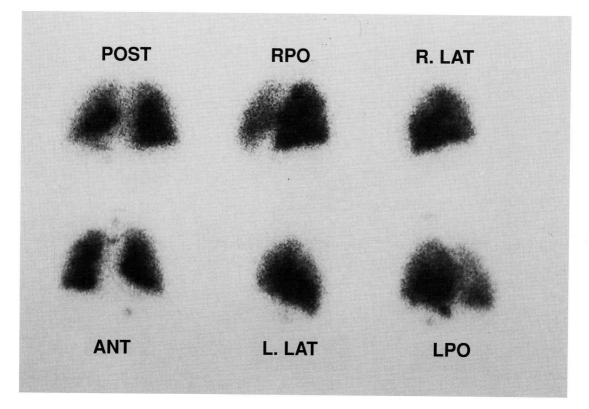

Figure 3. Technetium 99 aerosol ventilation scan showing a ventilation mismatch.

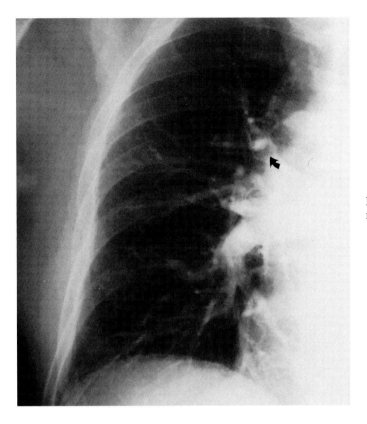

Figure 4. Pulmonary angiogram showing multiple emboli in the right lung.

CASE 25: Clinical Presentation – Chest Pain and Dyspnea

CLINICAL PRESENTATION

This 41-year-old woman came in complaining of chest pain and shortness of breath. She had had a similar episode 3 days before admission that came on quite suddenly and was followed by persistent dull chest pain felt in the retrosternal and epigastric regions. This was relieved somewhat by lying on her right side. She had no hemoptysis. Four months previously, she had a venographically proven deep-vein thrombosis and had been on anticoagulants for 3 months.

EXAMINATION

On examination, the blood pressure was 125/95, the pulse rate was 115, and the respiratory rate varied between 25 and 40. There was a loud friction rub at the left base, but otherwise her chest was clear. The cardiovascular system examination was normal. She had slight pitting edema in both lower legs.

INVESTIGATIONS

The chest x-ray was normal. The IPG was abnormal on the right. A V/Q scan showed multiple segmental per-fusion defects with ventilation mismatch (high probability). Angiography revealed extensive emboli in both lungs. Venography documented proximal deep-vein thrombosis in the right leg.

TREATMENT

She was treated with intravenous heparin and warfarin, but while on warfarin, she developed bleeding into the right hip. Anticoagulants were stopped and an inferior vena cava filter was inserted.

TEACHING POINT

This patient developed recurrent thromboembolism 1 month after discontinuing warfarin treatment for a previous deep vein thrombosis. There were no predisposing factors for the recurrence. Both the leg tests and lung studies revealed thromboembolism and treatment was commenced in the usual fashion. A surprising complication was bleeding into the hip joint and this required insertion of an inferior vena cava filter. Because of the high probability lung scan, pulmonary angiography is optional in this patient.

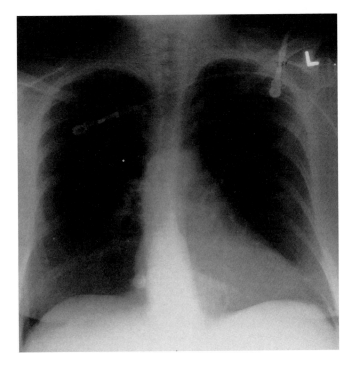

Figure 1. Negative chest x-ray.

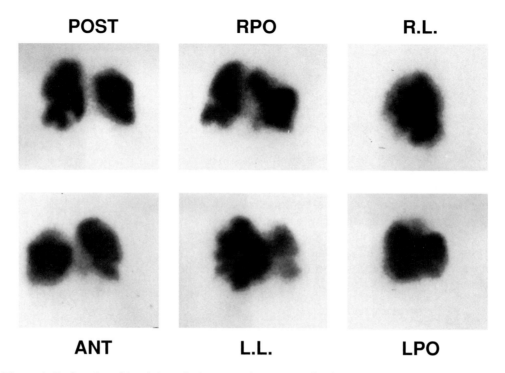

Figure 2. Technetium 99 mAA perfusion scan showing multiple segmental perfusion defects.

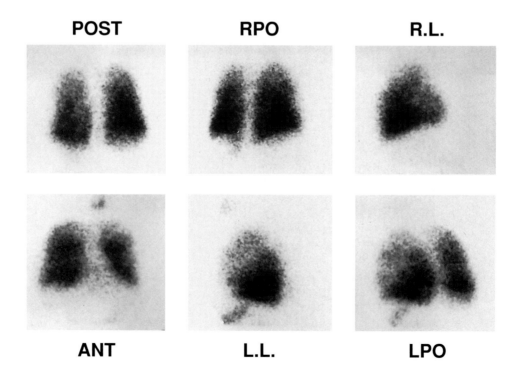

Figure 3. Technetium 99 aerosol ventilation scan show ventilation mismatch.

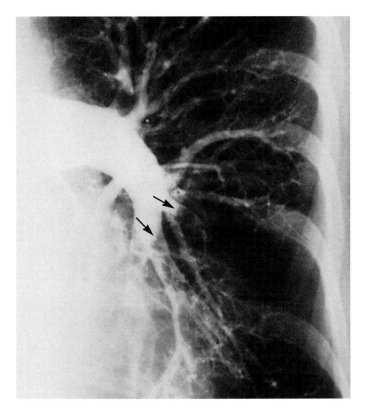

Figure 4. Pulmonary angiogram showing multiple pulmonary emboli in second- and third-order vessels in the left lung.

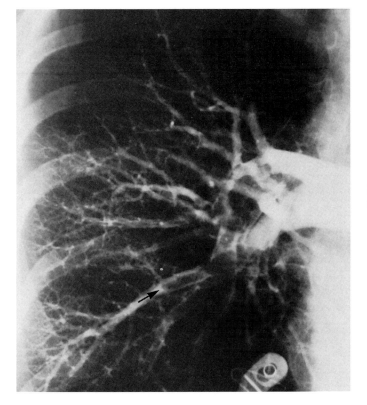

Figure 5. Pulmonary angiogram showing multiple pulmonary emboli in second and third-order vessels in the right lung.

Index

Acknowledgements

COLOUR
Heather Angel 51 (top), 51 (bottom), 106 (top right); Bruce Coleman Ltd./Jane Burton jacket front, 54 (bottom left), 54 (bottom right), 55 (top), 55 (bottom), 58 (top left), 58 (top right), 58 (bottom), 102 (top left), 103 (top), 106 (bottom), 146, 147 (top), 147 (bottom), 150 (top right), 150–151, 158–159, 158 (bottom), jacket back; A. Cupit 102 (top right), 107 (top), 150 (top left); A. van den Nieuwenhuizen 50 (top left), 50 (top right), 50 (bottom); Barry Pengilley 59 (bottom), 63 (bottom), 98 (bottom), 102 (bottom), 151 (top), 154 (bottom), 155, 159 (top); Photo Aquatics/S. Frank 59 (top), 99 (top), 103 (bottom), 111 (top); Photo Aquatics/Hansen 106 (top left); Photo Aquatics/R. Zukal 54 (top), 62 (top), 62 (bottom), 63 (top), 98 (top), 99 (bottom), 110, 154 (top), 159 (bottom); Wildlife Photos/B. Evans 107 (bottom), 111 (bottom).

BLACK AND WHITE
Heather Angel 17 (bottom), 71, 73 (bottom), 82 (top), 82 (bottom); Bruce Coleman Ltd./Jane Burton 44, 46, 68–69, 72, 78, 83, 92, 124–125, 127, 141, 166–167; Bruce Coleman Ltd./Russ Kinne 85, 88–89, 126, 128–129; Bruce Coleman Ltd./John Markham 68 (bottom), 69 (bottom), 74, 77, 122, 170; A. van den Nieuwenhuizen 11 (left), 11 (right); Laurence E. Perkins facing title-page, 15, 17 (top), 52, 53, 56–57, 61, 70, 73 (top), 75, 76, 79, 81, 86–87, 90, 91, 100–101, 118–119, 120–121, 132–133, 135, 136, 137, 138–139, 143, 144, 148–149, 152, 156 (top), 156 (bottom), 164–165, 168–169; Photo Aquatics/Jaroslav Elias 10, 64–65; Photo Aquatics/S. Frank title-page; Zoological Society of London 123.

The drawings on pages 21, 26 and 33 are by George Thompson (© The Hamlyn Publishing Group).